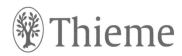

From Listening to Language

Comprehensive Intervention to Maximize Learning for Children and Adults with Hearing Loss

Editors

Jane R. Madell, PhD, CCC A/SLP, LSLS Cert AVT, FAAA
Pediatric Audiologist and Retired Director
Hearing and Learning and Cochlear Implant Centers
NYEE-Beth Israel Medical Center
New York, New York, USA

Joan G. Hewitt, AuD, CCC-A, TOD, FAAA
Pediatric Audiologist
Project TALK, Inc.
Encinitas, California
Faculty
California State University–San Marcos
San Marcos, California, USA

49 illustrations

Thieme
New York • Stuttgart • Delhi • Rio de Janeiro

Library of Congress Cataloging-in-Publication Data
is available from the publisher

Thieme Medical Publishers, Inc.
333 Seventh Avenue, 18th Floor
New York, NY 10001, USA
www.thieme.com
+1 800 782 3488, customerservice@thieme.com

Cover design: © Thieme
Cover image source: © Thieme
Typesetting by Prairie Papers

Printed in Germany by Beltz Grafische Betriebe

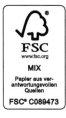

5 4 3 2 1

ISBN: 978-1-68420-251-5
Also available as an e-book:
eISBN (PDF): 978-1-68420-252-2
eISBN (epub): 978-1-63853-706-9

Contents

Video Contents

Foreword

The advancement of newborn hearing screening programs, early developmental research, and digital technologies have all transformed conversations about hearing loss. Historically, discussions about hearing loss have focused on the ear. But due to neurobiological research, today's conversations and interventions, such as those detailed in this book, focus on the brain.

How can today's children with hearing loss learn to listen, talk, and read? Our biology is that we hear with the brain. The brain, unlike any other organ, is essentially unformed when one is born; brain development is completely dependent on environmental experiences.

Conscious thought is represented as patterns of neural activities. Every sensory stimulus we encounter elicits its own unique response from a unique set of neurons across the brain. With regard to the auditory system, every specific sound we perceive is associated with its own similarly specific and unique pattern of firing neurons that are stimulated by and respond to the sound we perceive. That is why in the first three years of life, the neural foundation for all thinking and learning is built through parent talk and conversational interaction.

When speaking with families, we can talk about the ears as the doorway to the brain for sound/auditory information (e.g., "you hear the sound of birds chirping, and your brain, through exposure, experience, and practice, does the work of learning to associate the chirping sound with a bird"). Hearing loss means the ear doorway to the brain for sound/information is partially or completely closed. How thick/heavy that door is depends on the type and degree of hearing loss. Technology, such as hearing aids and cochlear implants, break through the doorway giving the child's brain access to all the sounds a child needs to develop their spoken language and to acquire knowledge. Chapters in this book explain how to access, spark, develop, and integrate a child's neural pathways for language, literacy, and social development.

With an emphasis on auditory neurobiology, we can describe a new population of children with hearing loss. This new population has the benefit of brain science, digital hearing technologies, language development research, and family systems research that can lead to spoken language and literacy outcomes consistent with hearing peers, when we do what it takes. This book clearly defines what it takes to attain that outcome in this day and age.

When listening and spoken language (LSL) are desired outcomes expressed by the family, then the child's auditory brain centers must be developed through the use of hearing devices and thoughtful, nurturing, family-focused auditory interventions. Delivering complete auditory information through the doorway to the brain, all day, each day, influences every aspect of a child's life. We are creating a hearing brain, and our conversations with families and children can focus attention on that fact.

Conversations with families and colleagues about the hearing brain can be practical and logical. Here are some suggestions for a conversational sequence. First, establish through counseling that the family has listening and spoken language (LSL) as desired outcomes for their child. Then, from the very start of intervention, discuss the concept that we hear, listen, and understand auditory information with the brain; the ears are the way in. Next, describe hearing loss as a doorway problem. Then, emphasize that the only purpose of wearing hearing technologies is to break through the (ear) doorway to deliver auditory information to the brain for neural integration and for the growth of knowledge. Stress that hearing technologies must be fit for maximum audibility and intelligibility; they must ensure that every speech sound reaches the brain at soft conversational levels. Next, it is imperative that hearing technologies are fit as early as possible in the first weeks of life and worn every waking moment for at least ten to twelve hours per day . . . eyes open, technology on . . . in order to reduce auditory neural deprivation. Critically, the child with a doorway problem must be in an enriched, family-focused auditory linguistic environment; the brain requires a great deal of auditory practice and auditory information in order to grow and integrate neural connections for the development of knowledge. Finally, it is suggested that audiologists, clinicians, and teachers refer repeatedly to the family's desired LSL outcome when explaining the reason for recommendations. For example, one can explain to the family that to increase the probability of attaining the family's desired outcome of LSL for their child, the child's technology (e.g., hearing aids, cochlear implants) must be worn at least ten to twelve hours per day in order to develop the auditory brain.

Professionals can include ongoing, embedded "brain conversations" with the child and family as part of every therapy session. Use the "brain" word many times during a session. For example, when talking about the child's technology, instead of saying, "put on your ears" when we put hearing aids and cochlear implants on the child, we can say, "put on your brain." When the child arrives at school wearing devices that are functioning well, we can offer a reinforcing comment to the child such as, "Good for you! Your brain is being fed with rich auditory information and is growing strong with knowledge." Even a very young child with hearing loss can learn the importance of growing the brain.

In this book, *From Listening to Language: Comprehensive Intervention to Maximize Learning for Children and Adults with Hearing Loss,* Jane R. Madell and Joan G. Hewitt have generously shared their wealth of experiences. They have assembled an impressive team of individual contributors, each a respected authority in family-focused hearing, listening, and spoken language development. Together, the authors cover virtually every dimension of comprehensive LSL intervention for all age groups, from speech acoustics, through access technologies, to telepractice and music therapy, and to executive functions and literacy. Each chapter has been written by an experienced and authoritative author. Coverage is broad, thorough, and complete. This will be an excellent textbook for graduate courses in audiology, speech-language pathology, early intervention, and deaf education, as well as a source book for experienced professionals and parents. I highly recommend adding this book to your course and to your library.

Carol Flexer, PhD, LSLS Cert AVT
Distinguished Professor Emeritus, Audiology
The University of Akron
Akron, Ohio, USA

Acknowledgments

We would like to thank the many families with whom we have had the honor to work who have taught us all we know about children with hearing loss. While they are too many to name, we want to thank all our brilliant teachers and mentors who guided us in the incredible task of learning to become master clinicians. We would also like to thank all the gifted clinicians we have worked with who have challenged us and helped us grow every day.

We cannot express enough thanks to the chapter authors who dedicated themselves to helping make this book the exceptional work it is. We also want to thank Bill Hewitt who patiently helped us design our cover house, which, we hope, illustrates our thought process in developing this book.

We want to thank our amazing families who have supported us over many years as our work distracted us from family activities. We thank with love husbands Rob Madell and Bill Hewitt; children Jody, Josh, Lee, and Brent; children-in-law James, Dawn, and Andy; and grandchildren Eva, Rose, Trixie and Clare. We love them beyond measure.

We want to thank the editors at Thieme who have supported us while we developed this book and especially Kenny Chumbley, without whose editing this task would have been much more difficult.

Jane R. Madell
Joan G. Hewitt

Contributors

Lyndsey Allen, BSc, LSLS Cert AVT
Nottingham, United Kingdom

Christine Barton, MM, MT-BC, Ret., Cert in Auditory Learning in Young Children
Developmental Music Specialist
St. Joseph Institute for the Deaf
Indianapolis, Indiana
Zionsville Community Schools
Zionsville, Indiana, USA

Becky Clem, MA, CCC-SLP, LSLS Cert AVT
Rehabilitation Services Education Coordinator
Cook Children's Medical Center
Fort Worth, Texas, USA

Michael Douglas, MA, CCC-SLP, LSLS Cert AVT
Consumer Engagement and Rehabilitation Program Manager
Consumer Engagement and Rehabilitation
MED-EL
San Marcos, Texas, USA

Sherri J. Fickenscher, MS, LSLS Cert AVEd
Education Support Specialist
Clarke Schools for Hearing and Speech
Philadelphia, Pennsylvania, USA

Paula E. Gross, EdD, CED
Assistant Professor
Communication Disorders and Deaf Education
Fontbonne University
St. Louis, Missouri, USA

Joan G. Hewitt, AuD, CCC-A, TOD, FAAA
Pediatric Audiologist
Project TALK, Inc.
Encinitas, California
Faculty
California State University–San Marcos
San Marcos, California, USA

Sarah Hogan, DPhil, MSc
Auditory Verbal United Kingdom
Chesterton, United Kingdom

Susan Lenihan, PhD
Professor Emerita
Communication Disorders and Deaf Education
Fontbonne University
St. Louis, Missouri, USA

Jane R. Madell, PhD, CCC A/SLP, LSLS Cert AVT, FAAA
Pediatric Audiologist and Retired Director
Hearing and Learning and Cochlear Implant Centers
NYEE-Beth Israel Medical Center
New York, New York, USA

Amy McConkey Robbins, MS, CCC-SLP, LSLS Cert AVT
Speech-Language Pathologist and Owner
Communication Consulting Services
Indianapolis, Indiana, USA

Lyn Robertson, PhD
Associate Professor Emerita
Department of Educational Studies
Denison University
Granville, Ohio, USA

Elizabeth A. Rosenzweig, PhD, CCC-SLP, LSLS Cert AVT
Assistant Professor of Practice and Director
Edward D. Mysak Clinic for Communication Disorders
Program in Communication Sciences and Disorders
Department of Biobehavioral Sciences
Teachers College, Columbia University
New York, New York, USA

Dan Salvucci, MED, EdM
Instructor and Director
Northeast Interdisciplinary Program
Communication Disorders and Deaf Education
Fontbonne University
St. Louis, Missouri, USA

Johnnie Sexton, AuD
Executive Director and Founder
The CARE Project
Raleigh, North Carolina, USA

Darcy L. Stowe, MS, CCC-SLP, LSLS Cert AVT
Chief of Listening and Spoken Language
Listening and Spoken Language
Hearts for Hearing
Oklahoma City, Oklahoma, USA

Gwen L. Suennen, MA Special Education
Auditory/Verbal Therapist
Deaf and Hard of Hearing Department
Poway Unified School District
San Diego, California, USA

Elizabeth Tippette, MSP, CCC-SLP, LSLS Cert AVT
Private Speech-Language Pathologist
Founder and Owner
Hear I Am! Speech Therapy
Winston-Salem, North Carolina, USA

Elizabeth Tyszkiewicz, LSLS Cert AVT
Birmingham, United Kingdom

Jenna M. Voss, PhD, CED, LSLS Cert AVEd
Associate Professor and Chair
Communication Disorders and Deaf Education
Fontbonne University
St. Louis, Missouri, USA

Ellie White, MS, MAEd, CED
Grant Mentor and Lecturer
Communication Disorders and Deaf Education
Fontbonne University
St. Louis, Missouri, USA

Elizabeth Ying, MA, SLP (Ret.)
Mount Vernon, New York, USA

Lindsay Zombek, MS, CCC-SLP
Supervisor of Speech Language Pathology
Ear, Nose, and Throat Institute
University Hospitals Cleveland Medical Center
Cleveland, Ohio, USA

I
Creating a Firm Foundation

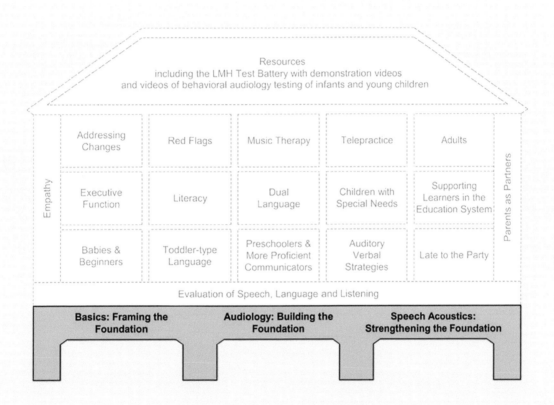

1 The Basics: Framing the Foundation

Joan G. Hewitt and Jane R. Madell

Summary

This chapter discusses the importance of auditory brain development and details the framework for this book. Auditory stimulation is critical in infants to develop the auditory brain. If the brain is not stimulated with clear sounds, it will get reorganized and there will not be another opportunity to develop the auditory brain. If children do not have a clear auditory signal, we cannot expect them to have good listening or spoken language skills. It would be wrong to conclude that a child born deaf can use sign language during the early years and still develop synaptic connections and neural networks in the auditory cortex that will be sufficient to foster auditory and spoken language development. In addition to having technology that provides good auditory access, children need to be exposed to intelligible speech and complex, high-level models of spoken language. If a child hears fewer words, either because of inability to hear words or because of reduced auditory stimulation and input, language and IQ will be affected. Families must understand that they are their baby's primary teachers and carefully choose the communication option that will enable them to create a language-rich environment for their child. Clinicians must ensure that appropriate technology is fitted and that intervention begins at the appropriate language stage, not chronological age.

Keywords

neurobiological hearing loss, early identification, synaptic pruning, communication options

Key Points

- Hearing loss in children is a neurological emergency.
- Auditory stimulation is essential for building a child's auditory brain.
- Early identification through newborn hearing screening, along with excellent technology, enables babies with hearing loss to learn with their typically hearing peers.
- Listening experience in infancy is critical for development of speech and language, and a strong auditory base in language is essential for reading and learning.
- The appropriate therapy starting point should be determined by a child's language level, not by chronological age.
- Language is best learned through hearing. Therapy that is auditory-based will be the most successful in helping children with hearing loss develop speech, language, and literacy skills.
- Families must understand that they are their baby's primary teachers.
- *All* spoken language development follows one very specific process ("hearer" to "listener" to "understander" to "speaker").

1.1 Building a House

Have you ever watched a house being built? Although it takes considerable time and skill, master builders take great care to lay a firm foundation, and only after the foundation is determined to be solid do they begin the processes of framing, adding stories, creating rooms, and so forth. Similar to building a house, speech and language development in children is a lengthy process, and it is built upon the foundation of hearing. For babies who are born with hearing, the foundation naturally exists for listening, receptive language, and expressive language to be built. However, for babies born with hearing loss, the foundation—hearing—is not firm or does not exist. Thus, hearing is where we must start if the goal is to develop spoken language in children with hearing loss.

1.2 Why Hearing Is the Foundation for Speech and Language Development in Children

There is substantial neurobiological evidence that hearing is the most effective sensory modality for developing spoken language and cognitive skills.[1,2,3,4,5,6,7] Children with typical hearing are born listening and have been listening for approximately 20 weeks in utero. They can recognize their mother's voice and can identify the important words in a sentence. In the first few months after birth a baby can discriminate various speech sounds. By their first birthday, babies' brains become reorganized so that they recognize speech sounds only in the language that they hear daily. By 6 months a child will recognize short phrases followed by familiar words, such as "Mommy has juice."[8]

In addition, hearing is the fastest sense. It gets information to the brain more rapidly than all the other senses. Moreover, while we can close our eyes and not see, we cannot close our ears; there are no "earlids." Thus, children with typical hearing are connected to their world through hearing 24 hours a day.

1.3 How Hearing Loss in Children Affects Speech and Language Development

Hearing loss in children is a neurological emergency. When a child is born with a hearing loss, that child has already had approximately 20 weeks of auditory deprivation in utero. Thus, time is of the essence. Hearing not only connects babies to the world around them, but the strong auditory base created by listening experience in infancy is essential for the development of language, which serves as the foundation for learning and reading (see Chapter 13). Even when children with hearing loss have appropriate technology, they still do not hear 24 hours a day. None of the technology available today is designed to be worn day and night. Nevertheless, the desire to connect auditorily to the world around us is so strong that parents often tell us their children want to keep hearing aids or cochlear implants on at night when they go to sleep.

So, for children with hearing loss, how do we start to frame the foundation?

1.4 Framing the Foundation: Current Research and Applications in Auditory Brain Development

Hearing occurs in the brain. Discussions about neurobiology of sensory input are really conversations about the brain. The brain is most plastic and has the most potential to create the detailed connections necessary when the child is youngest. Because the infant brain grows quickly, it is essential that we provide the infant's brain with good, clear auditory stimulation. In the absence of sound, the brain will reorganize itself. When the brain is stimulated with clear auditory signals, synapses develop to connect neurons to process those signals. If a part of the brain is not stimulated, the synapses that are not going to be used are eliminated from the neural pathways (synaptic pruning) so that the neurons can be put to some other use. While synaptic pruning occurs throughout the lifetime, the most significant synaptic pruning occurs during the first few years. If we do not provide clear auditory stimulation early, synaptic pruning in the auditory centers will occur, and the child will not get another opportunity to develop the auditory brain.[9,10]

For auditory stimulation, the ears are the doorway to the brain. Hearing loss interferes with sound reaching the brain by, essentially, closing the doorway to the brain. Technology, appropriately fitted, opens the closed doorway, enabling sound and spoken language inputs to reach the brain and develop the auditory pathways. The brain can only organize itself around the stimulation it receives. If it receives a complete auditory signal, the brain will be organized with detailed auditory connections. Research clearly shows that early identification of hearing loss and early fitting of technology can provide the essential early access to the brain that is critical for auditory learning.[11,12,13,14] If the brain receives an incomplete signal because of hearing loss, the brain will be organized differently. If a child does not receive a clear signal, both receptive and expressive speech and language as well as literacy will be affected. How children hear is how we can expect them to talk: in Michael Merzenich's phrase, "muddy in, muddy out."[15]

Pearl

If we don't provide auditory stimulation early, we do not get an opportunity later to develop the auditory brain.

Pearl

The purpose of technology is to get auditory information to the brain.

1.5 What Happens If There Is No Frame: Auditory Deprivation

There are a significant number of studies exploring brain activity in children with and without hearing loss. Research has demonstrated that auditory stimulation results in responses in the auditory cortex. Hand movements demonstrate activity in the occipital cortex but not the auditory cortex.

While long-deafened adults who have not used technology and have used sign language may be able to identify some gross sounds after receiving a cochlear implant, they cannot identify open-set speech information. Long-duration unamplified or poorly amplified deafness results in reorganization of the auditory cortex such that connections never develop to enable a listener to interpret sound and spoken language meaningfully. If auditory input is not delivered to the auditory cortex, then it cannot be distributed to the rest of the brain for the higher-order processing necessary to convey a meaningful auditory experience. If the secondary auditory cortex is not stimulated early, the visual cortex will take over the neurons that normally make up the secondary auditory cortex.

It would be wrong to conclude that a child born deaf can use sign language during the early years and later develop synaptic connections and neural networks in the auditory cortex that will be sufficient to foster strong auditory and spoken language development. The sole use of visual forms of communication during the first few years of life without auditory language stimulation results in the appropriation of the secondary auditory cortex by the visual cortex. In other words, what would have been the auditory portions of the brain will now be used for processing visual information, and it will not be possible to reverse this reallocation. If we do not provide auditory stimulation early, the auditory centers of the brain do not get developed, and children cannot learn to use audition to understand speech and language later.[16]

Sharma and colleagues[9] studied cortical auditory evoked responses and showed that children who received cochlear implants during the first 3 years of life had P1 latencies that were similar to those in children with normal hearing. Children who received cochlear implants after 3 years of age had delayed latencies. The researchers concluded that the P1 latency is a biomarker of auditory brain development. Thomas and Zwolan[16] demonstrated that children who receive auditory verbal therapy to develop the auditory centers of the brain have better language skills than children who use auditory-oral communication, and children who use total communication have even poorer language skills (for descriptions of these methods, see the later section "Framing Communication Options for Children with Hearing Loss" in this chapter). Furthermore, Geers and coworkers[2] showed that children who use sign language, even for a short period of time before receiving cochlear implants have poorer speech production, speech perception, and literacy skills than children who never use sign language. These studies demonstrate that if early and sufficient access to meaningful auditory stimulation is not provided during the early years of a child's life, the child's brain and auditory brain function will be forever altered, and as a result, auditory performance and spoken language will suffer for the rest of the child's life.

1.6 Framing Material 1: Consistent Auditory Access through Technology for Auditory Brain Development

Every day of auditory exposure counts. One might assume that, as long as children receive auditory access by age 3, they will have good speech, language, and literacy. However, Hart and Risley[17] demonstrated that the language abilities of typically hearing children who were exposed to 45 million words during their first few years far exceeded those of those who were exposed to a smaller number of words. While this research was conducted on children with typical hearing, the conclusion is the same: if a child hears fewer words, either because of inability to hear words or because of reduced auditory stimulation, language and IQ will be affected. McCreery and colleagues,[18] working with children who use hearing aids, have shown that children who used technology for 10 or more hours/day achieved mean language scores that were almost half a standard deviation higher than children who used hearing aids less than 10 hours/day. Moreover, research has also shown a strong correlation between the length of deprivation (or auditory brain reorganization) and the amount of time the child will need to catch up to hearing peers once hearing through technology has been established. Yoshinaga-Itano[19,20] found that children with hearing loss who received appropriate intervention before 6 months of age achieved speech and language outcomes commensurate with their hearing peers. However, children who did not receive rich auditory access until they were 13 to 24 months of age required 1 to 2 years of catch-up time in addition to the expected annual language growth to reach the level of their hearing peers. Even more concerning, children who did not receive optimal auditory access until after 24 months of age required more than 3 years of catch-up growth. Thus, for children with hearing loss, technology must be provided within the first few weeks and must be monitored at least once daily to ensure that it is providing sufficient auditory access.

Pearl

Technology must be monitored at least once a day to ensure that children are hearing what they need to hear.

1.7 Framing Material 2: High-Quality Input and Auditory Brain Development

In addition to having technology that provides good auditory access to the brain, children need to be exposed to intelligible speech and complex, high-level models of spoken language. Language exposure needs to include abstract concepts and questions about why something happens, not just naming items and asking simple yes/no or who/what/where questions. A great deal of research has demonstrated that children with hearing loss who are exposed to greater amounts of intelligible speech and complex language achieve higher spoken language outcomes than children with hearing loss who are not exposed to complex language and intelligible speech.[1,18,21] Other research has shown that visual stimulation, such as sign language, does not contribute to developing spoken language. In her extensive research on communication development of young children, Nittrouer[22] found that sign language does not promote spoken language development in typically hearing children or in children with hearing loss. Moreover, further research has shown that the more a child with hearing loss is exposed to sign language at the expense of spoken language, the less adept the auditory cortex will become at interpreting speech information, resulting in poorer listening, spoken language, and literacy skills.[1,2,23] Thus, families must be educated about how to provide not only a lot of language input, but also complex language input, including reading and singing. Early language learning will result in differences in learning and literacy. Children who have better language skills have better literacy skills. See Chapter 13 for more information about literacy.

1.8 Framing Deafness: How the Definition of Deafness Has Changed

The research we have now has resulted in a new view of deafness. Most families of children with hearing loss choose spoken language. When asked why, they often say that they want their child to go to school with siblings and with peers in the neighborhood. In addition, 95% of children with hearing loss are born to families with normal hearing[24] who do not know sign language and to whom attempting to learn a second language while parenting a newborn or toddler can seem overwhelming.

So, what do we need to do to ensure that children with hearing loss develop rich spoken language and have significantly better opportunities? Newborn hearing screening identifies babies at birth. Technology can and must be fitted within weeks of identifying hearing loss. Current hearing aids and implantable devices can provide children with the ability to hear. Families must understand that they are their baby's primary teachers and that they need to learn how to check technology and provide optimal language exposure. Words we used to describe hearing loss even 15 years ago are different from those we use to describe it now. We no longer assume that a child born with a severe or profound hearing loss will not be able to learn to listen and talk. We can honestly tell families that with early identification, optimal exposure to sound, and good listening and spoken language (LSL) therapy, we expect that their child will have the necessary tools for learning to listen and talk.

1.9 Framing Communication Options for Children with Hearing Loss

Different communication options are available for management of infants and children with hearing loss. The decisions about which communication option to choose and how to choose technology are overwhelming for families. Most families know nothing about hearing loss when they receive the diagnosis. If they know anyone with hearing loss, it is likely to be an older adult who hates their hearing aids and does not wear them consistently. We need to assist families by providing the information they need, but the decision about which option to choose is ultimately the families'.

1.9.1 What Are the Choices?

Table 1.1 describes the different communication options in the United States. When an infant or young child is identified with hearing loss, the audiologist and otologist who are working with the family will help the family understand the communication and education options. We ask the family what their goal for their child is. Where do they want the child to be in 3 years, 5 years, 10 years, and so on?

Families who want their children to use their native spoken language can choose LSL, also called auditory verbal therapy (AVT), which is auditory based, or auditory-oral, which uses audition and speech reading. If families choose the auditory-oral approach but feel the need for some additional assistance to have the child get speech reading information, they may add cued speech, which uses hand cues to distinguish between phonemes that look the same on the lips, such as /p/, /b/, and /m/. Families who use cued speech will need to learn to cue, and if the child is in a mainstream class, there will need to be a cued speech transliterator at school.[3]

Some families may choose a combination of spoken language and sign. Sign support relies on spoken language, with sign to fill in missing information. Total communication (TC) uses both spoken language and sign language and generally advocates for simultaneous communication, which uses both spoken language and sign at the same time. A sign system such as Signing Exact English, rather than American Sign Language (ASL), will be used in simultaneous communication. Signed English uses English

Table 1.1 Communication approaches from most auditory to least auditory

SPOKEN LANGUAGE APPROACHES	
Listening and Spoken Language (LSL), also called auditory-verbal therapy	This is an auditory-based approach that has listening and spoken language as the outcome. Infants and children are fitted with technology early, and families work with clinicians who assist them in being their child's primary therapist and in helping the children to use listening to develop speech, language, and literacy skills. The therapy is primarily an early childhood program but often continues into later years. Therapy is based on the 10 Principles of Auditory Verbal Practice available from AG Bell (Alexander Graham Bell Association for the Deaf and Hard of Hearing) and in the Resources chapter of this book. Children are mainstreamed in regular school programs.
Auditory-oral approach	This approach has spoken language as the outcome. Active listening is enhanced by technology, and speech-reading and listening are used in learning. Sign language is not used. Children may be educated in mainstream classes or in classrooms with other children with hearing loss who are being educated with the goal of spoken language. This is sometimes (less correctly) called auditory-verbal education.
COMBINED APPROACHES	
Cued speech	Cued speech is a supplement to spoken English in which hand signals are used to make spoken language fully visible, since about 60% of phonemes cannot be distinguished visually. For example, /p/, /b/, and /m/ all look the same when produced on the lips. Family members need to learn hand cues so that children can use them to distinguish between phonemes that look alike. Cued speech is easier to learn than sign language because it uses the same word order as the spoken language and the number of gestures to be learned is limited. If in a mainstream classroom, the child will need a cued speech transliterator.
Sign-supported speech	Signs are used to support spoken language when the child is confused. Signing is considered a bridge to learning spoken language. It may be useful in difficult situations such as in noise. Families will have to learn a form of sign language to be able to support their child's language and social development. If in a mainstream classroom, the child may need a sign language interpreter.
Simultaneous communication	This is a system in which spoken language and signing are used together. A sign system, not American Sign Language (ASL), will be used so that it agrees with the spoken language system. Families will need to become fluent in providing sign language while speaking to provide rich language stimulation to their children. If in a mainstream classroom, the child will need a sign language interpreter.
Total communication (TC)	Total communication is a system that uses sign, spoken language, and written language for communication. TC programs report that they use whatever is needed to foster communication. However, if a child is in a classroom where sign language is being used, they may have fewer opportunities to learn to use audition. Families will need to become fluent in a form of sign language to provide rich language input to their children. If in a mainstream classroom, the child will need a sign language interpreter.
VISUAL APPROACHES	
Bilingual-bicultural (BiBi)	A person who is fluent in ASL and English is bimodal. With young children, ASL is usually taught first and English taught second, primarily to develop literacy skills. If the child is not in an ASL classroom, the child will need an interpreter. Families will need to become fluent in ASL to provide rich language input and support their children. Some children who have been educated using listening and spoken language choose to learn ASL as young adults or teens, primarily to communicate with Deaf friends who do not use spoken language and to access communication in difficult listening situations.

language word order with endings (-ing, -ed, etc.) spelled out or marked. While both spoken language and visual language may both be presented at the same time, it is difficult for the child to attend to the auditory signal when there is a visual signal presented at the same time. In addition, it is difficult for the communication partner to simultaneously coordinate the fine motor timing and grammatical complexities of spoken language with the gross motor movements of a manual language.

ASL is not merely a sign system but a language in its own right that forms words and constructs phrases and sentences differently than English does. BiBi (Bilingual-Bicultural) is a system that uses ASL, usually learned first, and English learned later, for literacy.[3]

Pearl

The decision about what communication option to use is the family's. The family's decision guides us.

1.9.2 Factors to Consider in Making Decisions about Communication Mode

What is the family's desired outcome?

If the family wants a spoken language outcome, they will choose LSL (the auditory-verbal approach) or an auditory-oral approach. What languages does the family speak at home? Research in child development encourages families to speak to children in the language in which they are most comfortable so that they can provide complex language models. This means that, if parents wish to teach their child with hearing loss to speak their native language, those who use spoken language have the advantage of already knowing that language fully and being able to immerse their child in it.

If the parents choose a language such as ASL that they do not know, are they committed to becoming fluent in that language?

If parents wish to use a manual language like ASL with their child with hearing loss, they themselves must become as proficient as a native signer. This may mean immersing themselves in learning ASL while, at the same time, maintaining their work and home lives and dealing with the stresses of their child's special needs. Learning a new language such as ASL generally requires formal classes and interactions with native signers. The complexities of learning a second language, especially a manual one that is so different from spoken language, can make it very difficult for many parents to move past basic signs and into rich conversation with their child. Meyers and Bartee[25] studied parents of deaf children and found that only 73% knew "some sign language." Moreover, while the signing skills of hearing parents did improve over the years, only 18% to 29% said they could understand their children "all the time." Finally, if families do not know ASL, they can expect that it will take about 3 years to become fluent signers, during which time their child will not have good language exposure.[26]

Will all family members be able to communicate using the selected communication mode?

Will siblings and grandparents be able to communicate with the child?

Will the communication approach allow the child to feel part of the family?

If the child is learning sign at school but the family cannot use sign, how will the family communicate?

Is the selected communication approach appropriate for that family and child?

For example, if a child has a disability that makes fine motor movements of the hands or gross motor movements of the arms difficult, will a sign language approach be successful?

How will the child be equipped by school age to begin school?

Will the child have developed the communication abilities to converse, play, and learn with peers of the same age?

Pearl

When selecting a communication mode, the family should consider whether all family members will be able to communicate using the selected communication mode. Will siblings and grandparents be able to communicate with the child?

1.10 The Framework of This Book

This entire book is based upon one foundational premise: In every country in the world, and throughout all time, children's development of spoken language is built on one very specific design. In utero by the beginning of the third trimester, a baby's ears are fully formed and start to hear. This early stimulation begins to develop the auditory brain. In the first months after birth, babies begin attending to the sounds around them, analyzing them, finding patterns in them, and eventually assigning meaning to them. In this critical period, they move from simply being "hearers" to becoming "listeners." As "listeners," babies begin to recognize that the spoken sounds of their caregivers refer to specific items or actions, they start to "understand," and receptive language begins to develop. Once a child has amassed a sufficient repertoire of receptive language by developing auditory portions of the brain, expressive language will begin to emerge. This process from hearing to listening to understanding to speaking is universal . . . except with children with hearing loss. Children with untreated hearing loss are not "hearers," so they lack the most basic input to become "listeners," "understanders," and "speakers."

1.10.1 What Happens When Children Are Not "Hearers"?

Historically, children who were deaf or hard of hearing struggled to develop language and literacy skills commensurate with their typically hearing peers.[27] For centuries, the debate raged over whether children with hearing loss were best served by learning spoken language, manual sign language, or a combination of these (see **Table 1.1**). Proponents of both communication methods were faced with the reality that, no matter the communication method, the vast majority of children who were deaf or hard of hearing had significant language, literacy, and achievement deficits compared to their typically hearing peers. Even total communication, which purported to combine the best of both manual and spoken language, revealed results no better than the individual methods themselves.

1.10.2 Can Children Who Are Deaf or Hard of Hearing Become "Hearers"?

YES, children who are deaf or hard of hearing can become hearers! With the advent of newborn hearing screening, current technology options, and intensive early intervention services, we now have the ability to identify deaf or hard of hearing babies at birth and to reduce auditory deprivation and delay in treatment previously experienced by so many children with hearing loss. In addition, with digital hearing aids and cochlear implants, appropriate auditory access to the brain is now possible. With these technologies, children with hearing loss have the potential to develop spoken language through listening like their typically hearing peers. In other words, we now have the resources necessary to enable sound to reach the auditory portions of the brain and for children with even the most profound hearing losses to become "listeners," "understanders," and "talkers" just like their hearing peers.

Pearl

Children with even the most profound hearing losses can become "listeners" and "understanders" and "talkers" just like their hearing peers.

1.10.3 Why Is Spoken Language So Important to Parents?

Very simply, spoken language is important to parents because 92% to 96% of children with hearing loss are born to hearing parents.[24] This means that, in families with children with hearing loss, the native language of the home, extended family system, and community is overwhelmingly spoken language. Thus, if parents wish to teach their child with hearing loss their native language, those who use spoken language have the advantage of already knowing that language fully and being able to immerse their child in it. This also means that the majority of parents of children with hearing loss have little to no knowledge of or experience with sign language. Thus, if those same parents wish

to use a manual language like ASL with their child with hearing loss, they themselves must become as proficient as a native signer (almost instantly) if they wish to provide their child with language that is rich, varied, and complex. In summary, over 90% of children with hearing loss have hearing and speaking parents who are already prepared to immerse their children in their native, home language. With appropriate technology and therapy, those children can learn to speak like their typical hearing siblings and peers.

1.10.4 What Does It Take for a Child with Hearing Loss to Become a "Hearer," "Listener," "Understander," and "Speaker"?

That is exactly what this book is about!

We have very purposefully organized this book to guide the reader in understanding the necessary interventions for children with hearing loss and in identifying the specific starting place and considerations for each individual child.

Section 1: Creating a Firm Foundation

First, children with hearing loss must have the foundation for spoken language; they must become "hearers." **Chapter 2 (Audiology: Building the Foundation)** and **Chapter 3 (Speech Acoustics: Strengthening the Foundation)** explain the intervention that is needed for diagnosis of hearing loss, optimal fitting of technology, and appropriate auditory brain access to the sounds of speech and language.

Section 2: Framing a Strong Structure

Next, children with hearing loss must be surrounded by parents and caregivers who are fully invested in filling the child's world with speech and language. The integral partnership between parents, caregivers, and professionals provides the necessary support and framework for intervention and progress.

Chapters 4 (Empathy: Changing the Culture of Communication) and **5 (Parents as Partners)** help clinicians to understand the incredible importance of parent involvement and the support we can offer them while, at the same time, recognizing the parents' grief, perspectives, and unique journeys.

Chapter 6 (Evaluation of Speech, Language, and Listening in Children with Hearing Loss: Knowing the level at which children are functioning) explains the assessment necessary to determine where the child is in the process and where to begin the intervention.

Section 3: Building the First Floor

Once we have a foundation of hearing, the support of parents and caregivers, and an accurate assessment of the child's level of functioning, we can begin to build the first floor of listening, receptive language, and expressive language development. We must remember that building this first floor of "listeners," "understanders," and "talkers" creates the support for all other areas of development that are dependent upon language (cognition, academics, literacy, etc.).

Determining where to start: Remember that the foundational premise of this book is that *all* spoken language development follows one very specific process ("hearer" to "listener" to "understander" to "speaker"). Thus, it is absolutely essential that we determine where a child with hearing loss is in the process and start the intervention at that specific stage. It is the child's stage of language development, *not* the child's chronological age or academic grade, that determines the starting point for intervention.

Pearl

It is the child's stage of language development, not the child's chronological age or academic grade, that determines the starting point for intervention.

The stages are: **Chapter 7 (Babies and Beginners: Starting with Nothing and Building Up to Words)** is the starting point for babies and older children who are new to listening and language. **Chapter 8 (Toddler-Type Language: Putting Words Together and Moving Up to Simple Sentences)** is the place to start with children who have developed basic receptive and expressive vocabularies and are beginning to combine two words and move toward the use of simple sentences. **Chapter 9 (Preschoolers and More Proficient Communicators: Using Complex Language and Using Language to Think)** discusses the progression from simple sentences to complex utterances and complex thinking with language

Chapter 10 (Auditory Verbal Strategies to Build Listening and Spoken Language Skills) details the use of specific strategies that are essential to creating a language-rich environment and encouraging listening, receptive, and expressive language development.

Chapter 11 (Late to the Party: When Children Come Late to Listening and Spoken Language) addresses determining the appropriate stage and process for intervention for children who begin intervention at older ages or with significant delays.

Section 4: Adding the Second Floor

Once we have begun the process of building a strong first floor of language development, we can begin to consider those important aspects of intervention that form the second floor.

Chapter 12 (Executive Function Integrated into Auditory-Verbal Practice) is required reading for anyone doing therapy with children of any age and provides insight into the intertwined connections between language and executive function. **Chapter 13 (The Auditory-Verbal Approach and Literacy)** details how to encourage higher level cognition and literacy through listening and spoken language development.

Chapter 14 (Dual Language Assessment and Intervention for Children with Hearing Loss) and **Chapter 15 (Children with Special Needs and Additional Disabilities)** explore the unique needs of children with hearing loss who are learning multiple languages or who have further challenges in addition to hearing loss.

Chapter 16 (Supporting Children Who Are Deaf or Hard of Hearing in the Educational Setting) discusses the unique educational needs of children with hearing loss and considerations for ensuring appropriate support for academic success.

Section 5: Completing the Structure

This section discusses additional aspects of intervention that assist the clinician in identifying changes in hearing status, integrating advances into practice, and assisting adult hearing aid and cochlear implant recipients.

Chapter 17 (Addressing Changes in Auditory Access) and **Chapter 18 (Red Flags: Identifying and Managing Barriers to the Child's Optimal Auditory Development)** examine necessary steps and interventions when changes in hearing occur or when concerns about a child's auditory development arise.

Chapter 19 (Music Therapy for Children with Hearing Loss) discusses using music to help build language skills, and **Chapter 20 (Telepractice for Children with Hearing Loss)** discusses the advantages and challenges of telepractice for providing therapy and will help clinicians get started with telepractice.

Chapter 21 (Working with Adults) examines how the interventions in this book can be applied to older children and adults with hearing loss who are learning to listen through newly fitted hearing aids or cochlear implants.

Section 6: Storing Treasures in the Attic

Chapter 22 (Resources) provides clinicians with a wealth of resources for many aspects of intervention.

References

[1] Ching TYC, Dillon H. Major findings of the LOCHI study on children at 3 years of age and implications for audiological management. *Int J Audiol* 2013;52(0_2):S65–S68

[2] Geers AE, Strube MJ, Tobey EA, Pisoni DB, Moog JS. Epilogue: factors contributing to long-term outcomes of cochlear implantation in early childhood. *Ear Hear* 2011;32(1, Suppl):84S–92S

[3] Madell JR, Flexer C, Wolfe J, Schafer E. Pediatric Audiology: Diagnosis, Technology and Management. 3rd ed. New York, NY: Thieme; 2019

[4] Robertson L. Literacy and Deafness: Listening and Spoken Language. 2nd ed. San Diego, CA: Plural; 2014

[5] Sloutsky VM, Napolitano AC. Is a picture worth a thousand words? Preference for auditory modality in young children. *Child Dev* 2003;74(3):822–833

[6] Tallal P. Improving language and literacy is a matter of time. *Nat Rev Neurosci* 2004;5(9):721–728

[7] Zupan B, Sussman JE. Auditory preferences of young children with and without hearing loss for meaningful auditory–visual compound stimuli. *J Commun Disord* 2009;42:381–396

[8] Choi D, Black AK, Werker JF. Cascading and multisensory influences on speech perception development. *Mind Brain Educ* 2018;12(4):212–223

[9] Sharma A, Martin K, Roland P, et al. P1 latency as a biomarker for central auditory development in children with hearing loss. *J Am Acad Audiol* 2005;16(8):564–573

[10] Gifford R. Cochlear implants for infants and children. In: Madell JR, Flexer C, eds. Pediatric Audiology: Diagnosis, Technology, and Management. 2nd ed. Thieme; 2014:238–254

[11] Kral A. Maturation and plasticity of the auditory pathways. Paper presented at: 11th European Symposium on Paediatric Cochlear Implantation, 2013, Istanbul, Turkey

[12] Kral A, Eggermont JJ. What's to lose and what's to learn: development under auditory deprivation. *Brain Res Rev* 2007;56(1):259–269

[13] Kral A, Kronenberger WG, Pisoni DB, O'Donoghue GM. Neurocognitive factors in sensory restoration of early deafness: a connectome model. *Lancet Neurol* 2016;15(6):610–621

[14] Kraus N, Anderson S. Hearing matters: hearing with our brains. *Hear J* 2012;65(9):48

[15] Doidge N. The Brain That Changes Itself: Stories of Personal Triumph from the Frontiers of Brain Science. London, UK: Penguin; 2007:70

[16] Thomas ES, Zwolan TA. Communication mode and speech and language outcomes of young cochlear implant recipients: a comparison of auditory–verbal, oral communication, and total communication. *Otol Neurotol* 2019;*40*(10):e975–e983

[17] Hart B, Risley TR. The early catastrophe: the 30 million word gap by age 3. *Am Educator* 2003;*27*(1):4–9

[18] McCreery RW, Walker EA, Spratford M, et al. Longitudinal predictors of aided speech audibility in infants and children. *Ear Hear* 2015;*36*(Suppl 1):24S–37S

[19] Yoshinaga-Itano C, Abdula de Uzcategul C. Early identification and social-emotional factors of children with hearing loss. In: Lurtzer-White E, Luterman D, eds. Early Childhood Deafness. Baltimore, MD: York Press; 2001:13–28

[20] Yoshinaga-Itano C. From screening to early identification and intervention: discovering predictors to successful outcomes for children with significant hearing loss. *J Deaf Stud Deaf Educ* 2003;*8*(1):11–30

[21] Ambrose SE, Appenzeller M, Mai A, DesJardin JL. Beliefs and self-efficacy of parents of young children with hearing loss. *J Early Hear Detect Interv* 2020;*5*(1):73–85

[22] Nittrouer S. Early Development of Children with Hearing Loss. San Diego, CA: Plural Publishing; 2009

[23] Dettman SJ, Dowell RC, Choo D, et al. Long-term communication outcomes for children receiving cochlear implants younger than 12 months: a multicenter study. *Otol Neurotol* 2016;*37*(2):e82–e95

[24] Mitchell RE, Karchmer MA. Chasing the mythical ten percent: parental hearing status of deaf and hard of hearing students in the United States. *Sign Lang Stud* 2004;*4*(2):138–163

[25] Meyers JE, Bartee JW. Improvements in the signing skills of hearing parents of deaf children. *Am Ann Deaf* 1992;*137*(3):257–260

[26] Werker J, Yeung HH, Yoshida KA. How do infants become experts at native-speech perception? *Curr Dir Psychol Sci* 2012;*21*(4):221–226

[27] Qi S, Mitchell RE. "Large-scale academic achievement testing of deaf and hard-of-hearing students: past, present, and future. *J Deaf Stud Deaf Educ* 2011;*17*(1):1–18

2 Audiology: Building the Foundation

Jane R. Madell and Joan G. Hewitt

Summary

The first step in management of children with hearing loss is accurate diagnosis, which begins with the audiological evaluation. This chapter reviews different tests that are part of the audiological evaluation. Behavioral evaluation is the gold standard. Behavioral evaluation is used to determine degree and type of hearing loss and to monitor technology. The chapter discusses behavioral observation, visual reinforcement, and conditioned play audiometry in detail. Diagnosing type and degree of hearing loss is reviewed in detail. Speech perception testing is a critical measure of function and is reviewed in detail. Clinicians working with children with hearing loss need to understand types of technology and optimal use of different types of technology. The chapter discusses how to determine whether a child is a candidate for hearing aids, cochlear implants, osseointegrated implants, or remote microphones. The chapter helps clinicians understand how to use audiological information to determine whether a child is receiving sufficient auditory brain development with technology to use audition to learn language and develop literacy skills.

Keywords

screening and diagnostic testing, otoscopy, tympanometry, otoacoustic emissions, auditory brainstem response, auditory steady-state response, behavioral audiologic testing, behavioral observation audiometry, visual reinforcement audiometry, conditioned play audiometry, conductive hearing loss, sensorineural hearing loss, mixed hearing loss, configuration of hearing loss, unilateral and bilateral hearing loss, earmolds, hearing aids, cochlear implants, auditory brainstem implants, implantable hearing devices, remote microphone systems, speech string bean, speech perception testing

Key Points

- Hearing is the foundation for speech and language development. Thus, the auditory deprivation caused by hearing loss in children is a neurological emergency.
- Children cannot begin to construct a framework for spoken language until their auditory brains have access to speech and language through appropriate diagnosis, treatment, and hearing technology.
- Newborn hearing screening enables early identification and early and appropriate fitting of technology, which in turn enables children with hearing loss to learn to listen and talk.
- Digital hearing aids and cochlear implants have dramatically changed the ability to access the auditory brain and the expected outcomes for children who are deaf or hard of hearing.
- In order to maximize outcomes, practitioners and parents must be knowledgeable about hearing evaluations; the audiogram; interpretation of results; the effect of each hearing loss on auditory, speech, and language development; and hearing technologies.

2.1 Starting with the Basics

It is understandable, when starting to work with a child, to want to go directly to learning how to do therapy, but that is not necessarily the best approach. It would be like starting to build a structure by attempting to construct the second floor first. There is some basic building block information that is critical to understand before beginning to provide treatment for children with hearing loss. For example, for children with hearing loss to succeed, they need to hear well. We would like to think that, by the time children arrive at our doors, they are already hearing very well with their technology. Unfortunately, that is not always the case. If children are not hearing well, speech-language pathologists (SLPs), listening and spoken language (LSL) therapists, and teachers of the deaf (TODs) cannot successfully maximize the children's performance. It is critical that clinicians understand how to read audiology reports, how technology works, and, most importantly, how to determine how well a child is hearing with technology, including what specifically the child is *not* hearing. These are the basic building blocks that we began to discuss in Chapter 1 and continue to discuss in this chapter and in Chapter 3.

2.2 Diagnosis of Hearing Loss

Although many of us remember studying the eye in school, few of us remember studying the ear. For those who decide to specialize in working with children with hearing loss, it is important to have specific education about the ear and ways to assess it. However, many clinicians working with children with hearing loss have not had specialized education about how the ear works, what tests are used to evaluate hearing, and how to interpret those tests. If many clinicians have not had this education, then we must realize that even though parents have all the test results showing that their child does not hear, they will likely have little to no understanding of how the ear works and how or why their child's ear is not functioning. As clinicians, we must ensure that we ourselves are knowledgeable about the function of the ear and hearing testing, diligent about sharing this information with parents, and cognizant of the need to review it as often as necessary for parents to truly understand it.

2.2.1 Screening vs. Diagnostic Testing

Hearing can be tested through screening or diagnostic evaluations. For infants and children, screening tests are designed to assess the hearing of newborns or school-age children quickly and efficiently in order to determine who may need full diagnostic testing. On the other hand, diagnostic tests are used to fully evaluate babies or children with identified concerns and risk factors or known hearing loss. It is important to understand that screenings are designed to minimize unnecessary referrals and identify only patients who definitely need diagnostic follow-up. However, screening protocols often miss mild hearing loss. For this reason, some infants and children may pass a screening test even though they have some hearing loss. Passing a hearing screening does not ensure a newborn or child has hearing within the normal limits. Some of those mild hearing losses may progress to more severe hearing losses. When parents are concerned about development, or children present with speech and language delays, a diagnostic audiological evaluation should always be completed prior to beginning any type of intervention.

Pearl

Passing a hearing screening does not ensure that a newborn or child has hearing within the normal limits. When parents are concerned about development, or children present with speech and language delays, a diagnostic audiological evaluation should always be completed prior to beginning any type of intervention.

2.2.2 Case History

All diagnostic testing should begin with a thorough case history. Depending upon the child's age, the case history should include pregnancy history; the birth and developmental history; known risk factors for hearing loss or developmental delay; findings of other professionals; medications; speech, language, and education history; previous evaluations; family history of hearing loss or other developmental disabilities; and parent concerns.

2.2.3 Otoscopy

The audiologist should look in the child's ears with the otoscope to visualize the ear canal, eardrum, and middle ear features. Otoscopy is important in identifying obstructions such as earwax or disease such as a middle ear infection called otitis media.

2.2.4 Tympanometry

Tympanometry provides information about the movement of the eardrum. It is not a hearing test. It is useful in identifying middle ear disease, such as otitis media, noted during otoscopy. The audiologist places a small probe at the opening to the ear canal. The probe pushes air into and pulls air out of the canal and then records the eardrum's movement in response.

2.2.5 Otoacoustic Emissions Testing

Otoacoustic emission (OAE) testing is not a direct measure of hearing, but instead a measure of outer hair cell function.

When the outer hair cells in the cochlea are working, they create their own sound or echo, which can be recorded with OAE equipment. OAEs can be used as a screening or diagnostic test. For this testing, the audiologist places a probe in the opening to the ear canal. The probe generates a noise and then records whether an echo is received from the outer hair cells in the cochlea. The presence of an OAE indicates a hearing threshold at each frequency tested as better than 30 decibels (dB) hearing level (HL) to 35 dB HL. The absence of an OAE indicates hearing poorer than 30–35 dB HL at the tested frequency. As a result, OAE testing may miss mild hearing loss (20–30 dB HL), and hearing loss from auditory neuropathy spectrum disorder (ANSD) and cochlear nerve deficiency (CND). In addition, some people with normal hearing may lack OAEs.

2.2.6 Auditory Brainstem Response (ABR) and Auditory Steady-State Response (ASSR) Testing

Auditory brainstem response (ABR) and auditory steady-state response (ASSR) testing are electrophysiological tests. These tests can record electrical activity of the auditory system and provide objective information that does not require the cooperation of the patient. Electrophysiological testing is not a direct measure of hearing but can provide valuable information about the function of the ear and predicted hearing capabilities.

When the cochlea and auditory nerve (cochlear nerve, cochlear branch of the vestibulocochlear nerve) send nerve signals to the brain, the electrical impulses can be recorded and analyzed. Newborns may be tested in natural sleep, but older children may require sedation to be tested. While the child is sleeping, the audiologist places electrodes near the ears and on the forehead. Small earphones are placed on or in the child's ears and deliver clicks or tones into the ear. The electrodes then record the brainstem's response to the types and intensities of sounds presented to the ear. Automated ABR screening uses a click stimulus and indicates hearing thresholds better than 35 dB normalized hearing level (nHL), but since the signal is a broad-frequency signal, it is possible that a child could have hearing loss at some frequencies and not others and still pass the screening. Diagnostic ABR and ASSR can provide predicted hearing thresholds at different frequencies, but they are not a direct measure of hearing; they are a measure of the response of the auditory brainstem to auditory stimuli.

Diagnostic testing with ABR should include testing with click stimulus to identify whether auditory neuropathy spectrum disorder (ANSD) is present, as well as tests of tonal thresholds to determine hearing loss at different frequencies. While both ABR and ASSR are useful tests, ABR is still considered the gold standard of electrophysiological testing. It is useful to remember that electrophysiological testing tests only responses at the level of the auditory brainstem, not the entire auditory system.

2.2.7 Behavioral Audiological Testing

Behavioral testing is the gold standard of hearing testing because it measures the entire auditory system from the outer ear to the auditory cortex.[1] Calibrated sounds of varying intensity and frequency (pitch) are presented, and the child's behavioral responses are recorded. For tests other than screening tests, the child is seated in a sound booth. In behavioral testing, the audiologist follows a procedure to find and record the softest level at which a child can hear different frequencies across the speech spectrum.

For air conduction testing, which tests the entire system of the ear (outer, middle, and inner ear), sounds can be presented through speakers, insert earphones, or supraural earphones. Testing with a speaker will not provide ear-specific information, and the audiologist will be unable to determine the hearing thresholds of each individual ear. Preferably, sounds are presented through insert earphones placed at the opening to the ear canal. We strongly recommend the use of insert earphones, which enable us to test each ear individually, provide more accurate testing because the insert earphones often fit better than headphones, and avoid placing extra equipment on the heads of small children or children who are tactilely defensive. For children with hearing aids, their own earmolds can also be connected to the insert earphone cables and used if they are more comfortable.

Bone conduction testing bypasses the outer and middle ears and tests the best potential of the inner ear. For bone conduction testing, a bone conduction oscillator is placed behind the ear. When sound is presented through the oscillator, it will vibrate the skull and stimulate the inner ear (**Video 2.1**).

2.2.8 Behavioral Observation Audiometry

Behavioral observation audiometry (BOA) is the only direct measure of hearing available for infants cognitively less than 6 months of age.[1,2] BOA involves recording the audiologist's observations of the baby's response or changes in responses to sound presented (ideally through insert earphones or the baby's earmolds). The targeted response is cessation or starting of sucking in response to the stimulus (**Fig. 2.1**). While babies may show other responses such as quieting, eye widening, or startle, these are not threshold responses and should not be considered a threshold response (**Video 2.2**, **Video 2.3**).

2.2.9 Visual Reinforcement Audiometry

Visual reinforcement audiometry (VRA) is appropriate for children who are cognitively 6 months to 3 years of age. VRA is a behavioral audiological test for babies and young children who have the head control and cognitive ability to make a head turn in the direction a sound is coming from. With the visual reinforcers, the audiologist conditions the child to turn in the direction of the sound. When the child turns in the direction of the sound, an animated toy or video screen is activated to reinforce the head turn (**Fig. 2.2**). Once the child is conditioned, testing can begin.[1] For air conduction testing, sounds are ideally presented through the insert earphones to obtain ear-specific information or, less ideally, presented in the sound field (through loudspeakers), which will obtain only better-ear information, since sound is being presented to both ears at the same time. VRA testing can also be performed with a bone vibrator or in the sound field while the child is wearing technology—hearing aids (HAs), cochlear implants (CIs), osseointegrated devices, or remote microphone (RM) systems (**Video 2.4**, **Video 2.5**).

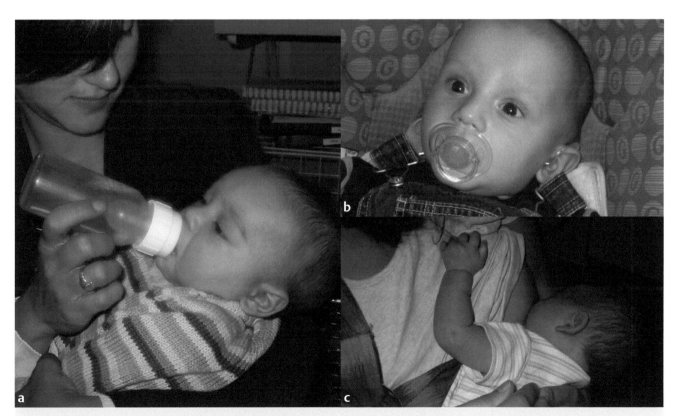

Fig. 2.1 Positioning the infant for testing: **(a)** using a bottle, **(b)** using a pacifier, **(c)** nursing at the breast.

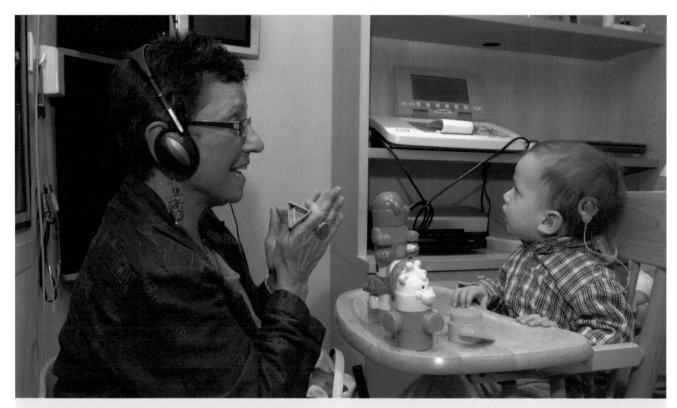

Fig. 2.2 VRA testing. Child with head turning toward the VRA toy.

2.2.10 Conditioned Play Audiometry

Conditioned play audiometry (CPA) is a behavioral test that is appropriate for children who are functioning at a cognitive level of approximately 2 to 5 years or older. Children are conditioned to play a listen-and-drop game in which they place a block in a bucket or pegs in holes each time they hear a sound presented through the insert earphones, through headphones, or in soundfield (**Fig. 2.3**). The audiologist records the softest intensities at different frequencies to which the child responds.[1] Video demonstrating hearing testing accompanies the textbook by Madell and coauthors (**Video 2.6**, **Video 2.7**).[1]

2.2.11 Standard Audiometry

Once children reach a developmental age of approximately 5 years old, they can participate in standard audiological testing. In standard audiometry, the children raise their hands or push a button each time they hear a sound. Again, the audiologist follows a procedure to find and record the softest level at which a child can hear each frequency across the speech spectrum.

Pearl

Behavioral testing is a critical part of hearing testing because it is the only test that evaluates the entire auditory system. Testing should not be considered complete until a behavioral evaluation is completed with testing in each ear.

2.2.12 Understanding Audiograms

The audiogram is simply a graph to record the patient's response or the data collected from testing. Across the top or x-axis of the graph are the frequencies (or pitches) that can be tested from low frequencies (125 Hz or 250 Hz) to high frequencies (8000 Hz or even 12000 Hz). Down the side or y-axis of the graph are the intensity levels from very soft (0 dB HL) to painfully loud (120 dB HL). The audiologist marks the child's best responses behavioral testing or thresholds estimated from ABR or ASSR results, at each frequency tested. A red circle indicates a right ear air conduction response (with earphones), and a blue X indicates a left ear air conduction response (with earphones). A left arrowhead or bracket (< or [) indicates a right ear bone conduction response, and a right arrowhead or bracket (> or]) indicates a left ear bone conduction response (obtained with the bone vibrator behind the child's ear).

In reviewing the audiogram, we can glean valuable information about the type, degree, configuration, and symmetry of the hearing thresholds. This information can help to shape our predictions of the specific listening, speech, and language challenges a particular hearing loss will cause. Testing will indicate what a child is hearing and, more importantly, what the child is not hearing. If a child has a moderate hearing loss, we can look at the Speech Banana, the Speech String Bean, or the count-the-dots audiogram (see Chapter 3) to predict what the child will be missing without technology as well as to check whether technology is providing optimal auditory access. This information will be very helpful in counseling families and, later, counseling older children about what they need to hear and what they are missing if they are not using technology.

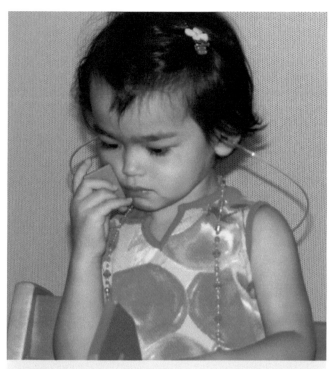

Fig. 2.3 Testing with conditioned play.

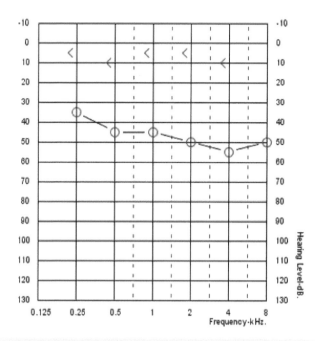

Fig. 2.4 Sample audiogram depicting conductive hearing loss.

2.3 Types of Hearing Loss

The ear is divided into three main parts: the outer ear, the middle ear, and the inner ear. Very simply, the outer ear is designed to direct sound to the middle ear. The middle ear is designed to amplify that sound and direct it to the inner ear. The hearing part of the inner ear, the cochlea, is designed to encode the sound and send the encoded messages via the auditory nerve to the brain for decoding. Thus, the main responsibilities of the outer and middle ears are to amplify and transmit the energy of the sound waves to the cochlea. Essentially, they are "conducting" mechanical vibrations, to be perceived as sound, to the inner ear. Thus, hearing loss stemming from the outer and/or middle ear is called *conductive* hearing loss. *Sensorineural* hearing loss may be due to damage to the cochlea or to the auditory nerve. The cochlea is the sensory portion of the system, and the nerve is the neural portion. The cochlea's main responsibilities are encoding the sound vibrations into neural signals to be transmitted to the brain. The auditory nerve transports the nerve signals representing sound from the cochlea to the brain.

2.3.1 Conductive Hearing Loss

Conductive hearing loss can stem from many sources. Familiar causes of conductive hearing loss are impacted wax in the ear canal, fluid in the middle ear, and perforations in the eardrum. However, conductive hearing loss can also result from congenital malformations of the ear such as microtia and atresia. Conductive hearing loss may be temporary and can often be treated medically. However, if the cause is structural malformations, medical treatment may not be able to cure the loss, but technology can be highly effective.

In audiological testing, conductive hearing loss is diagnosed when air conduction thresholds (those obtained through insert earphones, headphones, or soundfield speakers) show hearing loss but bone conduction thresholds (those obtained with the bone conduction oscillator on the mastoid bone behind the ear) are within normal limits (see **Fig. 2.4**). Air conduction results that show hearing loss, combined with bone conduction results that are within normal limits, indicate that the cochlea is functioning appropriately, but something is keeping the sound from conducting normally through the outer and/or middle ear. Results from otoscopy and tympanometry are often used to identify the source of the conductive loss more specifically.

Conductive hearing loss tends to affect low frequencies more than high frequencies. Also, while conductive hearing loss can significantly impact the amplification and transmission of sound through the outer and middle ears and lessen the information that reaches the inner ear, information that does reach the cochlea can still be encoded and transmitted. With appropriate hearing technology to aid in amplifying and transmitting sound to the cochlea, a patient with conductive hearing loss should be expected to have good perception of spoken language. Some research[3] has demonstrated speech perception problems for some children with middle ear disease.

2.3.2 Sensorineural Hearing Loss

Sensorineural hearing loss can stem from many sources. Familiar causes of sensorineural hearing loss are aging and exposure to loud noise. However, sensorineural hearing loss in children is often the result of genetic disorders that affect the function of the cochlea or malformations of the inner ear. Other causes include high fever, infections, and ingestion of medications that are toxic to the ear. Sensorineural hearing loss is permanent. Hearing loss caused by damage to the cochlea can usually be treated successfully with HAs or CIs. Hearing loss caused by damage to the auditory nerve, such as ANSD, is often less successfully treated with HAs but may do well with CIs.

In audiological testing, sensorineural hearing loss is diagnosed when air conduction thresholds and bone conduction thresholds are essentially the same (**Fig. 2.5**). These results indicate that bypassing the outer and middle ears does not improve the thresholds, so the loss is completely located within the inner ear.

Sensorineural hearing loss tends to affect high frequencies before low frequencies. Moreover, since sensorineural hearing loss creates difficulties in the inner ear with encoding and transmitting sound to the brain, only a partial or distorted signal may reach the auditory cortex. Even with appropriate hearing technology, a patient with sensorineural hearing loss may have difficulty perceiving some aspects of spoken language.

2.3.3 Mixed Hearing Loss

Patients can have both conductive and sensorineural hearing loss at the same time. This is called a mixed hearing loss. Mixed hearing loss generally occurs when a patient with sensorineural hearing loss experiences a conductive problem such as wax impaction or middle ear fluid or when there are some structural problems in the outer or middle ear in addition to the hearing loss in the cochlea. The addition of the conductive component reduces the amplification and transmission of sound to the already damaged cochlea, resulting in further hearing loss and less benefit from hearing technology. Medical intervention to treat the conductive component is essential to attempt to eliminate the additional hearing loss.

In audiological testing, mixed hearing loss is diagnosed when bone conduction thresholds are better than air conduction thresholds but are still not within normal limits, so both sets of results

show a hearing loss (**Fig. 2.6**). These results indicate a moderate loss with air conduction testing. However, bone conduction testing, which bypasses the outer and middle ears, shows a mild hearing loss and, thus, something in the outer and middle ears is contributing to the hearing loss. However, since the bone conduction results are not entirely within normal limits, the inner ear is also contributing to the loss. Again, otoscopy and tympanometry are often used to identify the source of the conductive component further.

Mixed hearing loss can impact any and all speech frequencies. Often, patients with sensorineural hearing loss who experience mixed hearing loss because of an additional conductive component from wax impaction or middle ear fluid will report that their hearing aid seems to be quiet or broken. Patients with mixed hearing loss need to receive both medical intervention to determine whether the conductive component can be treated and audiological intervention to determine the appropriate hearing technology for the sensorineural component.

2.4 Degrees of Hearing Loss

In order to quantify hearing loss, unaided audiological thresholds to tonal stimuli are evaluated to determine degree of hearing loss. For many years, the same degrees of hearing loss were used for both children and adults. However, in 1991 the guidelines for children were amended to reflect the fact that hearing loss has a greater impact on children because they are still developing speech and language.[4] Traditionally, degree of hearing loss was measured by averaging the hearing thresholds at 500, 1000, and 2000 Hz. Because of the importance of high frequencies, some audiologists now use a four-frequency average adding 4000 Hz. However, it is important to note that a child's hearing loss may not always fall neatly into one specific category and that averaging may underrepresent the actual impact of the loss. Thresholds can be better at some frequencies and much poorer

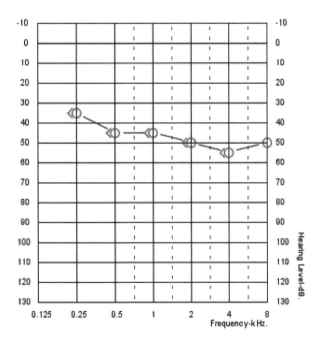

Fig. 2.5 Sample audiogram depicting sensorineural hearing loss.

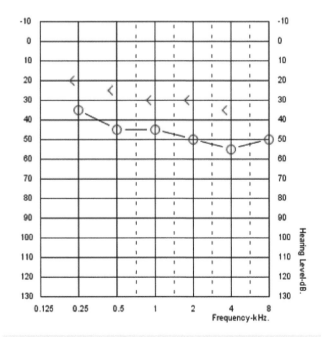

Fig. 2.6 Sample audiogram depicting mixed hearing loss.

at other frequencies, so we may need to use multiple categories to quantify the hearing loss. For instance, a loss may be described as within normal limits to moderate if the low frequencies are normal and the middle or high frequencies have moderate hearing loss, or mild to severe if the low frequencies have a mild hearing loss and the higher frequencies have a severe hearing loss. See **Table 2.1** for the degrees of hearing loss for children.

It is important to note that many public schools and pediatricians' offices screen at 25 dB HL or 30 dB HL. This means that children with thresholds in the slight/minimal or mild hearing loss ranges can pass a hearing screening even though they have a hearing loss. Passing a hearing screening does not ensure that a child has hearing within the normal limits. It is important to remember that even a slight or mild hearing loss will have educational implications. Children with speech and language delays should always have a complete audiological evaluation, not a screening, prior to beginning intervention.

Pearl

Passing a hearing screening does not ensure a child has hearing within normal limits. Even a slight or mild hearing loss will have educational implications.

By recognizing the degree of hearing loss, we are provided with general guidelines of how that hearing loss will impact the child's development. **Table 2.2** shows the predicted impact of the degree of hearing loss on a child's listening, articulation, and language development if the child is not fitted with technology. Again, it is important to remember that thresholds may fall into several different categories, so the impact may be more noticeable in some areas of development than in others.

2.5 Configuration of Hearing Loss

When we look at the audiogram, we also may note the shape of the thresholds on the graph. The configuration tells us which areas of the frequency range the child hears better and which areas are more difficult to hear. The configuration gives us an indication of the types of perception errors the child may make and may help us understand why a child's production has been impacted. (See **Table 2.3** and accompanying **Fig. 2.7**, **Fig. 2.8**, **Fig. 2.9**, **Fig. 2.10**, **Fig. 2.11**, **Fig. 2.12**)

2.6 Unilateral vs. Bilateral Hearing Loss

Children can have hearing loss in one ear (unilateral or single-sided; see **Fig. 2.13**, **Fig. 2.14**) or in both ears (bilateral). For many years, medical and audiological practitioners were under the

Table 2.1 Degrees of hearing loss for children

Degree of hearing loss	Threshold range (in dB HL)
Normal hearing	0 to 15
Slight/minimal	16 to 25
Mild	26 to 40
Moderate	41 to 55
Moderately severe	56 to 70
Severe	71 to 90
Profound	Over 90

Table 2.3 Basic audiological configurations and their effect on perception

Configuration of thresholds	Effect of configuration
Flat (similar thresholds across all frequencies; see **Fig. 2.7**)	Fairly consistent effect on perception of all phonemes
Sloping (poorer thresholds in high frequencies than at low frequencies; see **Fig. 2.8**)	More access to low-frequency phonemes (vowels/nasals) than to high-frequency phonemes (voiceless consonants)
Steeply sloping or **ski slope** (significantly poorer thresholds in high frequencies than at low frequencies; see **Fig. 2.9**)	Access to suprasegmentals and some low-frequency phonemes (vowels/nasals) with little or no access to high-frequency phonemes (voiceless consonants)
Reverse or **rising slope** (poorer thresholds in low frequencies than at high frequencies; see **Fig. 2.10**)	More access to high-frequency phonemes (voiceless consonants) than to low-frequency phonemes (vowels/nasals)
Cookie bite (poorer thresholds in the mid frequencies with better thresholds at the low and high frequencies; see **Fig. 2.11**)	More access to low- and high-frequency formants than to mid-frequency formants, which may result in unusual phoneme confusions
Left corner (low-frequency responses in severe to profound range with little or no high-frequency responses; see **Fig. 2.12**)	Severe to profound hearing loss with no access to speech, language, or even environmental sounds

Table 2.2 Predicted impact of degree of hearing loss on a child's listening, articulation, and language without hearing technology

	Slight / Minimal	Mild	Moderate	Moderately Severe	Severe and Profound
Hear soft sounds?	No	No	No	No	No
Vowel articulation?	Most likely unaffected	Most likely unaffected	Most likely unaffected	Affected	Limited or no development
Consonant articulation?	May be affected	Most likely affected	Affected	Limited or no development	No development
Receptive language?	May be affected	Delayed for age	Significantly delayed	Minimal development	No development
Expressive language?	May be affected	Delayed for age	Significantly delayed	Minimal development	No development
Processing time for spoken language?	May be affected	Noticeably longer	Awkwardly long	Longer, may not help	May not process even with visual support

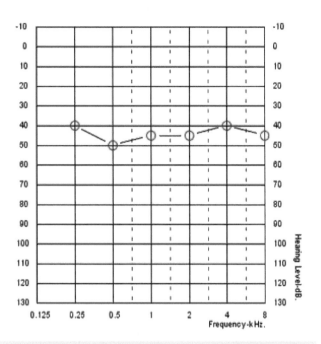

Fig. 2.7 Sample audiogram depicting flat hearing loss configuration.

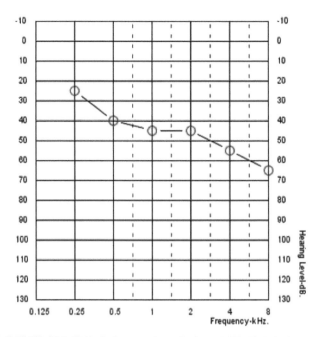

Fig. 2.8 Sample audiogram depicting sloping hearing loss configuration.

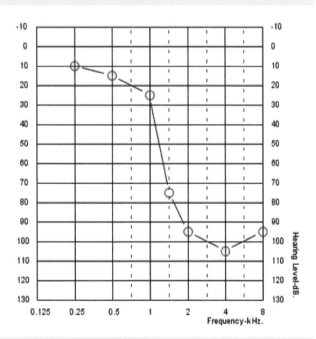

Fig. 2.9 Sample audiogram depicting steeply sloping / ski slope hearing loss configuration.

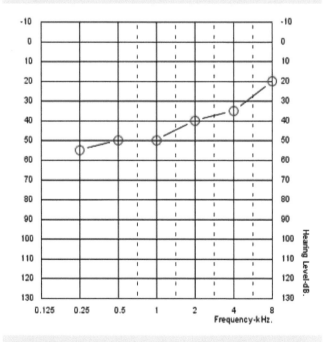

Fig. 2.10 Sample audiogram depicting reverse slope / rising hearing loss configuration.

misconception that hearing from one ear was "good enough." Vila and Lieu[5] summarize the significant body of research, which points to the challenges for children who must learn language and navigate the educational system with normal hearing in only one ear. In addition, Vila and Lieu discuss the permanent changes in the development of the auditory cortex that can occur in children when input from one ear is impaired or absent. We must remember that children with unilateral hearing loss are lacking basic binaural hearing benefits such as the ability to localize sound, increased perception of loudness from binaural summation, improved ability to hear in noise from binaural squelch, and increased access to input from binaural redundancy.

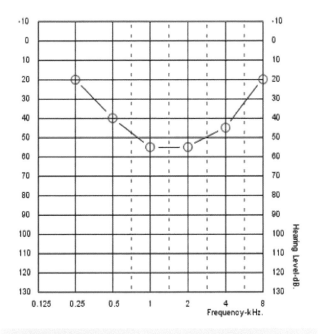

Fig. 2.11 Sample audiogram depicting cookie bite hearing loss configuration.

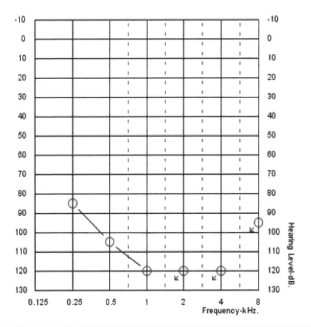

Fig. 2.12 Sample audiogram depicting left corner hearing loss configuration.

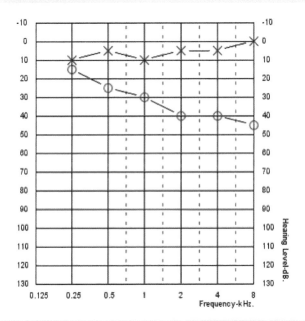

Fig. 2.13 Sample audiogram depicting unilateral hearing loss.

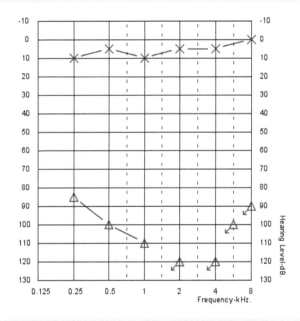

Fig. 2.14 Sample audiogram depicting single-sided deafness.

2.7 Symmetry of Hearing Loss

Finally, it is important to recognize whether the air conduction thresholds are symmetrical (the same in both ears) or asymmetrical (different between the ears). Our ears go everywhere together, so we would expect something that affected the hearing in one ear to affect the hearing in the other ear in the same way. However, this does not always happen. Some children may have asymmetrical hearing loss. This means that the type,

degree, and/or configuration of the hearing loss in one ear may differ slightly or even significantly from that in the other ear (see **Fig. 2.15**). It is important to verify the thresholds and perception of each ear independently to ensure that both can reach their best potential and that one is not so much poorer that it interferes with the abilities of the better ear. It is also important to remember that asymmetrical hearing loss can lessen the benefits of binaural hearing discussed previously.[5]

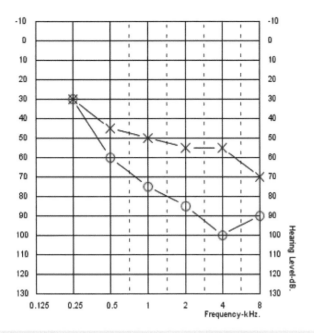 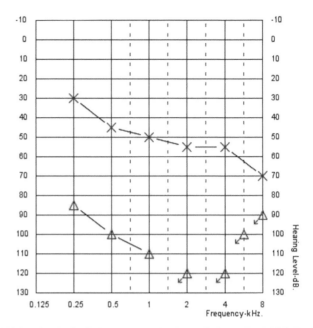

Fig. 2.15 (a,b) Sample audiograms depicting asymmetrical hearing loss.

2.8 Understanding Technology

Clinicians who work with children who are deaf or hard of hearing must understand, not only hearing loss, but also the available hearing technologies. Clinicians should be expected to converse knowledgeably with the parents about different technologies, demonstrate how to check and use the devices, evaluate the basic functions of the devices, and provide data about the benefit the devices provide.

Clinicians should also be keenly aware of the fact that all the electronic devices to be discussed in subsequent paragraphs require programming by the audiologist. When the devices are fitted and programmed optimally, our expectation is for the child to hear optimally and make optimal speech and language progress similar to that of their typically hearing peers. When the wrong devices are selected or the devices are not fitted and programmed optimally, we can expect to see issues that impact not only hearing, but speech, language, social, and educational development. Clinicians should understand that obtaining optimal programming requires input from professionals, parents, and caregivers. Audiologists have tools that can be used to program the hearing devices, but SLPs, TODs, listening and spoken language specialists (LSL), and parents observe the day-to-day results of the programming. The parent and clinician observations of technology performance and benefit with technology should be compiled and shared with the audiologist in order to optimize programming. Clinicians should recognize that programming can be an ongoing process in which their observations and input are invaluable. Families and clinicians should be encouraged to keep a notebook in which they record what sounds the child responds to in each ear separately and both ears together at close distance, at 3 feet (1 m), 6 feet (2 m), and 10 feet (3 m). For infants, families

should be encouraged to test one or two Ling-Madell-Hewitt (LMH) sounds[6] when the infant wakes, record responses with each hearing aid separately at close or far distances, and share this information with the audiologist, who will be able to use it to adjust technology settings. (See Chapter 3 for a discussion of the LMH test battery.) For example, if testing indicates at home that a child can hear /s/ and /i/ at 3 feet but not at 6 feet or 10 feet, then the audiologist can adjust high frequency or soft speech settings to improve hearing performance at a distance. As a child gets older, further testing, including perception of additional phonemes using the medial consonant test, should be added. (For a detailed discussion of identifying when programming of technology is not optimal, see Chapter 18).

2.8.1 Earmolds

The earmold is the plastic part, shaped like the bowl of outer ear, that connects to the hearing aid and fits into the ear canal. The earmold can be a custom mold made to the shape of the child's ear or can be a flexible dome. It is important for the clinician to check the earmolds regularly to ensure they are not cracked, broken, or occluded with earwax. The clinician should also verify that the earmold fits well. If the earmold keeps slipping out of the ear or the child is experiencing an increasing amount of feedback, then the child needs to be referred to the audiologist and the earmolds may need to be replaced. From birth to age 5, a child can have as many as 32 earmold changes. Infants may need earmolds every 4 to 6 weeks because of how quickly they grow. Children a little bit older may move to every 3 to 4 months before they need a new earmold. Even once a child's growing slows, the earmolds should still be changed every year for sanitary reasons and because they may become hard and uncomfortable.

2.8.2 Hearing Aids

Today's hearing aids (HAs) are sophisticated digital processors that can be programmed and customized to provide benefit for many degrees and configurations of hearing loss. HAs can be worn in the ear (ITE) or behind the ear (BTE). Generally, for pediatric patients BTE HAs are safer, more durable, and more reliable. Moreover, with BTE HAs, as the child grows, only the earmolds need to be remade instead of the entire HA casing with ITE hearing aids, which would leave the child without amplification during the recasing process and could significantly increase the cost.

All HAs contain a microphone, which picks up sound in the environment; an amplifier, which increases the intensity of the sound; and a receiver, which delivers the amplified sound into the ear. While all HAs contain these basic parts, it is important to understand that brands and models differ in their ability to fit specific hearing losses, the features they offer, and the quality of the sound. **Table 2.4** provides descriptions of different HA features and considerations for the use of each with children.

Table 2.4 Descriptions, pros, and cons of hearing aid features

Hearing Aid (HA) Feature	Description	Pros	Cons
Number of frequency channels	As channel number increases, allows HA to be programmed more specifically to configuration of hearing loss	May improve sound quality	May increase cost
Extended frequency bands	Allows access to greater speech frequencies	May improve access to and perception of high frequency phonemes	May increase feedback
Frequency shifting/lowering/compression	Shifts higher frequency sounds to lower frequencies where hearing may be better	May provide speech and language benefit for improved access to high frequency phonemes and sounds	Will distort "shifted" phonemes and sounds
Directional microphones	HA contains multiple microphones, which can focus to the front or in varying directions on the person speaking.	May focus on voice in front and reduce noise input from behind or to side of child	Works only for listeners old enough to face the speaker consistently. May limit access to speakers from behind or to the side
Noise reduction	Attempts to reduce noise without affecting speech signal	May reduce noise input	May also reduce sounds child needs to hear
Feedback cancellation	Identifies and eliminates HA feedback (squealing / whistling)	Eliminates annoying feedback	May reduce or eliminate output for high-frequency phonemes or environmental sounds (e.g., eliminating timer beep or reducing amplification for /s/)
Spatial sound features	Allows improved localization of sound	Improves localization of speakers and sounds in classroom and social settings	
Data logging	Records number of hours HA is used and may record HA setting changes and daily listening environments	Provides data that may be used for counseling about child's device use and listening environments	May provide inaccurate or incomplete data
Multiple programs	HA stores multiple preprogrammed settings that can be changed by the user	Allows program or setting changes in different listening environments, such as noisy places or when listening to music	Requires child or adult to be educated on when to change the program Often not used or not used correctly by listeners
Remote control/Phone Apps	Allows changes of settings and/or programs; may be used for troubleshooting or remote programming	Allows child or adult to change settings and/or programs without touching the HA; may provide troubleshooting and programming information for parent and clinician	Requires child or adult be educated on when to change the program Easily lost or misplaced or may not be accessible to someone without App
Rechargeable batteries	Uses charger and eliminates the need to change the battery	Does not require purchase of batteries	May render child unable to hear if battery dies and charging time is required and/or no charger is available
Wireless/Bluetooth connectivity	Allows HA to connect to cell phones and other Bluetooth devices	May allow connection to lessons and tests on tablets and other devices in school Allows social connections through phone	May not connect to all devices May permit student to stream without others knowing (e.g., listening to music on phone in class)
Direct digital modulation (DM) connectivity	Allows direct, wireless connection to DM microphones	Improves signal-to-noise ratio	Adds technology, which needs to be checked to ensure clear transmission
Direct audio input	Allows input from a receiver or cable	Allows direct connection to microphone systems, computers, tablets, and phones	Adds connectors, which needs to be checked to ensure clear transmission
Telecoil (Tcoil)	Allows reception of signals from Tcoil-compatible telephones and public induction loop systems	Allows access to remote microphone systems and induction loop systems in classrooms, theaters, churches, etc.	May reduce access to high frequency sounds Signal reception may be affected by head movement and loop placement Adds connectors, which need to be checked to ensure clear transmission

2.9 Implantable Hearing Devices

With advances in technology, a variety of hearing devices are now surgically implantable.

2.9.1 Implantable Middle Ear Hearing Devices

Implantable middle ear hearing devices are approved for patients with mild to severe sensorineural, mixed, or conductive hearing loss who cannot wear traditional hearing aid amplification for anatomical or physical reasons. These devices are implanted into the middle ear and connected to an external sound processor. Like conventional hearing aids just described, the sound processor has a microphone, amplifier, and receiver that deliver the sound to the middle ear device and may have the features described in **Table 2.4**. By directly moving the ossicles or vibrating the oval window membrane between the middle ear and cochlea, these devices are designed to increase the amplification of sound as it moves through the middle ear in order to deliver a stronger signal to the cochlea.

2.9.2 Osseointegrated Hearing Devices

Traditionally, osseointegrated devices are used for patients with conductive hearing loss; for those with mixed hearing loss with a large conductive component who cannot wear traditional hearing aid amplification because of anatomical or physical reasons; and, recently, for children with single-sided deafness. The osseointegrated sound processor is a sophisticated digital hearing aid that may have many of the features noted in **Table 2.4**.

For patients with atresia or microtia, osseointegrated devices bypass the abnormal anatomy and directly stimulate the inner ear. Initially, these devices are worn on a headband until a child is old enough for surgery. While on the headband, the device will vibrate the skull. However, amplification will be reduced if the headband and device are not in tight contact with the skull. When the device is surgically implanted, an abutment or implant is surgically placed on or in the skull. Once the surgical site is healed and the implant has integrated with the skull, an external processor is attached. Sound is collected by an external processor and delivered as vibrations to the skull. The vibration of the skull directly excites the fluid in the cochlea so that the hair cells are stimulated and respond. Osseointegrated devices surgically implanted or on a headband may also be used for children with single-sided deafness (SSD). The device is placed behind the nonfunctioning ear. The microphone picks up sound on that side of the head and, by vibrating the entire skull, delivers the sound to the functioning cochlea. However, it is important to understand that for children with SSD, an osseointegrated device does not restore hearing to the deaf ear or provide any binaural benefits. In addition, in some noisy settings, it can actually interfere with the listening abilities of the normal hearing ear.

2.9.3 Cochlear Implants

A cochlear implant (CI) is designed for patients with moderately severe to profound sensorineural hearing loss who do not receive sufficient benefit from traditional hearing aid amplification.[7,8,9] In cochlear implant surgery, a receiver/stimulator is placed under the skin behind the ear, and a channel is created so that the surgeon can place electrodes in the cochlea. An external sound processor is connected by a magnet to the internal device. The external processor may look like a hearing aid or may be a small disc placed on the head. The external processor has a microphone that receives sound, converts it to electrical impulses, and sends it to the internal device, which then directs the electrodes to fire and stimulate the neural tissue in the cochlea. Many hearing aid features listed on **Table 2.4** are also available with CI processors.

2.9.4 Auditory Brainstem Implant

An auditory brainstem implant is a surgically implanted device for patients who cannot benefit from an HA or a CI because of significant inner ear abnormalities such as cochlear aplasia (absence of the cochlea), cochlear nerve aplasia (absence of the auditory nerve), cochlear nerve hypoplasia (underdeveloped auditory nerve), ossification of the cochlea, or acoustic neuromas (tumors affecting the auditory nerve).

As with the CI, an internal receiver/stimulator is surgically placed under the skin behind the ear, but for an auditory brainstem implant the electrodes are placed on the brainstem to bypass the damaged or missing inner ear and nerve. Also as with the CI, when the implant is activated, an external processor is placed on the ear to connect to the internal device and stimulate the auditory brainstem. In many cases, the external processor is identical to that of a CI and has many of the same features.

2.10 Remote Microphone Systems

Two of the biggest issues with hearing loss, even with optimally fitted technology, are distance and noise. Microphones on hearing devices perform best when the talker is within 3 feet. As a speaker moves farther and farther from the hearing device microphone, the more difficulty the microphone has collecting the sound. For every doubling of the distance between the listener and the talker, the signal drops 6 dB (discussed in Chapter 3). Obviously, it would be impossible for every speaker to stay within 3 feet of the microphone on a child's device at all times. The problem of distance is compounded by the fact that children spend much of their day in noisy listening environments. Homes, daycares, classrooms, sports fields, and so forth are noisy places. Many times, the noise in the environment is sufficiently loud to mask or cover up what the child needs to hear. Thus, all day long, children with hearing loss are struggling to hear people talking who are at a distance and whose voices are embedded in the surrounding noise.

Remote microphone (RM) systems provide a way to bring the desired speaker's voice closer to the child. Remote microphones are designed to be worn about 6 inches from the speaker's mouth, so the voice is transmitted to the hearing technology as if the speaker were only 6 inches from the child's ear. By bringing the talker's voice closer, the voice naturally becomes louder, which helps to separate it from the background noise. By making the speaker's voice appear closer and louder, we improve the signal-to-noise ratio (SNR), which is the difference between the loudness of the signal we want to hear (speech) and the background noise. While remote microphone systems are routinely used in school, they should be considered for home use, especially for young children learning language, as well as for sports, dance class, religious instruction, and other activities. Every child with hearing loss needs a remote microphone system for use in all difficult listening situations or when more than 3 feet from the person speaking.

Remote microphone systems can be personally worn attached to or part of hearing aids or other technology, or they can be standalone soundfield systems.

2.10.1 Personal RM Systems

Remote microphone systems can deliver the parent's, teacher's, or other talker's voice directly to the hearing technology. This may necessitate a receiver connected via a port or additional connector to the hearing technology, or the receiver may be built into the hearing technology with no additional receiver needed. The child's audiologist will determine whether additional connectors or receivers are necessary for the specific technology the child uses.

2.10.2 Soundfield Systems

Soundfield systems involve a microphone worn by the teacher or speaker, which delivers the teacher's voice wirelessly by frequency-modulated (FM) radio to one or more loudspeakers placed within the room. This system is designed to amplify the speaker's voice so that it is louder than the noise and the SNR is improved. In addition, listeners in all parts of the room will have access to the speaker's voice regardless of how far away the teacher is standing. A soundfield system can be expected to improve the SNR by about 3 dB, meaning that it will raise the speaker's voice by about 3 dB. For children with normal hearing, the addition of the signal from the soundfield system will provide increased access to auditory information, making listening in the classroom easier. However, for a child with hearing loss, a soundfield system is not sufficient. Research by Shaefer and Kleineck,[10] Wolfe et al,[11] and others has shown that a soundfield FM will increase speech perception by 3.5%, but a personal wearable RM will increase speech perception by 38%.

Pearl

All children with hearing loss need a personal wearable RM system for use in all learning situations. A soundfield FM will increase speech perception by 3.5%, but a personal wearable RM will increase speech perception by 38%.

2.10.3 Pass-Around Microphones

Pass-around microphones are second remote microphones used in a classroom. Microphones worn by teachers will amplify their voices but will not enable the child with hearing loss to hear other children in the classroom as they answer questions or participate in discussion. The pass-around microphone will be passed around from child to child as they speak, to amplify children's voices when they ask and answer questions, give reports, and participate in discussions. In some systems, the teacher's microphone can be placed on a desk or table and used as a conference microphone for small-group work. Since personal RM systems deliver the speaker's voice as if it were approximately

6 inches away from the child's hearing technology, they can be expected to improve the SNR by up to 6 dB. (In many European countries, classrooms have multiple pass-around microphones, often one for each desk, ensuring that children hear everything. In the United States we have not progressed that far.) If there is a soundfield system in the classroom, the pass-around microphone can be connected or synched to the child's personal system as well as to the soundfield system, allowing all children in the classroom to benefit from the improved auditory signal.

2.11 Issues That Affect Auditory Learning

Therapy cannot proceed until the child is hearing with technology. Simply fitting a child with hearing aids or other technology does not guarantee that the child is hearing well enough. For a child to learn language through audition, the child needs to hear both normal and soft conversation. A child who hears well at normal conversational levels (45–50 dB HL) will be able to hear conversation at 6 feet away, but children also need to hear soft speech, which is at 30–35 dB HL. A child who hears soft speech can hear conversation at about 10 feet away. Soft speech is essential because 90% of what children learn, they learn incidentally, by overhearing conversation not directed at them. If children need to learn everything by having the talker sit directly in front of them, exposure to language will be significantly reduced. By overhearing conversations around them and hearing a parent talking from a distance, they have the opportunity for much more language exposure.

2.11.1 How to Know Whether a Child Is Hearing Well Enough

Never assume. Monitoring of hearing needs to be performed by the audiologist, the SLP, the LSLS, the TOD, and the parent. In other words, everyone working with a child with hearing loss is responsible for monitoring audition.

The audiologist will test hearing periodically. Testing will include testing hearing with and without technology. **Table 2.5** lists all the tests that should be conducted as part of an audiology

---

Table 2.5 Audiological test protocols

- Unaided testing
  - Threshold testing with earphones (500–8000 Hz) in each ear
  - Speech perception testing at 40 dB above pure tone average (PTA) or at comfortable listening level if 40 dB above PTA is too loud
  - Middle ear evaluation—tympanometry
  - Otoacoustic emissions
- Function testing (speech perception) for child without technology
  - In soundfield at 50 dB and 35 dB in quiet and at 50 dB HL +5 SNR
- Testing with technology
  - Aided thresholds in each ear 500–6000 Hz to assess access to soft speech
  - Speech perception testing
  - Normal conversation (50 dB HL) (right ear, left ear, binaural)
  - Soft conversation (35 dB HL) (binaural)
  - Normal conversation in noise (50 dB HL +5 SNR) (binaural)

evaluation. Some of the tests, such as speech perception testing, may not be performed on infants.

Fig. 2.16 shows an audiogram with the speech banana and the Speech String Bean[12] at the top of the speech banana. If children hear at the top of the speech banana, they will hear 90% of what is said. If they hear at the bottom of the speech banana, they will hear 10% of what is said.[13] Our goal is to have children hear as much of the auditory signal as possible. The blue line shows the level of normal conversation, and the red line shows the level of soft conversation. We want to be sure that children are hearing well enough to hear both normal and soft conversation. A child, for example, who is hearing with technology at 35 dB will not hear soft conversation.

By evaluating audiological test results, we will know what a child is hearing and what the child is not hearing. If threshold testing indicates that the child is not hearing high frequency sounds, we know the child will be missing high frequency phonemes such as sibilants and fricatives. This will significantly affect language learning (see Chapter 3 for more information).

2.11.2 Speech Perception Testing

Speech perception testing is probably the most important part of the audiological test battery, since the goal of technology is to provide access to speech and language. Testing is used to assess how well a child hears and understands what is being said. For children with hearing loss or with auditory processing disorders, speech perception testing will provide information about how much language they are being exposed to, and, if they are using technology, it will tell us how well the technology is working.[14]

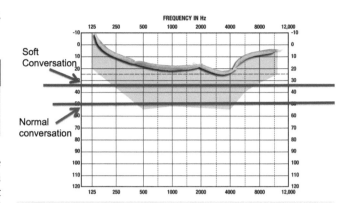

Fig. 2.16 Speech String Bean with normal and soft conversational levels.

We use speech perception testing to determine candidacy for technology. If unaided testing indicates that a child is not hearing sufficiently well, it makes the case for fitting the child with hearing aids. If we know that the hearing aids are working well but the child is not hearing well enough with hearing aids, that finding may indicate that it is time to change HAs or move from HAs to CIs. By evaluating specific perception errors, the audiologist can determine which part of the speech spectrum the child is missing and can adjust technology settings to provide improved input in those specific frequency bands. The Medial Consonant test[15] developed by Tyler, which is now part of the LMH Test Battery (see Chapter 3 for further discussion) is a very useful tool for evaluating perception of all consonants. Children are asked to repeat consonants embedded in vowels (*aba*, *afa*, etc.). The errors are recorded, and the confusions are evaluated. By looking at the frequency energy bands of the errors, the audiologist can determine how to change technology settings. **Table 2.7** lists speech perception tests by age.[16,17,18,19,20,21]

By monitoring performance over time, we will identify changes in performance that develop. We expect that speech perception will improve as children develop better auditory skills. If we

Table 2.6 Summary of testing protocols used with technology at different ages

	0–6 months	6–12 months	12–24 months	24–36 months	Over 36 months
RECD	✓	✓	✓	✓	✓
Cortical responses	✓	✓	✓	✓	✓
Aided thresholds 500–8K	✓	✓	✓	✓	✓
SAT – LMH sounds	✓	✓	✓		
SRT			✓	✓	✓
Speech perception 50 dB HL Quiet			✓ (R, L, B)	✓ (R, L, B)	✓ (R, L, B)
Speech perception 35 dB HL Quiet				✓ (B)	✓ (B)
Speech Perception 50 dB HL +5 SNR				✓ (B)	✓ (B)

Abbreviations: B, Binaural; L, left ear; R, right ear; RECD, real ear to coupler difference; SAT, speech awareness threshold; SRT, speech reception threshold.

Table 2.7 Speech perception tests by age

	0–6 months	6–12 months	12–18 months	18–24 months	24–36 months	3–5 yrs	6–8 yrs	8+ yrs
SAT	✓	✓	✓	✓				
SRT			✓	✓	✓	✓	✓	✓
ESP[16]	✓	✓	✓	✓				
NU CHIPS[17]				✓	✓	✓		
WIPI[18,19]						✓	✓	
PBK[20]						✓	✓	
NU 6/ CNC							✓	✓
HINT[21]							✓	✓
BabyBio							✓	✓
AzBio								✓

Abbreviations: **AzBio**, **AzBio** (Arizona Biomedical Institute) sentence lists (Auditory Potential LLC); Baby Bio, pediatric version of **AzBio** (Auditory Potential LLC); CNC, Maryland CNC word recognition test; ESP, Early Speech Perception test; HINT, Hearing in Noise Test; NU 6, Northwestern University Auditory Test No. 6 (Auditec, Inc.); NU CHIPS, Northwestern University—Children's Perception of Speech; PBK, Phonetically Balanced Kindergarten test; SAT, speech awareness threshold; SRT, speech reception threshold; WIPI, Word Intelligibility by Picture Identification.

notice a reduction in functioning, or a lack of improvement, there is a problem that needs to be identified. This might include equipment failure or may indicate that the child is not using technology full time (at least 10 hours/day). If the audiologist can ensure that the technology is working properly and that it is providing sufficient auditory access, then we need to look to the habilitation. It may indicate that the child is in need of more or improved auditory therapy (**Video 2.8**, **Video 2.9**, **Video 2.10**, **Video 2.11**, **Video 2.12**).

Pearl

Speech perception is a critical part of the audiological evaluation and will provide information about how a child is performing and assist in modifying technology settings and planning remediation.

2.11.3 Scoring Speech Perception Tests

Speech perception testing of children with hearing loss should be scored the same way we score speech perception testing of their typical hearing peers. Describing speech perception test results as "excellent" or "good" indicates that all is going well. Describing speech perception test results as "fair" or "poor"

Table 2.8 Evaluating Speech Perception Performance

Excellent	90–100%
Good	80–89%
Fair	70–79%
Poor	Less than 70%

indicates a problem that needs to be identified and corrected. We need to check technology first. If technology is found to be providing what it needs to provide, then the clinicians working on language and auditory development need to work on building skills. **Table 2.8** provides recommended scoring designation.[22] It is critical to be honest in the way we describe test results. If we describe a speech perception score of 64% as "good" speech perception, families and clinicians do not know when therapy or technology needs to be modified. Only by being honest in the way we describe test results can we expect that the children will receive the assistance they need.

2.11.4 What Technology Must Do to Meet the Criteria of Acoustic Accessibility

Children need to hear throughout the frequency range. Hearing 6000 and 8000 Hz really does matter. Missing high frequencies results in missing grammatical markers for pluralization and possessives and missing nonsalient morphemes (i.e., morphemes that are not stressed during conversation, such as prepositions). In addition, we need to be certain that the child is hearing soft speech. Soft speech is about 30–35 dB HL. If children cannot hear soft speech, they will not hear peers in the classroom or on the playground, nor "overhear" conversation, and thus they will have limited incidental learning, resulting in reduced language and literacy skills.

2.11.5 How Often Children Should Be Tested

Babies need to be tested often. They are not able to report problems hearing. Children under the age of 4 years should be tested every 3 months. Children older than 4 should be tested every 6 months. When children become teenagers and are better reporters of technology problems, they may be able to move to annual evaluations. Should the child, family, or clinicians working with a child become concerned about performance at any time, the child should be seen for a complete audiological evaluation.

2.12 Developing a Team and Working Collaboratively

It takes a village to raise a child with hearing loss. The child is always at the center, with family close by. In addition to the family, every child with hearing loss will require an audiologist, an auditory-based speech-language therapist, and medical provider (usually both a pediatrician and an otologist). A child with additional needs may have physical and/or occupational therapists on the team. As the child reaches school age, there will be one or more classroom teachers. Most children with hearing loss will benefit from a TOD to provide preview and review of vocabulary and concepts, advocacy training, and academic tutoring if necessary. An educational audiologist in the school will be an asset in monitoring classroom technology and helping school staff understand about the effect of hearing loss on learning. Unfortunately, many school districts no longer have educational audiologists. If there is no educational audiologist in the school district, the clinical audiologist will have to take over many of the responsibilities of the educational audiologist, including assisting and selecting RM systems and educating school staff about appropriate care and use of the child's technology and remote RM systems. (See Chapter 22 about roles of the educational audiologist, SLP, and TOD.) Members of the team will change as the child's needs change and as the child grows older.

2.12.1 The Team Coordinator

Someone needs to monitor how a child is progressing. The team coordinator will be responsible for coordinating with other members of the team to be sure that everyone knows what is happening, how the child is doing, and what, if any, areas of concern exist.

Initially the team coordinator will likely be the audiologist who is diagnosing the hearing loss and fitting technology. If there are significant medical issues, the team coordinator may be the physician. As the child moves into early intervention, the LSLS or SLP will likely be the coordinator. As the child moves into school, the TOD may become the coordinator. Eventually, the parents or the child may become the coordinator. As children grow older, they should become more responsible and take over.

It is critical that a system be developed for sharing information. In an ideal world, everyone on the team would meet periodically to discuss progress and concerns. This could be done in person or via a videoconference (e.g., Zoom call). If this is not possible, or in between team meetings, information can be shared via email, a joint web page for each individual child, or a notebook that is passed around. Different systems will work for different groups. It is very important that some system be developed, because if there is no system for communicating between team members, information will get lost and the child will suffer.

2.13 What the Audiology Report Needs to Include for Families and Clinicians

Families and clinicians often complain that they just can't read audiology reports. They are written in some "foreign language" and are not intelligible. Audiologists often write for other audiologists and for otolaryngologists. What information do they need to transmit to families and to other clinicians? If the necessary information is not included in the report, families and clinicians should request it.

2.13.1 Degree of Hearing Loss and Auditory Functioning

What does it mean to say a child has a moderate hearing loss? It would be good if, after describing the hearing loss (mild, moderate, etc.), the audiologist described how this degree of hearing loss will affect function in some detail. For example, with a moderate hearing loss:

> Without hearing technology, Ralph will be able to hear speech if the talker is standing next to him and speaking into his ear. He will not be able to overhear conversation when he is more than 2 feet away from the talker. This means he will have much less language exposure, which will result in poor language development and poor literacy skills.

This kind of information is much clearer. It helps the family understand why we need to move to using technology; helps the pediatrician, teacher, SLP, or other professional understand the interventions that need to be implemented; and helps the family accept both technology and therapy.

2.13.2 Is the Technology Providing Sufficient Auditory Access?

Once a child has technology, we need to know whether it is working well. It is not enough to say a child "has hearing aids." The question is how well they work. Audiology reports need to include information about what a child is hearing with the technology. Is the child hearing softly enough? For example, if aided thresholds are at 40 dB (moderate hearing loss levels), the report might say:

> With the current hearing aids, Clare is hearing at moderate hearing loss levels. She will not hear soft speech. This means she will have much less language exposure, which will result in reduced language development and poor literacy skills.

2.13.3 Does the Technology Provide Information throughout the Frequency Range?

Is the child hearing high frequencies with the technology? It is really important to hear high frequencies. So, if children hear well at low and middle frequencies but do not hear high frequencies, they will not hear /s/, /ʃ/, /f/, and so on. The report needs to state clearly what a child is and is not hearing with technology.

2.13.4 Can the Child Hear Soft Speech?

What exactly is the child hearing with technology? The audiology report should include tests of speech perception at normal and soft conversational levels in quiet and in competing noise. The report might say:

> Rosie has excellent speech perception at normal conversational levels, but speech perception is fair at soft conversation and poor in competing noise.

By clearly stating the facts, the audiologist can justify the need for therapy to improve auditory skills and for use of an RM system in school and in other difficult listening situations.

2.13.5 Justifying the Need for Auditory-Based Therapy

If a child is not doing well, audiological test results can justify the need for therapy. If audiology has done all that can be done with the technology, if we have provided sufficient auditory access, if it is working well, and if it is being used full time, then lack of progress in one or more areas indicates that we need to move to auditory-based therapy to help improve skills.

2.13.6 How Does This Help?

The foregoing test information helps everyone truly understand the child's auditory status. Audiologists are frequently reluctant to say that a child is doing poorly, but if the report does not clearly state that a child is not doing well, interventionists do not know that they must identify things to be done to improve performance.

Pearl

Only by working as a team can we provide children with all they need. It does "take a village." Team members need to find good ways to communicate.

2.14 What Information the Audiologist Needs from Families and Interventionists

Audiologists cannot do their job well without information from those who see these children more often than the audiologist does. Families, LSLSs, SLPs, and TODs are more likely to know whether the technology is working well or not. It is everyone's responsibility to share information.

2.14.1 How Many Hours a Day Is the Child Wearing the Technology?

It is obviously critical that children wear their technology all day long. If a child wears hearing aids only 4 hours per day, it will take 6 years to hear what a typically hearing child hears in one year. Research by Moeller[23] and others[7,24,25,26] has demonstrated that children who wear technology 10 hours/day or more can perform at the level of their typically hearing peers, and those who use technology less than 10 hours/day cannot. Families often overestimate how many hours/day a child is using technology. It is useful to probe a little: "Do you put it on as soon as he wakes up?" "How many hours a day do they nap?" "Do you keep it on when you go out for a walk? in the car? What about after the bath?" "What time does it come off for the night?" "What about with babysitters or grandparents?" By asking these kinds of probing questions, we can help families recognize when the child is not using the technology as much as they thought. In addition, most current HAs and CIs have technology (data logging) that enables the audiologist to know how many hours/day the technology is being used.

2.14.2 Does the Child Like the Technology?

Does the child want to put it on in the morning? Does it require a lot of coaxing to get it on? How often does the child take it off during the day? If the child does not want to wear the technology, do you know why? Is it too loud and, therefore, uncomfortable? Is it too soft and not providing the ability to hear well? Are there specific situations where the child does not want to wear it? The car? The playground? Is the child having problems tolerating the hearing devices in competing noise? Are there social issues that are making the child uncomfortable? Is the child getting teased at school about having to wear technology? The audiologist needs to know the answers to these questions.

A 12-year-old we know had had a CI for many years. While a successful auditory-oral communicator, the child still gave parents a problem about putting the implant on first thing in the morning. A new audiologist changed the CI program, and now the patient is hearing more clearly and more comfortably. Now the child reaches for the CI immediately on getting out of bed. The child just was not hearing well enough with the old CI program. The change in behavior happened overnight. *Never assume!*

2.14.3 What Kind of Noise Environment Is the Child In?

Is the child in a relatively quiet environment at home, or are there other children there all day? Are they in daycare, and, if yes, how many children and how many adults are in the room? If in school, what kind of class is it? How many children and teachers are in the classroom? How noisy is the room? Getting this kind of information can justify to families and others the need for an RM system very early. In addition, it can make a case for trying to arrange noise control in the classroom, such as placing footies on the chairs and tables, keeping doors and windows closed, and having only one person speak at a time.

2.14.4 Is There Any Evidence the Technology Is Not Working Well?

Sometimes when children reject a device or are not making progress, it is because they are not hearing well, so checking out how the child is using the device will help. Are the child's auditory skills progressing in development or maintaining as expected? Are skills deteriorating? If yes, it may indicate problems with the technology.

2.14.5 What Is the Child Hearing?

The family and others working with the child need to report to the audiologist whether the child is hearing all phonemes. Are there some consistently missed, or does the child hear only when sounds are loud? Are there perception errors the child is consistently making (e.g., *slipper* for *kipper*, missing the final /s/ in *boots*)? How far away can the child hear? To have optimal access to incidental language, we want a child to hear at 10 feet, at least in quiet.

2.14.6 Voice Quality

If a child has a gravelly, nasal, or other unusual voice quality with technology on, it may indicate that the child is not hearing well. Also, if parents report that the child's voice is consistently too loud or too soft, this may indicate a need to check technology settings.

2.14.7 Language Development

If children's language is age appropriate, they should be progressing at a rate of one year's development in one year's time. If children's language is delayed, they need to progress at a rate of *more* than one year's growth in one year's time, or they will not be able to close the gap between their language and their peers'. If a child is not making sufficient progress, it will be necessary to evaluate all the contributing factors and determine what needs to be done.

Pearl

If children's language is delayed, they need to progress at a rate of *more* than one year's growth in one year's time, or they will not be able to close the gap between their language and their peers'.

2.14.8 Using the Information

By collecting the information just discussed and acting on it, the team can modify the technology to ensure that children are hearing what they need to hear to be able to use audition to learn.

2.14.9 Listening to Each Other

Open communication among team members will positively impact the success of the child. If team members cannot successfully communicate with each other, they will negatively impact

the child's success. It is essential that we all understand that different members of the team have different areas of expertise, and each has an important contribution to make. Audiologists will learn a great deal by hearing from clinicians about what a child is hearing and what the child is missing. By actively listening, the audiologist can get useful information about what can be changed in technology settings. Clinicians doing auditory work can benefit from information the audiologist can provide about use of the technology and its limitations. For example, if the clinician is concerned that a child is not hearing well enough with HAs, the clinician and audiologist can brainstorm together how to approach the family to discuss moving to CIs. By respecting each other's contributions, team members can focus on the children, and the sky will be the limit, as it should be.

Pearl

By respecting each other's contributions, the team members can focus on the children, and the sky will be the limit, as it should be.

2.15 Summary

Audiology is the basis for auditory learning. For children with hearing loss to be successful in the development of speech and language, they need to hear well. To ensure that they are hearing well, audiological evaluations need to be accurate and complete, and technology needs to be appropriately fitted and providing access to both normal and soft conversation. Speech perception testing needs to ensure that we know how children hear with technology and that they hear well enough to understand speech in complex situations. We need to know whether children have problems hearing specific phonemes and, if they are missing something, what they are missing.

The entire team is responsible for monitoring auditory performance. The audiologist will do that in the audiology test booth. SLPs, LSLSs, TODs, and families must also monitor performance carefully and be able to report to each other and to the audiologist what the child is hearing and what the child is missing. By working together as a team, we are more likely to ensure the success of the children we work with.

References

[1] Madell JR. Behavioral evaluation of hearing in infants and children. In: Madell JR, Flexer C, Wolfe J, Schafer EC, eds., Pediatric Audiology: Diagnosis, Technology and Management. 3rd ed. New York, NY: Thieme; 2019:75–90

[2] Madell JR. Testing babies: You can do it! Behavioral observation audiometry (BOA). *Perspect Hear Hear Disord* 2011;21(2):59–65

[3] Madell JR. Impact of otitis media on auditory function. In: Rosenfeld RM, Bluestone CD, eds. *Evidence-Based Otitis Media.* New York, NY: Elsevier; 1999:337–350

[4] Northern JL, Downs MP. Hearing in Children. 4th ed. Baltimore, MD: Williams and Wilkins; 1991

[5] Vila P, Lieu JEC. Asymmetric and unilateral hearing loss in children. *Cell Tissue Res* 2015;361(1):271–278

[6] Madell JR, Hewitt JG. (2021) The LMH test for monitoring listening..Hearing Health & Technology Matters. https://hearinghealthmatters.org/hearingandkids/2021/3245/

[7] Ching TYC, Dillion H. Major findings of the LOCHI study on children at 3 years of age and implications for audiological management. *Int J Audiol* 2013;52(2):S65–S85

[8] Dettman SJ, Dowell RC, Choo D, et al. Long-term communication outcomes for children receiving cochlear implants younger than 12 months: a multicenter study. *Otol Neurotol* 2016;*37*(2):e82–e95

[9] Gifford R. Cochlear implants for infants and children. In: Madell JR, Flexer C, eds. In: *Pediatric Audiology: Diagnosis, Technology, and Management.* 2nd ed. New York, NY: Thieme; 2014:238–254

[10] 10. Schafer EC, Kleineck MP. Improvements in speech recognition using cochlear implants and three types of FM systems: a meta-analytic approach. *J Educ Audiol* 2009;*15*:4–14

[11] Wolfe J, Morais M, Nrumann M, et al. Evaluation of speech recognition with personal FM and classroom audio distribution systems. *J Educ Audiol* 2013;*19*:65–79

[12] Madell JR. The Speech String Bean. *Volta Voices* 2016;*23*(1):28–31

[13] Pasco D. An approach to hearing aid selection. *Hear Instrum* 1978;*29*:12–16

[14] Madell JR, Schafer E. Evaluation of speech perception in infants and children. In: Madell JR, Flexer C, Wolfe J, Schafer E, eds. *Pediatric Audiology: Diagnosis, Technology, and Management.* 3rd ed. New York, NY: Thieme; 2019:97–108

[15] Tyler R, Preece JP, Lowder MW. *The Iowa Cochlear Implant Test Battery.* Iowa City, IA: University of Iowa;1993

[16] Geers AE, Moog JS. *Early Speech Perception Test.* St. Louis, MO: Central Institute for the Deaf; 1990

[17] Katz J, Elliot L. Development of a new children's speech discrimination test. Paper presented at: American Speech and Hearing Association, 1978; San Francisco, CA

[18] Ross M, Lerman J. A picture identification test for hearing impaired children. *J Speech Hear Res* 1970;*13*:44–53

[19] Cienkowski KM, Ross M, Lerman J. The Word Intelligibility by Picture Identification (WIPI) test revisited. *J Educ Audiol* 2009;*15*:39–43

[20] Haskins H. A phonetically balanced test of speech discrimination for children [master's thesis]. Evanston, IL: Northwestern University; 1949

[21] Nilsson M, Soli SD, Sullivan JA. Development of the Hearing in Noise Test for the measurement of speech reception thresholds in quiet and in noise. *J Acoust Soc Am* 1994;*95*(2):1085–1099

[22] Madell JR, Batheja R, Klemp E, Hoffman R. Evaluating speech perception performance. *Audiol Today* 2011 Sept-Oct:52–56

[23] Ambrose SE, Walker EA, Unflat-Berry LM, Oleson JJ, Moeller MP. Quantity and quality of caregivers' linguistic input to 18-month and 3-year-old children who are hard of hearing. *Ear Hear* 2015;*36*(Suppl 1):48S–59S

[24] Boons T, Brokx JP, Dhooge I, et al. Predictors of spoken language development following pediatric cochlear implantation. *Ear Hear* 2012;*33*(5):617–639

[25] McCreery RW, Walker EA, Spratford M, et al. Longitudinal predictors of aided speech audibility in infants and children. *Ear Hear* 2015;*36*(Suppl 1):24S–37S

[26] Geers AE, Strube MJ, Tobey EA, Pisoni DB, Moog JS. Epilogue: factors contributing to long-term outcomes of cochlear implantation in early childhood. *Ear Hear* 2011; *32*(1, Suppl):84S–92S

3 Speech Acoustics: Strengthening the Foundation

Jane R. Madell and Joan G. Hewitt

Summary

Typically hearing children access speech and language through listening, but hearing loss affects the quantity and quality of the speech and language information received. In order to ensure appropriate technology fittings and plan aural habilitation, we must know what a child with hearing loss hears and does not hear. This chapter explains basic acoustic properties of sound, basic speech production, and their relationship to each other and to hearing loss. This chapter also discusses considerations for evaluating children to ensure that they are able to access all frequencies-and phonemes—across the speech spectrum—at soft, normal, soft and loud conversational levels.

Keywords

speech acoustics, intensity, frequency, duration, decibels (dB), suprasegmentals, segmentals, phonemes, phonation, resonance, consonants, vowels, vowel formants, consonant frequency bands, voicing, speech banana, speech string bean, audibility, intelligibility, speech bubble, Ling-Madell-Hewitt (LMH) Test Battery

Key Points

- Audition is the only sense capable of appreciating all aspects of speech.
- Hearing loss causes problems accessing spoken language.
- Understanding speech acoustics is critical to evaluating what children are hearing and what they are missing, which enables us to plan remediation.
- Vowels carry 90% of the energy of speech but only 10% of the information for understanding speech. Consonants carry only 10% of the energy of speech but 90% of the information for understanding speech. Accessing all phonemes is critical.
- Hearing is first. Once children hear, we can expect them to start listening. Once children are listening, they are ready to understand, and once they understand, they will start to talk, but auditory access must come first.

3.1 What Speech Acoustics Is and Why We Need to Know about Speech Acoustics

Speech acoustics is a way of analyzing speech information to understand better how it is transmitted and received. By understanding speech acoustics, we can evaluate what children

are hearing and what they are not able to hear and use this information to modify technology settings and to plan habilitation. Audition is the only sense capable of appreciating all aspects of speech. Daniel Ling[1] and others regard audition as potentially the most important sense and the only one directly capable of appreciating the primary characteristics of speech. Therefore, the greatest problem with having a hearing loss is the difficulty it causes in accessing listening and spoken language. The goal of technology and auditory-based therapy is to improve listening for children with hearing loss. By improving listening, we can improve language development, spoken language, and literacy. Different hearing losses affect access to spoken language differently. The more severe the hearing loss, the more access to spoken language will be affected. With hearing technology, we attempt to correct for the hearing loss. If children with hearing loss are to succeed in learning to listen and speak, then we need to understand how hearing loss affects their access to auditory information.

Listening is the basis of any auditory-based therapy program. We know that children learn language best when they hear language around them. We assume that children with typical hearing are hearing everything they need to hear. We cannot make the same assumption about children with hearing loss, even when they are using technology. By understanding speech acoustics, we can understand what sounds of speech children are hearing and what sounds they will not be able to hear. With that information we can better understand a child's speech perception and production and use that information to modify technology settings, adapt our strategies and techniques, and plan therapy. We need to know exactly what children are hearing. Speech acoustics gives us the answers to important questions such as: Are they hearing all the phonemes? If not, which phonemes are they missing, and which do they hear only in a distorted form? Where do these sounds fall on the child's audiogram? Are they hearing them? Do they hear some phonemes when standing close to the talker but not when 6 feet away? Are they hearing phonemes at normal conversational levels? Are they hearing phonemes at sufficiently soft levels that they can overhear conversation, which will enable them to benefit from incidental learning? What are their speech perception and production error patterns, and do these relate to what sounds they are or are not perceiving? *Never assume!* Just because a child has been fitted with technology does not mean that the technology is appropriately set. Only by ongoing evaluation and monitoring of performance can we know how well a child is hearing. This is a team effort requiring information from parents, audiologists, speech-language pathologists (SLPs), listening and spoken language (LSL) specialists (LSLS), and teachers of the deaf (TODs). Why is this important? As Ling said, "What they hear is what they say." By really understanding speech acoustics, we can better evaluate children's speech and language development, which will help us plan for the child.

Pearl

By really understanding speech acoustics, we can better evaluate children's speech and language development, which will help us plan.

By understanding what children with hearing loss are hearing and, more importantly, what they are not hearing, we can better manage their therapy. We can help the audiologist understand what technology settings need to be adjusted to improve speech perception. What exactly does this mean?

As we have said, children learn spoken language and speech through listening. Typically hearing babies have been hearing for about 20 weeks by the time they are born. At birth, they recognize their mom's voice and recognize their native language.[2,3] Infants who are deaf or hard of hearing have missed some auditory exposure during pregnancy and, depending on how long it takes for hearing aids to be fitted, may have an even longer time of auditory deprivation. If the technology is not appropriately set, additional time for auditory brain access and brain development is lost. All clinicians working with families need to be aware of what a child is and is not hearing so that technology settings can be adjusted with the goal of improving auditory perception and performance. If children miss time listening, they fall further behind and may have difficulty catching up.

The goal of newborn hearing screening is to identify children with hearing loss and fit them with technology as soon as possible so that their listening age and chronological age will be very close. The American Academy of Pediatrics (AAP) Joint Commission on Infant Hearing[4] recommendations are that babies be screened by 1 month of age, be diagnosed by 3 months of age, and begin remediation by 6 months of age ("1-3-6"). It is expected that the regulations will upgrade these goals to 1-2-3, which will provide access to auditory information sooner. If a baby is identified at birth and fitted appropriately with technology within weeks, the baby's listening age and chronological age will be essentially the same. If the child does not have appropriate technology settings until age 18 months, on the other hand, then at a chronological age of 2 years, the child's listening age will be only 6 months. This needs to be considered when we think about development and performance.

3.2 Describing Sound

Sound is described by intensity, frequency, and duration. Frequency is the correlate of the sensation of pitch. Low-frequency sounds are heard as low-pitched sounds (bass), and high-frequency sounds are heard as high-pitched sounds (treble). Intensity is correlated with the sensation of loudness. High-intensity sounds are loud, and sounds with low intensity are soft. Duration describes how long the sound signal continues. Is it a short sound like "ba" or long like "ahhhhh"?

3.2.1 Energy of Sounds

The energy of sounds is measured in decibels (dB). This measure is on a logarithmic scale. Doubling the intensity of a sound increases it by about 3 dB; multiplying the intensity tenfold increases it by 10 dB (one bel). The range between the softest and loudest speech sounds is about 30 decibels for speech at a given volume. The phoneme /θ/ as in *thin* is the least intense speech sound, and the most intense is the vowel /ɔ/ as in *more*. All other phonemes fall into the intensity range between those two.

Most of the energy of speech falls in the frequency region below 1000 Hz (also written as 1 kilohertz or kHz), but the highest concentration of information useful in distinguishing speech sounds from each other falls between 1000 and 3000 Hz, and additional useful information occurs above 3000 Hz.[5] Vowels and other low-frequency phonemes have high intensity and carry 90% of the acoustic energy of speech but only 10% of information necessary for understanding speech. Consonants have less intensity, carrying only 10% of the acoustic energy of speech but 90% of the information for understanding speech. In other words, vowels and low-frequency sounds may be loud and easy to hear, but they carry much less information for understanding speech. On the other hand, consonants can be very soft and much harder to hear, but they carry the vast majority of information needed for speech understanding.

Pearl

Vowels and other low-frequency phonemes are high-intensity and carry 90% of the acoustic energy of speech but only 10% of information for understanding speech. Consonants have much less intensity, carrying only 10% of the acoustic energy of speech but 90% of the information for understanding speech.

Examining speech acoustic information and comparing it to the audiogram and to the child's speech production and perception will provide insights into the child's access to acoustic cues, phonetic cues, and phonemes and will help us understand which phonemes are accessible with and without technology. Hearing aids (HAs) now provide good access through 6000 Hz or higher for children with mild to moderate hearing loss, but for children with severe and profound hearing loss, HAs frequently do not provide sufficient high-frequency information critical to the understanding of speech. Fortunately, cochlear implants (CIs) provide good access to the high-frequency sounds that are not available to children with severe and profound hearing loss when using HAs, which is why they are so important for children with severe and profound hearing loss.

3.3 Understanding Speech Features

Speech features are classified into two main categories: the suprasegmental and segmental. Suprasegmentals are described by duration, intensity, and pitch (DIP). They control and modify rate, rhythm, stress, and intonation. Segmentals are the consonants and vowels. Consonants are described by three dimensions: manner, place, and voicing. Manner is how the sound is produced (nasal, plosive, fricative, affricative, liquid). Place is where the sound is produced (bilabial, labiodental, linguadental, alveolar, palatal, velar, glottal). Voicing describes whether the vocal cords are vibrating when the sound is produced. When the vocal cords vibrate, the sound is voiced (/g/, for example), and when they are not vibrating, the sound is unvoiced or voiceless (/k/, for example). See **Table 3.1**.[1,6,7]

Speech sounds are analyzed by which frequencies carry the most energy for that sound. These are called energy bands or formants. **Table 3.2** shows speech features by frequency bands for consonants. Consonant formants are in four general frequency bands. Some consonants have energy in two frequency bands and some in more than two. **Fig. 3.1**[5] shows the amount of energy at half-octave intervals, demonstrating the importance of different frequencies for understanding speech.

By looking at **Table 3.2**, it is easy to see that many consonants have energy at 4000 Hz and above. This makes it clear how critical high-frequency sounds are to speech perception, production, and intelligibility. From **Fig. 3.1** we can see which frequencies have the most speech information. It is clear that the majority of speech information is between 1000 and 3000 Hz, but critical information is found above and below this area.

By looking at **Table 3.2** and **Fig. 3.1** we can evaluate children's errors and determine what they are not hearing. Some errors may be due to development of articulation. If we think that may be the case, we can test what they are hearing by using pictures so they can point to what they hear and not have to repeat it. This information enables us to consider their auditory access to the different sounds of speech and elements of language. We can look at some of the main features and show where they are on the audiogram

to get a basic understanding of the correlation between speech features and the audiogram. For example, if a child is not hearing /s/ and /ʃ/, the information from **Table 3.2** will let us know that the child is not hearing sufficiently at 4500 Hz and above. By checking whether the child is hearing other sounds that have energy at 4000 Hz and above, we can understand even more. In another example, if a child is confusing cognate (voiced vs. unvoiced) pairs (e.g., /p/ and /b/ or /k/ and /g/), we can look at **Table 3.2** and see where the energy for those sounds are. The phonemes /b/ and /g/ have low-frequency voicing components that their unvoiced counterparts /p/ and /k/ do not. We can conclude that the child either has insufficient access to the low-frequency information to perceive low frequencies or too much low-frequency sound, which is causing upward spread of masking that interferes with perception of the voiceless consonants.

Speech sounds have many features, and fortunately, these features provide redundancy to the speech signal, which enables us to determine what is being said even if we miss some elements of the sound.

3.4 Producing Sound

Sound is created by a complex speech mechanism that includes four systems: the respiration, phonation, resonation, and articulation systems. Sound is created as we modify air flow through these systems.[6,8] Phonation is first created when air is forced through the pharynx and larynx; whether or not the vocal folds are vibrating determines whether the sound will be voiced or voiceless. Resonance occurs when air is diverted to the nasal or oral cavities. Nasal sounds are produced when air is diverted through the nasal cavity. Nonnasal consonants are produced when air is diverted through the oral cavity alone. The mouth, teeth, tongue, and jaw, which are the components

Table 3.1 Manner, place, and voicing of consonants

- **Manner of production** (the way air moves through the vocal tract)
  - ○ Nasal: air resonates through the nasal cavity rather than the mouth
  - ○ Plosive or Stop: pressure is built up behind articulators in the mouth, then released with a burst
  - ○ Fricative: articulators partially block sound so air moves through narrow channel in the mouth
  - ○ Affricate: sound created when a plosive / stop is combined with a fricative
  - ○ Liquid: sound created when the tip of the tongue approaches articulators but does not come close enough to create turbulence
  - ○ Approximant or Glide or Semi-Vowels: sound created when 2 articulators come close together but not close enough to create turbulence

- **Place of Production** (the anatomical place where the sound is produced)
  - ○ Bilabial: both lips
  - ○ Labiodental: lower lip and upper front teeth
  - ○ Linguadental: tongue tip and teeth
  - ○ Alveolar: tongue tip and ridge behind upper front teeth
  - ○ Palatal: front of tongue and hard palate
  - ○ Lateral: linguadental, alveolar, or palatal but one or both sides of the mouth are open, allowing air to escape freely
  - ○ Velar: back of tongue and soft palate
  - ○ Glottal: originating at the vocal folds

- **Voicing**
  - ○ Voiced: vocal folds vibrating
  - ○ Unvoiced: vocal folds not vibrating

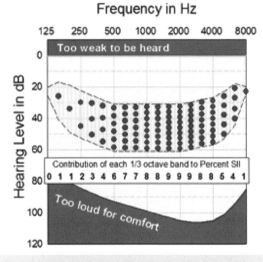

Fig. 3.1 The contribution of frequency to Speech Intelligibility Index represented by dots within the speech banana. (Reproduced with permission from Boothroyd.[5])

Table 3.2 Energy bands for consonants in English

	Bands		Consonant Energy Bands			
			1	2	3	4
Manner	Voiced	Voiceless	200–800	1000–1500	1500–3500	3500+
Plosives	b		300–400		2000–2500	
	d		300–400		2500–3000	
	g		200–300		1500–2500	
		p			1500–2000	
		t			2500–3500	
		k			2000–2500	
Nasals	m		250–350	1000–1500	2500–3500	
	n		250–350	1000–1500	2000–3000	
	ŋ[a]		250–400	1000–1500	2000–3000	
Fricatives	v		300–400			3500–4500
	z		200–300			4000–5000
	ʒ[b]		200–300			4000–4500
	ð[c]		250–350			4500–6000
		h			1500–2000	
		f				4000–5000
		s				5000–6000
		ʃ[d]			1500–2000	4500–5500
		θ[e]				~6000
Affricates		tʃ[f]			1500–2000	4000–5000
	dʒ[g]		200–300		2000–3000	
Liquids	r		600–800	1000–1500	1800–2400	
	l		250–400		2000–3000	

[a]The sound of *ng as in sing.*
[b]The sound of *3 measure or g in mirage.*
[c]The sound of *th in this.*
[d]The sound of *sh in shoot.*
[e]The sound of *th in thin.*
[f]The sound of *ch in chest.*
[g]The sound of *j in jest or g in passage.*

of the articulatory system, control the place of production and further modify the air flow and sound as it passes through the oral cavity.

3.5 Suprasegmentals

The suprasegmental elements of speech are duration, intensity, and pitch (DIP). They control and modify rate, rhythm, stress, and intonation as we speak. Suprasegmental features of speech are overlaid on utterances and can be applied to vowels, consonants, and even strings of sounds, words, or phrases.

3.6 Segmentals

Individual vowels and consonants form the segmental elements of speech. Segmentals are also called phonemes and can be analyzed individually.

3.6.1 Vowels

Vowels are produced as air passes through the larynx and open vocal tract. Vowels create resonances that produce energy clusters at specific frequencies which are referred to as energy bands or formants. Throat resonance is the first formant (F1) and has limited variability because it depends on the individual throat. The resonance which results from the mouth cavity is primarily shaped by tongue position; this creates the second formant (F2) and has wider variability. We change the vowel sound by varying the size and shape of the throat and mouth cavities. In **Fig. 3.2**, vowels of the English language are represented with their first and second formants and are arranged in an ascending order of frequencies for their F_2.[1,9]

While vowels are not easy to distinguish visually, they are auditorily accessible if a person has access to F_1 of all the vowels. However, to discriminate among vowels, it is necessary to have access to F_2. On **Fig. 3.2**, look at F1 for /u/ (as in who) and /i/ (as in see). Their F1s are essentially in the same place (they are both known to linguists as "high" vowels), so if you have access only to F1, you would not be able to determine which sound was being made. Only with access to F2 will you be able to make the distinction between the "front" vowel /i/ and the "back" vowel /u/.

Pearl

A child needs to hear from 200 Hz to 3000 Hz to be able to identify all the vowels.

3.6.2 Consonants

Consonants are produced when the air passing through the vocal tract is briefly stopped, impeded, or deflected at some point. As previously noted, consonants can be described by their place of production, manner of production, and voicing. Place of production refers to the specific parts of the mouth, or articulators, that are used to stop or restrict the airflow. Manner of production refers to the way in which the airflow is modified by the specific articulators. Voicing refers to whether or not the vocal folds are vibrating to produce sound as the airflow undergoes its alteration.

Like vowels, consonants produce their own bands of energy. As already discussed, **Table 3.2** depicts the energy bands of English consonants. You will note that voiced consonants have energy in the low-frequency energy band resulting from the movement of the vocal folds, but voiceless consonants do not have low-frequency energy bands because they result solely from the change in shape of the oral, nasal, and throat cavities. In comparing vowel and consonant energy, you may also notice that several consonants have energy at frequencies higher than those of vowels. Finally, it is evident that consonants have a significant amount of mid-frequency information that distinguishes one consonant

from another (e.g., /b/ from /d/). Thus, to have full access to all consonants, children with hearing loss must have optimal access to low-, mid-, and high-frequency information (even though they may be able to make some distinctions, such as between /b/ and /d/, visually).

3.7 The Speech Banana and the Speech String Bean

The speech banana is a description of where speech information falls on the audiogram graph. As we said above, speech sounds vary about 30 dB from the softest to the loudest phoneme. A child who hears at the top of the speech banana throughout the frequency range—at the level of the **Speech String Bean**[10]—will hear 90% of what is said. A child who hears at the bottom of the speech banana will hear only 10% of what is said.[11] Our goal is to have the child hearing close to the level of the Speech String Bean. If we plot the phonemes onto the speech banana, we can see where energy for specific phonemes lies. If you look at the speech banana with the String Bean in **Fig. 3.3,** you can graphically see that phonemes have energy (formants) in more than one place. We can use **Fig. 3.3** to see that /d/ has energy at about 300 Hz and 2500 Hz, and /t/ has energy at 2500 Hz. If those with hearing loss do not hear low-frequency sounds, they will be missing the voicing of /d/ and will confuse these two phonemes. Understanding where the energy is for each phoneme is essential to trying to understand what a child is missing and how to modify technology to try and improve auditory access. The point of placing phonemes on the speech banana is to get a general idea of where the formants of different phonemes fall. This also illustrates that phonemes in similar frequency bands can have differences in intensity. We can see that nasal formants are weaker than the formants of voiced consonants, though they are in the same octave bands. We can also observe that that second formants for vowels with a high-frequency component have less acoustic energy and are less intense than the turbulent

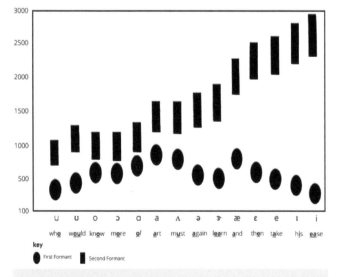

Fig. 3.2 Formants for English vowels.

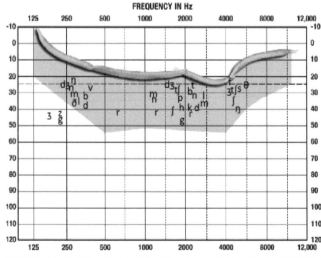

Fig. 3.3 Speech banana with Speech String Bean and phonemes.

energy of /ʃ/ and /tʃ/.[9] However, it is important to understand that the phoneme frequencies on the speech banana are estimates. Men's voices are lower in frequency than women's voices, while children's voices are even higher than women's, so the same phoneme spoken by men, women, and children will fall differently when plotted on the speech banana, but the relationship of one phoneme to another will remain the same.

3.8 Information Available in Different Frequency Bands

It is useful to know what information is available at different frequencies. Knowing this information can contribute to determining what a child is not hearing. These types of information are summarized in **Table 3.3**. If a child is not correctly using voicing or nasality cues, we can assume they are not hearing well at about 500 Hz. If they are demonstrating problems with place of articulation, we can assume they are having difficulty hearing at about 2000 Hz. This information, in addition to aided hearing and vowel and consonant formant information, can help plan remediation.

3.9 Audibility vs. Intelligibility

It is important to understand the difference between audibility and intelligibility. Very soft speech may be audible (meaning you can detect it), but that doesn't mean that it is intelligible (meaning that you understand what is being said). For example, a child may detect /m/ and /u/ but, without access to the third formant (2000–3000 Hz), may not be able to discriminate one from the other. Intelligibility is critical if we are to recognize the differences among words, which can sometimes be very subtle, and understand what is being said. Speech must be comfortably loud to be intelligible; however, if speech is too loud, it can become distorted. A child may be able to hear the difference between one syllable and two syllables (e.g., *book vs. airplane*) but not to discriminate finer differences between the words (e.g., *book and look*).

3.10 Hearing, Listening, Understanding

There are multiple steps that children have to take before they can begin to listen and talk. First, children have to hear. If they cannot hear, they will have no access to auditory brain development,

which is necessary for language and literacy development. Typically hearing children have easy access to sound because they hear. Children with hearing loss need to be appropriately fitted with technology before they can hear. Once children can hear, they can begin to listen. Even infants and very young children start paying attention and listening to things around them. A crying baby will often quiet on hearing mommy's voice. When little ones hear noises in the kitchen, they will crawl or walk that way. These children are listening to sounds around them and responding. Once children start to listen, and pay attention to what daddy says, they can begin to understand. If mommy says "*milk*" or "*bottle*" often, then the child begins to recognize that word and associate what mommy means when she says the word in a sentence: "*Here comes your bottle. Are you ready?*"

Hearing is first. Once children hear, we can expect them to start listening. Once children are listening, they are ready to understand. Once they understand they can start to speak—but auditory access must come first.

Pearl

Hearing/listening/understanding. Hearing comes first. Once children have good auditory access, they can begin to listen. When they can listen, they can start to understand. Once they understand, they can start to speak.

3.11 The 6-dB Rule

Clinicians, teachers, and families can implement the 6-dB rule to improve the access for the child by decreasing the distance between them and the child. An increase of 6 dB in the intensity of speech sound can make a significant difference for a listener, because it will be perceived as twice as loud by the child.[5] It is important to realize that, the intensity of speech will increase and decrease as the child moves closer to and farther from the speaker. **Fig. 3.4** demonstrates the effect of distance. The farther the talker is from the listener, the softer the sound. In fact, speech falls by 6 dB every time the distance is doubled. The reverse then follows: we are able to increase the intensity of the speech signal by decreasing the distance. For example, suppose speech is at 50 dB HL (a normal conversational level) when the child and the talker are 3 feet apart. If the child moves to a distance of 6 feet away, the intensity level of speech will drop to 44 dB HL. If the child moves closer to the talker (from 3 feet to 1.5 feet), the talker's speech will be increased from 50 dB to 56 dB.

Table 3.3 Speech Information availability at different frequency ranges

250 Hz	500 Hz	1000 Hz	2000 Hz	4000 Hz and above
First formant for high vowels Fundamental frequency for female and child voices Nasal murmur Stress, inflection, intonation	First formant for low vowels Voicing cues Nasality cues Stress, inflection, intonation Plosive bursts for /b/ and /d/	Acoustic cues for manner Second formants for back and central vowels Nasality cues Some plosive bursts Voicing cues Stress, inflection, intonation	Acoustic cues for place Second and third formants for front vowels Consonant-to-vowel transitions Plosive bursts Affricate bursts Fricative turbulence	Key frequency for /s/ and /z/, critical in English for plurals, idioms, auxiliaries, third person, questions

Source: Adapted from Ling and Ling.[9]

If we consider a normal conversational speech distance of about 6 feet, by approaching the child and decreasing the distance to 3 feet, we increase the sound by 6 dB and double the loudness perception. If we continue to halve the distance until we are next to the child's ear, about 4.5 inches away, we have increased the signal by a total of 24 dB This is a very significant increase in the loudness of the signal being presented to the child.

Pearl

By decreasing our distance from 6 feet away from the child to only 4.5 inches, we can add 24 dB to the signal the child is hearing.

3.12 The Speech Bubble

We all have difficulty hearing at a distance, so it stands to reason that children with hearing loss will have even more trouble hearing at a distance. Even with good technology, distance can be challenging. Families need to understand the distance at which their child can hear well. Anderson[12] developed the concept of the speech bubble to help clinicians and families understand the problems of distance. **Fig. 3.5a** shows a child who is sitting outside of the speech bubble, and **Fig. 3.5b** shows the child within the speech bubble. If children are sitting within the bubble, we expect them to have good auditory access, which will lead to building good language. The size of the listening bubble will depend on the degree of hearing loss and the use of technology. Without hearing technology, we would expect a child with a mild hearing loss to have a larger speech bubble than a child with a severe hearing loss. But once technology is appropriately fitted, we expect the child with a severe hearing loss to have good access to auditory information and a much larger speech bubble than before. If the speech bubble remains quite small or limited, a change in technology (e.g., from HAs to CIs) should be considered. The audiologist should be able to help understand what a particular child's speech bubble is by evaluating technology access and speech perception at different

intensity levels and can share this information with families and other clinicians. Families and clinicians will figure out what a child's speech bubble is by observing the child's responses during interactions. This is also why distance should be added to daily listening checks. We want to encourage families to be within their children's speech bubble as much as possible so that we can be sure that the children have good auditory access to language. When it is not possible to be within the child's speech bubble, a remote microphone (RM) system should be used (see Chapter 2).

3.13 All Sounds Not Created Equal: Vowels vs. Consonants

We know that vowels are primarily low-frequency sounds, and fricatives and affricates are high-frequency sounds. But some vowels (e.g., /i/) have both a low- and a high-frequency formant. Vowel sounds are louder (greater intensity) than consonants and have longer duration than most consonants. Nasals /m/ and /n/ and fricatives such as /f/, /ð/, /s/, and /ʃ/ have a longer duration than other consonants such as plosive consonants /p/, /t/, /b/. When someone is having difficulty hearing, our intuition is to speak in a louder voice or yell to be heard, but in fact, talking

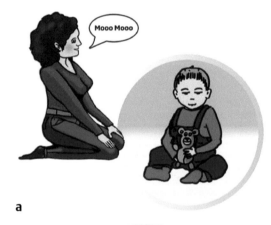

a

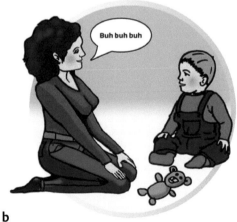

b

Fig. 3.5 (a) Parent outside of the child's speech bubble, so the child cannot hear what is being said. **(b)** Parent within the speech bubble, so the child will hear.

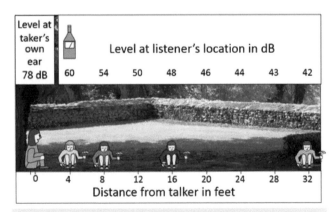

Fig. 3.4 The long-term average level of speech, in dB SPL, at various distances from an average talker. The talker is assumed to be speaking with conversational effort to the first child, who is 4 feet away. (Reproduced with permission from Boothroyd.[5])

louder has the opposite effect. Raising our voices makes vowels louder but does not improve accessibility to consonants. When we whisper syllables, words, or sentences, we decrease the vowels' acoustic energy and thereby provide more audibility to the quieter acoustic components of consonants. This strategy is known as acoustic highlighting (discussed in Chapter 10). These principles also affect listening when there is background noise. Since background noise and most environmental noises are low-frequency sounds, and since low frequencies carry significant energy, they have the ability to mask high-frequency consonants through "upward spread of masking," which means that they can spread energy and cover up higher-frequency sounds, making speech difficult to understand when it is noisy.

Pearl

When someone is having difficulty hearing, our intuition is to speak in a louder voice or yell to be heard, but in fact, this has the opposite effect. Raising our voices results in increasing the intensity of the voice, which makes vowels louder but does not improve accessibility to consonants.

3.14 The Ling–Madell–Hewitt (LMH) Test Battery

The LMH Test Battery[13] is a series of functional listening assessments that increase in difficulty as the child's speech perception and ability to respond grow.

The first test, the LMH 10–sound quick test, is a quick and easy way to check a child's detection ability across the speech spectrum. The original Ling test used six phonemes (/m/, /a/, /u/, /i/, /ʃ/, /s/),[14] but it did not sufficiently assess the mid-frequency access, which is critical for consonant identification. With digital HAs and CIs, we need to ensure that children have not only access across the speech frequencies, but also sufficient distinction of subtle differences between sounds. Madell and Hewitt therefore added four additional consonants (/z/, /h/, /n/, and /dʒ/), to correct this problem, forming the Ling–Madell–Hewitt (LMH) 10–sound quick test (**Fig. 3.6**). The abbreviation "LMH" can also be understood as Low–Medium–High frequencies.

The test is administered by a parent or a professional, who presents the sounds in random order and with varying intervals of silence between sounds. Each sound is presented three times in quick succession (e.g., a-a-a or z-z-z), and children indicate

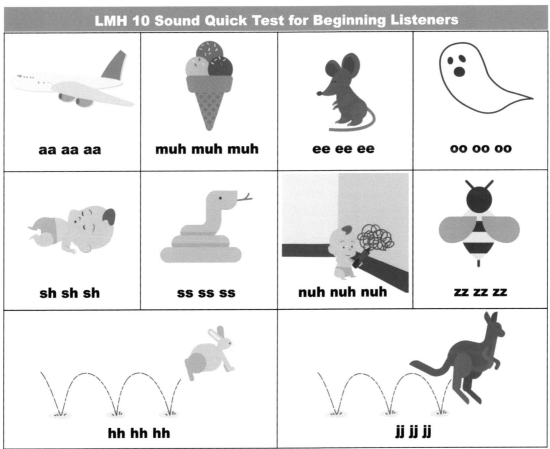

Madell and Hewitt, 2021

Fig. 3.6 The Ling–Madell–Hewitt (LMH) 10–sound quick test.

that they heard (or detected) the sound. It is important when presenting the sounds to produce each sound with the same duration so as to give no clues (e.g., don't make /ʃ/ shorter than /u/). It is also important to present the sounds at the level of normal conversation and not louder. For example, in normal conversation /s/ is much softer than the vowel /u/. We don't want to exaggerate the loudness of /s/, but rather present each sound at the same loudness in which it would normally be presented in general conversation, so that we are assessing how the child will hear it in general conversation. Testing begins with detection. Children may respond by dropping a block into a bucket, building a tower, or an infant may demonstrate by alerting or by starting or stopping sucking. As children develop their auditory skills, they move from detection to identification of the 10 sounds by either pointing to the appropriate picture or repeating the sound, and then to imitation (**Video 3.1**, **Video 3.2**, **Video 3.3**). By knowing which sounds are not audible or which are perceived incorrectly, we can predict which other sounds may not be audible and then move to modify technology settings to improve auditory access.

The LMH Test Battery does not end with the LMH 10–sound quick test. English has 42 phonemes. To truly understand how well a child hears all the phonemes, it is essential to begin testing every phoneme, not only the LMH 10. Evaluating perception of all consonants will enable clinicians to know what children hear and what they do not hear.

Children progressing from the LMH 10–sound quick test to all phonemes can be asked to imitate all phonemes using the same three quick presentations (e.g., /ba/, /ba/, /ba/ or /t/, /t/, /t/ or /f/, /f/, /f/) (**Video 3.4**). Practitioners and parents may be concerned about moving to this next step because a child cannot articulate all the phonemes yet. This concern should not deter professionals from introducing this next step. Errors that children make can provide significant information about their speech perception, even when the articulation is inaccurate. For instance, if a child does not yet know how to articulate /g/ or /k/ but produces /b/, /b/, /b/ for /g/, /g/, /g/ and a glottal /ʔ/, /ʔ/, /ʔ/ for /k/, /k/, /k/, we can have significant confidence that the child is hearing the voicing and frequency band of the /g/ and the voiceless stopping of the /k/. The errors are appropriate and point to good perception even though articulation is difficult. On the other hand, if the same child produces /m/, /m/, /m/ for /g/, /g/, /g/ and /hm/, /hm/, /hm/ for /k/, /k/, /k/, we have evidence that the presence of too much low-frequency information may be negatively impacting perception.

Once children's imitation skills have advanced to the point that they can imitate vowel-consonant-vowel (VCV) combinations, the LMH Test Battery moves to perception of all consonants in this manner (e.g., /aba/, /ata/, /afa/) (**Video 3.5**, **Video 3.6**, **Video 3.7**). In the author's experience, children with hearing loss as young as 2 years of age can begin to participate in this level of assessment, which provides the most realistic perception information. (See Chapter 2 for more information about the Medial Consonant test and other speech perception tests.)

Finally, while a child's perception needs to be checked every day, the LMH Test Battery advocates for moving assessment from professionals to parents as the child demonstrates the ability to complete each step. Thus, once a child begins showing detection of the LMH 10 quick sounds, the practitioner should be encouraging the parent to take responsibility for monitoring detection at home each day. The practitioner can then gather that daily detection information from the parents and, at the same time, be working to develop identification of the sounds through the use of the pictures. As the child learns to identify the sounds, the parents should be encouraged to check identification each day while the practitioner now begins encouraging imitation of the 10 sounds and then all sounds. The goal is for all children to able to complete the medial consonant (VCV) level of imitation within their home and clinical settings. Working through the LMH Test Battery as the child's skills grow provides invaluable information for the audiologist to optimize technology settings, for the practitioner to plan intervention, and for the parents to understand what their child hears (**Video 3.8**, **Video 3.9**).

Pearl

If a speech sound is not accessible (detectable), then the child cannot discriminate it from other sounds, develop it, or use it. It is critical that we know what a child can hear.

3.15 Planning Therapy Using Speech Acoustics Information

Through effective use of the aided audiogram and the Speech String Bean with phonemes and the tables with formant information, we can assist interventionists in bridging the gap from the theoretical to the practical. By using what we know of speech acoustics and combining that with what we understand about a child's aided auditory access, we can determine how to plan treatment. We combine information from a child's aided audiogram showing auditory access, and formant information of both vowels and consonants, to determine what children are hearing, what they are not hearing, and how to proceed with management.

3.16 Summary

Speech acoustics is the foundation on which all habilitation and rehabilitation to achieve listening and spoken language is based. By understanding the principles addressed throughout this chapter, clinicians can apply speech acoustics to intervention with children with hearing loss. The relationship between speech acoustics and speech and language is integral. Having discussed speech features and their correlates, the relationship to specific speech sounds and features, we can relate it specifically to difficulties in the development of speech production and development of language functions. When addressing speech production, it is useful to remember that if you don't have access to the sound, you don't hear it, won't understand it, and won't learn to produce it or use it in language.

Pearl

If you do not have access to a phoneme, you will not perceive, and will not easily learn to produce it or use it in language.

Discussion Questions

1. If a child has a cookie bite audiogram with hearing at mild hearing loss levels in the low and high frequencies and at moderately severe hearing loss levels in the mid frequencies, describe what the child will hear.

2. If a child is producing low-frequency consonants but not high-frequency consonants, what might that tell you?

References

[1] Ling D. *Speech and the Hearing-Impaired Child: Theory and Practice*. 2nd ed. Washington, DC: The Alexander Graham Bell Association for the Deaf; 2002

[2] Graven SN, Browne JV. Auditory development in the fetus and infant. *Newborn Infant Nurs Rev* 2008;8(4):187–193

[3] May L, Gervain J, Carreiras M, Werker JF. The specificity of the neural response to speech at birth. *Dev Sci* 2018;21(3):e12564

[4] Muse C, Harrison J, Yoshinaga-Itano C, et al; Joint Committee on Infant Hearing of the American Academy of Pediatrics. Supplement to the JCIH 2007 Position Statement: principles and guidelines for early intervention after confirmation that a child is deaf or hard of hearing. *Pediatrics* 2013;131(4):e1324–e1349

[5] Boothroyd A. The acoustic speech signal. In: Madell JR, Flexer C, Wolfe J, Schafer E, eds. *Pediatric Audiology: Diagnosis, Technology and Management*. 3rd ed. New York, NY: Thieme; 2019:185–192

[6] Ladefoged P. *A Course in Phonetics*. 5th ed. Boston, MA: Thomson Wadsworth; 2006

[7] Ling D. *Foundations of Spoken Language for Hearing-Impaired Children*. Washington DC: Alexander Graham Bell Association for the Deaf and Hard of Hearing; 1989

[8] Pickett JM. *The Acoustics of Speech Communication: Fundamentals, Speech Perception, Theory and Technology*. Boston, MA: Allyn and Bacon; 1999

[9] Ling D, Ling AH. *Aural Habilitation: The Foundations of Verbal Learning in Hearing-Impaired Children*. Washington DC: Alexander Graham Bell Association for the Deaf and Hard of Hearing; 1978

[10] Madell JR. The Speech String Bean. *Volta Voices* 2016;23:28–31

[11] Pasco D. An approach to hearing aid selection. *Hear Instrum* 1978;29:12–16

[12] Anderson K. Early Listening Function (ELF) parent involvment: the magic ingredient in successful child outcomes. *Hearing Review* n.d.;9(11):24–27, 56

[13] Madell JR, Hewitt JG. The LMH test for monitoring. Hearing Health & Technology Matters. August 3, 2021. https://hearinghealthmatters.org/hearingand-kids/2021/3245/

[14] Ling D. What is the Six Sound Test and why is it so important in auditory verbal therapy and education? In: Estabrooks W, ed. 101 *Frequently Asked Questions about Auditory-Verbal Practice*. Washington DC: Alexander Graham Bell Association for the Deaf and Hard of Hearing; 2012:58–62

II
Framing a Strong Structure

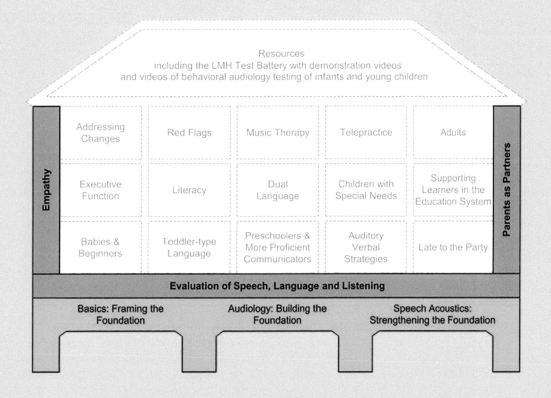

4 Empathy: Changing the Culture of Communication

Johnnie Sexton

Summary

This chapter focuses on the emotional journey of families and the importance of bringing a greater sensitivity to the attention of those professionals providing services to families. The emotional impact of working with families on professionals is also discussed. The grief process is discussed in detail. Strategies are shared on how to communicate differently and with greater empathy to ensure that families feel they are true partners in the care of their child.

Keywords

empathy, grief, networking, compassion, loyalty, unconscious bias, cultural competency, cultural humility, active listening, retreats, support groups

Key Points

- Most families go through a grieving process when they hear the unexpected news that their child has hearing loss.
- Grieving is cyclical and may occur at different points along the family's emotional journey when unexpected events occur.
- Professionals who work with families are often not trained for or comfortable with providing emotional support for families.
- Changing the culture of communication between parents and professionals is key to creating a true partnership to manage the child with hearing loss.
- Once parents have been able to accept their child's hearing loss, it is easier to advocate for the child's needs, and this can lead to parents becoming leaders.
- Bringing families together is one of the most impactful strategies used and will result in no parent or child ever feeling alone again.

4.1 Introduction

More than ever, the topic of empathy is discussed in professional arenas, social and mainstream media, and the general population. An adjacent and parallel discussion centers on the emotional journey of families with children who are deaf or hard of hearing (DHH). It is the author's belief that the latter cannot be addressed without addressing the former and that bringing about change in the culture of communication between parents and professionals is dependent on spending time understanding the emotional journey of families and deepening one's sense of empathy.

4.2 Understanding the Emotional Journey of Families

As a pediatric/educational audiologist for over 40 years, the author has seen many families along the way who have had unexpected news soon after the birth of a baby (or later in childhood) that their child has hearing loss. This unexpected news causes an immediate emotional reaction and often starts a process of grieving.

4.2.1 How the Journey Begins

A bond is established before birth between parent and child. They have many hopes and expectations that this baby will be beautiful, perfect, wonderful, healthy, and more. These expectations continue after the birth of the baby.[1]

As Dr. David Luterman stated in 2013,[2] parents who are expecting a baby live in a cloak of invincibility. It is a beautiful time in the life of a family, and the parents think that nothing can happen to them. However, in some cases when the baby is born, there is unexpected news, an emotional surprise.

Mandates for screening newborns for hearing loss are now in place across the United States and U.S. territories and in many other countries. Babies are required to have their hearing screened at birth before being discharged from the birthing facility. Should a newborn not pass the hearing screening, news is then delivered to the parents, who are usually not expecting to hear anything other than "all is well." When this occurs, professionals will immediately bombard the parents with lots of information, as is their responsibility. Parents need to be educated on what is happening, and yet parents often share that they usually do not get sufficient time to process the information and the emotional reaction that comes with receiving unexpected news. The questions must also be raised: are professionals trained and prepared to deliver information that results in an emotional response from new parents, and are they comfortable doing so?

4.2.2 Unexpected News

Luterman also reports that when faced with shocking news, humans go to a different place in the brain and memory function shuts down and information is not processed; parents often report not remembering the information beyond a diagnosis or screening outcome.[2]

This unexpected news can result in a variety of responses initially: sorrow, mourning, distress, deep emotional outpouring, but in some cases relief and even happiness (e.g., if the parents are themselves deaf or heard of hearing and look forward to their children sharing this identity). Parents may suppress their emotions initially and avoid the reality of what is happening. It is not unusual to have spousal conflicts arise, with one parent not being on the same page as the other parent in the processing of the new information and the emotions experienced. Many families isolate themselves because they are not comfortable sharing this news with extended family members, neighbors, and friends. These reactions are all ways in which parents try to understand what the impact of having a child with hearing loss really means.

Pitfall

Bombarding parents with too much information can result in parents feeling overwhelmed and not able to process everything they are given.

4.2.3 Experiencing Grief/Emotional Surprises

Grief is historically associated with death; however, in a broader sense, grief is the sense of unexpected loss of something in life. We refer to grief as "emotional surprises."

Grief is a process and is not "one-stop shopping" for an experience in life that brings about the feelings of grief. Grief is a part of life, everyone's life, and is common to all people. Grief comes and goes. One does not complete a grief experience, never to return. In fact, the reaction to emotional surprises years later will conjure up deep reactions. The grief experience affects people in different ways and impacts both families and professionals who work together. Grief can have a positive outcome because the human spirit can rebound and the destination becomes resilience.

Emotional surprises come in different forms. We do not intend to equate the following grief experiences, but these are examples of emotional surprises that could happen to anyone:

1. Critical illness diagnosis
2. Loss of a pet
3. Inability to have children
4. Body image issues
5. Divorce or breakup of a relationship
6. Failure at school and/or work
7. Loss of a job

Unexpected news about a newborn or young child will bring about an emotional reaction. This news can be associated with the outcome of newborn hearing screening if a baby does not pass the initial screening procedure and the second screen. Babies who do not pass the second screening are referred for a diagnostic evaluation. Many families have shared that the journey to diagnosis is very emotional. Not only are the parents in shock with the unexpected news of a potential for hearing loss, but they now must navigate a healthcare system that is likely very unfamiliar. Many parents have shared that getting a confirmed diagnosis may take weeks, maybe months, adding to the grieving process.

Soon after a hearing loss diagnosis, parents are contacted by early intervention specialists, speech-language pathologists (SLPs), and other professionals who are ready to step in and begin to work with the family. This barrage of attention can be overwhelming to the family. Usually, from birth to 3 years, children with hearing loss receive services from these agencies and professionals. In many states, these children are transitioned to public schools at age 3, and that change brings about another grief experience. Families and their professional service providers develop relationships over time, and the thought of suddenly 'handing off" their children to a new set of professionals results in feelings of grief resurfacing.

In the early days after a hearing loss diagnosis, parents are also faced with several decisions. Imagine knowing nothing about hearing technology and being told that one needs to select a hearing aid manufacturer/brand, model, color, and so on, immediately followed by a choice in earmolds (color, etc.). If the hearing loss is severe enough, there may be discussion about long-term use of technology, moving from hearing aids to cochlear implants. Going so quickly from the birth of their baby to making technology decisions often causes parents feelings of being overwhelmed, confused, frustrated, ambushed, and guilty. However, in some instances where the parents are themselves deaf, the news of hearing loss may make them happy, relieved, and even celebratory.

A final decision that parents are faced with early on is the communication option for their child: listening and spoken language, a visual mode of communication, or a combination of the two.

4.2.4 Stages of Grief/Emotional Surprises

The stages of grief have been described many ways by a variety of professionals who primarily have focused on grief caused by the death of a loved one. The author has developed a list of stages, shown in **Fig. 4.1**. Each parent may go through all these stages or some of them. There is no linear pattern that exists when it comes to the effects of emotional surprises in the life of a parent. One thing that does seem to hold true is that there are points along the emotional journey when the feelings of grief resurface or recycle after having receded.

The initial feeling of shock seems to be common to most parents when receiving unexpected news of hearing loss, followed by a period of denial. Parents and families cannot believe that this news is true and have significant emotional reactions as a result. Until a confirmed diagnosis is reached, parents often find themselves living in a state of denial because it isn't "true" or "real." It is not unusual for parents to think "this cannot be happening to me"

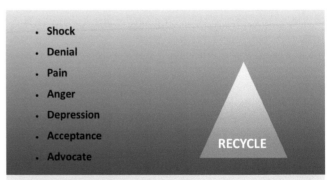

- Shock
- Denial
- Pain
- Anger
- Depression
- Acceptance
- Advocate

RECYCLE

Fig. 4.1 Emotional stages.

or "they must be wrong." Once the confirmed diagnosis is shared with parents, the truth begins to sink in, and they likely will go through a period of pain and hurt. The expectations they had for their child are suddenly altered, and the dreams they had for their child are no longer alive, at least for a period. Through pain, anger can surface. Parents often look for something or someone to blame for what is happening. Parents may blame each other in a search for a cause of the hearing loss. This blaming can fracture relationships, at least for a period of time. As the truth sinks in, parents often experience depression and sadness, mourning the loss of much more than the hearing of their child. The reality of what is happening may take some time to accept, but once acceptance occurs, the parents are able to begin to move forward on their emotional journey for the best interest of their child. A final stage on the journey is, or should be, advocacy. Parents become empowered through the acceptance of the hearing loss and work toward advocating for making sure that their child has every opportunity to be successful and the child's own ability to overcome adversity and barriers is realized. The parents come to realize that it is their own resilience that will carry them onward.

Because there are transitions and triggers along the journey, parents may very well experience recurrence or "recycling" of any or all of these stages of grief. Parents do not get a certificate of completion at the end of the first cycle of grief. In fact, emotions will get recycled when the child meets new service providers. At age 3 in many states, the child transitions from early intervention services to the public schools' preschool programs. The next transition point usually is when the child enters kindergarten. Parents become worried and afraid of what the next chapter in their child's journey may entail. The journey continues on to middle school, playing sports, high school, college, marriage, getting a job, and on through the rest of their lives. In addition to "time points" for the recurrence of grief, parents will also suffer grief, anxiety, and worry when they must make health-related decisions, such as which communication modality to follow, whether to go with a cochlear implant, what brand of technology, or even the color of the child's hearing aid or earmolds. While parents may not go through every stage of grief, some of those same emotions will surface throughout the life of the child.

Parents often report that they do not receive emotional support and sensitivity for their journey from professionals. Professionals are usually very capable of delivering information to parents and explaining test results and recommendations. Informational counseling is a long-standing traditional role played by professional service providers; however, emotional support counseling (also known as adjustment counseling) is greatly lacking. Very few graduate programs provide coursework about counseling and the emotional journey that parents need.

4.2.5 Emotional Impact on Professionals

Professionals also have an emotional reaction to the family's journey, experiencing internal feelings as they observe parents expressing grief. How do the professionals themselves deal with these emotions? The initial reaction is to continue to "dump" an overload of information on parents without any sensitivity to the need for time to process. Many professionals do know that there needs to be a correct balance between showing sensitivity and keeping a sense of professionalism as they work with the family. Professionals may be uncomfortable because they are inexperienced or untrained to provide the sensitivity necessary to give parents the emotional support in these situations. However, it is the author's belief that professionals cannot be truly successful working with families if they themselves are unable to acknowledge and support the emotions of the parents. Feelings just are and cannot be controlled; thus, the emotional support needed must be a critical part of what a professional demonstrates when working with families.

Pearl

When parents see that professional service providers also have emotional responses to what's happening, it humanizes everyone in the communication loop.

4.3 Background and Training for Professionals in Emotional Support Counseling

Are the professionals who immediately "dump" large amounts of information on parents trained, and do they have the time, to lend some emotional sensitivity in such situations, and are they comfortable doing so? Across the board, the answer is no in many cases. The author collected data over a 4-year period with 624 respondents from professionals working with families who have children born DHH. The respondent group consisted of audiologists, SLPs, teachers of the deaf (TODs), social workers, physicians, nurses, and school administrators. **Table 4.1** provides the results.

Across professions, over half of the respondents indicated that they were not trained in providing emotional support counseling for parents or children. Historically speaking, it was unheard of (for the most part) to have courses taught in providing counseling and emotional support for clients, parents, families, or children. There is a recommendation in the United States now to add such coursework for students enrolled in graduate programs in speech-language pathology and audiology, but the majority of training programs still do not have a course in place. Some of those who responded stated that they provided emotional support counseling for parents or children, but all commented that this came about through "on the job" training. No respondents disputed the fact that emotional support counseling has importance, but many were not academically trained to provide it. It was also of interest to question the comfort level of professionals who provide emotional support counseling, as that relates to the emotional reaction of the professional providing such support. As seen in **Table 4.1**, only 55% of the respondents indicated that they were comfortable doing so.

The final request in the survey was for respondents to rate their emotional support counseling skills as absent, emerging, present, developed, or consistent. It is interesting to note that only 9% of the respondents indicated that they had developed counseling skills that were consistently used in their professional work (**Fig. 4.2**).

Table 4.1 Responses of Professionals working with children who are deaf or hard of hearing to questions about education in providing emotional support

Question Related to Emotional Support Counseling	YES (%)	NO (%)
Experience with parents	50	50
Trained to work with parents	35	65
Importance of counseling parents	100	0
Comfortable counseling parents	55	45
Trained to counsel children	40	60
Importance of counseling children	100	0
Comfortable providing support for children	55	45

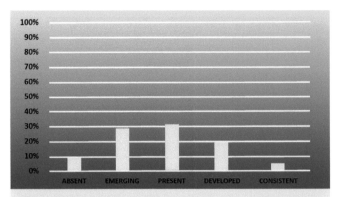

Fig. 4.2 Counseling skills ratings. Data collected by the author, 2012–2016 (unpublished).

4.4 Bringing about Change in How Professionals and Parents Communicate

Over the years, professionals and parents have not always had a balanced communication exchange. In the traditional role, professionals are the authorities on a particular topic/diagnosis/treatment and convey information in a unilateral, one-dimensional manner. Most professionals come from a medical/clinical perspective, and parents don't often feel as if they are able to express their emotions and ask questions. Parents report that they are not often made to feel that they are partners in the care plans for their children. What makes the difference is making sure that parents and professionals gain a greater sensitivity about each other's journey and open up the opportunities to communicate with each other in a fair and balanced manner.

How can parents and professionals change the culture of how they communicate with each other? A first step can be to examine the question "Why do you do what you do?" By gaining a deeper understand of self, it is likely that a deeper understanding of others may result. A significant part of that exploration is for parents to truly understand the emotional journey of professionals and for professionals to truly understand that journey for parents. Most people know *what* they do and *how* they do it, but do they fully know and understand the *why*— the purpose, cause, or belief that drives every one of us?[3]

Pearl

Professionals must take the time to understand why they do what they do in order to truly embrace the families with whom they work.

Who initiates this change in communication? Parents? Professionals? Both? In an effort to achieve balance and equality, it is important that professionals give parents the permission to speak up, speak out, and speak often. Parents also have to step up and advocate for their child with the professional and not be afraid to speak up. Both have a role in making this change happen. If parents do not sense that their professional service provider is open to making this change, they have to be brave, speak up, and ask for it.

4.4.1 Empathy

So, what is empathy? Brené Brown defines *empathy* as connecting with the emotions another person is experiencing, rather than to that person's experience itself.[4] Therefore, it does not require that we have experienced the same situation they are going through. Tchiki Davis of the Berkeley Well-Being Institute states that empathy is the ability to sense other people's emotions (affective empathy) coupled with the ability to imagine what someone else might be thinking or feeling (cognitive empathy).[5]

To fully realize empathy, it is important to understand the emotional journey of others, therefore enabling an individual to know what it is like to be in someone else's shoes, to live in their skin, so to speak. In life, all people are on their own individual emotional journeys experiencing highs and lows, experiencing grief as related to those "emotional surprises." It is a part of the human experience.

The topic of empathy is somewhat abstract for many people. Typical questions include "Do you have it?" "How do you know you have it?" "Can you talk about it?" "Can you demonstrate it?" There are several key components in exploring one's empathy: compassion, loyalty, cultural humility, and recognition of unconscious bias.

4.4.2 Compassion

Compassion is looking for what you have in common with others rather than focusing on differences. In a TEDx talk, Betty Hart talks about canceling "cancel culture" with compassion: rather than rejecting others who have profound differences with us, we should reach out to them. Finding understanding and common ground, as ideologically opposite Supreme Court Justices Ginsburg and Scalia did and as Hart and her father did, will lead to greater compassion, which is on the path to empathy.[6]

4.4.3 Loyalty

Loyalty is a direct result of building relationships over time. People feel loyal to friends, family members, and professionals who provide services to them. Developing loyalty is a common occurrence with parents of young children and their early interventionists. Loyalty occurs in all people in all walks of life.

Loyalty is rooted in emotion and is a component in the ability to understand the feelings of others, helping people connect with others on an emotional level.

In the late 1990s, Melanie Tervalon and Jann Murray-García created a discussion of *cultural competence* versus *cultural humility*. They considered cultural competence, understood as "a detached mastery of a theoretically finite body of knowledge," to be setting a standard that is not realistic, placing professionals on a level of "all knowing and all powerful." In contrast, cultural humility is defined as "a lifelong commitment to self-evaluation and critique, to redressing power imbalances . . . and to developing mutually beneficial and non-paternalistic partnerships with communities on behalf of individuals and defined populations."[7]

4.4.4 Cultural Humility

Cultural humility focuses on the fact that patients/clients/parents are not being heard and that has to change. This groundbreaking distinction is essential in working to remove clinician–client (professional–parent) imbalances. Tervalon encourages all professional caregivers to recognize that everyone is a complicated individual and that there are key tenets to achieving cultural humility.

The first tenet is lifelong learning for everyone. In this mindset, professional service providers must keep themselves open to learning new and different information, must admit mistakes, and must never assume that there is nothing else to know or learn. As time moves forward, everyone must engage in critical self-reflection in order to be able to constantly evolve. The key is the realization that individuals don't know everything there is to know about any given subject matter.

The second tenet is to recognize and challenge power imbalances. As discussed earlier in this chapter, both professionals and parents must give each other permission to have open dialogue and to share equally in the communication exchange, respecting partnerships. And finally, institutions must reflect the same values and goals as staff when it comes to these issues.

Pitfall

Not recognizing power imbalances between professional service providers and parents will create a one-dimensional relationship and not bode well for progress.

4.4.5 Recognition of Unconscious Bias

Unconscious bias, also known as implicit bias, is often thought of as the beliefs that a person holds without being conscious of them but that affect the person's thoughts and judgments. In order to understand unconscious bias, individuals must look inward to discover and dissect themselves. Unconscious bias is based on one's upbringing and life experiences. Addressing unconscious bias is an important task for both professionals and parents. Recognizing that someone has it does not mean that they are a bad person, but it does challenge individuals to better understand themselves and others.

The author developed the Unconscious Bias Exercise Tool (UBET) in 2020 (see **Appendix A**) in an effort to help professionals and parents take a closer look at themselves and those who are not like them. It was designed to provide means of opening up a discussion on biases that may exist towards others, especially in the context of professional service providers working with families.

There are a number of categories that can be used to describe oneself, and the same categories are to be used to describe someone else who may be the opposite.

When describing oneself, one can bring to one's conscious mind aspects of previous experiences that shape one's response to another person based on what one sees or hears. For example, someone may see others who are not like them through the lens of stereotypes and, as a result, make judgments based on those biases. A heterosexual male may anticipate that a gay male hired into his workplace will exhibit effeminate behaviors because the heterosexual male doesn't know any gay men personally. A younger, tech-savvy manager at a software company may pass over older team members because of the assumption that older people are not tech savvy, only younger people. A person who is deaf and uses ASL as their mode of communication may assume that the audiologist presenting to the facility where they work is against Deaf culture and very much against use of ASL. While none of these may be true, they can all seem true based on the biases that precede the situation.

Why is this important when professionals meet parents? Automatic conclusions are reached and assumptions made based on what is "seen" initially. An early interventionist who is white and who visits the home of a family with a newly identified child with hearing loss may make judgments about the family because it is a family of color or a biracial family, only to learn immediately that the family is no different from the interventionist's own family. Or, if a black male audiology graduate student is doing an externship in a white, upper middle-class suburb of a major city, older white patients may form opinions of him based on the color of his skin rather than the abilities he brings to the work environment. For professionals and parents to work together in harmony and effectively, it is important to engage early on in a discussion to address any issues of unconscious bias. This discussion will also help ensure that there are no misunderstandings and no misperceptions on the part of either the parent or the professional. By discussing these issues early, they may feel that they can bring up concerns as they develop over time.

4.5 Strategies

4.5.1 Encourage

The family's emotional journey begins with unexpected news that usually brings about grief. It is the role of professionals to move the family forward on their journey with a destination of resilience. The American Psychological Association (APA) defines resilience as "the process of adapting well in the face of adversity, trauma, tragedy, threats, or significant sources of stress."[8] In a sense, resilience is a hardiness, a mental toughness and a resourcefulness. No matter how bad something may seem, tomorrow will be better for most people. Getting up each day and moving forward is resilience.

The APA has several resources with ways to build resilience. The overall theme is to be encouraging. Professionals can easily provide words of encouragement with every encounter they may have with families. Connecting families with each other is a very impactful way to make families feel that they are not alone. Opportunities for self-discovery are great assignments for families to venture out on their own to meet and interact with other families. For example, in many places such as museums and aquariums, there are "deaf awareness days."

Accepting and managing change is a huge step for families. Nevertheless, there is one thing that cannot be changed: the fact that a child has a hearing loss. Once that is accepted, the management becomes far less stressful, and parents can begin to recognize that there are many positive things about their child. Encouraging parents to keep things in perspective will assist them with focusing on the overall family routine and recognizing there is more going on in the family than managing a hearing loss. In fact, hearing loss is only one of the many things that families are dealing with daily. One of the hardest things for parents to do in some instances is to take decisive actions. For example, when a recommendation is made for a child to receive a cochlear implant, parents often are initially focusing on the surgical aspect. Some parents are concerned about how rapidly the technology is changing and, therefore, worry their child's implant processor will soon be outdated. A great way to encourage parents in these situations is to ask them how long they are willing to wait to have the implant surgery and what will certainly be lost as a result of delays. Most professionals will work with parents to establish goals. Encouraging families to work continuously toward those goals is essential.

Overall, encouragement can center on taking good care of one's self, being positive, nurturing self-esteem, and never seeing anything as impossible to overcome.

4.5.2 Listening

Becoming a good listener will make a person more empathetic. Active listening puts a person more closely in the shoes of others, which is the pathway to a deeper sense of empathy.

Some strategies that help engage a professional in active listening with parents:

1. Don't respond with information all the time.
2. Be the "other adult" in the room; it's completely acceptable to say nothing.
3. Acknowledge and validate what is said by parents/family members.
4. Guide toward discussion.
5. Don't lecture.
6. Don't tell parents what you would do if it were you.
7. Don't create co-dependencies.

Nonverbal Listening Strategies

1. Allow the parents to talk and let them finish what they are saying.
2. Always maintain eye contact. Don't look away or be distracted by computers, phones, beepers, and so on. Let the parents know that you want to communicate with them.

3. Display openness with body language. Be sure not to place barriers between you and the parent when meeting/talking.

Verbal Listening Strategies

1. Give the parents feedback on what they shared with you. Paraphrase or restate what you thought you heard. For example, "Mrs. Jones, it sounds like you are upset today because your husband cannot be here with you today." The parent might immediately respond with, "No, I am not upset at all with my husband for not being here. He has to work. I am upset because I now have to go home and try to remember what you have said to me in terms that I don't really know or understand." By using this strategy, the professional has instant feedback on whether understanding has been improved or not.
2. Be very encouraging of parents to relax when meeting. Don't have physical barriers in place between parent and professional. For example, make sure there are no tables dividing parents and professionals. Sit in a comfortable configuration in order to make sure everyone involved can feel relaxed.

4.5.3 HEAR

Donna Wilson and Marcus Conyers[9] developed a tool that makes clear what active listening is all about:

- **H**alt: Stop internal dialogue.
- **E**ngage: Focus on the speaker.
- **A**nticipate: Look forward to what is to be said.
- **R**eplay: Think about what is said, analyze and paraphrase it.

Pearl

Active listening will greatly enhance empathy.

4.5.4 Be Mindful

With every encounter a professional has with parents/families, it is important to be present and to be mindful. Professionals are humans with many things going on in their own lives. If needed, walk away and take a few minutes alone. Close your eyes and take three deep breaths. At the end of each day, reflect on the day's experiences to gain insight into working with families. Make sure you encourage families to find something to celebrate each day. In fact, professionals should do the same thing. Don't focus on the negatives but find the positives.

4.5.5 Hit the Pause Button

One strategy learned by this author in working with families is to "hit the pause button." Parents have reported time and again that they were never given enough time to process information shared with them, whether it be during the diagnosis phase or along the way with therapies, interventions, and so forth. Take time to ask parents what they need. Do they need an extra day to understand everything? Some parents will need more time than others. Don't leave parents hanging if they ask for more time. Check in periodically to see how they are doing. Always follow up, no matter what the circumstances. Be sure to allow enough time to pass before delivering more and more information.

Pearl

Hitting the pause button is a key tool for success when professionals are delivering information to parents.

4.5.6 Probe

Rather than assume that parents have retained all of the information along the way, it is important to check in on a regular basis with some basic questions:

1. Ask parents whether they understand everything about their child's hearing loss. It isn't uncommon for parents to share that they barely remember that initial description of their child's audiogram and remember nothing since. Take time to go over the audiogram again and again and make it more and more meaningful.
2. Ask parents whether they understand their child's technology. Technology can be complicated and overwhelming, according to many parents. Check in to make sure that the parents know how the technology operates, how to check it to make sure it is properly functioning, how to change or charge the batteries, and how to use any assistive technologies that may connect with the primary devices. Ask parents whether they are having any difficulty changing batteries or putting in earmolds. Opening the question can help families ask for assistance.
3. Ask parents whether they have good resources for support. Many families may encounter times when they need assistance and don't know where to turn. Asking a parent how they are managing with the cost of technologies, repairs, and so on may open a dialogue to address some of their needs that directly relates to the child's needs. For example, the child may need new hearing aids and the parents don't have the resources to purchase them.
4. Ask parents whether they can talk with others about their child, their child's hearing loss, and their child's technology. Early on, parents may tend to isolate and not feel comfortable sharing what's happening with their child in terms of hearing loss and managing hearing loss. It is important to ask whether the parents have shared the news with extended family, daycare workers, school personnel, neighbors, and friends. Asking this question will open up a valuable dialogue that is necessary for the family on the emotional journey to move forward with confidence.
5. Ask parents to describe their day-to-day lives.
6. Ask parents to share how their day may be different from that of a parent of a child with typical hearing.
7. Ask parents to share what makes a great visit with the audiologist, SLP, or early interventionist.
8. Ask parents what they worry the most about.
9. Ask parents to share what they can celebrate.

All of these probes will open up discussions that will greatly assist them in gaining a greater sense of themselves and their journey.

4.5.7 Support Groups

No one can do as much for a family as another family on the same or similar journey. That is why support groups are so important for parents, children with hearing loss, and siblings. Parent support groups are most successful when parent leaders are identified to organize and manage these groups. First, find a reason to meet. Identify a topic or theme to advertise and reach out to local communities to bring parents together. Offering a meal or snacks is another strategy that may bring more families to a support group meeting. Make sure that there is a reason offered to help individuals talk in the group. Icebreaker activities have been very successful in facilitating open discussion and sharing. Just the simple question "Why are you here?" can be enough to stimulate dialogue. A follow up icebreaker can be "Tell everyone about your family." Another activity that has real success is to pair up parents who do not know each other and instruct the pairs to tell each other three things about their family that have nothing to do with hearing loss. When the assigned task is completed, each person then reports to the entire group what they learned about their "new friend." These strategies alone can account for several hours of sharing in a group of approximately 20 parents. After the first meeting, find a reason for everyone to return and get the group to provide input on that decision.

Children with hearing loss also need to feel connected to other children "like them." Depending on the ages of the children, play activities can be designed to enable the children to be together for no other reason than to have fun together. Group discussions can start as young as 7 or 8 years. Asking kids to tell something "funny" about having a hearing loss is a good icebreaker. It is also useful to ask the kids to list problems they experience from having a hearing loss. Once the list is developed, the whole group can make suggestions about how to solve the problem. Other children who are peers are more likely to be able to provide support and suggestions that will be helpful, from how to talk to the teacher when one can't hear to how to talk to parents. Peers may also help children who are rejecting technology to rethink the rejection. Teens and tweens will enjoy more structured activities and guest speakers. Of course, all activities for children 18 years and younger need to be properly supervised and managed. Organizing a group of volunteers is a key component of having a successful event for children. One resource for volunteers that has been successful for the author is local university students in degree programs related to audiology, speech-language pathology, and Teachers of the DHH education.

Siblings also need their own time together. Many professionals across the country help organize "sib shops" or sibling groups. These groups bring together the brothers and sisters for peer-to-peer support. Often siblings feel left out or uninvolved in a family with a child who is DHH (or who has any disability); the people they can most closely relate to are those who are on the same journey. Sib groups can be scheduled to meet in person or virtually. They can plan field trips and other outings to bring them together. Simply having a "fun" event to bring them together for a meal (pizza, hot dogs, etc.) may be enough to give the siblings the opportunity they need to share and process their own emotions about what is happening in their respective families.

Pitfall

When families are not connected to other families, they tend not to feel a part of a community that can support them.

4.5.8 Family Retreats

Bringing groups of families together for a weekend or even a day has such huge impact on their emotional state and journey. The single most common comment by parents and children after a retreat experience: "I don't feel alone anymore."

The mission of a retreat is to:

1. Provide families with opportunities to work through the grieving process individually and together
2. Enable families to confront and solve their issues of grief to the point of sharing their journey with other families
3. Assist parents on their journey to arrive at a place of acceptance and advocacy with compassion
4. Allow kids who are DHH to connect with each other
5. Allow siblings to spend time together

Although family retreats are very effective for families early on in their emotional journeys, there is positive impact for families with children of any age and at any stage of their emotional journey.

Family retreats do require that a budget be developed, and funds sought to cover the costs of the entire weekend experience. Costs such as housing, food, and transportation can be overwhelming but not impossible to manage. Seeking grant funding, local business sponsorships, and donations can make the family retreat possible.

A good solid plan for a family retreat is important to ensure success, and the planning should begin 3 to 6 months in advance of the retreat experience. Volunteers are needed for a variety of functions during the retreat, which is typically a long weekend. The volunteer pool can consist of audiologists, SLPs, teachers, graduate and undergraduate students from university programs, DHH young adults, older siblings, and parents. Another necessary component is to have in place a leadership team consisting of:

1. Retreat director
2. Childcare coordinators
3. Volunteer coordinators
4. Speaker coordinator
5. Mentor family (a family that has been on the emotional journey longer and participated in retreats in the past)
6. Food coordinator

A family retreat has many components, and to make sure all goes well, a solid team in place can then plan the retreat agenda. A sample agenda may include:

1. Free time for families with children
2. Kids' group
3. Dads' group
4. Moms' group
5. Sibs' group

6. Family picnic without volunteers (bonding time)
7. Group dinner with volunteers and families
8. Empowerment seminars (parents only)
   a. Emotional journey
   b. Audiology
   c. Communication
   d. Technology
   e. Panels with young adults who are DHH
   f. Resources
9. Planned children's activities
   a. Field trips, learning songs, art/crafts, etc.
10. Filming parent stories
    a. Parents only; no children present
    b. Voluntary
    c. Private opportunity to share
    d. Emotional breakthroughs occur

Although traditionally family retreats have been over a weekend, it is also possible to have impact in a single day retreat, which can be much more cost-effective with an abbreviated agenda. In recent times, family retreats have been successfully transitioned to virtual platforms in an effort to continue to reach more and more families.

4.5.9 Journaling

The idea of journaling is not new, by any means. Using what the author refers to as "Journals to Resilience" has been a very effective tool for parents in their emotional journeys. Journals are traditionally written either in a computer document or on paper (in a journal book, for example). There are several benefits:

1. Record thoughts on any given day
2. Review those thoughts later for reflection
3. Help solve problems
4. Gain clarity
5. Verify progress over time
6. Gain perspective in realizing that on any given day, circumstances may seem overwhelming and even insurmountable, but reviewing later helps one realize that very important process called resilience

Prompts for parents when writing in a journal might include:

1. What happened?
2. How did you feel about it?
3. What did you do about it?

These are simple to follow and should not create any challenges for anyone who is attempting to record their thoughts. Professionals may invite parents to share their journal entries with them about the emotional journey as it relates to having a child with hearing loss.

It is important that any professionals review their own professional scope of practice on the topic of counseling. Audiologists, for example, are not mental health counselors, but counseling for a patient or family as it relates to a hearing loss is within their scope of practice. Sharing the journal entries with the professional service provider can allow for review and interaction, stimulate discussion, and even strengthen the professional-parent relationship. Sharing the journal entries can occur in person, via email, or virtually.

Video journaling has become more and more commonplace now that most people have cell phones with a video camera function. Encouraging parents to take a few minutes to record their thoughts on any given day may be an easier strategy and result in a higher success rate for completing the journaling task.

Pearl

When parents take time to record their thoughts and emotions on a regular basis, they have the ability to review and reflect on their journeys in a positive way.

4.5.10 Community Involvement

There are different things we can do to explore new ways to communicate more effectively and to change the culture of communication. The key element for achieving this goal is to bring parents, children, and professionals together for a common cause or community event. Working together on a committee takes away the traditional roles of professional service provider and parent/patient/child. Some examples of activities include movie night; partnering with community arts programs including theater productions, art openings, and theater shows; and fundraisers for hearing loss activities including awareness campaigns, Walk4Hearing, and local galas.

Being involved in these community events will allow everyone on a team to spend time together working on a project that may have nothing to do with hearing loss or at least take everyone out of the traditional roles and environments.

4.5.11 Parent-Professional Collaboratives

The parent-professional collaborative is designed to directly enable work to be done between parents and professionals on how to change the culture of communication. This event (whether in person or virtual) is designed to bring parents and professionals together for a two-day experience with no children present. An agenda is developed that will allow time for the two groups to be together to address topics of mutual interest as well as time for breakout groups. The primary focus is to examine the emotional journey of families *and* professionals. The desired outcome is to overcome barriers to effective communication between the two groups.

4.6 Summary

Throughout this chapter, the emotional journeys of families and professionals have been discussed in quest of greater understanding of the obstacles to effective communication. Moving through the emotional journey stages will deepen and strengthen the sense of empathy on the part of all parties. Strategies were discussed and centered around key yet simple terms including building resilience; practicing active listening; using the pause button; asking probe questions; creating support groups and retreats for families, DHH children, and siblings; journaling; and parent-professional collaboratives.

It is important to remember that, when professionals show empathy for families, both become empowered. Knowing that they are not alone, and feeling supported, are the most desired outcomes for families. And finally, always remember that hearing loss is only one among many issues that families deal with daily.

Discussion Questions

1. Does everyone experience grief in some form? Give examples.
2. Describe the grief journey in stages.
3. How is empathy strengthened? Share strategies.
4. How can the UBET be implemented in the workplace?
5. What are key strategies that can change the culture of communication?
6. What are the key components discussed for empathy building?
7. How can families benefit from discussing their emotional journeys with other families?

References

[1] Salehi K, Kohan S. Maternal-fetal attachment: what we know and what we need to know. *Int J Pregn & Chi Birth* 2017;2(5):146–148 10.15406/ipcb.2017.02.00038
[2] Luterman D. Lecture, North Carolina Speech, Hearing, Language Association Annual Convention; 2013
[3] Sinek S. *Start with why: how great leaders inspire everyone to take action.* New York, NY: Portfolio; 2009
[4] Brown B. The Dare to Lead glossary: key language, skills, tools, and practices. https://daretolead.brenebrown.com/wp-content/uploads/2018/10/Glossary-of-Key-Language-Skills-and-Tools-from-DTL.pdf. Published October 2018. Accessed December 21, 2021
[5] Davis T. Empathy: definition, examples, and explanations. https://www.berkeleywellbeing.com/empathy.html. Accessed December 21, 2021
[6] Hart B. Canceling cancel culture with compassion. TEDxCherryCreekWomen. https://www.ted.com/talks/betty_hart_canceling_cancel_culture_with_compassion?utm_campaign=tedspread&utm_medium=referral&utm_source=tedcomshare. November 2020. Accessed December 21, 2021
[7] Tervalon M, Murray-García J. Cultural humility versus cultural competence: a critical distinction in defining physician training outcomes in multicultural education. *J Health Care Poor Underserved* 1998;9(2):117–125
[8] American Psychological Association. Building your resilience. https://www.apa.org/topics/resilience/. Updated February 1, 2020. Accessed December 21, 2021
[9] Wilson D, Conyers M. 4 proven strategies for teaching empathy. https://www.edutopia.org/article/4-proven-strategies-teaching-empathy-donna-wilson-marcus-conyers. January 4, 2017. Accessed December 21, 2021

Appendix A: Unconscious Bias Exercise Tool (UBET) Individual Version

Intent

Understanding others, gaining insight, experiencing greater empathy

Background

Unconscious bias is a neutral term, the beliefs held outside of a person's consciousness.

Overview

The Unconscious Bias Exercise Tool (UBET) is designed to allow individuals completing it to look inward at how they define themselves based on upbringing, background, and life experiences. In addition, the exercise is designed to take the individual completing it to a different or even opposite perspective, allowing a closer look at how individuals view those who are not like them.

The desired outcome is to gain a deeper and broader perspective of oneself and others.

Instructions

Please complete the first section (YOU), listing things about YOU.

Then go to the next section (DIFFERENT FROM YOU) and describe someone who is or could be different than you in terms of background, upbringing, etc., using the same categories.

Please know that you are not required to answer any item with which you are uncomfortable. Thanks.

Section 1

- **YOU**
  - Race/ethnicity _____
  - Gender _____
  - Sexual identity _____
  - Age _____
  - Children
    - Yes
    - No
  - Hearing status
    - Deaf
    - Hearing
    - Hard of hearing
  - Communication mode
    - Spoken language
    - Visual language
    - Combined spoken and visual language
  - Parents
    - Living
    - Deceased
  - Siblings
    - Yes, if so, how many? _____
    - No
  - Educational level
    - High school
    - College
    - Graduate Degree
    - Doctoral Degree
  - Religion
  - Socioeconomic status
  - Geography
    - Where did you grow up?
    - Where do you currently live?
  - Marital status _____
  - Occupation _____

Please share how completing this section made you feel about yourself.

_____
_____
_____

Section 2

- **DIFFERENT FROM YOU: Using the same categories above, describe a person who is the opposite of you, different from you, not you.**
  - Race/ethnicity _____
  - Gender _____
  - Sexual identity _____
  - Age _____
  - Children
    - Yes
    - No
  - Hearing status
    - Deaf
    - Hearing
    - Hard of hearing
  - Communication mode
    - Spoken language
    - Visual language
    - Combined spoken and visual language
  - Parents
    - Living
    - Deceased
  - Siblings
    - Yes, if so, how many? _____
    - No
  - Educational level
    - High school
    - College
    - Graduate Degree
    - Doctoral Degree
  - Religion
  - Socioeconomic status
  - Geography
    - Where did you grow up?
    - Where do you currently live?
  - Marital status _____
  - Occupation _____

Take time to consider how you felt about this person, who is different from you. Was there any part of this that upset you? Did anything make you feel glad that you are not this person? If so, why? Be honest and write your feelings below. _____

_____
_____
_____

Please share any additional comments.

_____
_____
_____

5 The Parent as a Critical Team Member: Creating a Partnership for Learning

Gwen L. Suennen

Summary

This chapter discusses recognizing and understanding the grief process for families with children who have a hearing loss. Family-centered therapeutic strategies are shared for establishing a good relationship with the parents and enabling them to become the primary language facilitators of their child's listening and spoken language. Home visits and teletherapy can provide the clinician a snapshot of the child's home environment and family life to enable home routines and play-based teaching. Ideas for presenting and communicating information with parents are shared. Factors that can negatively impact attention and auditory development are discussed. Strategies to improve listening, language, and cognitive skills through play, reading, and questions are presented.

Keywords

guiding parents, grief, denial, acceptance, primary language facilitator, emotional and educational family support, family dynamics, family-centered therapeutic strategies, cognitive development, open-ended question, consistent communication, developmentally appropriate, positive reinforcement, desired outcome, auditory brain development, normal language development, language experience books, sensory integration, auditory fatigue

Key Points

- The purpose of coaching parents in a clinic setting, in an educational environment, or in homes is to enable them to become their child's primary listening and spoken language teachers.
- Understanding family dynamics, the grieving process, and the emotional state of the family members is essential to helping establish a good relationship and assisting them in becoming their child's primary language facilitators.
- Demonstrating teaching through play involves engaging parents in the play with the child, modeling listening and language through using toys interactively, discussing types of toys, and discussing with parents why we may be using a specific toy (language target).
- Home visits enable the therapist to gain an understanding of the home environment, the child's family life, and the natural interaction of family members. They can serve as a high-interest opportunity to teach listening and language through home routines.
- Motivating and guiding parents to read aloud and sing to their children successfully is critical for the development of listening, language, and cognition.

- Determining parent needs in working with older children with hearing loss may require the clinician to initiate communication to probe for areas of concern. Continued education for personal care of amplification, cognitive development, reading, home organization for homework, understanding of individualized education programs (IEPs) and individualized family service plans (IFSPs), as well as audiograms may be needed.
- Parents of children whose hearing loss is identified at preschool or school age may miss crucial parent education and coaching.

5.1 Parents as Partners: Building the Partnership

Children spend much more of their day in the presence of their parents than they do in the presence of a teacher of the deaf (TOD), speech-language pathologist (SLP), or listening and spoken language specialist (LSLS). Therefore, these professionals' role is to coach parents into becoming the primary facilitators in helping their child use hearing to develop listening skills and spoken language. This can be achieved through active, consistent parent participation in individualized auditory-verbal therapy and by guiding parents to create environments that support listening and spoken language throughout the child's daily activities. Since parent commitment, training, and follow-through are essential to the success of auditory-verbal therapy, the entire team must ensure that barriers do not interfere with parents' ability to become their children's primary language facilitators.

5.1.1 Understanding Individual Family Demographics

As practitioners who work with children with hearing loss, we must consider how best to connect with our clients' families to provide them the emotional and educational support they need to become their child's primary language teachers. The deaf and hard of hearing population ranges from rural to inner city, including every racial, ethnic, and socioeconomic group. Children with hearing loss can be adopted, fostered, or born into their families; they can be only children or have many siblings. Their parents may be single, married, divorced, or widowed. Children may be raised by other family members such as grandparents. The parents may each be working part time, working long hours at a full-time job, or a stay-at-home caregiver. A parent may have minimal family support from a partner/spouse or may live with extended family members who take an active role in childcare and language modeling and/or who speak multiple languages in the home. Each of these factors can have an impact on the parents' emotional response to their child's hearing loss and our ability to provide services.

The auditory-verbal therapy approach focuses on the partnership with the parent(s) of the child with hearing loss. Clinicians must invest the time to understand the family structure, gain the trust of the family members, and develop family-centered therapeutic strategies and goals. Studies show that the level of parents' education, the strength of the family's commitment, the level of parents' involvement in their child's education, and the family's ability to delegate roles toward attaining their child's goals are all correlated with outcomes for children with hearing loss.[1] Yucel found that most parents who had a higher level of education needed less information in any field than those with less education did. Additionally, the parents' needs decreased as the level of the parents' economic status increased. Moreover, additional studies found a correlation between low socioeconomic status, low levels of awareness of the families, and a delay in obtaining personal amplification.[1] This could possibly be caused by economic limitations. A parent needs questionnaire may be useful in creating an appropriate educational environment for considering individualized needs. One example of a parent needs checklist is the Comfort Level Checklist for Auditory-Verbal Families, which provides parents' comfort levels with areas such as troubleshooting technology, understanding their child's audiogram and IEP terminology, calling attention to sound and using target language with home routines.[2] In addition, Dana Suskind's book *Thirty Million Words: Building a Child's Brain*[3] is an excellent resource to help families in low-income communities to build language.

5.1.2 Recognizing Grief

It is not uncommon for practitioners working with young children with hearing loss, in a desire to address this neurological emergency, to plan and implement lessons without taking into account where the parent may be emotionally. It is imperative that the educator carefully consider each of the previously mentioned factors in an effort to meet the parents at their emotional level.

Parents imagine what their child will be like when they are expecting a newborn. Upon learning that their child has a hearing loss, these dreams may temporarily become shattered, resulting in a grieving process. Grief is a natural reaction to a sense of loss. Parents may be concerned that something they did may have caused the hearing loss. The parents might be coping with the emotionally laden thoughts that their perfect child might not hear the lullaby they want to sing to him, play the violin that her sisters play, or listen to the birds chirping. Parents may think that their child with hearing loss might never talk or sing. As professionals, being aware of the various stages of grieving such as denial, anger, guilt, depression, bargaining, hope, and acceptance can help us assist the parents with the understanding and counseling they may need.[4] Parents may go through one or all these stages in the process of accepting their child's hearing loss. We must keep in mind that the grieving process is an ongoing one. Grieving happens in stages, but it is not a one-way progression. While parents may seem to be accepting the hearing loss and doing well at one moment, an event such as starting school, participating in a sport, or watching other children making progress can bring back an "earlier" stage of grief. (See Chapter 4 for further discussion on grief and emotional growth in families.) This means the parents will experience emotionally difficult times related to a series of experiences throughout their child's development (e.g., mainstreaming, friendships, sports) that will each once again highlight that their perfect child has a hearing loss. Some describe it as a grief roller coaster! Without support to cope through the grief process, parents often have difficulty understanding the needs of their child, the hearing technology available, or the educational process involved in raising their child.

Pitfall

Without support to cope through the grief process, parents often have difficulty understanding the needs of their child, the hearing technology available, or the educational process involved in raising their child.

The relationship between the parents of a child with hearing loss and the hearing health professional has a powerful impact on the effectiveness of the (re)habilitation process.[5] It is our job as professionals to recognize when parents are grieving and to provide the emotional support they need to make appropriate decisions. As the parents work through their grief and begin to accept their child's hearing loss, they may begin to explore, hope, and invest instead of focusing on their emotions. For parents of children with hearing loss, the pressure of time to act quickly to optimize the child's listening and communication skills can complicate the grieving process. Presenting a model of a grieving process such as Karen Martin's Pathways Through Grief model to the parents may be helpful.[6] If parents are having significant difficulty coming to terms with their child's hearing loss, a recommendation of professional support and counseling is appropriate.

Denial is the first stage of grieving; some parents initially will not admit or accept their child's hearing loss, so they seek second or third opinions from other audiologists. They may *bargain* or postpone getting appropriate technology, believing their child does not need hearing devices right away. Although not common, some families wait several months or even 1 to 2 years after diagnosis and recommendations for intervention before they decide to proceed with amplification and intervention for their child. In these cases cultural differences, spousal opposition, or lack of family support may be factors that create roadblocks to getting the child hearing aids (HAs) or cochlear implants (CIs). Inquiring about the parents' reasoning for delaying intervention can lead to productive discussions and can guide the clinician to clarify misinformation, provide additional information, and/or connect the family with other families who have children with hearing loss. Continuing to see the family, just for counseling, can speed up the process. The parents' reasons may be financial, aesthetic, fear of surgery, family or community cultural issues, or self-protective (denial that their child has a hearing loss). We also need to be cognizant that, since the parents we work with come from a variety of socioeconomic backgrounds, some families may not have insurance or the financial resources to assist in obtaining hearing technology or therapy for their child. We should be able to provide parents with a list of agencies that give scholarships or grants for hearing technology if finances are an issue and provide them with assistance making contact if necessary. If the reason for not obtaining hearing technology is aesthetic, it may be helpful for the parents to meet children wearing the devices, to view photos of the recommended devices on young children, connect with other families, and discuss additional information from the audiologist if needed. If the parent is in denial that their child has a hearing loss, it can be helpful to review the audiogram with familiar sounds, discuss the effect of brain development when children do not have access to sound, share notes from therapy logs/classroom observations, and communicate with other service providers such as the physical therapist (PT), occupational therapist (OT), and resource specialist (RSP) to demonstrate how the child is missing critical information for learning language and developing the auditory brain. Having the parent in the audiology test booth to see and hear what the child is missing can be particularly helpful. If acceptance is delayed, and denial continues, some parents may seek alternative approaches as "cures" for their child's hearing loss, thereby delaying or preventing the child from becoming comfortable with their own hearing loss.

5.1.3 Creating a Safe Place

It is critical that, as professionals, we listen to parents' concerns and display empathy. Consistently checking in with the parents by asking questions (such as "How are you doing/feeling?" or "How are things going?") during conversations not only nurtures the parent/clinician relationship but allows parents to feel open to discussing their feelings. Without a safe environment to share feelings, the parents may decide not to talk about how they feel regarding their child's hearing loss, which can create additional stress for the family.

Along with an empathetic style, using an open-ended questioning style helps foster parental input into the rehabilitative process. In an effort to understand how best to provide family support, it is important that we inquire regarding parental concerns on an ongoing basis (e.g., "Do you have any new concerns?"). This simple question keeps you, as the therapist, connected to what is happening in the home and opens discussions. The parent may be concerned about their child's sleep issues, challenging behavior, difficulty making friends, or future mainstreaming. The Question Prompt List (QPL)[7] is very helpful. With this resource, parents can look at a list of possible questions that may prompt them to discuss issues that are concerning them with the practitioner.

Families can feel isolated and overwhelmed when vast amounts of new information are presented to them after diagnosis. Parents have stated that speaking with other parents who are raising children with hearing loss can be a great source of support. Providing families with contact information of other families who are willing to share their stories and time, or introducing them to other families in the waiting room or therapy room, can be most beneficial. We must remember that many parents may not feel comfortable discussing concerns or their personal/family life until the parent/interventionist relationship has been well established and solidified. A skilled therapist knows that it takes patience, understanding, and multiple attempts at opening communication before parents become comfortable sharing.

Pearl

A skilled therapist knows that it takes patience, understanding, and multiple attempts at opening communication before parents become comfortable sharing.

5.1.4 Recognizing Unique Family Member Roles

Family psychotherapists tell us that, because the members of a family are interconnected, when a child is diagnosed with a hearing loss, we have an entire family system affected with a hearing problem.[8] Unexpressed anger can be unintentionally displaced on another family member, and unacknowledged guilt can lead to intense dedication to and overprotection of the child with the hearing loss, leaving little time for siblings or the marriage.[7]

Professionals need to understand how the family dynamics affect the success of the child from diagnosis through mainstreaming. To enable the child with a hearing loss to be successful, all family members need to have a stake in developing a unit that nurtures and functions as optimally as possible.[8] To understand the family as well as the family dynamics, it is imperative to foster a positive relationship with all the involved members of the family. This can be achieved by asking about how the parents, grandparents, siblings, and caregivers as *individuals* are doing and within these discussions, attempting to ascertain the stressors in the family. Areas of stress within the family may stem from long hours in a job situation, sibling rivalry, marital stress, difficulty handling the home routine, responses of the extended family members to the hearing loss, responsibility for caring of an extended family member, or the health of a spouse. Stress may have existed before the hearing loss was diagnosed and may be exacerbated by the diagnosis and all that is involved in having a child with a disability. When both parents must work, they may feel additional guilt in not being available to spend time with their child encouraging language development. Find out what kind of family support the parents have, such as extended family living nearby or relatives taking care of the child several days per week. Again, in addition to the informal counseling provided in therapy sessions, if it appears that professional counseling for the family would be beneficial, have references available to share.

Keep in mind that mothers and fathers may handle the acceptance of the hearing loss and overall stress differently. Fathers tend to deny the need to learn about hearing impairment and are less inclined than mothers to develop constructive coping strategies to deal with their stress.[9] Grandparents may be afraid to say how they are feeling as a result of the hurt they feel for their child and grandchild.[8] Grandparents may also resist using technology when they are babysitting if they do not fully understand the need. Although we come to therapy with our lesson plans and goals in mind, be aware that taking the time to be a good listener to family members creates positive relationships and may be critical to helping families learn to navigate the challenges they face. When parents feel isolated with no appropriate avenue to process their feelings, it can lead to anger and possible avoidance of staff.[5]

Pearl

Mothers and fathers may handle the acceptance of the hearing loss and overall stress differently.

Inviting extended family members to therapy sessions is helpful so that the child can have multiple language facilitators in his or her world. Encourage both the mothers and the fathers to attend therapy sessions, along with a grandparent (if they live in the home or see the child often) and other involved relatives or family friends (if they are caregivers). Siblings can join for portions of intervention sessions as well. If family members cannot attend due to scheduling conflicts, record therapy sessions or have family join in virtually.

Pearl

Inviting extended family members to therapy sessions is helpful so that the child can have multiple language facilitators in his or her world.

5.1.5 Navigating the Many Modes of Therapy

In the last few years, we have seen dramatic changes in delivery models for intervention. As clinicians, we may prefer one delivery model over another, but we may be forced to use an unfamiliar or uncomfortable model. First, it is important to recognize and be honest about our training, comfort levels, strengths, and weaknesses. It is also important to reach out for training and mentoring when we are faced with a delivery model that is unfamiliar or uncomfortable. HearingFirst.org is an excellent resource for clinicians facing new delivery models.

Some early intervention programs provide services for children with hearing loss within the home setting. With the advent of distance learning, we can now go into the home via the computer and view the child's skills, the parents' expectations, the discipline style, and the child's self-help skills. Home visits and teletherapy (see Chapter 20) can give the clinician a snapshot of the child's home environment and family life, along with the natural interaction of family members. While we make the best attempt to provide an educational and fun environment in a therapy setting for our students to listen and learn spoken language, entering into the home environment personally or virtually can give the clinician insight into the kind of books and toys available in the home, the number of screens used during the day, as well as any interfering background noise or reverberation that could impede learning. In addition, observations can be made regarding how the child communicates with family members. Do they attend to verbal interactions at home? How do speech and language differ at home from therapy sessions? Do parents or siblings talk for them?

If noise or reverberation is an issue, it is important to give a gentle awareness of how the noise in the home (e.g., television, radio, dishwasher, or washing machine) can impact listening and language development. A visual handout can help demonstrate the impact of noise upon listening and language development,[10] or a sound level meter phone app (e.g., Decibel X[11]) can help the parents monitor various levels of sound in their home as well as various other environments. Homes with very little carpet and high ceilings may have reverberation that can be reduced with the aid of fabric such as rugs, curtains, or additional towels. Visiting the families in their home, whether in person or via the internet, helps create an understanding of home life and establish a good connection between the parents and the clinician.

During an in-person home visit, take the time to notice simple, but often overlooked opportunities for listening and language such as feeding and talking about the fish in the fishbowl, cutting a flower from the garden and putting it into a vase, waiting for the mail truck or garbage truck, or watching an animal run across the lawn. Take time to go through the daily routine of the child. Is the parent giving the child choices and talking about those choices when the child is getting dressed? Interact with the child using the child's toys. Some homes are filled with an abundance of toys, and suggestions can be made for rotating them so that the child is excited to play with and learn from them. Others may have sparse options for interactive play items, but parents may be open to suggestions of additional toys for their child.

During an in-person home or teletherapy visit with a family, it is easy to reinforce the goal of working on two- or three step play sequences and listening. For example, in a situation with a toy kitchen that lacks any plastic food or dishes for the child to engage in pretend play, we might improvise by using real items from the kitchen. The conversation with the parents can then explain how having a child's own play items in the toy kitchen would enable him to initiate play as well as conversation with his siblings or other family members. Always be mindful of the varying socioeconomic statuses of the families, and make suggestions for second-hand stores, yard sales, discount stores, and clearance sales if appropriate. As children outgrow toys, encourage parents to donate them to the center or other families of younger children so that they can continue to be used and loved. For additional information on teletherapy, see Chapter 20.

5.1.6 Providing Information

There is an abundant amount of information we need to present to parents when working with young children with hearing loss. As stated above, we must recognize that parents who have just learned their child's diagnosis are first processing this emotionally. They are trying to understand the testing, technology, and habilitation while rearranging their schedules to accommodate medical, audiological, and therapy appointments and adjusting how they communicate with their child.

Depending on where they live, traveling to appointments can take a long time. In our efforts to assist the parents to become our partners and to learn how to become their child's primary language teacher at home, we need to research, gather, and organize a vast amount of educational material and ideas. As therapists and educators, we must proceed cautiously with our presentation of the information, as an overload of material can paralyze the parent and create indecisiveness. Although parents need and want information, the style and manner with which the information is provided may be critical to its acceptance and integration by the parents.[9]

Pitfall

As therapists and educators, we must proceed cautiously with our presentation of the information, as an overload of material can paralyze the parent and create indecisiveness.

Providing help in organizing this new information is instrumental for ongoing educational purposes. One very effective strategy for sharing information with parents is creating a *parent notebook* with subject tabs such as "audiology," "listening," "language," "IFSP" or "IEP," "home routines," "behavior," "resources," "reading," and "other issues." This enables the clinician to share information in smaller increments, as the notebook keeps it organized and it can be easily shared with other family members and other clinicians. Another method to assist parents with the influx of information is to develop a filing system or demonstrate how to create separate folders for emails and important papers. If handouts are presented in a therapy session or discussion, follow up by inquiring whether the new materials are helpful: "Did you have a chance to read the handout?" "What are your thoughts about . . . ?" "Did you learn anything new from the article?" "Were you able to share this with Dad?"

5.1.7 Consistently Communicating

Consistent communication with parents is also essential for success when working with children of all ages who are deaf or hard of hearing. Find out what mode of contact is preferred by the parents, whether by phone, email, texting, or a combination. What is the preferred language of the parents? Is it English or another language? Do the parents use spoken language, American Sign Language (ASL), or some other form of signing? Do they need an interpreter? How well do the parents read?

To achieve optimal success with the child, the clinician should discover or ask the parents' learning style to best present information. Do they process information best through auditory, visual, or kinesthetic means? Many parents acquire and use information more easily if it is presented in multiple forms. Providing written along with verbal instructions allows parents a backup if they cannot recall or did not correctly process the verbal information that was presented. Video recording parts of therapy sessions may provide clarification of concepts as well.

Once the child attends preschool, consistent communication between the parents and all service providers is critical for success. The parent may primarily communicate with you as the hearing specialist, and education for all service providers will most likely depend on the clinician initiating conversations. However, it is the therapist's role to teach and empower parents to become their child's advocate by gradually learning to communicate effectively with educators themselves. Classroom teachers and other service providers need to be in-serviced at the beginning of the school year about needs related to hearing loss, expectations for what the child can and cannot hear/understand, IEP accommodations, soundfield, and/or personal remote microphone (RM) technology. Continuity of care among staff is maintained through frequent check-ins with providers, classroom observations, and communications regarding any changes with technology or listening skills.

Prior to triennial evaluations, reminders may need to be sent to all staff administering tests, stating that the child needs to wear functioning hearing technology for the evaluations to be valid, that testing is best accomplished in a quiet room with few distractions, and that, if personal RM equipment is used, it needs to be worn during testing. If oral directions are given, it is essential that the child be able to see and hear the testing presenter. If the child is accessing an evaluation via the internet, he or she may need to utilize a computer cord with his or her personal RM system and may need captioning. For additional information, see Chapters 2 and 16.

In addition to communicating with parents regarding hearing technology and listening in therapy/classroom, touch base with them periodically following an observation, noting the child's attention, participation, pragmatic skills, interactive play, speech, and use of expressive language. This will keep the parents abreast of how their child is developing. If the therapist is meeting with both the parent and the child, it can be a good time to share a short story of an observation of their child during the preschool class, such as the child offering to share a book, raising her hand to lead the song, or joining in playtime at the kitchen center. In our efforts to be supportive, even when communicating a concern with a parent, keep in mind to begin the conversation with a positive comment if possible.

5.2 Parents as Their Child's Primary Language Facilitators: Setting Expectations

5.2.1 Therapy through Parent Involvement

The importance of parent involvement has already been discussed, but this is where we begin with the actual implementation and integration of the parents into the process as part of the foundation for developing the child's listening and spoken language abilities. The premise of involving parents and other caregivers in therapy sessions is to empower them as the child's primary language teacher. Our job is to ensure the parents' understanding of their critical role in the child's success through integrated, daily carryover at home. Be aware that this is not a clearly understood concept in all areas of education and speech-language pathology. Parents spend many more hours each day with their child than clinicians do. If parents can become the child's primary teachers, the intensiveness of the intervention and chances of success are far greater. In a few schools and private practices, structuring the therapy sessions with parents as partners is the norm. It is expected that the parent sit with the child and the clinician at the table or on the floor, take turns, contribute as an interactive part of the session, and continue the learning at home. Unfortunately, because implementing this type of partnership is challenging, many school settings and private practices do not recognize the incredible potential and value of parents as primary facilitators. Administrators and school staff on the early intervention or preschool assessment team may need to be educated about the value and role of including a caregiver in therapy sessions. However, with exposure to this model, professionals will eventually begin to see the benefits of focusing on having therapy extend beyond the clinic walls and centering on the goal of mainstreaming the child as soon as possible. Educating coworkers is worth the time and energy, as it creates consistent intervention, which enables the families to extend the learning for their children with hearing loss outside of the therapy setting.

Pitfall

Unfortunately, because implementing the parent/clinician partnership is challenging, many school settings and private practices do not recognize the incredible potential and value of parents as the primary language facilitators.

5.2.2 Preparing Parents

The auditory-verbal therapy model begins with the assumption that the parents' desired outcome is listening and spoken language (LSL). The effectiveness of this therapy model depends on the parents' commitment to being active and consistent participants and the clinician's ability to guide/coach them to be the primary facilitators of their child's LSL development. Parents of a child with a hearing loss need to be made aware that aside from some minor modifications, this process has more similarities to than differences from facilitating language with typically developing children. We model and explain that listening and spoken language are what they do with their child all the time. Every parent-child interaction, whether changing their diapers, dressing them, washing their hands, brushing teeth, grocery shopping, preparing meals, helping with homework, or reading stories, is a part of daily living that has listening and language as the foundation. We encourage parents to respond with interest to whatever their child is telling them, verbally or nonverbally. Parents need to talk frequently at a level that the child can understand about things of interest to the child, using repetition of novel vocabulary and concepts to ensure learning.

Clinicians must understand that parents will begin auditory-verbal therapy at widely differing levels of parenting readiness and experience. This may be the parents' first child, so they may be struggling with basic feeding and diapering and are now dealing with hearing loss. This may be a second child, so the parents have experience but are now struggling with how to manage two children. This may be a third or fourth child, so the parents are very experienced but must juggle the needs of children at significantly different ages. They may be working parents who rely on caregivers for eight or more hours per day.

Working with parents and caregivers with varying degrees of readiness and experience means that clinicians must be prepared to coach concerning not only listening, speech, and language development but also all basic parenting skills. It helps to be aware that parents may be struggling with parenting skills such as dealing with sibling rivalry, discontinuing use of a pacifier, or juggling bedtime routines. Clinicians should be prepared to demonstrate and provide written resources or video resources (e.g., YouTube videos) to develop basic parenting skills.

5.2.3 Understanding Hearing Loss

For parents and caregivers to be the primary facilitators of language with a child with hearing loss, they must first understand the hearing loss and the implications of that loss. As we discussed earlier, although the audiologist presents this information during the diagnostic process, shock, grief, and lack of knowledge of hearing loss often interfere with parents' ability to truly understand and retain this information. Moreover, certain aspects of hearing loss can seem irrelevant for a newborn who is always within arms' reach but be crucial for a toddler who is running away. While the audiologist should be reviewing this information with parents at each visit, clinicians will have more regular contact with the family and should be reviewing and applying this information at every visit.

5.2.4 Ensuring the Use of Appropriately Functioning Technology

In addition to the hearing loss and its implications, parents and caregivers must also understand and take responsibility for the child's hearing technology. It is critical that both clinicians and parents perform regular technology listening checks to determine whether the child is accessing auditory information through appropriately functioning hearing technology. Although the audiologist counsels the parents on care of the child's personal hearing devices, clinicians need to understand how technology works, since they may need to help educate parents, caregivers, school staff, and others regarding how to complete a listening check, how and how often to clean earmolds, how to secure technology on the child's head, how to use an electronic drying device (e.g., Dry & Store[12]) consistently when the hearing devices are intermittent or sound distorted, and how to verify connection to a personal RM system.

Providing feedback to parents on a consistent basis regarding functioning of technology is not only essential to listening, speech, and language development; it provides consistent communication with the family. Obviously, parents of babies and young children must be trained to assume responsibility for daily checking and securing of the hearing technology. Some parents want their preschool or school-age child to assume responsibility for the care of their hearing devices soon after they receive them. It is helpful to advise parents to assist with the technology until their children become good reporters of when their hearing devices are not functioning properly. In some families, the likelihood of personal care increases if specific IFSP or IEP goals are written for care of hearing technology. In any case, frequent interactions among the clinician, the child, and the parents are often required before consistent device care is maintained.

When working with a child who is able to self-report, asking open-ended questions such as "How are you taking care of your hearing aids at home?" can lead to specific information, leading the therapist to educate both the child and the parent on the proper care of the technology devices. With consistent monitoring and communication, the clinician and family can provide the audiologist with feedback about the benefit of the HA/CI programming as well as the consistency of wearing. If the clinician or parent notes that the child is, for example, using an increased voice volume, omitting final consonants, asking for clarification more often, struggling to attend, or showing changes in behavior, the audiologist will be able to make any modifications necessary for successful listening, speech, and language growth.

Pearl

If the clinician or parent notes that the child is, for example, using an increased voice volume, omitting final consonants, asking for clarification more often, struggling to attend, or showing changes in behavior, the audiologist will be able to make any modifications necessary for successful listening, speech, and language growth.

Pearl

Asking parents, "If your child did not have a hearing loss, would this behavior have been allowed?" is a reminder that their child is a child first and has hearing loss second.

5.2.5 Expecting Typical Development and Behaviors

Understanding Typical Development

As discussed earlier, parents of a child with hearing loss may have significant parenting experience or may have no parenting experience. Those with significant parenting experience may have realistic expectations of how their child should be learning and growing. On the other hand, first-time parents may not be familiar with all the developmental milestones their child should be achieving. In addition, if the child with the hearing loss is the youngest child in the family, parents may want to "prolong" the baby stage and may think less mature behavior is "cute." For all families, but especially those in which the child has no older siblings, it can be helpful to briefly review and share resources detailing normal child development as well as language development. *By the Ages*[13] and *Ages and Stages*[14] are two publications that are still very informative.

Expecting Developmentally Appropriate Behavior

The majority of parents raising young children encounter challenging behavioral issues that can be difficult to deal with and manage, but these challenges can be magnified when the child has a hearing loss. Although teaching and training children is the primary responsibility, joy, and privilege of the parents, difficulties such as failing to set boundaries due to guilt, language delays, and educational challenges often lead to behavior problems. Although it is normal for a child to resist at times, parental guilt or differing caregiver expectations may blur these boundaries and create difficulty distinguishing between normal development and effects of the disability.[8] It is the parents' responsibility to expect developmentally appropriate behavior, model resilience and independence, teach conflict resolution, and gradually reward self-responsibility with more freedom until the child reaches adulthood. Asking parents "If your child did not have a hearing loss, would this behavior have been allowed?" is a reminder that their child is a child first and has hearing loss second.

Moreover, parents often feel that discipline equates to punishment; however, the word *discipline* means training or teaching children how to behave using both positive and negative techniques.[15] When parents understand that children are more comfortable when they are aware of their boundaries, then parents are more willing to set limitations and follow through. Asking parents "Are you comfortable saying 'no' to your child?" helps to determine whether they are ready to set boundaries. A worthy resource that has been utilized by many parents is *Good Behavior Made* Easy.[15] This publication is filled with ideas such as focusing on one behavior at a time, using behavior charts, knowing how to reward/praise, setting time limits, understanding how to implement time outs, and establishing routines.

Clinicians should feel comfortable modeling how to implement natural consequences, such as removing a toy after the child throws it, and how to incorporate a variety of positive reinforcement strategies to shape a behavior during a therapy session. For example, during a teaching session, therapists can use a variety of intermittent praise phrases ("I like that," "Nice work," "Good job," "You're listening!") to reinforce behavior positively or use frequent rewards on a behavior chart to demonstrate to a parent how to improve motivation and repeat performance. Clear boundaries can be demonstrated in therapy by stating rules in a simple way and with visual referents if needed. Behavior can be shaped by ignoring undesired behaviors, using realistic consequences, or appropriately using time out. It is important that parents and clinicians relate to children in a positive way. Too much negative or critical actions make children feel inadequate and less likely to want to work cooperatively.

Setting Realistic Listening and Language Goals

It is important to clarify the parents' long-term goals for their child with hearing loss during one of the initial therapeutic sessions, as parents may have unrealistic expectations, or they may have limited expectations. They might assume that, after children receive their personal amplification devices, they will immediately begin to respond to sound, localize the sound source, start to babble, respond to their name, and behave like other children of the same chronological age. On the other end of the spectrum, we may encounter parents who have low expectations and are satisfied with slow, incremental progress. It is essential to ask the parents what their desired outcomes are for their child. They may need help in formulating what their expectations are and could be, and as clinicians, we can help guide them. If the long-term goal for their child is to listen and talk and be educated with their typically hearing peers, then we can discuss consistent auditory access and development of listening skills. The IFSP or IEP goals may need to be reviewed periodically if the parents' focus begins to waver or if it becomes necessary to demonstrate how the therapy and home activities are supporting their long-term plans.

When working with young children, frequently share with parents that one of our primary long-term goals will be conversation, not simply words. When children are able to converse, they will be exhibiting listening skills, reciprocal turn taking, good connected oral language, and appropriate social skills. Parent education must include the importance of auditory brain development related to typical stages of speech and language development. If the parent has realistic and appropriate expectations, the carryover from therapy into the home should be easier.

Since we know that children with hearing loss can acquire language following a similar timetable as hearing children, we can use rating scales based on normal language development. The Cottage Acquisition Scales for Listening, Language & Speech (CASLLS)[16] is an excellent tool for this, providing a sequence of listening, language, and play in a visual display for the therapist to utilize and share. These rating scales can be reviewed with the parents over subsequent time periods, so they can gain an understanding of their child's progress as well as therapy targets. See Chapter 4 for additional assessment information.

Maintaining a Predictable Routine

All children, especially children with hearing loss, function better with routine and predictability in their life.[17] Teachers will verify this: when their daily schedule is interrupted, the students can be out of sorts. When engaging in distance learning, parents who have not kept their children with hearing loss on a schedule report having more behavior issues at home. Helping the parent implement a schedule or routine in the home can improve their child's comfort level and consequently improve behavior through the predictability that it provides. Use of a chart with picture pockets enables parents to insert photos of daily routines such as getting dressed, going to school, snack time, and homework, which can be placed in the appropriate order to demonstrate the day's events to the child.

Pearl

Helping the parent implement a schedule or routine in the home can improve their child's comfort level and consequently improve behavior through the predictability that it provides.

5.2.6 Recognizing Factors That Can Adversely Affect the Child's Auditory Development

When the parent or the clinician has difficulty sustaining the child's attention, several factors need to be evaluated. First and foremost, clinicians need to determine whether the child is hearing. Has there been a listening check with the technology? All team members should be monitoring the personal technology to ensure that the child is consistently wearing it and understanding speech well with it. An important role of the clinician is to teach the parents, caregivers, and school staff to perform daily listening checks at home and school. If listening checks

indicate that the child is not hearing everything up close and at a distance, consult with audiologists to determine whether this may be a cause of inattention.

Another difficulty with attention in young children with hearing loss may stem from lack of sleep. Discussing multiple issues regarding sleep patterns such as bedtime routines, fear of darkness, trouble falling asleep, getting up during the night, possible inadvertent "rewards" for the child for waking up too early (such as being allowed to climb into the parents' bed) can help parents identify and change habits in order to support a more well-rested child. Since children with hearing loss work harder than their hearing peers, they typically require more sleep. To help educate parents on this topic, refer to a sleep chart based on age, in addition to a good reference on sleeping issues such as *Solve Your Child's Sleep Problems*.[18]

A child's diet may need to be addressed if hunger or malnutrition is affecting attention or the ability to retain learned information. Since morning or after school is often the best time to work with children with hearing loss, we may see them early in the day, when they have yet to eat or drink anything, or late in the afternoon, when they have not recently eaten. In such cases, it may be necessary to have discussions with parents who bring their child to therapy about providing healthy meals/snacks prior to therapy and sharing the benefits of water to hydrate the brain.

Two other factors that can negatively impact auditory development when working with young children are allergies and otitis media. It is our job to educate parents on the effects of possible fluctuation of hearing loss due to allergies, fluid, or negative pressure in the middle ear. We must direct them to seek appropriate medical advice and follow up with them to learn the outcome.

Research/studies have found that excessive use of television or electronic screens may adversely affect attention and language.[19] Because the majority of screen time is passive and young children need to be learning through active formal/informal teaching situations as well as interactive play, clinical recommendations for limiting or minimizing screen times should be shared with parents.

Another topic typically overlooked but deserving of parental discussion when auditory development is an issue is that of auditory fatigue. Children with unilateral or bilateral hearing loss exhibit auditory fatigue from the listening effort involved in daily activities as well as curriculum.[20] Parents and classroom teachers are often unaware of how much energy children with hearing loss are expending just to listen. It is essential that classroom teachers and parents be given information about auditory fatigue so that they can understand and provide listening breaks to support the child.

Some children who have a sensorineural hearing loss may also have challenges in attending due to sensory integration dysfunction (SID). SID is the brain's inability to process and organize information received through the senses in order to interact effectively with the environment. Learning to recognize the signs (unusually high or low activity; poor balance; inability to calm oneself; over- or undersensitivity to touch; avoidance of textures, some foods, and clothing tags) and referring to an occupational therapist who specializes in sensory integration can help the family with not only focus and attention issues, but behavior as well. A sensory profile questionnaire such as the Sensory Integration Screening Questionnaire[21] can be completed by caregivers to determine at-risk behaviors. Sharing strategies to promote sensory processing can be incorporated into therapy session. More in-depth information can be found in *The Out-of-Sync Child*[22] and *The Out-of-Sync Child Has Fun*.[23]

If a child with hearing loss has additional handicapping conditions or medical needs, it is imperative that the therapist stay informed and communicate consistently with the parents, nurse, and other professionals working with the child. Parents of children with additional handicapping conditions can become overwhelmed with information and, as a result, may forget or may be inhibited about disclosing relevant details pertaining to their child. More information on assisting children with multiple challenges can be found in Chapter 15.

5.2.7 Integrating Listening into Daily Life to Develop Spoken Language

Listening and Language through Daily Routines

When teaching parents to facilitate their child's language development, focus on the importance of developing the auditory part of the brain by demonstrating how listening is connected to immersing their child in language. We can demonstrate this through utilizing three tips for family conversation, known as the three Ts.[24] The first tip is *Tune in* to the child's interests and follow that lead or get the child interested in what you are doing. The second one is *Talk more:* talk about what the child is doing and what you are doing. Studies have shown that when the child hears more words prior to kindergarten, it makes a significant and positive impact on a child's vocabulary knowledge and ability to read.[25] The third T is *Take turns* with talking so that we begin to model what conversation looks like. The parent talks, then pauses, looks at the child, and waits for a response. Engage in back and forth turn taking.[24]

When engaging with the parent and child with hearing loss, the most meaningful way to incorporate listening and language into daily life is to center learning around natural home routines. As clinicians, we model behavior we expect from parents and then ask parents to use what we have demonstrated in working with their children. We begin by using the child's home routines; we have the parents show us what they do with each routine, and we help them modify it for their child's language level. For babies and toddlers, many activities happen multiple times each day (e.g., changing diapers or having a snack) or regularly from one day to the next (e.g., eating dinner or taking a bath). Helping parents to develop a language-rich narrative for each activity and then to expand that narrative as the child's receptive understanding grows creates a fun, interesting auditory environment that bathes the child in language. Through parent-clinician discussions, the most important routines for the family can be identified and targeted first. Initially, clinicians may need to brainstorm appropriate language with parents and model ways to gain the child's attention auditorily in order to input language, but as the parents and caregivers become more comfortable talking through routines, the emphasis should shift to increased parent modeling with the assistance of clinician input. An early intervention program that professionals can use with parents of early language learners with routines is Learn to Talk Around the Clock by Karen Rossi.[26] It contains thematic units such as "On the Go," "Bathtime," and

"In the Garden," which contain worksheets for modeling, self-talk, parallel talk, ideas and expanding language, ideas for books/props, planning grids, and behavior checklists.

Once children become mobile, they love to help their parents. Using more interactive, everyday routines—such as putting toys away, riding in a car, unloading the dishwasher, helping with laundry or unloading groceries—can still form the basis of abundant, auditorily based learning experiences. For example, with early language learners, helping their parents set the table can provide many opportunities to listen, follow verbal directions, and reinforce language targets: "Where are the forks?" "Put Mommy's plate on the table," "Here is Daddy's plate," "Put your plate next to Daddy's," "Put the napkins next to the plates."

During demonstrations of home routines, parents may be surprised when their child does not know some of the vocabulary presented by the clinician, such as *toothbrush*, *toothpaste*, *cap*, *faucet*, and *rinse*, although the child has participated in the activity repeatedly. Often, children with hearing loss may call a toothbrush a "brush your teeth" because this is what they have heard their parents say, in place of naming the toothbrush itself. Clinicians should encourage parents to tune in to specific vocabulary and to reinforce unfamiliar words when deficits are noted.

Pitfall

During demonstrations of home routines, parents may be surprised when their child does not know some of the vocabulary presented by the therapist such as **toothbrush**, **toothpaste**, **cap**, **faucet**, and **rinse**, although the child has participated in the activity repeatedly. Children may call a toothbrush a "brush your teeth" because this is what they have heard the parents say, in place of naming the toothbrush itself.

Listening and Language through Play

Most parents do not realize that play is a representation of and a way to practice conversation and that many children with hearing loss (and some children with typical hearing) might need to be taught how to play. Modeling how to play, demonstrating what types of toys promote interactive play, and encouraging turn taking/conversation during therapy sessions are essential to listening, speech, and language development. Play can evolve from hiding toys under a napkin while the child is in the highchair to setting up a make-believe flower shop with artificial flowers, vases, a grocery with toy food, and a cash register.

With the ever-expanding supply of electronic and screen-based toys, many parents may not understand the benefits of "old-time" imaginative toys and may not know how to use these toys to elicit play and language. In selecting toys for use with children with hearing loss, be aware that because of the nature of the interaction taking place during play, "noisy" toys will compete with the verbal input of the parent or the therapist. The therapist may need to model choosing quiet toys, to encourage optimal auditory development, for parents in a therapy session. Additionally, games played on the tablet, phone, or computer generally have limited benefit for developing listening and language.

It's important to share with parents the reason a particular toy is being utilized in a therapy session so that they understand speech/language targets and to demonstrate attributes of toys that may be appropriate for their child. To help model conversation through play, it is helpful to have a collection of character toys (e.g., Little People, realistic dolls, loving family) that can be used in large toy vehicles, in a farm or zoo model, or with building blocks. Use the parent to help model dialogue while interacting with a toy kitchen, making creations with Play-Doh, setting up a birthday party for the teddy bear, or pretending to grocery shop.

Parents of school-age children, particularly those late identified or those with progressive hearing loss, may need to understand the importance of play, not just academic intervention. These children may have missed out on critical stages of language and pragmatic skill development, which are essential to forming friendships and interacting in a variety of social scenarios at school as well as bonding with their siblings. Checking in with parents by asking questions such as "What kind of outdoor games does she like to engage in?" "Does he have some favorite board games?" "What does she like to play with when her friends come to the house?" "What do he and his brother do together?" can provide the therapist with valuable information pertaining to the child's ability to initiate and interact with others in play.

If the therapy sessions primarily take place outside of the home, do not assume the parent is able to transfer the listening and spoken language involved in play learned with the toys in therapy to the ones at home. It can be beneficial for the parents to bring in some of their child's favorite toys to a few sessions for practice or to engage in play through a few teletherapy sessions.

Listening and Language through Reading to Children

All parents want their child to become a good reader. As with normally hearing children, we begin as parents by having our babies and toddlers listen to us read aloud to them. With our knowledge of auditory brain development, we know that the listening experience in young children is critical for the development of speech and language, and a strong auditory language base is essential for reading.[27] *Jim Trelease's Read Aloud Handbook* discusses the importance of reading aloud and talking in relation to the child's ability to read and write: "The listening vocabulary is the reservoir of words that feeds the speaking vocabulary, the reading vocabulary and the writing vocabulary, all at the same time."[28] Thus, listening to stories read aloud contributes to a child's auditory development, overall background knowledge, and understanding of language, all of which are prerequisites to learning to read. (See Chapter 13 for more information.)

To create a literacy-rich environment, parents should be encouraged to model sustained silent reading at home and have books readily available in multiple places where the child spends time. A basket of picture books in the car, containers of books in the family room, and shelves of books in the bedroom are just a few examples. Parents often benefit from lists of appropriate book suggestions for different ages.

As professionals, we can also share additional ideas of ways to promote reading at home to further develop early literacy skills such as singing songs, reciting nursery rhymes, doing fingerplays, making connections with text by pointing out environmental print, playing with rhyming words, pointing out words with similar initial sounds of words, isolating sound ("What sound does this word start with?"), blending sounds, guiding visual tracking, providing writing opportunities such as writing letters to Grandmas, making a shopping list, and reading a recipe when baking.

Some parents state that their children with hearing loss will not attend when they read books to them. Parents need clinicians to model strategies to use when reading aloud to early listeners such as using simple, repetitive sentences; using lots of inflection in your voice; pausing after sentences; talking about the pictures instead of reading the text; verbally cueing the child to turn the page; prompting the child to point out something on the page; choosing an easier book; or shortening the story. Provide a written handout that parents can share with all other family members who read to the child. Have parents bring in some of the books from home to have them practice. If the books are too challenging or the pictures too busy, make suggestions for easier books at this stage of learning.

Making language experience books is an exceptionally high-interest way to stimulate listening, language, and an interest in books. Language experience books demonstrate to the child that what we say, we can write, and what we write, we can read. These books are made by parents (initially with clinician help) and are often read repeatedly, becoming the child's first reader. Demonstrate this technique for parents by taking photos during an activity and making a sequenced language experience book with them in therapy: painting a pumpkin, building a zoo with animals and blocks, giving a doll a bath, etc. The *All About Me*, language experience book might include photos of each family member and written sentences regarding the routine of the child's day such as getting dressed, brushing his/her teeth, reading with Daddy, playing in the sandbox, etc. A *Places We Go* book, includes photos of the outsides of a familiar place (i.e. school, store, park, Grandma's house) and photos showing the activities inside or at the place. Many parents like to keep a copy of this book in the car after reading it at home so they can use it when they get into the car, as it provides the child with a visual reference when the parent states, "We're going to ____". Language experience books are a great way for a child with limited language to share with Mommy, Daddy, siblings, or grandparents about activities that happened when the family members were not present.

It is essential that parents understand that the power of reading aloud does not stop when their children begin to learn to read. To enable the child with hearing loss to progress with auditory and language development as well as comprehension of more complex inferential question forms, it is imperative that clinicians encourage parents to continue reading to their child even after they can read to themselves and to actively choose books at a slightly higher level than the children can read themselves. See Chapter 13 for more information.

Listening and Language to Build Cognition

We often think that goal of listening and language is to be able to get our needs met, but stating our needs is only the beginning of language development. What sets humans apart is our ability to understand and share abstract ideas through our use of language.

As clinicians, we must help parents and caregivers recognize the endless opportunities to expand not only children's language but also their thinking.

In an effort to improve the deaf or hard-of-hearing child's understanding of reasoning skills (cognitive development) and understanding of inferential questions, it is important to model higher-level thinking skills in the activities we present in therapy. These higher-level thinking skills include observation, association, sorting, classification, estimating, part-to-whole, estimating, patterning, sequencing, problem solving, predicting, inferring, mapping, cause and effect, and evaluation. Parents can assist the child with cognitive development through the use of questioning strategies that guide the expansion of critical thinking skills. Model for parents how to move away from "yes/no" and simple Wh- (who, what, when, where) questions and begin using open-ended and lifting questions, which expand thinking skills. We must help parents to understand that lifting questions encourage the child to think beyond simple Wh questions and to analyze events and relationships more deeply. In the same way, open ended questions do not have one right answer but provide the child with the opportunities to learn that, in many situations, multiple different responses and solutions are possible. For more specific suggestions regarding question forms, see the Cognitive Skills Chart in Chapter 22.

Pearl

We must help parents to understand that lifting questions encourage the child to think beyond simple Wh questions and to analyze events and relationships more deeply. In the same way, open-ended questions do not have one right answer, but provide the child with the opportunities to learn that, in many situations, multiple different responses and solutions are possible.

5.3 Clinicians as Coaches: Effectively Empowering Parents and Caregivers

It is not enough for the parents to observe the therapist engaging with the child during the session. Inviting the parent to participate in play and eventually lead play by way of turn taking is of utmost importance if listening and spoken language development is to extend to the home. If parents initially resist, continue to encourage and model play with their child. It may be helpful to visually display the listening or language targets of the activity you are focusing on and to allow the parents to observe a few turns of the back-and-forth game or engagement in the activity, and then have them join in, always with encouragement. When playing with a familiar toy that the family has at home, first inquire how they engage with it and talk about it at home. "Can you describe how he plays with cars?" "Are there any toy characters that could 'talk' and ride on them?" "How do you play with the toy kitchen?" "Can you give me an example of what he does with the food?"

Pearl

It is not enough for the parents to observe the therapist engaging with the child during the session. Inviting the parent to participate in play by way of turn taking is of utmost importance if listening and spoken language development is to extend to the home.

Parents often need ideas for how to play and what to say when interacting with toys. For example, when playing with foam blocks, the parent might input "up, up, up" and "fall down" during play. This is an opportunity to expand cognitive thinking as well as receptive and expressive language: for example, to ask "What could this be?" while beginning to build something: maybe a bridge, a fence for toy animals, train tracks and a toy train, a tunnel with a car, or a house. The parent listens to the therapist describe what she is doing (*self-talk*) such as "The tigers need a fence," "I can put the blocks together," or "This will be a door." The clinician demonstrates *parallel talk* by describing what the child is doing, such as "You have another one," "It goes on top," or "Oops! It fell down." Then the parent joins in and builds something with her blocks and/or adds onto the child's creation.

When playing with a baby doll, the following could be a sample play/therapy scenario with the parent, therapist, and child: "The baby is dirty," states the therapist. "What should we do?" The child points to the bathtub. "Yes, let's put him in the bathtub." Child says "bath." The therapist continues, "Uh-oh, the bathtub is empty. What do we need?" The child replies "water," and the therapist asks, "Mommy, can you help us?" Mommy pours the water into the bathtub without talking and the therapist states, "Mommy is pouring the water," -prompting the parent to repeat, "I'm pouring the water." The therapist continues with prompting the child to listen and imitate "wash the feet," "wash the face," "wash the tummy," and so on. Mommy is encouraged to take turns giving similar verbal directions or language input, such as "You're washing the baby's hair," "Take the baby out," "Let's dry the baby." Therapy continues with drying, dressing, brushing his hair, feeding, brushing his teeth, while the child listens to verbal directions and language input by the parent or therapist, and all engage in play with the baby doll. As play continues, the parent is encouraged to provide more and more of the dialogue and narration, and the child is encouraged to use key phrases appropriately in turn taking.

5.4 Additional Support for Families

Providing parents with family support and additional education through parent group meetings has numerous advantages. Families can feel isolated and have a desire to connect with other families of deaf and hard-of-hearing children. During discussions within a group, new shared concerns may come to the forefront that need addressing. Parent meetings can be held weekly, monthly, bimonthly, or periodically on some other schedule, with topics predetermined by the staff or derived from parent suggestions. See Chapter 4 for more information about providing parent support.

5.5 Working with Older Students

Although parent participation may look different as the child enters the mainstream environment, the communication between parent and clinician continues throughout the student's educational process. Parents may not feel they need to be as involved, yet their knowledge of the clinician's work and support in the school remains critical to the success of their child. Fostering a good relationship with the family may involve more emails, phone calls, and attendance at parent conferences. The therapist consults with the child's teachers and any additional service providers, ensuring that feedback is given to the parent. Parents should be encouraged to be a part of the team by communicating with staff and working collaboratively. This role of the clinician demonstrates a willingness to be involved with their child and reflects professional competence. Since most teachers and other service providers do not have the background knowledge or expertise to work with students with hearing loss, it is our role as a clinician not only to provide in-services and regularly consult with staff, but to empower parents (as well as the student) to advocate whenever an educational, technological, social, or emotional issue arises.

Since some of our older students with hearing loss continue to struggle with literacy and cognitive skills, we need to assist their parents with reading aloud at home (it does not stop in preschool), choosing appropriate books (provide book lists), and stressing the importance of reading daily, including chapter books that may be at a level above the child's reading level. Parents of older children may need ideas for interactive games including board or card games, particularly for those students whose pragmatics skills may not be commensurate with their hearing peers. Clinicians may suggest language and cognitively rich games to play at home or with friends such as Apple to Apples, Scattergories, Outburst, Life, or Never Ending Stories.

When a child with hearing loss is having difficulty in the educational environment, the clinician may need to initiate communication with parents about areas of need. One topic of concern that arises often with older deaf and hard-of-hearing students is the need for assistance with time management at home for completing homework. Other challenges that can impact learning and may need a clinician's guidance include routines/schedules, workspace organization, snack times, auditory fatigue, and sleep schedules. Parents are most appreciative to receive sample schedules, ideas for color-coding, multisensory learning strategies, and organizational tips. Although the parent may not be attending regular therapy sessions, be sure to invite them periodically to share an idea or strategy: "I wonder if you can attend your son's therapy next week so I can demonstrate a strategy we're using with his reading fluency skills, which can be practiced at home."

If a student is in a mainstreamed environment and is the only one with a hearing loss or one of only a few at the school, he or she can feel isolated. Since parents may have limited contact with other families who have a child with a hearing loss, connecting them with other families who have children with similar needs is helpful for emotional and educational purposes.

As a child with hearing loss becomes older, the needs, accommodations, and goals change. It is our role as clinicians to be certain that parents have a clear understanding of the information used to determine when goals are met, why modifications of current goals may be necessary, and what baselines for new goals indicate. When parents understand their role as part of the IEP team and feel comfortable sharing information, the clinician gains more useful information for writing an appropriate IEP document as well as working with the family.

Older students with hearing loss and their parents will continue to need education and communication regarding care of their personal technology. Older children have to be responsible for managing their own technology. Clinicians need to be sure they know how to do it with the assistance of their family. Children need to learn to advocate for themselves. Teach parents and children to model self-advocacy phrases such as, "I didn't hear you," "Say it again, please," or "What did you say?" to show that it is normal for all to ask for clarification of auditory information. More sophisticated self-advocacy phrases such as "I don't know what that word means," "I heard you say '. . . ,' but I didn't hear the beginning," or "I didn't hear the last part of your question" should be practiced in therapy or in class with the clinician or at home with the parents. We want to encourage students to use these more sophisticated phrases because they will generally receive a warmer, more positive response to these than to "What did you say?" or "Can you repeat that?" Educate parents, as well as the students, about possible barriers to auditory access such as earwax impeding sound, poorly fitted earmolds, or ramifications of an inconsistent use of a an HA/CI dehumidifier. It is the clinician's responsibility to help educate the child and parents regarding troubleshooting technology as well as understanding the impact of the audiogram with understanding of speech to ensure more consistent use of amplification devices.

For students whose hearing loss is later identified, who have not had good audiological management, or who have other handicapping conditions, auditory and spoken language support services will most likely be needed. Parental involvement and support are particularly important with this group to ensure that these children are meeting age-appropriate linguistic milestones. Since we know that listening and language are foundational to reading, when our students with hearing loss have delays in auditory development and have language gaps, it is often reflected in their reading, writing, and cognitive abilities. Proper evaluation will provide a baseline in helping guide the parents as well as the IEP team members with necessary support for the development of appropriate auditory, speech, language, and cognitive skills. Encourage parents to provide data from their experiences to assist in recording progress and determining ongoing needs/goals. For example, parents may have concerns regarding changes in listening or attention, difficulties with behavior in certain environments, social interactions with friends, or recent speech/language observations.

For older students with lower language skills, a good way to help parents understand language, vocabulary, and pragmatic progress is to take periodic language samples for comparison over time. As mentioned previously, comparing the deaf or hard-of-hearing student's language to a similar timetable as that of hearing children with the use of the CASLLS can demonstrate to parent where listening and language development may have been interrupted or compromised. If the gaps in the child's auditory skills and language are not addressed, delays lengthen as the academic demands increase. In cases where parents want to place primary educational emphasis on their child's academic skills, it is our role to educate them on the importance of filling in any auditory, language, pragmatic, and vocabulary gaps.

Pearl

In cases where parents want to place primary educational emphasis on their child's academic skills, it is our role to educate them on the importance of filling in any auditory, language, pragmatic, and vocabulary gaps.

Our role in helping parents with the development of critical thinking skills continues as the child with hearing loss gets older. Many deaf and hard-of-hearing students may have challenges with reasoning skills. Assessments can help identify areas of need such as inference, problem solving, prediction, negative questions, and sequencing. To identify possible gaps in language and cognitive skills, three outstanding assessment tools can be utilized for evaluating hearing-impaired students (ages 6+): the Listening Comprehension Test–2 (LCT-2)[29] and Listening Comprehension Test—Adolescent: Normative Update (LCT-A:NU),[30] which assess the ability to identify main ideas and details, reasoning, vocabulary, and understanding messages, and the Test of Problem Solving—Elementary, Third Edition, Normative Update (TOPS-3E:NU),[31] which assesses inference, problem solving, prediction, negative questions, determines causes, and sequencing. These assessments are normed on hearing peers and provide the clinician with a good amount of information regarding how children with hearing loss are utilizing their auditory, language, and cognitive skills. If a student has challenges with negative questions, additional exposure to these question forms in a variety of situations improves learning, such as "Why didn't . . . ?" "Why won't . . . ?" "Why can't . . . ?" Or a student who has difficulty with inferences can be exposed to questions such as "How does he feel?" "Why did he think the house was on fire?" "How do you know that . . . ?", "When do you think this happened?" "Why didn't she tell her Mom?" Or a student challenged by problem solving might be drilled on questions such as "What could she do to solve the problem?" "What do we need if we are going to . . . ?" Providing parents with lists of sample cognitive questions to ask at home helps their child improve higher-level thinking skills as well as aiding carryover into inferential reading comprehension skills. Some excellent resources for additional cognitive work with older students include *Manual of Exercises for Expressive Reasoning (MEER)*[32] and *Handbook of Exercises for Language Processing (HELP)*.[33] Refer to **Table 5.1** in Resources for more in-depth cognitive levels, sample cognitive questions, and suggested activities to promote reasoning skills.

5.6 Summary

It is our role as clinicians and educators of children with hearing loss to guide and coach parents to become their child's primary listening and spoken language teachers. Understanding the grieving process, the emotional state, and the family dynamics helps form a positive relationship with the parents and supports the educational process. Parents and students often feel isolated and enjoy being connected with other families who have children with hearing loss. Providing organized educational information to parents in small increments and communicating in ways that

the parents can best understand are key to helping the family process and retain new skills. Group meetings are another way to share information with parents regarding a multitude of concerns/issues. Areas of concern that may need to be addressed with parents are attention, technology issues, sleep, auditory fatigue, sensory integration, and behavior. Attention, in turn, may be affected by allergies, diet, and screen time. We enlist parents as our partners when we demonstrate teaching listening, language and cognition through play activities and through a variety of daily home routines. Modeling reading strategies and creating language experience books can assist parents in the development of early language skills. Parents of older children with hearing loss may need guidance with continuation of technology troubleshooting, behavior listening checks, use of self-advocacy phrases, pragmatic skills, and prompting critical thinking skills.

Discussion Questions

1. What are several ways we can assist parents to become the primary language facilitators of their child with hearing loss?

2. How can the grieving process affect the parents' decisions and relationship with their child with hearing loss?

3. As a clinician, what are several methods/styles you could use to encourage parents to participate and share concerns?

4. It is important to share information with parents. However, why should we avoid overloading them? How might we be able to tell that we are reaching the point of overload?

5. When providing family support, what are three possible areas of concern you may need to address with the parents, either on an individual basis or in a group meeting?

6. Why is it important for parents to meet other families with children with hearing loss?

7. Give some examples of toys that promote interactive play for both early language learners and older children with hearing loss. Why is it important for parents to learn how to participate in play with their child?

References

[1] Yucel E, Derim D, Celik D. The needs of hearing impaired children's parents who attend to auditory verbal therapy-counseling program. *Int J Pediatr Otorhinolaryngol* 2008;*72*(7):1097–1111

[2] Sunshine Cottage School for Deaf Children. Comfort Level Checklist for Auditory Verbal Families. San Antonio, TX: Sunshine Cottage School for Deaf Children; 2004

[3] Suskind D. *Thirty Million Words: Building a Child's Brain*. New York, NY: Penguin Random House; 2015

[4] Epstein S. Coping with grief. *Volta Voices* 2005;*12*:46–47

[5] Bader JL, Robbins R, Feld S. Good Grief! [VHS tape]. Denver, CO: Hear at Home; 2001

[6] Martin K, Ritter K. Navigating the emotional impact of diagnosis. *Volta Voices* 2011;*18*(3):14–16

[7] Sonova USA. Childhood Hearing Loss Question Prompt List (QPL) for Parents. Phonak. https://www.phonakpro.com/content/dam/phonakpro/gc_hq/en/resources/counseling_tools/documents/phonak-pediatric_fcc_qpl.pdf Accessed January 19, 2022

[8] Luterman DM, ed. *Children with Hearing Loss: a Family Guide*. Sedona, AZ: Auricle Ink; 2006

[9] Pratt SR. Post-fitting issues: a need for parent counseling and instruction. *Trends Amplif* 1999;*4*(2):103–107

[10] Sindrey D. Good & Not So Good Sounds. The Listening Room. https://advancedbionics.com/content/dam/advancedbionics/Documents/libraries/Tools-for-Toddlers/tools-for-parents/Good-and-Not-So-Good-Sounds.pdf Accessed January 21, 2022

[11] SkyPaw Co, Ltd. Decibel X Pro Sound Meter. https://skypaw.com/decibelx.html Accessed January 21, 2022

[12] Ear Technology Corporation. Dry & Store. https://dryandstore.com/ Accessed January 22, 2022

[13] Allen KE, Marotz LR. *By the Ages: Behavior & Development of Children Pre-Birth through Eight.* Clifton Park, NY: Delmar Thomson Learning; 2000

[14] Miller K. *Ages and Stages: Developmental Descriptions and Activities, Birth through Eight Years.* Rev. ed. Owings Mills, MD: Telshare; 2001

[15] Garber SW, Garber MD, Spizman RF. *Good Behavior Made Easy Handbook: Over 1200 Sensible Solutions to Your Child's Problems from Birth to Age Twelve.* 2nd ed. Glastonbury, CT: Great Pond; 1993

[16] Wilkes EM. *Cottage Acquisition for Listening, Language and Speech: User's Guide.* San Antonio, TX: Sunshine Cottage School for Deaf Children; 2001

[17] Voss J, White E. *Small Talk: Bringing Listening and Spoken Language to Your Young Child with Hearing Loss.* St. Louis, MO: Central Institute for the Deaf; 2015

[18] Ferber R. *Solve Your Child's Sleep Problems.* London, UK: Vermilion; 2013

[19] Lin L-Y, Cherng R-J, Chen Y-J, Chen Y-J, Yang H-M. Effects of television exposure on developmental skills among young children. *Infant Behav Dev* 2015;*38*:20–26

[20] Davis H, Schlundt D, Bonnet K, Camarata S, Hornsby B, Bess FH. Listening-related fatigue in children with hearing loss: perspectives of children, parents, and school professionals. *Am J Audiol* 2021;*30*(4):929–940

[21] Becker-Weidman A. Sensory Integration Screening Questionnaire. Tampa, FL: Center for Family Development. https://www.center4familydevelop.com/Sensory-Integration%20Checklist-2.pdf Accessed January 22, 2022

[22] Kranowitz CS. *The Out-of-Sync Child: Recognizing and Coping with Sensory Processing Disorder.* Rev. ed. New York, NY: TarcherPerigee; 2006

[23] Kranowitz CS. *The Out-of-Sync Child Has Fun: Activities for Kids with Sensory Processing Disorder.* Rev. ed. New York, NY: Perigee Books; 2007

[24] Flexer C. How to grow a young child's listening brain. Continued Early Childhood Education. https://www.continued.com/early-childhood-education/articles/to-grow-young-child-listening-22841 Accessed December 30, 2021

[25] Hart B, Risley TR. The early catastrophe: the 30 million word gap by age 3. *Am Educator* 2003 Spring;4–9 https://www.aft.org/ae/spring2003/hart_risley Accessed January 22, 2022

[26] Rossi K. *Learn to Talk Around the Clock: A Professional's Early Intervention Toolbox.* Washington, DC: Alexander Graham Bell Association for the Deaf; 2003

[27] Cole E, Flexer C. *Children with Hearing Loss: Developing Listening and Talking, Birth to Six.* 4th ed. San Diego, CA: Plural; 2019

[28] Trelease J, Giorgis C. *Jim Trelease's Read-Aloud Handbook.* 8th ed. New York, NY: Penguin Books; 2019

[29] Bowers L, Huisingh R, LoGiudice C. *The Listening Comprehension Test—2.* East Moline, IL: Linguisystems; 2006

[30] Bowers L, Huisingh R, LoGiudice C. *The Listening Comprehension Test—Adolescent: Normative Update.* Austin, TX: Pro-Ed Linguisystems; 2018

[31] Bowers L, Huisingh R, LoGiudice C. *Test of Problem Solving—Elementary.* 3rd ed. Normative Update. Austin, TX: Pro-Ed Linguisystems; 2018

[32] Zachman L. *MEER 1: Manual of Exercises for Expressive Reasoning.* East Moline, IL: Linguisystems; 1982

[33] Lazzari AM, Peters PM. *HELP 5: Handbook of Exercises for Language Processing.* East Moline, IL: LinguiSystems; 1991

6 Evaluation of Speech, Language, and Listening in Children with Hearing Loss: Knowing the Level at Which Children Are Functioning

Elizabeth Ying

Summary

Advances in technology options, as well as the increased availability of parent-child-focused early intervention programs that emphasize auditory skill development and the comprehension and use of spoken language, have significantly improved function and performance in children with varying degrees of hearing loss. As a result, SLPs and Listening and Spoken Language Specialist (LSLS) professionals are now challenged to obtain quantifiable evidence with which to determine the effectiveness of the hearing habilitation and rehabilitation programs they provide across the ages. This chapter is structured to provide a rationale and framework for conducting comprehensive diagnostic and therapeutic management of children who are deaf or hard of hearing. It details the components of a speech-language evaluation/functional listening assessment, including a descriptive analysis of potential testing protocol applicable to four developmental populations (infants, preschool, school-aged and teenage). In addition, important considerations (specifically active parental involvement) are highlighted to facilitate the formulation and implementation of effective training to develop a reliance on listening for spoken language learning.

Keywords

speech-language specialist (SLS), universal newborn screening, functional listening assessment, listening check (technology), phonemic awareness, detection, discrimination, identification, comprehension, receptive language, expressive language, pragmatic functioning, early intervention, aural habilitation, aural rehabilitation, incidental learning, telepractice, active parental involvement

Key Points

- The diagnostic role of a speech-language pathologist in evaluating a child with hearing loss should be guided by aided audiological functioning, the reason for testing as well as the child's everyday communicative demands.
- The comprehensive evaluation of the communication skills of a child with hearing loss must include assessment of functional listening that simulates the demands of everyday listening environments.
- Responsiveness to spoken language via audition alone must be assessed given that audition is the most effective and efficient modality for acquiring and monitoring spoken language.

- Due to the young age of early diagnosis and amplification fitting, the evaluation of infants and toddlers should encompass both informal and formal diagnostic protocols.
- The use of formal diagnostic measures that are normal on typically developing peers are appropriate for use with children with hearing loss, given that children with hearing loss can be expected to acquire functionally adequate listening and age-appropriate spoken language skills.
- Feedback from the functional listening assessment/speech-language evaluation should be shared with the audiologist, interventionist, and teachers to provide optimal continuity of care for a child with a diagnosed hearing loss.
- The authorization of telehealth options has created a need to incorporate alternative strategies to conduct valid and comprehensive communication evaluation for children with hearing loss.

Any degree of conductive or sensorineural hearing loss (HL) is considered to be an acceptable "diagnosed medical condition" ensuring eligibility for services through early intervention and public-school programs across the United States. However, to determine the frequency and nature of the allowable services will heavily depend on findings from a comprehensive speech-language and functional listening assessment. In a 2007 position statement, the Joint Commission on Infant Hearing (JCIH) stated that *"All families of infants with any degree of bilateral or unilateral permanent hearing loss should be considered eligible for early intervention service."*[1] Pediatric healthcare providers were, in turn, advised that *"Abnormal hearing test results (in infants and older children) require intervention and clinically appropriate referral, including otolaryngology, audiology, speech-language pathology, genetics, and early intervention."*[2]

This chapter will present the components of the speech-language and functional listening assessment protocol across age ranges. Ideally, this assessment should be conducted only after the child with a confirmed hearing loss has been appropriately fitted with technology. However, regulatory time mandates from early intervention or Board of Education requirements might necessitate the evaluation to take place prior to the fitting of amplification. In such instances, obtained findings must be documented as being "incomplete," affording merely a baseline of the child's performance prior to receiving necessary and/or appropriate hearing technology.

The diagnostic protocol used for the assessment of a child with hearing loss should, in turn, be tailored to reflect the primary purpose of the evaluation, as follows:

1. *Eligibility Evaluation:* To determine eligibility for services or enrollment into a habilitation program or educational placement
2. *Establish Intervention Plan:* To assess the child's present level of functioning to establish specific training objectives
3. *Progress Assessment:* To determine progress and needs for future intervention

6.1 Who Should Conduct the Assessment?

Due to its comprehensive nature, the speech-language and functional listening assessment falls within the scope of practice of a licensed speech-language pathologist (SLP), preferably one who has training in evaluating and developing auditory skills in children with hearing loss.[2] *Formulating and implementing aural habilitation/rehabilitation training also fall within the professional domain of the SLP.[1]* The limited availability of a local SLP, experienced with the impact of hearing loss on language learning and overall communicative interactions, may necessitate that this evaluation be conducted by either an audiologist or teacher of the deaf and hard of hearing (TOD) with a specialized certification in listening and spoken language (LSLS certified).

Pitfall

Aural habilitation/rehabilitation coursework is limited or optional in the majority of graduate programs in speech-language pathology. When offered, these courses are frequently taught by audiologists as opposed to SLPs, resulting in a greater focus on amplification fitting and technology as opposed to the assessment and treatment of communication-related effects of hearing loss. ASHA no longer requires previously needed "audiological screening hours" so it is conceivable that more recent graduating SLPs may never have even interacted directly with a child with hearing loss. However, it is inevitable that a child or adult with hearing loss will be encountered by an SLP in any future work setting. Fortunately, virtual and in-person continuing education courses can assist the novice or motivated SLP to expand their knowledge base and skills in providing services to children with hearing loss.

6.2 Test Conditions

Traditionally, speech-language and functional listening assessments have been conducted in facility-based settings (including clinics, hospitals, and schools). Increasingly, however, home-based assessments are being requested and/or mandated in accordance with recommendations from the JCIH stating; *"In response to a previous emphasis 'natural environments,' the JCIH recommends that both home-based and center-based intervention options be offered."*[1]

In addition, there is a growing need, particularly heightened by the Covid-19 pandemic, for virtual assessments, as a component of the telehealth expansion in the US and internationally.

The availability of HIPPA-compliant telehealth platforms enables families that reside in rural or less developed communities, with fewer resources and qualified professionals, to have access to the same high quality of care available in better resourced urban environments.

Regardless of the setting, care should be taken to ensure that the evaluation is conducted in a well-lit environment with few visual or auditory distractions. Use of an acoustic hoop (an embroidery hoop covered with speaker fabric) permitting sound to be presented without degradation of intensity or clarity, is necessary to fully assess the audibility of speech directed to the child.

6.3 Background Information and Case History

Prior to or at the start of the speech-language/functional listening assessment detailed information about the prenatal, birth, and perinatal development of the child diagnosed with hearing loss should be gathered. Gathering this information in a culturally sensitive and understandable manner has been strongly advocated by state coordinators within the national Early Hearing Detection and Intervention (EHDI). While it is also paramount that the SLP in partnership with the referring audiologist have an understanding of the child's unaided hearing loss, even more valuable is understanding of the child's aided hearing performance. Such information is critically needed to fully interpret how the child responds to sounds and speech directed to or occurring around him during the speech-language/functional listening evaluation. In addition, prior to starting any testing with the child, the SLP must perform a listening check of the child's technology (e.g., hearing aid, cochlear implant, osteointegrated system) to ensure it is working optimally and that the child has auditory access to the information presented during the assessment.

Additional information provided during the case history or parent interview will provide a more complete diagnostic profile and will impact on the decision-making regarding management needs for the child and/or his family (**Table 6.1**).[3,4,5]

It is also essential to have knowledge about the everyday "communicative demands" of the child being evaluated. For example, the toddler that spends his day in a daycare setting interacting with several caretakers and a group of typically developing peers has different demands to listen and speak than the child spending his day at home with a parent or a full-time nanny. The listening experiences and spoken language directed to the child has impact on auditory skill emergence as well as the trajectory of the child's speech and language acquisition and use.

Pitfall

Underlying the interpretation of results obtained from a Functional Listening Assessment (FLA) is a thorough understanding of the four auditory processes listed from the most basic to the most sophisticated response, as follows: Detection, Discrimination, Identification, and Comprehension. (See appendix A for classification of skills in each domain).

Table 6.1 Supplemental queries

Information	Clinical Clues	Diagnostic Implications
Additional medical conditions	Prematurity[3]	Etiology of hearing loss Possible developmental delays
	Jaundice[4]	Etiology of hearing loss Closer monitoring for possible progression
	Cleft palate and other craniofacial anomalies[5]	Impact on speech production
	Syndrome related[4]	Impact on global motor development (including speech as a motor function)
Feeding related issues	Poor sucking Poor swallowing	Failure to thrive concerns Impact on speech production
Results of UNHS	Referred for one or both ears	Audiological follow-up and management Need for ENT follow-up
Fitting and use of amplification	Parental comfort	Device use Care and maintenance of equipment
Family history of hearing loss	Parental prior experience with and/or acceptance of the diagnosis of hearing loss	Audiological or genetic follow-up Selection of training options Realistic expectations
Parent-Child Interaction	Identify comfort level of interactions with the child and facilitative behaviors supportive of listening and spoken language	Establish training needs and specific parental behaviors to be reinforced and expanded on within a family-centered intervention model
Family support	Parental comfort level with diagnosis	Habilitation/rehabilitation training options
Preferred communication mode	Parent-child interactions	Habilitation/rehabilitation training options

6.4 Functional Listening Assessment

There is wide variability in the functional listening skills and linguistic competency of two children with identical etiology and degree of hearing loss. Numerous child-specific variables (including age of diagnosis, socioeconomic status, and even the number of words spoken in the home on a daily basis) contribute to the rate and nature of listening and spoken language skill acquisition among children with similar hearing sensitivity levels. Nevertheless, what most distinguishes the speech and language evaluation of a child with hearing loss and one with normal hearing is the need to assess responsiveness to sounds and speech, within quiet and adverse listening conditions. In addition, findings obtained during the functional listening assessment should support the results from objective or behavioral hearing testing. Gross disparities in performance warrant collaboration between the audiologist and diagnostic SLP and could signal the need for more immediate audiological testing, perhaps earlier than planned, and/or the necessity for reprogramming of the technology fitting.

Pearl

Consideration should be given to the disparity between the child's Chronologic Age (age since birth) vs. "Hearing Age" (interval since first fitted with amplification) vs. "Listening Age" (Interval since child received sufficient auditory access from amplification to support language learning.)

6.5 Suggested Test Options

No single test or testing protocol addresses the needs of all children regardless of age or degree of hearing loss. The selected protocol should reflect the purpose of the evaluation. Clinical guidelines from the American Speech Language Hearing Association[6] state that "the primary goals of evaluation and assessment by an SLP are to obtain an adequate and representative sample of behaviors from which to make inferences concerning the child's speech, language and communication behaviors." It is also considered best clinical practice to use a combination of standardized measures and informal inventories comprised of both direct observation and parent/caregiver report.

The remainder of this chapter will detail the specific components, administration and clinical value for a range of informal and standardized diagnostic tools. These tools are not intended to be exhaustive in nature. However, they currently are among the most commonly used measures for the assessment of listening and spoken language skills in infants, preschoolers, and school-aged children with hearing loss.

6.6 Informal Functional Listening Assessment

Evidence-based clinical practice obligates speech-language pathologists to establish accountability standards for the services they provide. To implement quality listening and spoken language intervention for infants and toddlers with newly identified hearing loss, it is advised that the early interventionist sample a range of behaviors. Descriptive observation of the behaviors exhibited in response to speech stimuli and systematically selected noisemakers is the appropriate "starting point" for the formulation of developmentally appropriate training objectives, for infants and toddlers with a recent diagnosis of hearing loss.

These detection/discrimination level sampling techniques should be meaningful, measurable, and repeatable to document the infant's or toddler's progress over time in acquiring more consistent and higher-level auditory responsiveness.

Although there are many longitudinal auditory checklists that provide a hierarchy of auditory skill emergence to track a child's progress over time, few of these checklists provide a task-specific structure for sampling or eliciting the particular behaviors.

Having to determine "present level of auditory functioning" of an infant referred following newborn hearing screening, oftentimes within a limited time span of a one-hour evaluation, may be stressful, particularly for the novice SLP with limited experience with this population.

The challenge of obtaining auditory performance data about a 2- to 6-month old child with hearing loss during a single testing session requires understanding of auditory skill progression, typical child development, as well as refined observational skills. The following "informal auditory checklist" (**Table 6.2**) has been compiled from years of clinical use and is being shared in this text to provide a framework for sampling specific auditory responses.

Obtained findings should then serve as baseline performance data with which to measure and monitor progress over time.

Table 6.2   Test: *Informal Auditory Checklist* *

Structure	Samples functional listening skills in the nonverbal or barely talking child with hearing loss, using play-based tasks and toys (see Appendix A)
Results	While attentive and actively engaged, noisemakers and speech spanning the speech frequency range are introduced to assess detection, discrimination, and identification level responses
Clinical Clues	• Yields information about the child's detection level response to speech and environmental sounds in quiet vs. noisy listening conditions as well as when presented from different directions or distances • Permits assessment of present level of functioning • Guides the formulation of training objectives • Tracking of skill emergence over time
Age Range	Infant through preschool ages (for older children with multiple involvement)

*For more information see Appendix B.

6.7   Questionnaires

The use of a parent questionnaire format serves a two-fold purpose in the diagnostic process of evaluating the auditory skill emergence in newly diagnosed infants, toddlers and preschoolers that have recently been fit with amplification. Parental responses on such questionnaires provide important information about specific behavioral responses observed when speech or sounds unexpectedly occur or are deliberately introduced within every-day routines within the home (**Table 6.3, Table 6.4, Table 6.5**).[7,8,9] The breadth of the questions, in turn, provide parents with a

better understanding of the behaviors they should be looking for. In conjunction with clinician observation, parents can gain a broader understanding of how hearing loss impacts future language learning and social-communicative interactions.

Table 6.3   TEST: *Infant-Toddler Meaningful Auditory Integration Scale (IT-MAIS)*[7]

Structure	10-item parent questionnaire assesses a child's nonverbal and vocal/ verbal responsiveness to auditory stimulation within everyday routines
Results	Test items are scored by frequency of occurrence (0%, 25%, 50%, 75%, 100%) that corresponds to a point score, with a possible score of 40
Clinical Clues	• Yields information about the child's detection level response to speech and environmental sounds in quiet vs. noisy listening conditions • Yields information about basic discrimination level of speech vs music, speaker's voices and emotional states • Permits assessment of present level of functioning and tracking of skill emergence over time
Age Range	Infant through preschool ages
Availability	Advanced Bionics

Table 6.4   TEST: *LittlEARS Auditory Questionnaire*[8]

Structure	35 question parent report inventory samples the emergence of auditory development in the first two years after the fitting of amplification (ceiling hearing age of 2 years)
Results	A response of "yes" credits the behavior as occurring at least once
Clinical Clues	• Directs training objectives • Permits assessment of present level of functioning • Tracks skill emergence over time
Age Range	Infants through preschool ages
Availability	MED-EL Worldwide, Innsbruck, Austria

Table 6.5   TEST: *Functional Auditory Performance Indicators (FAPI)*

Structure	Samples a range of auditory behaviors in varying listening conditions (close vs. distant, with vs. without visual clues, quiet vs. noisy, and prompted vs. spontaneous), either through direct observation or parent report
Results	Provides a hierarchical profile of frequency of occurrence of auditory skills in 7 sampled domains, yielding scores ranging from (NP) *not present*, (E) *emerging*, (P) *in process* to (A) *acquired* (based on frequency of occurrence from 0–10% for NP to 80–100% for A)
Clinical Clues	• Behavioral responses classified hierarchically as: (1) Sound awareness (2) Sound is meaningful (3) Auditory feedback (4) Localization (5) Auditory discrimination (6) Auditory sequential memory (7) Linguistic auditory processing • Identifies presence/absence of skill • Directs training objectives • Tracks skill emergence over time
Age Range	Infants through preschool years
Availability	Texas School for the Blind and Visually Impaired

6.8 Diagnostic Tests

6.8.1 Phoneme Level

The normal developmental progression of phonemic development indicates that vowel elements emerge earlier than consonant sounds. Due to their acoustic properties (loud audibility within the low frequency speech range), even children with more significant severe to profound hearing loss demonstrate increased attention, discrimination and identification of vowels elements at early ages in infancy.[10] Consonants vary more widely in both their intensity and the frequency characteristics required for their accurate audibility and recognition. It should further be noted that consonant perception is also influenced by the child's cognitive development and the ability to grasp regularities underlying phonological principles governing his native language.

Employing a feature analysis for observed misperception of consonants at any age is a valuable means of determining whether a child's consonant perception is following a normal developmental progression as well as whether it is appropriate for their degree of aided hearing. Each consonant in the English language can be classified according to three articulatory features: voicing, manner. and place (where in the mouth the sound is made). (See Chapter 3 for more detailed information). These features correspond respectively to low-, mid- to high-, and high-frequency acoustic cues. Consonant confusions or misperceptions are determined by changes in an ongoing behavior or a behavioral choice made (by the non-verbal or barely talking child) or by the repeat back response given (by the verbal child) in response to sounds presented to them (**Table 6.6, Table 6.7, Table 6.8**). The errors obtained are subsequently analyzed in terms of the number of features of the target consonant exhibited in the error consonant. Consonant confusion, in turn, can then be classified as ""good" vs. "bad" mistakes; with a good mistake exhibiting only 1 missing feature as compared to a "bad mistake" with 2 or more features undetected or unidentified.

Table 6.7 TEST: *Ling Sound Test*[11]

Structure	Consists of 3 vowels (ah, oo, ee) and 3 consonants (m, sh, s) that span the speech frequency range; sampling detection (presence vs. absence), discrimination (change/no change) and identification (closed vs. open set) level responses
Results	Provides critical information about auditory access to speech across the frequency range and can be directly compared to findings obtained with these same sounds during hearing testing in the booth
Clinical Clues	• Documents progression and identifies problems with technology • Guides future training • Identifies modifications needed in the re-programming of amplification devices: specifically signals when the child has insufficient access to high frequency sounds (confusing oo with ee or failing to detect sh or s), needs a loudness boost (due to confusion of oo and m), or simply the disparity between a child's responsiveness to low- through high-frequency sounds vs. speech
Age Range	Across the ages from infancy through adulthood
Availability	Advanced Bionics (see Chapter 2, Audiology)

Table 6.8 TEST: *Iowa Medial Consonant Test*[12]

Structure	Samples consonant identification via repeat back of each English consonant within a medial word position with the vowel ah (a ___a)
Results	Provides critical information about consonant confusions (by voicing, manner or frequency categories) at differing distances
Clinical Clues	• Identifies specific consonant confusions to guide future training • Identifies modifications needed in the reprogramming of technology • Documents progress over time
Age Range	Preschool through school-aged to adulthood
Availability	https://successforkidswithhearingloss.com/

Table 6.6 TEST: *Change/No Change Informal Sampling Task*

Structure	Suprasegmental contrasts (ah produced in prolonged vs. short, repeated patterns) or segmental level stimuli (2 different vowel elements) can be presented within a "habituation test" paradigm as follows: Observe the child's response to the presentation of the habituation target, ex: "ee-ee-ee-e", then randomly insert the novel target "oo" then resuming to produce the target "ee-e-e". Accept any change in behavior (such as eyes widening or shifting, searching, increased activity, etc.) as indication that the child detected the change and/or discriminated between the two auditory targets.
Results	Gains information about the child's basic detection and discrimination of auditory stimuli
Clinical Clues	• Documents progress over time • Directs modifications needed in training • Provides information to share with audiologist about audibility of sound with present amplification program and possible need for changes in technology settings
Age Range	Infancy through adulthood

6.8.2 Word Level

Diagnostic measures that present two or more options to choose from are classified as closed-set listening tasks. Closed-set measures require a more simplistic auditory judgment compared to open-set identification tasks with an infinite number of possible responses.

Traditionally, audiologist use both closed and open set measures, depending on the age of the child, to obtain a percent correct score. These "speech discrimination" scores are then used to determine the appropriateness of the technology fitting for an individual child.

However, judgments regarding the "functional adequacy" of such scores remains arbitrary, and more often than not, audiologists tend to err in accordance with more objective verifying data from measurement of the output of the hearing aid and how well it matches the manufacturers specification for that hearing aid. (See Chapter 2 for more information.) Madell and Flexer[13] and Madell et al[14] attempted to establish uniform standards for determining the adequacy of aided speech discrimination testing by audiologists, as follows:

"We may not always get it, but it has to be our goal. Excellent speech perception is 90 to 100%. Good speech perception is 80 to 89%, fair speech perception is 70 to 79% and poor speech perception is less than 70%."

The aspect of "cognitive load" is another variable that influences a child's response accuracy during speech discrimination testing particularly at the word and sentence levels. Familiarity with the vocabulary of the test administered to a child can have both positive and negative effects. Error responses and test taking difficulties could be reflective of how much focus can be directed to discriminating between similar sounding sounds when they occur in familiar vs. novel words (**Table 6.11**). Several researchers have documented that in infants with normal hearing, difficulties are usually attributed to the fact that infants' attention to the phonetic detail in novel words is attenuated when they must allocate additional cognitive resources demanded by novel word learning tasks.[14]

As a result, the audiologist, like the SLP, systematically selects from a battery of speech reception tools to obtain a valid assessment of the child's auditory performance (**Table 6.9, Table 6.10, Table 6.11, Table 6.12, Table 6.13, Table 6.14, Table 6.15, Table 6.16**).[15,16,17,18,19,20,21,22]

Table 6.9   TEST: *Early Speech Perception (ESP)*[15]

Structure	Evaluates the speech perception abilities of very young children through closed-set object selection (for the younger child) or picture pointing (for older children)
Results	Skills areas sampled ranging from pattern perception (involving 1, 2 and 3 syllable words) to word-identification based on vowel elements. There is a spondee word subtest, consisting of evenly stressed words like toothbrush, airplane, cupcake and lunchbox, which can be compared to speech reception testing conducted during routine audiological testing. The monosyllable subtest is comprised of words with the initial consonant /b/ and differing vowel contexts, including bat, belt, boat, boot, etc. Compiled scores across subtests yields a ranking from Category 1 (No Speech Perception) to 4 (Open-set Speech Perception.
Clinical Clues	• Provides a structure for sampling suprasegmental and phonemic level skills • Guides formulation of training objectives • Systematic means of monitoring basic auditory emergence over time, particularly for the older child transitioning from receiving minimal benefit from hearing aids to being fitted with cochlear implants
Age Range	Preschool through school-aged
Availability	Central Institute for the Deaf and Hard of Hearing, St.Louis, MO

Table 6.10   TEST: *AB Lists Computer Assisted Speech Perception Assessment (CASPA)*[16]

Structure	List of 10 monosyllabic words/nonsense words that are phonemically balanced and comprised of phonemes that span the speech frequency range, presented via audition alone (or for comparative purposes presented with supplemental visual clues), in quiet and/or noisy listening environments
Results	Provides word correct response accuracy under bimodal/bilateral and separate ear listening conditions as well as a phonemic analysis of the error patterns of all vowel and consonant confusions
Clinical Clues	Identifies specific needs for future device re-programming and guides the formulation of more appropriate word level training objectives to resolve confusion errors
Age Range	Preschool through adulthood
Availability	Journal of American Academy of Audiology

Table 6.11   TEST: *Lexical Neighborhood Test (LNT)*[17]

Structure	List of 50 monosyllabic words composed of phonemes that span the speech frequency range, divided into 25 "easy" and 25 lexically "hard" words (determined by the number of similar-sounding words with which the target word might be confused).
Results	Provides word correct and phoneme correct scores when presented under best aided (bilateral/bimodal) and separate ear listening conditions. Also, permits a phonemic analysis of the error patterns of all consonant confusions
Clinical Clues	• Identifies specific needs for future device re-programming, particularly if phoneme scored according to acoustic features perceived or confused • Yields critical information about how the lexical neighborhood of the presented vocabulary impacts on overall word identification • Can provide a comparison of response accuracy to recorded stimuli vs. when presented via live voice, e.g., valuable information in light of the increased use of digital technology within classroom instruction and during remote learning routines. • Permits monitoring of skill progression over time
Age Range	Preschool through adulthood
Availability	Auditec, St. Louis, MO

6.8.3 Sentence Level

Table 6.12   TEST: *Mr. Potato Head Test*[18]

Structure	This modified open-set measure has 2 forms with 10 items each; requiring the child to manipulate the potato head toy in accordance with simple verbal directions, presented via audition alone. Specifically, they are asked to choose from a closed set of 30 items to put on a body part/clothing item or to perform an action with the toy, such as: "give Mr. Potato Head his pink ears" or "Make Mr. Potato Head wash his hands."
Results	Scores reported as percentage of key words and sentences correctly identified.
Clinical Clues	• Word identification via audition alone, under best aided listening condition and/or in quiet vs. in noise • Attention to task with a large set of alternatives to select from • Vocabulary acquisition for concepts frequently encountered in the daily routines of preschool aged children
Age Range	Preschool through early school-aged
Availability	Indiana University School of Medicine, DeVault Otologic Research Laboratory

Table 6.13   TEST: *Common Phrases*[19]

Structure	List of 10 simple statements and questions frequently encountered in the daily routines of preschool-aged children, presented via addition alone under best-aided condition (in quiet and noise) as well as under separate ear listening conditions
Results	In order to be credited for a correct response, the child is required to repeat back the test item verbatim. Scores are reported in terms of the percentage of the sentences correctly identified.
Clinical Clues	• Accuracy of sentence identification in contrasting listening conditions • Provides information about a child's sustained attention for the completion of a multi-word utterance. • In addition, yields information about whether a child perceives only the key words as opposed to the unstressed linguistic elements (articles, prepositions) within simple statements and questions. • Monitor improvement over time.
Age Range	Preschool through early school-aged
Availability	Indiana University School of Medicine, DeVault Otologic Research Laboratory

Table 6.14   TEST: *Hearing in Noise Test (HINT-C)*[20]

Structure	Samples open-set speech reception of 10 simple sentences (with 4–6 words), presented via audition alone and requiring repeat-back responses. Test items contain less common and/or predictable vocabulary.
Results	Provides word correct and sentence correct scores of auditory performance under different listening conditions (bilateral quiet, bilateral noise, right ear alone, and left ear alone)
Clinical Clues	• As this test is also commonly used by audiologists during speech discrimination testing in the booth, it affords a comparison of performance via recorded vs. live voice presentation and can guide modifications for device re-programming • Provides information regarding access to stressed vs unstressed linguistic elements, e.g., key words vs. function words, respectively • Identifies accuracy of sustained attention and response accuracy for sentence level material • Guides future training objectives to improve on speech reception of less frequently encountered statements and questions, which are semantically highly predictable. • Monitor improvement over time
Age Range	School-aged to adulthood
Availability	Auditec, St. Louis, MO

Table 6.15   TEST: *Pediatric/Adult Az Bio Sentence Test (Az Bio)*[21]

Structure	List of 20 simple and complex sentences, presented via audition alone, requiring a repeat-back response.
Results	Provides percent-correct scores for words and sentences, in contrasting listening conditions (bilateral quiet, bilateral noise, right ear alone, and left ear alone).
Clinical Clues	• As this test is also commonly used by audiologists during speech discrimination testing in the booth, it affords a comparison of performance via recorded vs. live voice presentation and can guide modifications for device re-programming • Identifies accuracy of sustained attention and response accuracy for sentence level material • Direct future training to improve on response accuracy (especially auditory closure skills) for longer and less predictable sentences, like those encountered within classroom instruction • Monitor progress over time.
Age Range	School-aged to adulthood
Availability	Auditory Potential, LLC

6.8.4 Paragraph Level

Table 6.16 TEST: *Clinical Evaluation of Language Functioning–5 (CELF-5)/ Paragraph Subtest*[22]

Structure	Paragraph level material is read followed by a list of related WH-questions, sampling the child's comprehension of the age-appropriate material presented. While this is not one of the core language subtests of the diagnostic test, its administration is valuable in the assessment of how a child with hearing loss responds to longer and more complex paragraph level material.
Results	Performance is assessed by the standard score, percentile ranking and age-equivalent scores calculated from the raw score obtained. As there are multiple paragraphs for each age level it is possible to administer linguistically comparable paragraphs in different listening conditions (quiet vs. noise or binaural vs. under separate ear listening conditions).
Clinical Clues	• Provides critical information for future training needs in terms of attention, sequential memory, auditory processing, and comprehension • Also, provides information about understanding and contingent response to WH-questions and inferential elements • Useful in monitoring progress over time
Age Range	School-aged to adulthood
Availability	Pearson, San Antonio, TX

Pearl

Using an assortment of subtests from various tests may yield a more representative sample of the child's level of functioning and management needs, rather than using one prescribed test completely (**Table 6.9, Table 6.10, Table 6.11, Table 6.12, Table 6.13, Table 6.14, Table 6.15, Table 6.16**). Tests normed on children with typical hearing are preferred, given that an increasing number of children with hearing loss attend general education vs. special education school placements. Using tests normed on children with hearing loss often yields ceiling-effect scores and an inflated view of the child's present level of functioning.

6.9 Receptive-Expressive Language Assessment

The wide variability observed in the vocabulary and language skills of children with hearing loss reflects a combination of factors. Perhaps one of the most important variables is insufficient exposure to enriched speech and language models within the child's everyday environment. In contrast to their normally hearing peers, there is some period during which the speech was not sufficiently audible to the child with hearing loss. As a result, some degree of structured language exposure is needed to overcome the effects of auditory deprivation that negatively affected the child's ability to fully access and learn from the auditory experiences within their everyday interactions.

Depending on the child's age, selected diagnostic protocols may encompass informal and formal measures. These measures might involve criterion-referenced or norm-referenced tools.

The advantage of norm-referenced diagnostic measures is that they permit comparison of the child's performance data to those of typically developing peers. With the expansion of early diagnosis and treatment, it is no longer atypical but rather routine, that a child with hearing loss achieves language competency and performance comparable to that of his normal hearing peers. The selected diagnostic measure should reflect the purpose of the test administration, (e.g., to determine eligibility for services, document present strengths and weakness, monitor growth in acquiring novel skills, or document the readiness for discontinuation of services.) The tests included in this text are not exhaustive of all commercially available diagnostic measures in the field of speech-language pathology. However, they are representative of widely used options for gathering comprehensive information within a time-constrained assessment.

Suggested testing has been categorized into the following domains:

• Receptive language—encompasses assessment of the understanding words and word combinations as well as the contingent response to spoken language, including acting on directions and questions by performing actions, manipulating objects, pointing to pictures, or verbally responding (**Table 6.17, Table 6.18, Table 6.19, Table 6.20, Table 6.22, Table 6.23, Table 6.25**)[23,24,25,26,27,28,29]

• Expressive language—encompasses the assessment of nonverbal and verbal behaviors exhibited to convey meaning intentionally (**Table 6.17, Table 6.18, Table 6.19, Table 6.21, Table 6.22, Table 6.23, Table 6.24, Table 6.25**)[23,24,25,26,28,29,30]

• Speech production—encompasses the assessment of speech intelligibility from the articulation of speech sounds in isolation, repeated and alternated syllables, words, and word combinations as well as overall voice quality, prosody, and intonational characteristics (**Table 6.26, Table 6.27**)[31]

• Pragmatic functioning—encompasses the assessment of how spoken language is used for various communicative purposes, such as labeling, commenting, requesting, directing, and questioning (**Table 6.25**)[29]

6.10 Suggested Test Protocol

6.10.1 Global

Table 6.17 TEST: *Rossetti Infant-Toddler Language Scale*[23]

Structure	Criterion-referenced inventory of preverbal and verbal behaviors underlying the development of spoken language
Results	Samples behaviors, via parent report or direct elicitation, in the following skill domains: interaction-attachment, gestures, play, language comprehension, and language expression. Responses are reported in terms of consistency of observation, yielding an index of emerging vs. mastered skills.
Clinical Clues	• Tracking of prerequisite skill emergence over time • Establishing more appropriate training objectives • Parent education and counseling
Age Range	Infants and Toddlers 0–36 Months
Availability	Super-Duper Publications, Greenville, SC

Table 6.18 TEST: *Receptive-Expressive Emergent Language Test—Third Edition (REEL-3)*[24]

Structure	Checklist of early nonverbal/verbal receptive and expressive communication behaviors based on parent report and/or clinical observation
Results	Raw scores in receptive and expressive language domain are converted to age equivalent, language ability scores and percentile rankings, compared to typically developing peers with normal hearing. A composite language ability score and percentile ranking is also obtained. Subtest and composite ability scores are further assigned a "description" ranging from poor to very superior.
Clinical Clues	• When administered to young infants, the behaviors elicited can provide more than a can or can't do. Rather, samples critical prerequisite behaviors that support the ultimate development of functional listening and spoken language skills • When used with older infants and toddlers, identifies stability of specific skills (for example attention to speaker), as well as addresses attention in developmental progression • Parent education and counseling • Guides future training needs • Affords a baseline with which to measure progress over time
Age Range	Infants and Toddlers 0–36 Months
Availability	Pro-Ed, Austin, TX

6.10.2 Vocabulary

Table 6.19 TEST: *MacArthur-Bates Communicative Development Inventory (MCDI)*[25]

Form: Words and Gestures

Structure	This is a parent questionnaire that assesses a child's early emerging receptive and expressive vocabulary. There are two versions, Words and Gestures (ages 8–18 months) and Words in Sentences. (ages 18–37 months). Individual test items of the Words and Gestures version, sample the understanding of social phrases, including; " Don't touch", "Let's go bye-bye" and "Throw the ball" as well as sound associations (meow, moo, yum-yum) and real words across a wide range of semantic categories, e.g., people, food, verbs, household objects, etc. Further samples spontaneous vs. imitative production of everyday gestures (waving) and play skill emergence (using a stick for a spoon or pretending to talk on the phone).
Results	Provides information about word learning across numerous semantic categories. In addition, can readily compare receptive understanding vs. production of individual test items. Responses yield a score that translates into percentile ranking relative to same-aged peers with normal hearing.
Clinical Clues	• Parent education and counseling tool • Guides the establishment of appropriate training objectives • Monitor progress over time
Age Range	Infants and Toddlers 8–30 Months
Availability	Paul H. Brookes Publishing Co., Baltimore, MD

Table 6.20 TEST: *Peabody Picture Vocabulary Test-5 (PPVT-5)*[26]

Structure	Samples receptive vocabulary for single words presented within a closed-set format, obligating a picture-pointing response. (By having the child with a hearing loss repeat-back the test prompt, the evaluator can ensure that the child accurately heard the test item and is not being penalized by an error in perception.)
Results	The raw score obtained reflects the number of correct responses and is used to calculate a standard score, percentile ranking, and an equivalent score relative to a normative group of typically developing peers with normal hearing
Clinical Clues	• Identify vocabulary delays to determine present level of functioning and/or progress over time in closing the gap between chronological age and lexical skills • Determine adequacy of receptive word knowledge to handle the instructional demands of current or future educational placement • Guide training in this domain
Age Range	Preschool through adulthood
Availability	Pearson, San Antonio, TX

Table 6.21 TEST: *Expressive One Word Picture Vocabulary Test (EOWPVT)*[30]

Structure	Samples expressive vocabulary and word retrieval skills by obligating the child to spontaneously label pictures. Verbal prompts ranging from "What do you call this?" to "What do you call the sharp things on the stem of a rose?"; allowing for alternate responses on many items
Results	Correct responses yield a raw score that is calculated into a standard score, percentile ranking and an age-equivalent score relative to typically developing peers with normal hearing
Clinical Clues	• There is some controversy about whether the expressive vocabulary score obtained on this test is more representative of the child's word repertoire than single word receptive vocabulary testing, as it allows for greater selectivity by the child in formulating a response. For the child with hearing loss, there is often wide disparity in vocabulary test scores on receptive vs. expressive measures; with the expressive score more inflated. It is perhaps more important to accept that both sampling techniques are valid, but likely provide different information about word learning and retrieval. For the child with hearing loss, they are not penalized for misperceiving or not hearing the test prompt accurately • Guides future training objectives in this domain and permits tracking of change over time
Age Range	Preschool through school-aged
Availability	Pearson, San Antonio, TX

6.10.3 Syntax and Grammar

Table 6.22 TEST: *Preschool Language Scale-5 (PLS-5)*[28]

Structure	Global receptive and expressive language assessment identifying delays or disorders of attention, gesture, play, vocal development, social communication, vocabulary, concepts, language structure, integrative language, and emergent literacy
Results	Yields a raw score for two domains (Auditory Comprehension and Expressive Communication) as well as a Total Language Score that can be used to calculate a standard score, percentile ranking and an age-equivalent score relative to typically developing peers with normal hearing
Clinical Clues	• Identifies present level of functioning relative to same-aged peers with normal hearing • Guides training needs for specific skills • Determines progress over time
Age Range	Infants to early school-aged
Availability	Pearson, San Antonio, TX

Table 6.23 TEST: *Clinical Evaluation of Language Fundamentals–5th Edition (CELF-5)*[22]

Structure	Norm-referenced assessment that provides a *core language* score that reflects global receptive and expressive language abilities, available in 3 forms for different age groups (Preschool, Ages 5–8, and Ages 9–21)
Results	Core language subtests include: *Sentence Comprehension* assesses the ability to comprehend specific grammatical forms within increasingly longer and more complex sentences by selecting the pictures that illustrate the meaning of the sentences *Word Structure* assesses the student's ability to apply grammar rules (including inflections, derivations, comparison, and pronouns) by filling in target words in sentences relating to pictures *Recalling Sentences* obligates the child to repeat-back verbatim progressively longer and more complex sentences, presented verbally with both auditory and speechreading cues *Formulated Sentences* samples the ability to formulate complete, semantically and grammatically correct spoken sentences in response to a picture prompt. The student is asked to formulate a sentence using a provided word or phrase
Clinical Clues	• Identifies present level of functioning relative to same-aged peers with normal hearing • Guides training needs for specific skills • Determines progress over time
Age Range	Preschool through adulthood
Availability	Pearson, San Antonio, TX

Table 6.24 TEST: *Structured Photographic Expressive Language Test (SPELT-3)*[29]

Structure	Samples expressive syntax and grammar formulation in response to a verbal prompt posed about a photograph
Results	The child is shown a photograph accompanied by a verbal prompt to provide a verbal response, "What's happening/What is he doing?" associated with a picture of a boy drawing. Such prompts are designed to elicit the formulation and use of a specific syntax or grammar form. In the example, present progressive verb. The test samples 53 linguistic elements, including negation, locatives, possessive nouns/pronouns, past tense copula usage, yes/no and WH-questions, passive voice, etc. Correct responses result in a raw score that can be calculated in terms of a standard score, percentile ranking and an age-equivalent score
Clinical Clues	• Provides several opportunities to elicit a selected language structure • Gives information about emergence vs. mastery • Identifies present level of functioning in terms of both attention to and understanding of a verbal prompt • Guides future training needs and monitors progress over time
Age Range	Preschool through school-aged
Availability	Janelle Publications, DeKalb, IL

6.10.4 Pragmatic Language

Table 6.25 TEST: *Test of Narrative Language-2nd Edition (TNL-2)* REFERENCE[29]

Structure	Norm-referenced test of pragmatic language assessed by sampling the ability to understand and spontaneously formulate 3 types of stories; a script, a personal narrative, and a fictional story
Results	The test is divided into a receptive (comprehension) and expressive (production) subtests. Following the reading of a short narrative, the child is obligated to answer related factual or inferential questions about what was read. Expressively, picture prompts are used to elicit a story from the child (after listening to a story told by the examiner). Testing sessions are recorded to facilitate accurate and easy scoring of key elements. A narrative language score is calculated on the basis of the response accuracy to the questions as well as the narrative elements included, such as plot, characters, sequential order, and use of conventions such as conjunctions. Standard score and percentile rankings permit comparison to a peer group with normal hearing.
Clinical Clues	• Establish more appropriate training objectives for facilitation of functionally adequate social communication skills • Identify the level of dependence on contextual support vs. linguistic clues to ensure understanding of longer narratives • Determine the need for developing more specific clarification strategies to resolve instances of communicative breakdown • Guide future training objectives of both semantic and structural verbal response to conversational, factual or fictional narratives presented within meaningful social contexts • Identify the need for establishing better strategies for launching and maintaining conversational topics • Document improvement over time
Age Range	Preschool to Teenage (4–15 Years)
Availability	Pro-Ed, Austin, TX

Pitfall

Formal diagnostic measures can only be validly re-administered within a specific time frame, e.g., within six-month intervals. For most children with hearing loss, there are multiple professionals involved in their management and care who must perform periodic assessment of a child's present level of functioning. Fortunately, there are numerous commercially available diagnostic measures such that progress monitoring can be conducted without duplication or the invalidation of test/retest standards.

6.11 Speech Production Assessment

Table 6.26 Informal observation (examples of possible comments)

Intentional Vocalizations	Louisa's primarily simple sentence constructs were characterized by frequent grammar errors, and she used statement constructs to question and request
Intelligibility	Good to the unfamiliar listener without a need for contextual support, despite occasional substitution errors.
Voice Quality	Natural-sounding with variability in intonational contour
Resonance	Generally oral in nature
Prosody	Often arrhythmic and evenly stressed
Vowels	Articulatory precise
Consonants	Articulatory precise with the exception of voiced and voiceless fricatives in all word positions

6.11.1 Formal Articulation Test

Table 6.27 TEST: *Goldman-Fristoe Test of Articulation-2 (GFTA-3) Sounds or Words*[31]

Structure	Samples the production of English consonants and consonant blends as they occur in single words
Results	The child verbally labels objects in pictures and the articulatory precision of the production of targeted speech sounds in the initial, medial, and final position of single words is assessed.; eliciting a raw score that can be used to calculate a standard score, percentile ranking and an age equivalent score relative to same-aged peers with normal hearing
Clinical Clues	• Affords information regarding spontaneous vs. imitative productions • Permits distinctive feature analysis highlighting the interdependency between perception and production • Identifies deletions, distortions, and substitution errors • Guides training objectives • Monitors progress over time
Age Range	Preschool through adulthood
Availability	Pearson, San Antonio, TX

77

6.11.2 Telepratice Option

Telepractice, using Web-based technology that permits two-way simultaneous communication at a distance, is now a clinical reality rather than an idealistic expansion idea discussed in strategic administrative planning sessions. With the Covid-19 pandemic, remote learning and teleintervention requirements challenged educators and therapists to think out of the box in how to address the instructional needs of all children, even those with hearing loss. At the early intervention level, this was a natural fit for auditory-based training approaches, as inherent in this training is active parental involvement through embedded coaching techniques. For the older school-aged student with hearing loss, they could have the same instructional experiences as their classmates, after resolving issues of connectivity to the auditory signal (through FM, CommPilot, or mini-microphone devices). While this service delivery option has been suggested as a means of addressing the lack of qualified professionals in communities with limited auditory-verbal resources,[14] conducting diagnostic speech-language evaluations and functional listening assessments via telepractice was not considered to be potentially feasible until it became a "requirement." The observational structure and use of parent-report questionnaires within the diagnostic evaluations of involving children with hearing loss readily lends itself to a telepractice model. For the school-aged, teleintervention experience has verified strategies for conducting the listening component of the assessment. Several of the previously cited formal speech-language tests are now available in digital form. However, in-person evaluations will likely be preferable for most SLPs and Listening and Spoken Language Specialists working with children with diagnosed hearing loss.

6.12 Conclusions

Monitoring auditory skill emergence and speech-language progression over time should continue to be a component of any aural habilitation/rehabilitation intervention for any aged child with hearing loss. There is a diverse body of longitudinal research documenting that children whose hearing loss is early identified, receive early amplification, and are enrolled in auditory-based early intervention achieve age-level listening and spoken language skills by preschool or early elementary school years.[32] Like their typically developing peers, children with hearing loss have to learn from the enriched and varied language models encountered at home, in classroom instruction, as well as within incidental everyday social-communicative interactions. Essential to this normalizing trajectory is the dynamic, ongoing collaboration between the audiologist and the interventionist. Empowering parents to remain actively involved in all aspects of the child's "hearing journey" cannot be under-valued; until the child is old enough to self-advocate and "own" his or her hearing loss.

References

[1] American Academy of Pediatrics, Joint Committee on Infant Hearing. Year 2007 position statement: Principles and guidelines for early hearing detection and intervention programs. *Pediatrics* 2007;*120*(4):898–921

[2] Buz Harlor AD, Bower C. Committee on practice and ambulatory medicine and; the section on otolaryngology. *Head and Neck Surgery Pediatrics* 2009;*124*(4):1252–1263

[3] Frezza S, Catenazzi P, Gallus R, et al. Hearing loss in very preterm infants: should we wait or treat? *Acta Otorhinolaryngol Ital* 2019;*39*(4):257–262

[4] Aradhya GH, Gaddam S. Co relationship between brainstem evoked studies and severe hyperbilirubinemia in high risk neonates. *Int J Sci Res* 2019;*8*:51–52

[5] Audiology Clinical Practice Guideline Cleft Palate/Craniofacial and Syndromic Patients. (2012), British Columbia Children's Hospital, Vancouver, BC

[6] American Speech-Language-Hearing Association. (2008). *Guidelines for Evaluations* [Guidelines]

[7] Zimmerman-Phillips S, Osberger M, Robbins A. IT-MAIS: Infant-Toddler Meaningful Auditory Integration Scale. Valencia, CA: Advanced Bionics LLC; 2001

[8] Kuehn-Inacker H, Weichbold V, Tsiakpini L, Coninx F, D'Haese P. Littlears auditory questionnaire manual—parent questionnaire to assess auditory behaviour in young children. Innsbruck, Austria: MED-EL; 2003

[9] Stredler-Brown A, Johnson DC. Functional auditory performance indicators: an integrated approach to auditory development. Denver, Colorado Department of Education, (2003), Special Education Services Unit. http://www.tsbvi.edu/attachments/FunctionalAuditoryPerformanceIndicators.pdf. Accessed January 3, 2018

[10] Curtin S, Fennell C, Escudero P. Weighting of vowel cues explains patterns of word-object associative learning. *Dev Sci* 2009;*12*(5):725–731

[11] Ling D. Speech and the hearing impaired child. Washington, DC: AGBell; 1976

[12] Tyler RS, Preece JP, Lowder MW. The Iowa Cochlear Implant Test Battery: Iowa City, IA: University of Iowa; 1983

[13] Madell J, Flexer C. Beyond ANSI standards: acoustic accessibility for children with hearing loss. Audiology Online; 2012

[14] Madell J, Batheja R, Klemp E, Hoffman R. Evaluating speech perception performance. *Audiology Today* 2011; (September–October):52–56

[15] Moog JS, Geers AE. Early Speech Perception Test for Profoundly Hearing-Impaired Children. St. Louis, MO: Central Institute for the Deaf and Hard of Hearing; 1990

[16] Mackersie CL, Boothroyd A, Minniear D. Evaluation of the Computer-assisted Speech Perception Assessment Test (CASPA). *J Am Acad Audiol* 2001;*12*(8):390–396

[17] Kirk KI, Pisoni DB, Osberger MJ. Lexical effects on spoken word recognition by pediatric cochlear implant users. *Ear Hear* 1995;*16*(5):470–481

[18] Robbins A. The Mr. Potato Head Task. Indianapolis, IN: Indiana University School of Medicine; 1994

[19] Robbins A, Renshaw J, Osberger M. *Common Phrases Test*. Indianapolis, IN: Indiana University School of Medicine; 1995

[20] Nilsson M, Soli SD, Sullivan JA. Development of the Hearing in Noise Test for the measurement of speech reception thresholds in quiet and in noise. *J Acoust Soc Am* 1994;*95*(2):1085–1099

[21] *AzBio Sentences*. Tempe, AZ: Auditory Potential, LLC; 2013

[22] Semel-Mintz E, Wiig E, Secord W. Clinical Evaluation of Language Fundamentals, Fifth Edition (CELF-5). San Antonio, TX: Pearson; 2003

[23] Rossetti L. The Rosetti Infant-Toddler Language Scale: A Measure of Communication and Interaction – Birth -Three. East Moline, IL: LinguiSystems; 2006

[24] Bzoch KR, League R, Brown, VR. Receptive-Expressive Emergent Language Test, Third Edition. San Antonio, TX: Psychological Corporation;1993

[25] Fenson L, Marchman VA, Thal DJ, Dale PS, Reznick JS, Bates E. MacArthur-Bates Communicative Development Inventories User's Guide and Technical Manual. 2nd ed. Baltimore, MD: Brookes Publishing; 2006

[26] Dunn LM, Dunn DM, Lenhard A. Peabody Picture Vocabulary Test. 5th ed. (PPVT-5). San Antonio, TX: Pearson; 2015

[27] Martin, N., Brownell, R, Expressive One Word Picture Vocabulary Test, Fourth Edition. Pro-Ed. Austin, TX; 2011

[28] Zimmerman IL, Steiner VG, Pond RE. Preschool Language Scales. 5th Edition. (PLS-5). San Antonio, TX: Pearson; 2001

6.13   Appendix A

Classification of auditory responses

Auditory Process	Underlying Skill	Auditory Demand
Detection	Presence or absence of sound	Auditory awareness Auditory attention Distance listening Localization
Discrimination	Distinguishes between two or more sounds	Change vs. No Change Same vs. Different
Identification	Recognition of what is heard and is able to repeat it back	Auditory association Auditory analysis Sound-blending Sequential memory
Comprehension	Demonstrates understanding and able to act on what is said	Auditory processing Auditory comprehension Auditory closure

6.14   Appendix B

Informal auditory checklist

Detection	Sampling task: While visually attentive to parent and/or while actively engaged, noisemakers and speech will be introduced to assess detection level responses	
Noisemakers	Loud	Soft
Clacker or Banging on drum (low)	__ of 3	__ of 3
Musical Toy (Mid)	__ of 3	__ of 3
Bell or Squeaky toy (High)	__ of 3	__ of 3
Discrimination		
Duration	Sampling task: Pushing a vehicle, spinning a toy, shaking a scarf or burp cloth in prolong vs. short durational patterns, while producing the low-frequency vowel "ah"	
Intensity	Sampling task: Can determine from response to above detection level noisemakers	
Syllable Number	Sampling task: Shaking burp cloth/scarf or bouncing the child or a stuffed animal in accordance with varying syllabic patterns, while producing the syllabic sequence "bah"	
Ling Vowels	ah, ee, oo Sampling Task: Observe any change in ongoing behavior indicative of detection of these vowel sounds when presented from both the right and left side. For older infants and toddlers, may elicit imitation of these vowels, suggesting identification level response.	
Ling Consonants	sh, s, m Sampling Task: Observe any change in ongoing behavior indicative of detection of these consonant sounds when presented from both the right and left side. For older infants and toddlers, may elicit imitation of these vowels, suggesting identification level response	
Sustained Attention	Sampling Task: Observe any searching behaviors for the sound source	
Localization	Sampling Task: Observe any searching behaviors for the sound source	
Onset of voicing	Sampling Task: Pretend play with a stuffed animal and a blanket or burp cloth. Pretend to rock and put the stuffed animal to sleep. Cover the toy and wait a bit before moving your mouth with reduplicated pattern of "bah-bah-bah"(without voicing), then add voicing while simultaneously removing the blanket. Sample 3 times. Confirm the consistency of response to the onset of voicing with responsiveness observed during the assessment when baby is talked to.	
Conditioned Response	Sampling Task: Observe and comment on whether the child has a "listen and drop" response; can hold a toy and wait for a speech stimuli before making a response (like putting cookies into the mouth of a cookie Monster toy in response to Ling sounds or "yum-yum".	

6.15 Appendix C

6.15.1 Speech-Language Evaluation/ Functional Listening Assessment

Preschool case		
Name: Female	Age: 2 months	Date of Evaluation
Address:	ICD10 Code:	Technology: RE: BTE HA
	Procedure Code:	LE: BTE HA

Purpose of Evaluation: To document present level of functioning to determine eligibility for services through the state's Early Intervention Program.

Background Information: Baby was born full term following a normal pregnancy and delivery. She was referred following Universal Newborn Hearing Screening (UNHS) of both ears. Two follow-up ABRs(Auditory Branstem Response) tests suggested a moderate sensorineural hearing loss (SNL) in right ear and a moderately severe loss in left ear. She had been fitted with binaural BTE hearing aids for only two weeks at the time of this evaluation.

FUNCTIONAL LISTENING ASSESSMENT

Informal Auditory Checklist

Detection	Sampling task: While visually attentive to parent and/or while actively engaged, noisemakers and speech were introduced to assess detection level responses	
Noisemakers	Loud	Soft
Clacker (low)	3 of 3	1 of 3
Musical Toy (Mid)	2 of 3	0 of 3
Bell (High)	1 of 3	0 of 3

Discrimination	
Duration	Not yet observed due to young age
Intensity	Not yet observed due to young age
Syllable Number	Not yet observed due to young age
Ling Vowels	ah, ee, and oo (oo after second exposure)
Ling Consonants	sh, s, and m (m after second exposure)

Sustained Attention: Sustained and sufficient to benefit from structured learning routines

Localization: Not expected at such a young age, but beginning to observe that child seems to search for sound

Onset of voicing: Consistently responsive to voice in the absence of being able to visually attend to the speaker

Conditioned Response: NA due to young age

Interpretation: Present level of functioning suggests that the infant is detecting loud noisemakers and speech across the frequency range. She was least accurate in responding to higher frequency noisemakers (musical toys or bells) as well as to softer noisemakers. The lack of detection or confusion of m and oo is often observed and might be attributed to insufficient loudness in the early programming of amplification devices. Her attention to the speaker is also sufficient to expect that she will benefit from structured therapy intervention at this time.

IT-MAIS	Total Score: 10 out of 40
> Vocalizations with vs. w/out HAs	0%—Not yet observed to alter vocalizations but more attuned to/ interested in people since fitted with her hearing aids
> Speech-like vocalizations	25%—Makes more sound since fitted with her hearing aids, including cooing, and other vowel productions
Detection	
Name in quiet	25%—Consistently detects speech even when she can't see the speaker
Name in noise	0%—Not yet observed
Sounds in quiet	100%—Observed to startle to loud sounds (like the phone ringing or other noises) and to be soothed by softer sounds (like singing or the music from her mobile)

Sounds in noise	0%—Not yet observed
Associates Sounds w/ sources	0%—Not yet observed due to young age
Discrimination	
Different Speakers	100%—Definitely observed to respond to familiar speakers (especially to her father's voice)
Difference between speech/Non-Speech	0% - Although seems to enjoy music from mobile,
Different emotional states	0% - Not yet observed

Interpretation: The infant was credited for consistent detection level responses to both soft and loud environmental sounds and speech, within a quiet listening environment. This performance is considered commensurate with her young age and the fact that she has only recently been fit with bilateral hearing aids. Today's score will serve as a baseline with which to measure the baby's progress in acquiring more functional listening skills as she adjusts to hearing aids and is involved in family-centered, auditory-based speech and language training

COMMUNICATIVE FUNCTIONING

Informal Observation of Prerequisite Behaviors underlying the Development o Spoken Language

Attention-Getting	Primarily cries to gain the attention of others, which is appropriate for her young age
Joint-Attention	Sustained and sufficient for structured learning routines
Turn-Taking	Though not expected for her young age; but observed to vocalize in response to being talked to
Communicative Intent	Mother and caregiver report that the baby is beginning to note differences in her crying when hungry, wet, tired, etc.

Interpretation: Exhibited behaviors are considered appropriate for her age. There is nothing to predict that she should not acquire functionally adequate listening and spoken language skills.

REEL-3

	Raw Score	Age Equivalent	Ability Score	%ile Rank
Receptive Language	11	1 months	95 (Average)	37th
Expressive Language	11	2 months	100 (Average)	50th
	Composite Language Score: 97			
	Composite %ile Score: 42nd			
	Descriptive Rating: Average			

Interpretation: The baby's composite score of 97 on this global test of receptive and expressive language skills fall within the "average" range relative to her same-aged peers with normal hearing. She is presently functioning as well as or better than 42% of her peers. On the receptive items, she was credited for startling to loud sounds stopping actions in response to sound and being soothed by her mother's singing to her. She is also visually attentive to speech directed to or around her. Expressively, the baby is credited for making sounds other than crying (including primarily vowel-like productions and an occasional "speech-like" imitation following an adult model). It should be noted that the skills sampled at her young age on their formal diagnostic measure may not fully predict how her diagnosed hearing loss will impact on her future speech and language development

Informal Observation of Phonemic Production/Speech Intelligibility

Intentional Vocalizations	NA due to her young age
Intelligibility	NA due to young age and restricted sample
Voice Quality	Natural-sounding and variable
Resonance	Insufficient sample to fully determine due to young age
Prosody	Although limited sample, definitive variability noted
Vowels	ah, eh, uh, ae (as in "hat"), ai (as in "hi")
Consonants	Not yet observed due to young age

Interpretation: The baby was relatively vocal throughout the evaluation, which was unexpected given her young age, her diagnosed hearing loss, and the fact that she has only worn HAs for two weeks. She exhibited sustained attention to speech directed to her by her mother, caregiver, and the evaluators, particularly at a close distance and when she could see the speaker's face

RECOMMENDATIONS

This diagnostic profile supports the baby's need for: 1) Continued audiological testing to monitor the stability of her hearing loss and her need for modifications in the programming of her technology 2) Weekly individual auditory-based speech and language training 3). Participation in a weekly parent-child group affording opportunities for the parent and child to interact and learn from other families with hearing loss

School-aged case

Name Male			Age 9.6	Date of Evaluation
Address:	Technology RE: BTE HA	ICD 10 Code		Mode of Communication Oral
	LE: BTE HA	Procedure Code		Educational Setting Regular 3rd grade w/o related services

Purpose of Evaluation: Assess performance w/alternative HAs and needs for LSL therapy intervention

Background Information: Hearing loss detected at birth and aided by 1 month. Received AVT until 5 ½ years old.
Drop in hearing over the past year and cochlear implants previously recommended, but parents declined to pursue.
Most recent audiological testing revealed child HAs maxed out with word recognition scores at 58% and 32% respectively for RE vs LE.

FUNCTIONAL LISTENING PERFORMANCE

	Listen Alone (Quiet)		Listen Alone (Noise)	
Linguistic Level		Binaural		Binaural
Ling Sound Test (Phonemes)	ah, oo, ee, m, sh, s		ah, oo, ee, m, sh, s	
Personal HA	ALL	6 of 6	NR s, sh	4 of 6
HA 2	ALL	6 of 6	NR oo, m	4 of 6
HA 3	NR s	5 of 6	NR oo, m	4 of 6

Interpretation: Personal HAs providing insufficient high frequency access; HA 2 and 3 insufficient loudness

AB List (Word Level)	Binaural (Quiet)			Binaural (Noise)		
Word Correct	Initial	Vowel	Final	Initial	Vowel	Final
Personal HA 80% (Q)/70% (N)	90%	90%	70%	80%	100%	90%
HA 2 40% (Q)/60% (N)	60%	90%	70%	80%	80%	70%
HA 3 10% (Q)/70% (N)	30%	100%	60%	90%	100%	60%

Interpretation: Child expressed definite preference for input provided by personal HAs. This was not atypical given the child has been wearing these HAs for the past 3.5 years. 80% response accuracy in quiet suggests that the child likely follows everyday conversation with a need for repetition, struggling more in noisy environments. Test sequence likely affected performance with HA3. However, in what he perceived to be more difficult listening condition (e.g. noise), response accuracy with HA3 was comparable to performance with personal aids. Analysis of errors further revealed that more consonant confusions with HA2 were "better mistakes" than with personal aids or HA3.

HINT-C (Sentence level)	RE Words	LE Words	Binaural	RE Sentences	LE Sentences	Binaural
	90%	96%	DNT	90%	70%	DNT

Interpretation: Under separate ear conditions, there was a substantial disparity in the child's sentence identification with his LE vs. his RE despite obtaining a comparable percentage of words.

Pediatric AZ-Bio (Sentence level)	Quiet			Noise		
Personal HA	DNT	89%	96%	80%	70%	96%
HA 2	DNT	90%	100%	80%	70%	90%
HA 3	DNT	80%	90%	90%	80%	60%

Interpretation: Open-set word and sentence identification with either device functionally adequate to meet everyday conversational demands. Evident that response accuracy decreases in the presence of competing background noise, with all devices. The disparity in his word identification at sentence level, compared to the above-cited open-set word level testing, supports the child's reliance on contextual clues to enhance his overall word identification.

Speech-language evaluation

PPVT-5 (Vocabulary)	Raw Score	Standard Score	%ile Ranking	Age-Equivalent Score
	104	75	5	6-4

Interpretation: SS reveals receptive vocabulary skills for single words fall below the average range relative to same-aged peers with normal hearing. Likely has difficulty meeting the instructional demands of 3rd grade curriculum.

SPELT-3 (Sentence Level) Expressive Syntax/Grammar	Raw Score	Standard Score	%ile Ranking	Age-Equivalent Score
	49 of 53	107	71	8.0 to 9.11

Interpretation: Performance falls within the average range relative to same-aged peers with normal hearing. Noted to use inappropriate lexical choices to describe pictures (e.g. "The lady's milking the baby" for "The lady's feeding the baby"); reflective of his persisting vocabulary deficit.

CELF-5 (Sentence Level)	Raw Score	Standard Score	%ile Ranking	Age-Equivalent Score
Recalling Sentences	15	9	37	5-10
Formulating Sentences	7	5	15	3-8

Interpretation: Under optimal conditions (with both auditory and speech reading clues), response accuracy was comparable to sentence identification via audition alone (cited above). Although his scores fall within the average range relative to his age-matched peers with normal hearing, persisting vocabulary delays negatively impacted his performance; as evidenced by his omission or substitution of key words within test items. Similarly, while the child exhibits adequately developed expressive syntax and grammar skills to meet daily conversational demands, his persisting vocabulary deficit most affected his ability to formulate grammatically well-structured sentences for more abstract concepts, on the expressive Formulating Sentences subtest.

GFTA-3 (Word Level) Speech Production Error	Raw Score	Standard Score	%ile Ranking	Age-Equivalent Score
	7	86	16	5.3

Interpretation: Production errors closely mirror perception errors; exhibiting frequent substitution of voiceless fricatives and affricatives in all word positions. Informal assessment judged overall speech intelligibility to be readily understood by the unfamiliar listener without a need for contextual support. Unable to self-monitor his own error production to self-correct them in the absence of an adult model to imitate.

RECOMMENDATIONS:

Subsequent to audiological reprogramming of HA2, in light of the child's sentence level identification and phonemic confusions at the word level with that device, it was recommended that a trial with full-time use of bilaterally fit HA2 would be initiated. In conjunction with that trial, weekly auditory-based structured listening training was advised. Emphasis was directed toward improved phonemic identification at the word level under separate ear conditions as well as binaurally in both quiet and noise. After an 8-week trial, these aids were purchased and the child has transitioned to bi-monthly therapy sessions, with a continued focus on vocabulary expansion and improved speech reception in the presence of competing background noise. Close monitoring of his progress over time is needed to assist the family in monitoring any change in hearing status that would warrant referral for cochlear implantation.

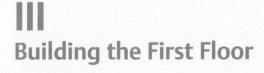

III
Building the First Floor

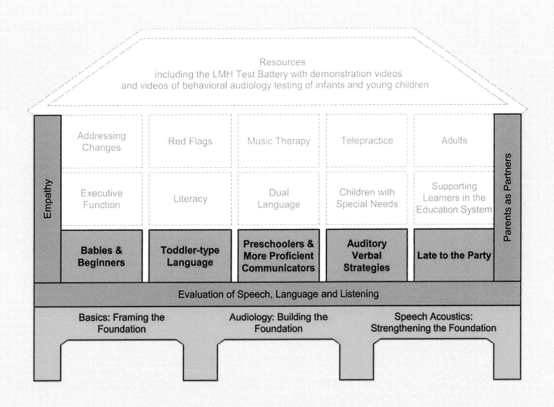

7 Babies and Beginners: Starting with Nothing and Building up to Words

Becky Clem and Elizabeth Tippette

Summary

This chapter discusses the significance of rapidly establishing auditory, speech, and language intervention following identification of hearing loss in infants and young children. When the family's goal for their child with hearing loss is to listen and speak, frequently and consistently exploiting audition, with maximum access to intelligible speech, is critical.

Keywords

hearing loss, early intervention, listening and spoken language (LSL), neuroplasticity, critical window, child development, audition, receptive language, expressive language, speech production, parent-coaching, family involvement, assessment, cognition, play skills, attachment, chronological age, listening age

Key Points

- All children with hearing loss who are first learning to listen fall into the "baby" stage regardless of the child's chronological age.
- Practitioners and caregivers exploit audition through rich, meaningful, functional, and redundant activities.
- Creating partnerships with families leads to better listening and spoken language outcomes as well as stronger infant-caregiver attachment.
- Natural sounding speech is facilitated through audition.
- Auditory comprehension precedes talking.

7.1 Characteristics of the Baby Stage in Listening and Spoken Language

Babies are synonymous with beginnings. Newborns, infants only a few hours old, arrive in the world completely dependent on adults for every aspect of life. Caregivers have the remarkable and overwhelming task of supplying the physical, emotional, and intellectual needs of newborns from the first moment of life. The first 3 months of life with a new baby are full of routines for feeding, sleeping, bathing, diapering, and bonding with caregivers. Babies communicate by crying for hunger, pain, distress, or feeling alone. Newborns are exposed to a world of speech and noise as their brains begin to sort and attach meaning to sounds. Over the first 18 months, babies will: smile, laugh, babble, use facial expressions, imitate others, dance to music, sit up, crawl, start walking, learn that sound is meaningful, follow some directions, play, and start learning to talk. As babies grow, they develop relationships with their caregivers and family. As their personalities develop, we see meltdowns and temper tantrums as they exert their will on the world. At this stage, they communicate with their behavior more than with words.

Babies with hearing loss (BHL) miss the early auditory communication input from caregivers. The hearing loss results in a barrier between the world and the baby's potential auditory brain development. The arcuate fasciculus is a fiber tract connecting the temporal lobe and the inferior parietal lobe to portions of the frontal lobe. Stimulation to the auditory cortex, which is housed in the temporal lobe, does not remain solely in that region. As such, a lack of stimulation in the form of auditory deprivation does not impact solely the child's development of speech and language. Forty percent of children with hearing loss (CHL) are thought to also have sensory processing difficulties.[1] Because the parietal lobe is responsible for the perception and integration of information from the five senses (hearing, smell, sight, taste, and touch), an absence of hearing stimuli creates a disorganized sensory system. Further, CHL are more likely to experience weaknesses in processes the frontal cortex controls. This is because of the missing sensory component sent by nerve fibers to that region. These processes include self-regulation and executive functioning, which are covered in-depth in Chapter 12.

7.1.1 LSL Services for Babies Before Fitting Technology

Auditory deprivation and the ensuing ramifications are halted when early detection procedures are heeded and when follow-up is timely and inclusive of necessary practitioners. Families and other practitioners may ask: Why do we need to begin listening and spoken language (LSL) services prior to the baby receiving hearing aids? How will the baby benefit from LSL services when we know the hearing aids aren't providing optimal access to speech? Why can't we wait until after the baby receives a cochlear implant? The response we must give is rooted in hearing science. Beginning LSL intervention with babies and beginning listeners:

- stimulates auditory pathways and teaches that sound has meaning
- takes advantage of what residual hearing a baby does have so that they can develop sound awareness and vocalizations within the range that they can hear
- decreases the amount of time a baby goes without any auditory information to the brain
- helps parents and family connect with their child through beginning communicative interactions and routines

- provides, if possible (depending on auditory access), evidence to parents and caregivers of their child's auditory responses so that they can facilitate learning to listen at home
- prepares parents and caregivers, even when the baby does not yet benefit due to lack of auditory access

Put simply, the goal of very early hearing loss identification, aggressive audiological management with appropriate amplification fitting, and family-centered listening and spoken language intervention is to mitigate the effects of hearing loss on the child's speech, language, listening, and learning development.

Pitfall

Babies with hearing loss (BHL) miss the early auditory communication input from caregivers. The hearing loss results in a barrier between the world and the baby's potential auditory brain development.

7.1.2 What the "Baby Stage" Looks Like for Older Children Who Are Beginning Listeners

As neuroplasticity is greatest within the first 3.5 years of life, for the purposes of this chapter, we consider "older children" as being greater than 3.5 years. However, we must remember that any child who does not begin the listening and language process during the first year of life will be delayed and will be considered a beginner even if the child is no longer a baby. Characteristics of late starters are[2]:

- having an incomplete auditory signal for learning spoken language
- possibly being dependent on visual input for learning language and communicating
- receiving a cochlear implant after several years of decreased auditory access .
- having inconsistent, incorrect, or no amplification
- having a longer period of auditory deprivation
- acquiring new or sudden hearing loss secondary to illness or accident
- being from a non-English-speaking home
- not having LSL services or inconsistent services despite early hearing loss identification
- receiving some input in both a visual and a spoken language, but without sufficient quantity or quality in either one
- having early identification, yet not receiving services, or receiving inconsistent services
- being impacted by COVID-19 (hearing loss not being considered an essential service; school and clinic closures; no access to telepractice services; delayed cochlear implant surgeries; supply chain delays for hearing technology)

Listening and spoken language intervention for the older child starts at the beginning with learning to listen in the same developmental stages as babies: detection, discrimination, identification, and comprehension of auditory information. Learning to listen and developing receptive language precede spoken expressive language. Learning sound awareness, attaching meaning to sound, and growing receptive language are the foundation for spoken expressive language.

Pearl

Learning to listen and developing receptive language precede spoken expressive language.

7.2 Important/Special Factors to Consider with This Stage

Decades of research on neural plasticity—the brain's ability to change in response to experiences—provide a clarion call to practitioners who work with CHL: there is great urgency to provide these babies access to the sounds of speech. Flexer states, "We should think of the early stimulation of the infant's brain with auditory information as a neuro-developmental emergency."[3] When not appropriately stimulated early in life, the brain reorganizes in a phenomenon known as cross-modal plasticity. In the absence of auditory stimulation, the auditory cortex begins to take on other functions, such as those typically performed by the areas of the brain responsible for visual and tactile processing.

Research from the ground-breaking Longitudinal Outcomes of Children with Hearing Impairment (LOCHI) study showed that better receptive and expressive language outcomes resulted from earlier access to technology (hearing aid fitting or cochlear implantation).[4]

Pitfall

When not appropriately stimulated, the brain reorganizes in a phenomenon known as cross-modal plasticity. In the absence of auditory stimulation, the auditory cortex begins to take on other functions, such as those typically performed by the areas of the brain responsible for visual and tactile processing.

7.3 Parent Involvement in Therapy: It's All About the Family

Family-practitioner partnerships provide support, guidance, coaching, and tools to achieve optimal LSL outcomes for the child. In addition to supplying the brain with access to sound, bringing a baby and their family to LSL intervention as quickly as possible after a hearing loss is identified lays the groundwork for strong communication and literacy outcomes through:

- facilitating positive caregiver-baby interactions and supporting families emotionally, while identifying needs for referrals to social work, financial support networks, and infant mental health experts (this topic is covered in-depth in Chapter 5)
- caregiver-coaching
- appropriate assessment and diagnostic intervention that is family-centered
- implementing a strong home program and daily routines steeped in language stimulation

7.3.1 Involving Parents: What Does Caregiver-Coaching Look Like?

At the start of an intervention session, the practitioner uses open-ended questions and makes inviting statements to help caregivers know they are in a judgment-free zone. This gives caregivers the opportunity to express their struggles, needs, and desires. We, as practitioners, gather keen insight on how to best meet caregivers where they are in their journey. Some examples include:

- "Tell me about your week!"
- "What is your favorite thing about your baby?"
- "What was the most challenging thing about the past few days?"
- "What are you celebrating?"
- "How are you feeling?"
- "Would you be willing to share with me what it was like finding out about your baby's hearing loss? I would like to know your story."

Caraway described the hallmarks of caregiver-coaching as ten distinct strategies. Those are summarized here and adapted with examples specific to the discussion of babies and beginning listeners.[5]

1. *At the request of the practitioner, the caregiver models skills or challenges they're experiencing:* "Show me what it looks like when you're singing 'Twinkle, Twinkle Little Star' to him. When he doesn't seem to become still and listen to you, what do you do?"
2. *Practice turn-taking between practitioner and caregiver:* "I'm going to model how to use the airplane sound while moving the toy along with my voice, and then I'll hand it off to you to give it a try."
3. *Practitioner invites the caregiver to engage:* "After you've heard me sing this little song a few times and you feel comfortable, please join me!"
4. *Practitioner teaches the caregiver directly:* "After we have filled up her brain with the repetition of the cow sound, we need to give her wait time and a nice quiet space with an expectant look to invite her to vocalize."
5. *Practitioner sets the stage for the caregiver to predict what might happen if a particular tactic is explored:* "What do you think would happen if we left the peekaboo cloth on his face this time for a moment instead of pulling it down for him?"
6. *During observation, the practitioner narrates actions or skills performed by the caregiver to reinforce them:* "You are so aware of her listening bubble. I noticed you used a soft voice right into her hearing aid when you read that book to her—that helps maximize the amount of speech she can hear clearly."
7. *Practitioner tells the caregiver information about what will occur in the session and why it is done:* "To begin to work on a skill you mentioned was very important to you and your family, looking when he hears his name called, we are going to practice first getting his attention through listening with noisemakers. This is a skill that typically develops before a baby responds to his name."
8. *A purposeful "mess-up" by the practitioner provides a teachable moment for the caregiver:* "Oh rats! Did you see me pull out the round-and-round toy without singing the song first? I completely forgot to focus her attention on listening first before I showed the visual!"
9. *Practitioner gives a "secret message" to the caregiver through a subtle verbal or nonverbal cue or a whisper:* [holding up a pointer-finger while whispering] "Good—now wait and lean in, let your eyes get really big…!"
10. *Practitioner pulls it all together to summarize key learning points and takeaways to reinforce skills and promote the home program:* "It was so powerful watching you respond to his raspberry lip-sounds today by blowing them back to him and then expanding that to a new skill of hand-to-mouth vocal play! When do you see yourself doing this in the week ahead? Who in your family are you excited to show this trick to?"

When parents cannot physically attend appointments, telepractice brings the LSL practitioner to the family and child, wherever they are. Teletherapy has grown in popularity, quite out of necessity, during the COVID-19 pandemic.[6] LSL intervention conducted via telepractice gives practitioners the opportunity to dive into the very essence of the LSL/auditory-verbal therapy (AVT) approach. Caregiver-coached and -led sessions in which the practitioner is not physically present help the caregiver learn to manipulate therapy toys and assist with the young child's behavior. Moreover, telepractice requires the practitioner to relinquish control of the session to the caregiver, thereby facilitating true carry-over of strategies, activities, and goals to the home environment.

7.3.2 Assessment and Intervention

When infants receive access to speech, whether optimally through properly fitted hearing aids, or only partially as they wait for cochlear implantation, our job as LSL practitioners is to lay a strong foundation. Babies' brains are, in the words of English philosopher John Locke, *tabula rasa*, a blank slate. Constantly stimulating the very young brain with rich language input through audition is key in ensuring limitless potential for babies with hearing loss. All LSL intervention for babies and beginning listeners must chiefly impact the caregivers who are present to provide that critical stimulation morning, noon, and night.

Assessment

Practitioners for the birth to 18-month-old population require a strong, working knowledge of typical infant and early child development to provide initial assessment and ongoing diagnostic therapy. **Table 7.1** describes the hallmarks of neurotypical listening and spoken language development within the first year of the neurotypical infant's life.[7] For infants or children

Table 7.1 Communication skills and red flags

Developmental age	Listening and communication skills of typically hearing infants *Red flags for a possible hearing loss in infants*
1–3 months	Begins to develop auditory awareness and auditory attention Startles to sounds (Moro's Reflex) Quiets when hearing mother's voice Makes cooing sounds Looks for sounds with eyes Enjoys listening to music Begins to inhibit sounds that are not meaningful Calms to music Laughs and smiles starting at 3 to 4 months Changes in sucking can indicate responses to sounds[8] *Does not startle to loud sounds* *Shows minimal or complete lack of response to familiar voices* *Does not vocalize* *Is unable to be calmed by soothing sounds*
4–6 months	Begins developing auditory discrimination Starts to develop auditory feedback loop (enjoys hearing own voice, vocalizes repeatedly, vocal turn taking with caregiver) Begins to localize to sound sources with head movement (coincides with sitting up) Laughs Makes cooing noises and/or calms with music and singing Starts babbling towards the end of this age level Makes at least 4 different sounds, primarily first vowels early and then early developing consonants Enjoys noise making toys Uses vocalizations for emotions (happy, upset, fussy, hurting, content) *Does not enjoy making noises with objects or noise makers* *Lacks babbling and abundant vocalizations* *Does not react to tone of voice (e.g., not responsive to "NO!" or "STOP!," or angry versus loving voices)* *Does not show interest in vocal exchanges with caregivers* *Does not respond to music or noises*
7–9 months	Babbles abundantly with at least 2 different syllables Localizes more consistently Starts to respond to own name (typically 8–9 months) Changes pitch from high to low and low to high in vocalizations Uses all suprasegmentals in vocalizations (duration, intensity, pitch) Loves to hear own voice May recognize familiar songs and attempt to make motions (8–9 months) Holds out objects to show people *Produces reduced amount of babbling or babbles with only one sound* *Is not localizing, or localizes to just one side* *Has not acquired many different speech sounds* *Uses primarily neutral vowels or vibrotactile sounds and minimal to no consonants* *Is unresponsive to loud environmental sounds* *Lacks attention to music* *Does not laugh at peek-a-boo and speech games (example: peek-a-boo, How big is baby?—soooo big!, Ride a little horsey up and down)*
10–12 months	The world of auditory comprehension begins to explode Makes connections between objects, people, actions, and words Develops meaningful auditory memory through repetition (example: does the unique motions for different songs; demonstrates understanding of onomatopoeia sounds, such as "moo" = cow) Begins to understand several words and familiar requests Shakes head NO Starts to wave "Hi" and "Bye-bye" Uses voice with music Babbles often and abundantly May have 1–3 true words Starts to use conversational like jargon with suprasegmentals Understands rituals through sound (nighttime and mealtime routines) Attends for short time to reading aloud Loves touchy-feely books *Does not respond to name* *Does not respond to sound from a distance* *Lacks progress in speech sound development* *May stop babbling* *Requires physical touch to get attention* *Responds to music when feeling vibrations instead of through listening*
13–15 months	Starts using single words May use single words in only one situation (e.g., "go" when going on a walk but not when going in the car) Uses communication for a reason: to request, interact, protest, label, greet, direct, show personal needs Initiates speech games Uses jargon with some true words *Uses behavior, not words to communicate*

Data from Tuohy J, Brown J, Mercer-Moseley C. *St. Gabriel's Curriculum for the Development of Audition, Language, Speech, Cognition, Early Communication, Social Interaction, Fine Motor Skills, Gross Motor Skills: A Guide for Professionals Working with Children who are Hearing- Impaired (Birth to Six Years)*. 2nd ed. Sydney: St. Gabriel's Auditory-Verbal Early Intervention Centre; 2005.

with hearing loss, we would look at these milestones starting not from the chronological age (CA based on their date of birth), but from the time they began to access sound optimally and consistently through use of hearing technology. This perspective on development is often referred to as a child's "listening age." When calculating listening age, we must consider both the child's aided hearing data and also wear-time. If children are not able to completely hear the full range of speech sound information or they are not wearing their hearing aids all waking hours, then these are critical considerations for determining how much and how long a child has been hearing. To illustrate this point, think about a 12-month-old baby with a moderate hearing loss who received hearing aids at 3 months old but did not begin wearing the hearing aids all waking hours until 3 months later (at chronological age 6 months old). This child's listening age is only 6 months old because that is the duration of time the child has had exposure to and practice with listening all waking hours.

Additionally, **Table 7.1** lists "*red flags*" or behaviors that may be observed by adults who are active in the lives of young children, such as parents, practitioners, primary physicians, early interventionists, and daycare providers. These behaviors noted in *italics* are warning signs for babies who have not been diagnosed with hearing loss.

Just like any dependable GPS system, we must know where we are starting and where we are going to reach our desired destination. Our starting point is determined by the evaluation data we collect at our initial assessment session(s). We then set goals with the family based on the infant's functional hearing, vocalizations, cognition, and language. Standardized speech, language, and learning assessments, such as the Receptive-Expressive Emergent Language Test, Fourth Edition and the Preschool Language Scale, Fifth Edition, may not provide a full picture of babies' and toddlers' needs. Thus, we rely on developmental and criterion-referenced guides of speech, language, listening, and cognition to measure the baby's baseline and subsequent progress. The following list for early language assessments and developmental inventories is not exhaustive.

- The Rossetti Infant-Toddler Language Scale[9]
- Guide to Communication Milestones, from Linguisystems[10]
- Cottage Acquisition Scales for Listening, Language & Speech (CASLLS)[11]
- MacArthur-Bates Communicative Development Inventories[12]
- Track a Listening Child[13]
- Integrated Scales of Development[14]

Caregiving-coaching begins in the moments following the description and explanation of the test results, when we invite parents immediately to reflect on the information we have shared with them through statements such as "I realize that I've given you a lot to think about and it may be overwhelming. What questions do you have so far?" As the caregiver vocalizes their reactions and feelings, it is especially important for the LSL practitioner to use reflexive listening and validation.

Intervention

Synthesizing all developmental data in one place assists with writing goals so that children with hearing loss make appropriate progress and close the gap between their current skills and those expected for their chronological age. Practitioners must recognize that a child is constantly aging while therapy goals are being targeted. To fully "close the gap," not only do we need to calculate the number of months the child is behind with developing LSL skills compared to their chronological age, but we must also determine the age the child will be at the targeted endpoint of the short-term objectives. For example, if a 12-month-old child has LSL skills at the 6-month-old level on today's date, and we plan to measure progress in 3-month intervals, then our goals must be strategically written to reach LSL skills like that of a 15-month-old (the age the child will be 3 months from now). For a child who is meeting typical cognitive/play, self-help, social-emotional, and motor milestones, it is reasonable for practitioners to strive to make 9 months of progress (the amount of delay currently *plus* the amount of aging the child will do chronologically) in 3 months' time. When additional delays are present, the practitioner and caregiver may need to adjust short- and long-term objectives to match the child's unique rate of progress and overall developmental functioning. (See Chapter 15.)

The Current Level of Functioning (CLF)[15] gives a snapshot of the baby's or beginning listener's present status of meeting milestones across developmental domains, with particular focus on audition, receptive and expressive language, and speech skills. This tool is formatted into Pre-Verbal and Verbal levels, both of which appear in the Resources section of this chapter.

The Pre-Verbal CLF is utilized prior to the baby or young child's first meaningful word (e.g., "No!" while turning the head away from an undesired food; or "Mama!" at the sight of the mother approaching from the other room). The Verbal CLF is utilized when the child begins saying spontaneous, meaningful single words. The LSL practitioner fills out the CLF form based on assessment data using the highest level of skill demonstrated by the child for each area listed. It is most helpful to use a hierarchy such as Track a Listening Child, Integrated Scales of Development or CASLLS to determine specific sub-skills for each age range and to assign an age-equivalent to the baby's or very young listener's performance.

Pearl

The Current Level of Functioning (CLF) gives a snapshot of the baby's or beginning listener's present status of meeting milestones across developmental domains, with particular focus on audition, receptive and expressive language, and speech skills.

For the Ling-Madell-Hewitt/Low-Mid-High (LMH) 10-Sound Test portion of the CLF, write which of the listening check sounds the child can detect, identify, or imitate, and at which distance(s). For the Audition section, write how the child is responding to auditory stimuli through sound awareness, matching of syllable patterns, and suprasegmentals (duration, intensity, and pitch). For the Receptive Language/Early Learning to Listen Sounds sections of the Pre-Verbal CLF, quantify how many of those sounds the baby/young listener understands through tasks such as pointing or item-selection. Likewise, for the Expressive Language/Early Learning to Listen Sounds sections, list how many sounds the baby uses as a label for an animal or object ("moo-moo" for a cow; "aaaaahh" for an airplane). Simply follow the directions described on the Verbal CLF to complete that form. The concept is the same, but for a developmentally older child.

Remember for each section, we want to provide a brief yet informative portrayal of the skills the child can perform. The boxes on the left column prompt the practitioner to assign an age-equivalent score or range to the listener based on what skills have been observed. The domains outside of LSL give important information about the child's global development so we can suggest additional evaluations or therapies, as needed. They also help to gauge the extent of developmental synchrony, how far away the child is from developing milestones in the typical sequence. Those additional areas are not included, however, in the CLF Age calculation for the final box at the bottom left side of the page.

Now that the parents have gained insight into their baby's development, we must involve them in writing and targeting objectives that are meaningful to them and to their everyday life with their infant or beginning listener. Bringing caregivers into a partnership with the practitioner gives them ownership of the process and holds them accountable for doing the hard work outside of the treatment session that is required for the baby or beginning listener to make appropriate progress. We invite this partnership by simply asking, "What are you excited to see your little one do?" "In the next month, what are the top three skills you want to help your child develop?" We guide caregivers to set realistic goals by using our knowledge of child development, supplemented by no-cost, parent-friendly visuals, such as those found online at Child Mind Institute, Zero to Three, and the Centers for Disease Control and Prevention (CDC).

LSL intervention for babies and beginning listeners follows the BHL's or CHL's lead and focuses on what is most salient for the family. The top ten guidelines for intervention are:

1. Always check equipment and do a listening check (e.g., the LMH Test)—ALWAYS.
2. Look at the audiogram.
3. Compare the audiogram to what's possible with learning to listen sounds, linguistic and speech information.
4. Use what you know about auditory access.
5. Plan your intervention based on auditory access.
6. Do developmentally appropriate, FUN, and functional activities.
7. KNOW infant and young child development and apply it specifically to each child.
8. Guide and coach families to be successful.
9. Keep at it even when there is a plateau.
10. Adjust your models of care, tailoring frequency of sessions to family's needs.

Fig. 7.1a,b depicts a lesson plan for a child who has been listening for 13 months with bilateral hearing aids and who is chronologically 16 months old. This plan was created for use in telepractice so the practitioner requested input from the little one's mother to include manipulatives and toys from around the home. For an older child who is beginning to listen, the goals may be the same, but the activities and materials would be specific to their cognitive and play skills and targeted toward their CA.

7.3.3 Keeping It Simple: The Home Program

For a baby or beginning listener to make appropriate progress in listening and spoken language, practitioners must help cultivate activities and real-life scenarios that require little to no thought to carry out during a normal, hectic day in the life of a caregiver. Whether a parent works outside the home or is the stay-at-home parent with their child(ren) during the day, life is busy and logistically complicated.

Literally and figuratively "meeting a family where they are" means doing all we can as practitioners to bring the therapy session to the family. Many private practice agencies are able to go into the daycares and homes of the infant or young child with hearing loss. When in the home environment, the practitioner is able to authentically discover each family's culture and ecosystem. In daycare, the practitioner must include the daycare provider on the child's team. The daycare providers can learn LSL strategies to facilitate developing LSL. Scheduling parent participation sessions at daycare, home, or clinic, emphasizes the caregiver as the primary language model and driver facilitating listening and talking for their child. Additionally, incorporating grandparents, nannies, babysitters, siblings, and neighbors into LSL sessions promotes integrating LSL principles into every facet of the baby's world.

How do we ensure parents work on goals outside of the therapy session? We ask them to brainstorm with us functional, easy, no-fuss activities that they can do with little to no planning! We ask them to walk us through their daily routines; to add up the amount of time they spend in a car-rider line dropping off and picking up an older sibling; to tell us about their work demands and the child's care provider schedule; to describe the chaos of the evenings with older siblings' soccer practice and dinner on-the-go; to detail diaper changing, bath, and bedtime routines. We discuss this information with parents so they may envision and inspire how listening and spoken language will easily fit into their baby's day. Listening and talking are what we do, all day long, regardless of how busy we are!

Caregivers help shape a little listener into a future talker by:

- Singing songs—the classics and the ones made up about baby's needs (e.g., to the tune of "Frere Jacques": "Stinky poopy, stinky poopy, oh-oh-no, oh-oh-no; get a fresh diaper, get a fresh diaper; off we go! off we go!").
- Adding a small cloth book or board book to the baby's diaper bag for on-the-go read-alouds or making up stories about the baby and her environment (e.g., "Once there was a beautiful little baby with big blue eyes! She loved to play patty-cake with her Mommy and go for walks around the neighborhood…"). For an older child who is new to listening, a small tote with a few books can be placed in the car for outings to help keep the child entertained while riding in the car, grocery-shopping, or dining.
- Babywear—by using a wrap or a papoose to keep baby close while a caregiver talks during household chores like laundry and cleaning or while shopping.
- Using a remote microphone during commutes and time in the car so that the baby can hear the parent's voice over road noise and distance. Older children who are much more physically active than babies will benefit tremendously from use of a remote microphone throughout the day so that they can hear what their caregivers say when they are out of earshot.

Lesson plan for: C. Chronological Age: 16 mo.
Listening Age: 13 mo.

GOAL	ACTIVITY/PROCEDURE	DATA	STRATEGIES/TIPS NEXT GOALS	HOME IDEAS
Parent Report: **Listening Check: Ling-Madell-Hewitt/ LMH 10** (C. will detect or identify via imitation each sound at 3 feet or greater):	____ a ____ u ____ m ____ s ____ sh ____ i ____ "J" ____ n ____ z ____ h {conducted via tele-therapy}	Practitioner's Self-Goal for the session: coach C's mother to achieve success with self-talk.	~20 hours prior to session, practitioner sent email to C.'s mother asking if the following manipulatives could be on-hand: pretend food, listening check toys, book options, a puzzle, and any other activities or toys generally enjoyed by C.	
Phoneme Level/Speech Babble C. will imitate all suprasegmentals, vowels and diphthongs, and age-appropriate consonant sounds through Learning to Listen Sounds and word-approximations via babble.	**Materials:** stuffed animals, pictures in book(s), puzzles **Procedure:** provide input via audition of new LLS • Lion or bear = "roar" or "grr" (low-pitched, loud) • Cow = "moo" (long) • Chicken = "cluck-cluck" (short) • ??based on toys (high-pitched and/or short)		• Select stimuli that are different acoustically to provide as much contrast as possible given C.'s degree of hearing loss	
Listening/ Conversation/Auditory processing of connected speech C. will participate in songs, play, and daily routines (simulated in therapy and actual) while responding with gestures, following directions, and vocalizations that show she understands: a. 1-step commands	a) **Materials:** Song with Farm Toy manipulatives, puzzle, or book **Procedure:** input of song *The Farmer in the Dell* …milks the cow …feeds the pig …plants the seeds …gathers eggs …picks the corn		• Give at least 2 full exposures to the song; then, on the 3rd time through, explore cloze / wait-time to see C.'s response	• Make a sock or paper bag puppet to be the farmer and act out various actions with animal toys (cow, pig) and real-life foods (eggs, corn)

Fig. 7.1 (a) A lesson plan for a young toddler, featuring a listening check, practitioner self-goal, and phonetic speech and audition goals, as well as activities, LSL strategies, and home program ideas.

GOAL	ACTIVITY/PROCEDURE	DATA	STRATEGIES/TIPS NEXT GOALS	HOME IDEAS
b. Stereotypical/common phrases c. 150 words/Learning to Listen Sounds **[this is also her (receptive) Vocabulary goal]**	b) **Materials:** puzzle **Procedure:** input of common phrases • "turn it over/around" • "Where's the ____?" • "I see ____." • "You found it!" c) **Materials:** puzzle, book, farm toy, song, pretend food **Procedure:** model/elicit imitation of • Lion or bear = "roar" or "grr" • Cow = "moo" • Chicken = "cluck-cluck" • others??based on toys • food names • food (noun), eat (verb), yummy/good (adjective), sharp (adjective), cut (verb), knife (noun)		• follow child's lead with the puzzle • give child choices between 2 objects (e.g. do you want the __ or the __?)	• Since she wears her hearing aids for a portion of bathtime, this could be a fun search-and-find game in the tub for bath objects
Language [this includes her (expressive) Vocabulary goal] C. will use words mixed with sentence intonation (jargon) in at least 80% of daily vocalizations.	**Materials:** pretend food **Procedure:** • food names • SINGLE WORDS: food (noun), eat (verb), yummy/good (adjective), sharp (adjective), cut (verb), knife (noun)		• Self-talk • Bathe the child in language • Wait-time/expectant look to encourage imitation	• Allow her to use her pretend food at her highchair while you prepare a real meal
Cognition/Other Mother will elicit imitation without use of "say…"	• Ongoing in the session; especially during language goals		• Take turns with mother to practice the skill	
Other/Spontaneous language				

Fig. 7.1 (b) A lesson plan for a young toddler, featuring receptive and expressive language, vocabulary, and parent goals, as well as activities, LSL strategies, and home program ideas.

Pearl

For a baby or beginning listener to make appropriate progress in listening and spoken language, practitioners must help cultivate activities and real-life scenarios that require little to no thought to carry out during a normal, hectic day in the life of a caregiver.

7.4 The Focus of Auditory Development at This Stage

During the first 18 months, babies develop from reflexive behaviors to intentional actions along with auditory comprehension and first words. By looking at and learning neurotypical listening and spoken language development alongside cognitive development, we can begin to formulate how to exploit listening for CHL. This proves to be true for older children who are beginning listeners: we start at the beginning of learning to listen.

7.4.1 Start at Diagnosis

Intervention can and should start quickly after diagnosis of hearing loss. Starting intervention before amplification provides families with some early strategies. For babies who are cochlear implant candidates, hearing aids are fitted before implantation. Currently, the U.S. Food and Drug Administration (FDA) approves cochlear implants by Cochlear Corporation for children at 9 months. Both MED-EL and Advanced Bionics have FDA approval for age 12 months. There are several states that have Medicaid authorization to implant as young as 9 months. Realizing the need to minimize the gap between hearing loss identification and access to speech for learning to listen and speak, a number of cochlear implant teams routinely implant children who are younger than the 9-month FDA guidelines. Along with fitting infants with amplification, ideally within the first 3 months of life, there are several essential elements needed in the infant's life for learning to listen and speak.[16]

7.4.2 Provide a Quiet Listening Environment

(For in-depth information about optimal listening environments and hearing technology see Chapter 2.)

In our modern world, the biggest culprits of noise pollution are transportation, everyday sounds (TV, radio, appliances, telephones, landscape equipment), workplace noise, and population growth.[17] There is evidence that young children have challenges learning words when there is too much background noise.[18] The subjects of both these studies were children with typical hearing. The impact of a noisy environment is exponentially worse as the infant with hearing loss has poorer access to speech. Some strategies to reduce home noise include the following suggestions:

- Turn off the TV, smart speaker, or radio if not in use.
- Move away from noisy appliances and use them during sleep time (e.g., run the dishwasher at night).

- Establish quiet listening spaces at home for reading and playing with baby.
- Use carpets, rugs, and pillows to help absorb sound.
- Walk through the home and identify noise sources to avoid.
- Use a sound-level meter app on smart phones to measure noise levels.

How can we help caregivers appreciate the impact of their baby's hearing loss? Using a familiar sounds audiogram (examples: John Tracy Center, https://www.jtc.org/hearing-loss; Hearing First, https://www.hearingfirst.org/m/resources/7734) to illustrate the loudness of many common sound sources helps caregivers learn about their child's hearing loss. By overlaying the baby's audiogram onto the familiar sounds audiogram, caregivers have a picture of their baby's hearing loss and how it impacts listening and language. We can also encourage parents and caregivers to try a "hearing loss simulation" in which they wear earplugs for several hours. While typically hearing adults will have, at most, a mild hearing loss when using earplugs, the simulation should help them experience some of the real-life challenges of navigating the world with hearing loss. Another way is to use internet videos that simulate different types of hearing loss. Examples of plain language hearing loss simulations include (this is not an exhaustive list):

- Flintstones Hearing Loss—https://youtube/zHWZ-iBhz-4
- Phonak hearing loss simulation—https://www.phonak.com/us/en/hearing-loss/signs-of-hearing-loss-and-what-to-do/hearing-loss-simulation.html
- Success for Kids with Hearing Loss: https://successforkidswithhearingloss.com/demonstrations-simulated-listening-with-hearing-loss-devices/#Loss

7.4.3 Establish Consistent Hearing Technology Use and Strategies to Access Sound

Besides reducing noise, parents and caregivers can use strategies to provide optimal access to any audible speech signal. First and foremost, infants must wear their hearing technology, in working order, with appropriate settings for all waking hours. The mantra "eyes open, hearing technology on" sets the tone for the best auditory brain stimulation. Keeping hearing technology on infants and toddlers is an arduous task for caregivers. Practitioners can partner with caregivers through teaching, counseling, and providing resources to increase wear time, thus giving the baby's brain auditory stimulation. Creating an environment for successful hearing aid retention includes:

- well-fitted earmolds
- quiet listening environment
- options for hearing aid retention
- family and professional support system
- caregiver commitment
- partnering with childcare for hearing technology retention
- visible success with hearing aids

Families with dual working parents may find hearing technology retention in a daycare, nursery school, or home-based care setting difficult. Parents worry about childcare personnel losing the devices, not replacing dead batteries, putting devices on incorrectly, and not putting them on the child. Childcare workers are anxious about losing the devices, financial responsibility, another child taking them, battery ingestion, and other hazards. Some tips from "Keeping Hearing Technology On: Support from Your Child's Caregivers"[19] include:

- Arrive at daycare with technology on and working.
- Teach caregivers how to check that the devices are working and how to put them on.
- Have a technology supply kit for daycare.
- Enlist other professionals to partner with daycare for intervention carry-over.

Oticon publishes *Meeting the Challenge: Keeping Hearing Devices on Young Children*,[20] an easy-to-follow, research-based guide for practitioners to share with families. This resource features pictures of infants and toddlers wearing various retention devices and briefly and powerfully expresses the "why" and "when" of young children's hearing aid needs. The authors break down the age ranges of children from birth to age 5 and provide specific developmental features of each age group. The document outlines the challenges caregivers typically face during those ages for hearing aid retention and strategies for mitigating those struggles. Finally, the resource summarizes ratings of each main type of hearing aid retention device based on the results of the Children's Hearing Aid Retention Survey by Anderson and Madell.

7.4.4 Strategies for Facilitating Auditory Development

Listening Bubble

For infants and toddlers to have maximum access to sound, their caregivers need to be inside their listening bubble (**Fig. 7.2a,b**). The listening bubble concept is also true for older children learning to listen. To establish a listening bubble, caregivers present sounds at different distances from the baby (with technology on) and observe responses. Initially we use any speech sounds for input: singing, animal noises, babbling. Later, when the child has more listening experience, we obtain low-, mid-, and high-frequency responses with the Ling-Madell-Hewitt test.[21] The distance where the child responds to speech sounds sets the boundaries for optimal auditory input. For a child with hearing aids, we can use the listening bubble to monitor hearing loss. For example, a child with an aided benefit at 20 dB

Pearl

The mantra "eyes open, hearing technology on" sets the tone for the best auditory brain stimulation.

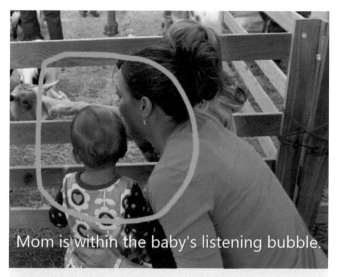

Fig. 7.2 (a) A photograph of a baby and her mother at an outing. Mom's positioning within the baby's listening bubble provides maximum auditory input for developing listening and spoken language outcomes.

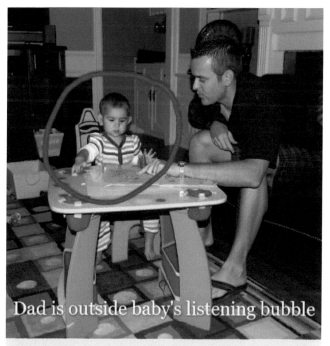

Fig. 7.2 (b) A photograph of a baby and her father during play at home. The dad is outside the baby's listening bubble. She will not have maximum auditory input. Dad can use the strategy of positioning for maximum auditory input and move closer to her. That will allow him to provide her the best listening experience for developing listening and spoken language outcomes.

imitates "shhh" at 3 feet. Three months later, mom reports that the child cannot imitate "shhh" at 1 foot or 3 feet and does not respond to that sound. That is a red flag for technology trouble, middle ear disease, and/or possibly a progression in the child's hearing loss.

Talking, reading, and singing to babies within that listening bubble exploit listening intentionally. Within that listening bubble, strategies to help maximize listening for the baby or older beginning listener include the following:

- Using a normal conversational loudness level—get closer, not louder
- Calling attention to sound and attaching meaning to it
- Singing
- Reading aloud
- Talking to the child in a quiet environment

Parentese

A newborn baby's first entry into the world is filled with sound. Although the auditory system is immature and the middle ear may have fluid post-delivery, typically hearing infants hear rather clearly at birth. They prefer infant-directed speech. Most often, adults naturally use "motherese" or "parentese" when they talk to babies. This "parentese" is higher in pitch and contains greater melodic contour; there is greater variation separating the highest and lowest pitches. Phrases are shortened, the rate is slower, vowels tend to be exaggerated, and specific words may have emphasis over others. For example, a parent might talk to the baby saying, "*Baby is soooooooo BIG!*" in lieu of "*Baby is so big!*" This infant-directed speech captures babies' attention through listening. These infant-directed speech activities stimulate the auditory cortex, and thus the baby embarks on beginning to learn speech and language through listening. For the neurotypical child with typical hearing, the first 12 months is the "learning to listen year"[22] with thousands of hours of listening experience. For BHL and older beginning listeners, their auditory systems need intentional, redundant, and meaningful auditory input. We want to capture their attention through listening. To do that we must exploit the auditory information by providing maximum auditory input.

7.5 The Focus of Language Development at This Stage

7.5.1 Receptive Language

Voices, reading aloud, music, and relevant environmental sounds facilitate auditory brain development.[23] What are the most relevant, meaningful sounds for the baby to hear in utero? Hearing the parents' voices is the most significant sound for babies. Babies recognize voices during the last trimester and can recognize those voices at birth.[24] For BHL, their auditory development, and thus their receptive language development, is at a disadvantage before birth. As they grow, the disadvantage is exponential. Babies with typical hearing need a minimum of 10–12 months of learning to listen and understand language before beginning to talk and another 12 months to acquire use of a 200–to 300–word

vocabulary.[10] By the age of 5, typically hearing children understand at least 10,000 words[25] and use about 2,000–2,500 words. That is, a child will possess a minimum of 4 to 5 times more receptive vocabulary than expressive vocabulary. These facts and figures again highlight the urgency to identify BHL, fit them with amplification, and initiate a partnership with parents for facilitating listening and spoken language.

With beginning listeners, regardless of their age, auditory development for receptive language is foundational for conversational competence, natural-sounding and intelligible speech production, and literacy skills. Receptive language, also known as auditory comprehension, is the result of auditory brain development and always precedes spoken expressive language. Yes, children need to be able to express their wants and needs, but they cannot do this until they have words firmly cemented in their receptive knowledge. Think about trying to request something in a language you do not know. You do not know the word for what you want, and even if someone prompts you with the word, it means nothing to you. In the same way, with all children, but especially with older children, working on expressive language before receptive language results in poor outcomes for developing conversational competence and academic success. When we have children imitate without word knowledge, they lack meaningful understanding of spoken language. Therefore, regardless of a child's CA, when there is a hearing loss and lack of auditory development, we start intervention at the beginning of the auditory hierarchy to develop a foundation for receptive language. (See Chapter 11 for more information.)

Pitfall

With all children, but especially with older children, working on expressive language before receptive language results in poor outcomes for developing conversational competence and academic success. When we have children imitate without word knowledge, they lack meaningful understanding of spoken language.

Pearl

Regardless of a child's chronological age, when there is a hearing loss and lack of auditory development, we start intervention at the beginning of the auditory hierarchy.

For babies and beginning listeners to develop a strong foundation of receptive language, their auditory brain development must progress through the auditory hierarchy from basic awareness of sound through multiple steps to finally arrive at auditory comprehension. Interventionists and caregivers alike should have a clear understanding of the progression of auditory skill development and the current level of the child. Two well-known, evidence-based hierarchies of auditory skill development are those of Erber[26] (**Fig. 7.3**) and Pollack[22] (**Fig. 7.4**). These are the same auditory hierarchies with different nomenclature.

Resources for other auditory development hierarchies (not an exhaustive list):

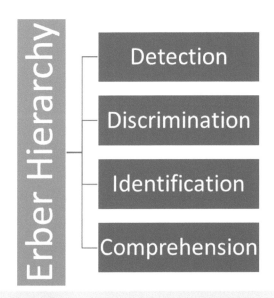

Fig. 7.3 The Erber Hierarchy of auditory skills development, adapted. Data from Erber N. *Auditory Training*. Washington DC: Alexander Graham Bell Association; 1982: 92–94.

- Auditory Learning Guide[27]
- Cottage Acquisition Scales for Listening, Language, and Speech (CASLLS)[11]
- The Shepherd Centre Functional Listening Index[28]
- Listening Skills Scale for Auditory-Verbal Therapy (LSSAVT)[29]
- Track a Listening Child[13]

Strategies for Facilitating Receptive Language Development

How do we focus on receptive language intervention during that first learning-to-listen year? Using Erber's hierarchy (detection, discrimination, identification, comprehension) as the framework for intervention, we make sure the baby or older beginning listener has appropriately fit hearing technology, a quiet listening environment, and caregivers within the BHL/CHL's listening bubble. Babies and beginning listeners are usually starting at detection and moving to beginning comprehension in the first year. During the first year for a baby with hearing loss, progress is dependent on access to speech information. For example, a baby who is a cochlear implant candidate and who only has access to speech information at 40 dB from 250 Hz through 1500 Hz with hearing aids will have a different (and much slower) rate of progress than a baby with aided benefit at 20 dB from 250 Hz through 8000 Hz. These differences in progress should not lower our expectations for the child with poor access to speech information but should be a catalyst for us to advocate for optimal auditory access as quickly as possible.

Detection: For detection, we want to start with rich auditory experiences. Some ways to facilitate sound detection are:

- Use noisemakers (rattles, squeaky toys, musical toys) as part of play for fun, transitions, or song props.[30] Get the baby's attention through the noisemaker sound and then talk about

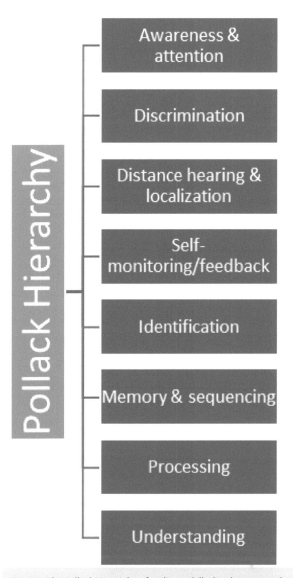

Fig. 7.4 The Pollack Hierarchy of auditory skills development, adapted. Data from Pollack D, Goldberg D, Caleffe-Schenck N. *Educational Audiology for the Limited-Hearing Infant and Preschooler: An Auditory-Verbal Program*. 3rd ed. Springfield, IL: Charles C. Thomas; 1997.

it. By talking about it, we attach meaning to the noisemaker. Noisemakers alone are not meaningful and become uninteresting quickly if they are used over and over again to "test" the baby's hearing.

- Model pointing to the ear and saying, "I hear that" when important environmental sounds and voices are detected.
- Use the LMH Test. For a baby with hearing loss, we want to know the "listening bubble" range for the LMH sounds. What phonemes result in a listening behavior response? What phonemes are not heard? At what distance does the child respond to each sound?
- Make animal sounds with toy animals using dramatic inflections, repetitions, and prolonging the sounds. Make the animal sound as if you were wearing the animal's costume and performing in a play!

- Sing songs and observe for behavior that shows the baby hears the sounds. By looking at the baby's audiogram and keeping in mind the listening bubble concept, determine songs that are accessible to the baby. For example, a baby with more auditory information in lower frequencies is more likely to detect "Old MacDonald Had a Farm" with the animal noises "moo," "baa," and "quack," versus "The Itsy Bitsy Spider" with its high frequency information in multiple /s/ words ("spider," "sun," "so," "itsy," "bitsy," "spout").
- Reading aloud using props to call attention to sound. In Bill Martin Jr.'s "Brown Bear, Brown Bear, What Do You See?" have the animal props out of the baby's sight. Make an animal's sound and watch for detection behaviors. When you observe those behaviors, bring out the animal, match it to the book page, and read.
- Using the onomatopoeia for Learning to Listen sounds (LtL) that have acoustic specific information consistent with the available speech access.[31,32] For example, a child with aided benefit of 30 dB at 250 Hz through 1000 Hz should detect "mmmmm" for ice cream, "oooo" for train, "wheeeee" for slide, "ahhhhh" for airplane, "bu bu bu bu" for bus, and "zzzzzz" for the bee.

Discrimination: For discrimination, we are looking for the baby to discern the difference between, for example, music versus speech versus knocking on the door. We can observe for progress in this area by:

- using music and encouraging dancing and movement; observe the baby's response to music in comparison to the response to speech or environmental sounds
- turning music on and off while observing the baby's responses to sound-on and sound-off
- continuing to use LtL sounds that have different acoustic qualities can also facilitate discrimination; an example is how the baby responds to the long duration of "mmmmmmm" for ice cream in comparison to "bu bu bu" for bus
- coloring with the child and making different sounds for different coloring patterns to see whether the child's motions change (for instance, coloring in continuous circles or spirals can be accompanied by "woo woo woo" while tapping the crayon to make dots can be accompanied by "bu bu bu"; when the child is coloring in circles, change from saying "woo woo woo" to "bu bu bu" and observe whether the child begins tapping the crayon)

Auditory Identification: Before children can comprehend chunks of information such as following directions, retelling a story, or answering questions, they need to attach specific, unique meaning to words and sounds. This is auditory identification. The identification level includes speech sound imitation. When children connect a sound to something specific or imitate a speech sound they hear, we know that they can identify that sound based on their action or imitation.

- Use the pictures of the LMH Test to see if the child points to the correct pictures when a sound is made.
- As soon as children can imitate, listen for imitation of the phonemes in the LMH Test. If the child's imitation matches the phoneme presented, then phoneme identification is confirmed. If the phoneme is produced differently from the model, the errored production gives us clues as to what the child may and may not be hearing. (See Chapter 3.)
- Observe identification behaviors in the environment. If the doorbell rings, does the child go to the door? If a phone rings, does a child look to a phone?
- Use the LtL sounds and observe identifications the child makes. For instance, if we say "moo," does the child look to or pick up the cow?

Comprehension: Early comprehension through listening is somewhat dependent on the child's aided benefit for speech information. Again, by comparing the baby's audiogram with the Speech String Bean and the Familiar Sounds Audiogram, we can determine how best to facilitate comprehension.[32,33] With audition alone, typically hearing children ages 9–18 months can:

- respond to "Wave bye-bye," "clap your hands," "peek-a-boo"
- show understanding of firm tone of voice for "No" and "Stop"
- understand family members' and pets' names (points, looks, moves to indicate understanding)
- follow simple, familiar commands, i.e., "Give it to me," "Let's go," "Get your shoes," "Sit down," "Come here"
- make choices, e.g., "Do you want milk or water?"
- point to pictures in books when named, e.g., "Where's the cow?"
- identify up to 4 body parts when named
- bring something familiar from another part of the house, e.g., "Go get your bunny"

How can we determine what to target for comprehension when the child is entering this stage? The easiest receptive language to observe is through the use of commands. If we tell a child to do something without any visual prompts and the child does it, then we have a good indication of auditory comprehension. For a child with access to all speech information through hearing technology (hearing aids or cochlear implants), we collaborate with parents about what would be most helpful for their child to understand at home. For some families understanding "sit down," "stop!" "Be careful" may be important for safety reasons. For more independent beginning listeners, commands related to routines may be the first priority (e.g., "brush your teeth," "wash your hands," "time for night-night"). When the child has access to all speech information at the Speech String Bean, then comprehending familiar commands with varying acoustic qualities is possible.

For a child with aided benefit for speech information at 30–40 dB from 250 Hz through 1000 Hz and 50 dB or poorer at 2000 Hz and above, we need to be creative to determine what commands might fit within the audible range. Although the child may be scheduled for cochlear implant surgery, that does not stop us from working on auditory comprehension in advance. For this child, we could target familiar commands with low- and mid-frequency information such as:

- "Let's go night-night" (access to the /n/, F_1 of /ai/ and duration suprasegmental)
- "Knock-knock" for knocking on doors, boxes, etc., in routines (access to /n/, F_1 of /a/, duration suprasegmental)

- "Go bye-bye" (access to F_1 for /b/, F_1 of /ai/, duration suprasegmental)

Similarly for an older child, we find familiar commands/phrases/requests that are relevant to their age and lower language level. For example, a 5-year-old with 1 year of listening experience with aided benefit at the "Speech String Bean," we could target frequent caregiver requests for a 5-year-old. These could include: "Get your backpack," "Wash your hands," "Put your plate in the sink," "Brush your teeth."

For a child with a profound, bilateral sensorineural hearing loss awaiting cochlear implantation, detection and discrimination may be the limits of auditory development before the implant. Those two steps may seem insignificant, but they ready the auditory system for more input after implantation. Detection and discrimination lay the foundation for attaching specific meaning to sound for identification and auditory comprehension.

Even though auditory comprehension is easiest to observe using commands, clinicians and parents need to ensure they are not overusing commands in their communication with a beginning listener. While babies begin to understand simple one-step commands by 12 to 15 months, at the same time, they should be developing receptive vocabulary which, at this age, is made up primarily of nouns (e.g., family names, toys, foods, body parts).[10] If we use primarily commands, we run the risk that children will begin to think of these commands as nouns. For example, many children with hearing loss have been observed to call a toothbrush a "brush your teeth." To avoid this, we need to help parents understand that babies and beginning listeners do not know that people, items, and actions have names. What is so clear to us—because we know language—is absolutely foreign to babies and beginning listeners. It is estimated that a baby will need to hear a word 1,000 times before comprehension of the word is cemented in the auditory brain. By toddlerhood, children may only need to hear a word 50 times to auditorily comprehend it and add it to their receptive vocabulary, but those first words need lots and lots and lots of repetition for babies. This need for tremendous repetition is no different for older beginning listeners.

Thus, we need to coach parents to use the names of people and objects in simple but clear statements, questions, and commands as they talk to their baby or beginning listener. Think about the difference between *"Let's put your shirt on. Do you want the shirt with the rainbow or the shirt with the bow? You picked the rainbow shirt. Pull your shirt over your head."* and *"Time to get dressed. Which one do you want? Pick one. Put it on."* The first communication allows the child to hear the word *"shirt"* a number of times to encourage comprehension and storage of this word in the auditory brain. The first communication also provides simple but rich language in each sentence to allow the child to hear additional receptive vocabulary. The second communication lacks specificity in every utterance. With this type of non-specific communication, while children may learn to understand *"time to get dressed"* or *"put it on,"* they will have limited opportunities to hear important vocabulary repeated over and over again and will not begin to comprehend critical words in an utterance (e.g., "Put your *shirt* on" vs. "Put your *pants* on.")

Questions are another excellent way to build auditory comprehension by providing opportunities to hear words over and over again. While parents and clinicians may be tempted to ask yes/no questions at this stage, asking questions with a choice allows us to input vocabulary and encourage auditory comprehension. Think about the difference between asking *"Do you want to put your shirt on?"* and *"Do you want to put on your shirt or your pants?"* The first question requires little to no understanding, but the second question provides the opportunity to hear two nouns (*shirt, pants*) and encourages the child to begin comprehending that each word refers to something different.

Finally, books are also an excellent way to expose a baby or beginning listener to receptive language over and over again. Most of us may have only a toy cow at home, but reading a book about cows allows us to show the child photographs of a cow and encourage comprehension of the word "cow" by using it over and over again. In the same way, language experience books, which have photographs and narration of the child's activities (see Chapters 5 and 13) enable us to repeat the language of the park every day, even when it is too rainy or cold for a visit.

We must always be cognizant of the fact that receptive language is the foundation for expressive language development and that babies and beginning listeners need significant repetition of words—1,000 times for the first words—to develop auditory comprehension of them. Only by exposing the child to a variety of language-rich commands, statements, and questions can we begin to develop a strong foundation of auditory comprehension/receptive language.

7.5.2 Expressive Language

How do babies communicate expressively? From birth, babies are tiny communicators. Crying is their primary means of communication for the first 5 months. They cry when hungry, tired, uncomfortable, hurting, needing a diaper change, and for no reason at all. When caregivers talk to babies, they may become quiet, smile, make excited body movements, or change their sucking patterns.[8] During these first 5 months, babies start smiling and discover their voice. They start making vowel sounds, cooing, and making noises such as gurgling and blowing raspberries. Caregivers can hear differences in the baby's vocalizations with laughing, fussing, and squealing. Babies may try to imitate facial expressions and coo back to caregivers who talk to them.

During the 6–11 months stage, the baby's communication expands beyond crying with some early reduplicated or canonical babbling such as "ba-ba-ba." The baby will take turns back and forth making sounds with a caregiver or do "serve and return." We begin to see imitation, starting with hand and body movements along with imitating some early developing speech sounds. Typically hearing babies at this stage love singing and music. You will hear dramatic changes in their suprasegmentals of duration, intensity, and pitch. Towards the end of this period, you may see or hear the baby do head shaking for "no," make some animal sounds, try to "sing" with songs, and point to an object or person with a vocalization. Towards the end of the second 6 months, babies will participate in social games. Playing *peek-a-boo, how big is baby? baby is soooo big, touchdown!* are easy, familiar, and fun speech games and fingerplays leading to communicative engagement between caregivers and babies.

As babies approach their first year, they start imitating adult speech sounds and patterns, pointing to something they want or want to show, making specific sounds for specific toys or objects (cars, animals), waving "bye-bye," and calling parents "mama" or "dada" or other word approximation. Their expressive communication becomes more specific.

Moving into the second year (12–18 months), we see babies use more jargon-like vocalizations with changing suprasegmentals. The jargon starts sounding as if it is a conversation and may have a few true words in the mix. When caregivers ask, "What's that?" babies in this stage start answering with a label such as "dog," "ball," "cookie." More true words appear along with some word combinations: "more juice," "shoes off," "hi mama." One hears rising inflections for questioning and the beginning use of "What's that?" By the end of the first 18 months, typically hearing babies have 20–100 or more words.[10]

Strategies for Facilitating Expressive Language Development through Listening

What about babies with hearing loss and beginning listeners? How do we facilitate expressive language development through listening? Children with typical hearing learn to listen and speak through incidental learning. They overhear words thousands of times, learn what sounds go with what objects/actions/feelings, and learn from listening to and engaging with others. For CHL, we must intentionally teach spoken language through listening. CHL may learn some through incidental listening as their auditory development progresses, but early on, practitioners and caregivers use intentional strategies and activities to facilitate spoken language.

The optimal way to work on expressive language is to embed LSL strategies within daily routines. Remember that receptive language is the foundation for expressive language. Babies learn to talk because they hear language around them, begin to comprehend the words, then—and only then—begin to use them expressively. We know from evidence and research that the number and quality of words that children hear the first 3 years impacts their later expressive vocabulary and reading success.[34] The greater the variety of words a child hears, the larger the expressive vocabulary later. According to Carol Flexer, CHL need "multiple, redundant, extrinsic practice opportunities to develop those auditory brain centers."[35] One of the best ways for children to learn expressive language is by hearing caregivers talk about what they are doing and by listening to caregivers read aloud. Daily life as a family with routines and activities provides the best opportunity for children to learn language. When practitioners partner with caregivers to teach and coach them about using LSL strategies throughout the day, babies and beginning listeners get that extrinsic practice often and with redundancy.

Expressive language strategies (see also Chapter 10) to use with babies and beginning listeners include the following:

- Expectant look—using a facial expression (raised eyebrows, surprised look, questioning look) to show the child you expect a response
- Joint attention—sharing a common focus with the child or following the child's lead
- Modeling—talking to a baby or child about what is happening using rich, grammatically-correct language

- Motherese or parentese—using a singsong voice when talking to babies. (video example can be found at https://www.youtube.com/watch?v=eZclOL7vIQQ)
- Serve and return—encouraging the back-and-forth communication and interaction between baby and caregiver (video example can be found at https://developingchild.harvard.edu/science/key-concepts/serve-and-return/)[36]
- Wait time or pausing—providing input or interacting with the baby or beginning listener and waiting expectantly for a response; giving the child auditory processing time and expecting a response
- Repetition—repeating information in a salient, highlighted manner. For example, *"I'm going to pick you up, up, up! Up, up, up you go! Daddy is going to pick you up, up, up to go bye-bye!"*
- Acoustic highlighting—using your voice as a highlighter for a word, phrase, or sound. For example, *"mmmmmmmmmm, that is soooooooo yummy,"* is highlighting by prolonging sounds in a word.

Additional Strategies for Facilitating Spoken Expressive Language for a Beginning Listener

Although some clinicians and many parents want older, beginning listeners to quickly learn to express themselves, we must use the same strategies as with a baby, but with different activities and routines. Beginning listeners, especially those with minimal vocalizations and minimal to no auditory experience, need highly successful, functional, and fun auditory and speech experiences. Before we can expect beginning listeners to talk, they need multiple, redundant, and extrinsic practice opportunities to develop auditory pathways. (See Chapter 11). Abundant use of vocalization is the first step in developing expressive language as we facilitate developing auditory function.[23] Encourage abundant vocalization in beginning listeners through:

- Using music and singing
- Playing hand-clapping games
- Reading-aloud and using vocal sound effects for the child to imitate
- Humming
- Vocalizing for requests
- Prompting to get "UH-OH!" and "OW!" to develop as early meaningful, intelligible expressions
- Modeling whispering
- Using an auditory sandwich strategy, starting with audition, followed by vibro-tactile or visual (have child touch your throat to feel vibration or see your lips during an utterance), and ending with audition only

Pearl

One of the best ways for children to learn expressive language is by hearing caregivers talk about what they are doing and reading aloud. Daily life as a family with routines and activities provides the best opportunity for children to learn language.

7.6 The Focus of Speech Development at This Stage

How do neurotypical, hearing infants develop speech for their language? As they grow, they develop abilities in producing and controlling speech sounds. Whether we are discussing a typically hearing infant or a baby who has hearing loss and is optimally fit with technology, the vocal behaviors they exhibit reflect their speech development. For children who are later-identified with hearing loss and do not receive optimum access to the full range of speech frequencies until they are older, we view speech development as truly beginning when consistent use of optimal hearing technology is established, rather than what is expected for that child's CA. To ensure speech milestones are met in a developmentally appropriate way, we follow guides like those shown in **Table 7.2** which describes the most foundational speech skills in the first year to year-and-a-half of life.[10,37,38,39] As we carefully plan intervention, consulting the developmental speech hierarchy reminds us that each new skill targeted must develop on the preceding skill(s). A 3-year-old with a moderately-severe hearing loss being fit with hearing aids for the first time should not be expected to master age-appropriate phonemes such as /f/ until

after we have ensured the child is able to imitate and then use all suprasegmentals, vowels, and early developing consonants. We are ever mindful to view babies, toddlers, preschoolers, or even school-aged children by their length and consistency of listening experiences, their access to all speech frequencies, and their current developmental level.

Daniel Ling described 7 states of speech acquisition for phonetic and phonologic levels,[40] adapted in **Table 7.3**. The phonetic level relates to human sounds. The phonologic level relates to how humans use those sounds in a specific language. The levels provide a structure for remediating speech disorders secondary to hearing loss. In working with CHL 0–18 months, facilitating natural sounding speech happens through providing an acoustically salient speech model during play and daily routines via the developmental model. Children who receive amplification later in life may need a remedial model based on the developmental hierarchy of acquiring speech. Developing a working knowledge and practice in early vocal development and speech acquisition is the foundation for facilitating natural sounding, highly intelligible speech in CHL. A famous adage of Dr. Daniel Ling is "We speak how we hear." As an example, depending on the degree

Table 7.2 Speech developmental milestones

Birth–3 months	Cries automatically and makes vegetative sounds such as burping, sneezing, coughing, releasing gas
2–5 months	Coos, smiles Becomes more social, laughs in interactions with caregivers Begins to make back consonants and vowels /uuu/ and /aaaa/
4–8 months	Starts performing vocal play Blows raspberries and squeals Increases vocalizations with more vowel and consonant variety Displays growing speech sound inventory
6–9 months	Displays canonical babbling (repeats same sound sequence such as /nanana/) Begins early consonant production of /b, p, m, n, d/
9–12 months	Performs non-reduplicated babbling—repetition of consonant-vowel (CV) combinations that are not repeated such as /ma–ba–ga/ Produces larger variation of consonants, abundant suprasegmental features Uses jargon Produces native language sounds with more specificity
9–14 months	Says words and uses word approximations, including some invented words such as "baba" for "bottle" Uses some true words having CV, VC, and CVC syllable structures
10–18 months	Continues to develop a wider range of consonants and vowels with suprasegmental use Begins to use sounds and words for wants, rejection, continuing activity, greetings, comments, and exchanging objects with adults Produces onomatopoeia sounds Points with question inflection Says "no" Vocalizes to songs, nursery rhymes and may have auditory closure for those

Data from Lanza JR, Flahive LK. *Guide to Communication Milestones: Concepts, Feeding, Morphology, Literacy, Mean Length of Utterance, Phonological Awareness, Pragmatics, Pronouns, Questions, Speech Sound Acquisition, Vocabulary.* East Moline, IL: LinguiSystems; 2008. Carson L. Stages of Early Vocal Development. http://talkingtogether.com.au/wp-content/uploads/2018/08/stages-of-early-vocal-development.pdf. Published 2018. Accessed November 6, 2021. NIDCD. "Speech and Language Developmental Milestones." https://www.nidcd.nih.gov/health/speech-and-language. Accessed November 6, 2021. Your Child's Development: Age-Based Tips From Birth to 36 Months. https://www.zerotothree.org/resources/series/your-child-s-development-age-based-tips-from-birth-to-36-months. Published 2008. Accessed November 6, 2021.

Table 7.3 Ling's phonetic-phonologic levels of speech acquisition

Phonetic level	Phonologic level
Uses voice abundantly	Vocalizes on purpose
Produces suprasegmentals (duration, intensity, pitch)	Communicates with vocal patterns
Produces vowels and diphthongs	Starts to approximate words with vowels and diphthongs
Produces consonants that differ by manner	Uses some true, clear words with natural voice quality
Produces consonants that differ by voice	Has clear sentences with natural voice quality
Produces consonants that differ by place	Uses clear phrases with natural voice quality
Produces blends	Produces intelligible speech with natural voice quality

Data from Ling D. *Foundations of Spoken Language for Hearing-Impaired Children.* Washington, DC: Alexander Graham Bell Association for the Deaf; 1988.

and configuration of the child's hearing loss, babble may lack complexity and the speech sound repertoire within babble may be limited.

When working with babies with hearing loss who have goals for natural voice quality with highly intelligible speech, the practitioner is to address developing speech through listening from the onset of evaluation and intervention. Speech production is an integrated part of the intervention plan. By using the developmental hierarchy and observing behaviors, along with the Ling phonetic-phonologic levels as a reference for remediation, practitioners have a foundation for teaching natural-sounding speech through listening. Natural-sounding, intelligible speech through listening is only possible when the child has maximum access to all speech frequencies during all waking hours. For those children who are cochlear implant candidates, their "all speech frequencies" access will not be possible pre-implantation. That does not preclude practitioners from addressing speech through listening, pre-cochlear implantation. Providing auditory input within the baby's accessible hearing is the key to stimulating auditory pathways, developing sound awareness, and learning that sound is meaningful.

We learn to speak based on what we hear. For example, a 12-month-old child with bilateral cochlear implants was the youngest of 4 children in a family that immigrated from Pakistan and spoke Urdu. The older siblings and parents were fluent in English. The parents' English had an accent consistent with their native Urdu. The parents desired that their child with hearing loss learn English as a first language. The child's primary language facilitator was the mother. From the onset of intervention, the mother provided rich listening and spoken language to her child in English, with an Urdu accent. As the child progressed and began talking, she used early English words, with an Urdu accent. This child learned to speak with the same vocal quality as her family.

Pearl

We learn to speak based on what we hear.

7.6.1 Strategies for Facilitating Speech Development

In an LSL approach, working on speech happens throughout the session and in the child's daily life. The desired outcome is natural-sounding speech with rich suprasegmentals, coarticulation, and a high level of conversational intelligibility. Encourage caregivers and family members to practice strategies in modeling speech to develop automaticity. Coach caregivers to consistently model the correct speech production when a child makes an error. We want the child to hear the correct production. The child may not imitate or correct the error, and that is okay! The purpose of the correct production is for the child to hear the accurate sounds. Specific strategies (see Chapter 10) to promote this outcome are listed in the following paragraph. It may seem inappropriate to use parentese with a 6-year-old beginning listener. The acoustic features of parentese may still be necessary and beneficial for the older child who is new to listening. We cannot start with the articulation of consonants that we would typically expect in an older child. This 6-year-old who is a beginning listener still needs a rich, salient, meaningful speech model starting with abundant vocalizations, suprasegmentals, and vowels for developing speech through listening.

Where do we start with a beginning listener who is not a baby? We start with successful vocalization experiences. Many older beginning listeners have poor experiences using speech (e.g., highly unintelligible speech, bullying at school because of voice quality, preferring gestures/signs to speaking, etc.). Using fun, high-interest, low-level activities is key to improving speech for older beginning listeners. The Ling Phonetic-Phonologic Model (**Table 7.3**) is a framework for intervention. For example, a beginning listener with bilateral cochlear implants activated at age 5 years vocalizes purposefully. The child is producing speech with durational changes (ahhhhhhhhhhhhhh versus u–u–u–u) with a loud intensity. The next step in speech work would be producing pitch changes and intensity changes with vowels. Use parentese with dramatic vocal changes to model vocal quality for the child. Motor movements replicating up and down while modeling pitch changes can be effective in facilitating pitch changes:

- Going up and down stairs when working on pitch
- Using pictures representing loud and soft sounds or high- and low-pitched sounds
- Using a sound-level meter app on smart phones to demonstrate real time biofeedback related to loudness levels
- Songs and speech games with movements or characters that lend themselves to incorporating pitch changes (e.g., "The Grand Old Duke of York," https://www.songsforteaching.com/folk/nobledukeofyork.php; "Baby Shark," https://www.today-sparent.com/baby/baby-development/baby-shark-lyrics/; "Go Bananas," https://genius.com/Little-big-go-bananas-lyrics)

Beginning listeners often enjoy these activities to facilitate early and frequent vocalizations:

- Making a comb kazoo. This is a comb with wax paper. Press your lips to the comb and vocalize. The voice makes the paper vibrate and changes the voice.

- Using musical instruments that require breath (flute, kazoo, horn)
- Using a microphone or a whisper phone (such as that found at https://www.learning-loft.com) and having the child makes sounds into it

Strategies to maximize speech development include employment of:

- Audition first
- Changing rate
- Modeling correct production
- Parentese
- Positioning for maximum auditory input
- Repetition

Pearl

If the child has poor experiences with using speech (e.g., highly unintelligible speech, bullying at school because of voice quality, preferring gestures/signs to speaking, etc.), using fun, high-interest, low-level activities is key to improving speech for older beginning listeners.

Pitfall

With an older child who is new to listening, we cannot start with the articulation of consonants that we would typically expect in an older child. A beginning listener who is older still needs a rich, salient, meaningful speech model starting with abundant vocalizations, suprasegmentals, and vowels for developing speech through listening.

7.7 The Focus of Cognition, Pragmatics, and Play at This Stage

Piaget best describes cognitive development in young children. During the first 18–24 months, babies develop through their senses and motor activity: the sensorimotor period. The most significant aspect of this stage is a baby's understanding of object permanence. Babies learn that objects are in their world and are separate from their own actions on them. For example, when babies play peek-a-boo with a caregiver, they know that the caregiver is still there despite being hidden. Babies enjoy dropping things from the bed or table. They learn that the object is still in the world even though they cannot see it. Object permanence is the precursor to the next stage of preoperational development.

Leading up to object permanence development, Piaget described substages occurring from birth to 18 months, during which infants' behaviors and interactions with their own body and objects in the environment move from reflexive to intentional.[41] These substages are outlined in **Table 7.4**.

Every aspect of cognitive development during the first 18 months is an opportunity to exploit audition in meaningful ways. Being close to the baby during the first several months gives maximum auditory access to what speech sounds are available for audition. Babies with hearing loss need abundant and meaningful input.

With beginning listeners who are older, integrating language into cognition, pragmatics, and play can be challenging but is critical to these children's development. Even with no spoken language development, we would expect a 2-year-old whose profound hearing loss has just been identified to understand object permanence and to be able to perform all the activities in **Table 7.4**. Naturally, we would also expect a 2-year-old beginning listener to be much more independent than a newborn beginning listener. With a baby, parents have many opportunities to infuse language as they put the child's socks on and as they teach the child to stack blocks, but a 2-year-old may already know how to put socks on and stack blocks without adult assistance. In therapy sessions and at home, LSL practitioners must work with caregivers to create a structure that encourages age-appropriate play and cognition. At the same time, practitioners set the expectation that parents will fully participate in the child's activities to provide the language for all the developing skills.

Table 7.4 Piaget's substages of cognitive development in the sensorimotor period

Piaget's Substage	Age of occurrence	Behavior of the infant
Reflexive actions	1st month of life	Reflexively sucks in response to brushing or touching the baby's lips
Primary circular reactions	1–4 months	Intentionally wiggles toes, sucks fingers, kicks legs for fun (not reflexively)
Secondary circular reactions	4–8 months	Intentionally performs actions with objects such as shaking a rattle, batting a toy, putting something in mouth
Coordination of secondary circular reactions	8–12 months	Intentionally crawls to get a toy from farther away Moves a blanket off a toy Initiates peek-a-boo with blanket
Tertiary circular reactions	12–18 months	Knocks down and stacks blocks Takes rings off a stack and tries to put them back on Assembles nesting cups Tries new activities with toys and objects

Data from Piaget J. Part 1: Cognitive development in children: Piaget development and learning. *J Res Sci Teach* 1964;2(3):176–186.

Slowing down and entering into an older child's routines and play can be incredibly challenging. Some parents will say, *"My child knows how to put on socks."* This is true, but beginning listeners, no matter how old they are, do not know that those things they are putting on are called *socks* and that they go on things called *feet* and that socks go on before things called *shoes*. In the same way, an older child who is a new listener can stack blocks but does not know they are called *blocks* and the one called *the big one* must go in the place called *the bottom*. Too often we see that older beginning listeners are too independent and are working too quickly for parents to input the necessary language. Moreover, many older beginning listeners have become accustomed to using gestures as pragmatic communication and pay little attention to spoken language as they go through their day. As clinicians, one of our main responsibilities is helping parents understand that without rich receptive and expressive language, progress in the development of cognition, play, and pragmatics will plateau at an immature level. As children's language grows, they begin to think with words, to engage in elaborate pretend play with words, and to share their thoughts and ideas with others through words. For our older new listeners to have the necessary language growth to do these things, we must demonstrate for parents and coach them on how to incorporate beginning listening and auditory comprehension into all the child's age-appropriate play and routines. We also must demonstrate for parents how they may need to stop understanding their child's gestures and anticipating their child's thoughts to create the need for the child to speak. Finally, we must also help parents to recognize that academics are not the same as cognition, play, and pragmatics. Parents of old beginning listeners often become focused on academics; we must help them to understand that, without a rich language foundation that allows children to think, play, and share with their words, academic progress will be adversely affected. (See Chapter 11 for more information.)

7.8 The Focus of Literacy at This Stage

Chapter 13 provides in-depth information about the development of reading and writing within the framework of LSL. We will just touch on the subject in this chapter.

Jim Trelease, author of *The Read-Aloud Handbook*, states: "If a child is old enough to talk to, she's old enough to read to. It's the same language."[42] Infants enter the world primed for listening to speech and also to literature in its most basic forms. Babies will first enjoy interactive books that are squeezable and chewable, soft and squishy, made of wipeable plastic or washable cloth. Books for babies have contrasting prints, such as black and white patterns, vibrant colors, and simple pictures or illustrations. Babies love looking at other babies and themselves! Books with baby faces and reflective surfaces that act as mirrors hold little ones' attention and help them begin to understand themselves and their world. Lift-the-flap books contain the element of surprise and keep beginning listeners engaged.

Young listeners who are toddler- or preschool-aged are engaged by books with repeatable lines, such as *Brown Bear, Brown Bear, What Do You See?* (Martin, B.), *The Napping House* (Wood, A.) and *We're Going on a Bear Hunt* (Rosen, M. & Oxenbury, H.). Hearing

First has compiled a resource on this topic featuring over 100 books with memorable text that is excellent for engaging little ones and building vocabulary, auditory memory, and prosody. That handout is found at https://www.hearingfirst.org/m/resources/227.

By incorporating a read-aloud activity into every LSL session, the practitioner gives caregivers an opportunity to build their confidence with this routine so it will occur more frequently at home. As with any skill in the LSL toolkit, reading aloud may come naturally to some caregivers and feel intimidating to others. Practitioners can empower caregivers to embrace reading to their beginning listener by:

- modeling a read-aloud with the child for the caregiver to observe
- using props along with the story
- providing a snack for the baby while reading aloud
- taking turns, page-by-page with the caregiver during a read-aloud
- assisting caregivers with getting a library card
- linking caregivers with the Dolly Parton Imagination Library, which sends a free, age-appropriate book monthly to children in most areas across the United States, from birth until age 5 years
- encouraging caregivers to place books in baskets throughout the house and on low shelves that are easy for little ones to access
- asking caregivers to bring a book to an LSL session to help guide them in appropriate book choice and read-aloud strategies

7.9 The Focus of Intervention at This Stage

Envision an LSL practitioner as bringing to every therapy session an invisible bag full of ready-to-implement tools. Auditory strategies, in conjunction with optimally fitted hearing devices in a quiet listening environment, ensure that speech information gets to the CHL's brain. Savvy caregiver coaching methods educate and empower the most important person in the CHL's life, the caregiver. (See Chapter 5 for more information.) A hearty dose of empathy enables the practitioner to walk sensitively with the caregiver through the stages of grief and to recognize that progress toward therapy objectives will most likely be impacted when caregivers are experiencing difficult circumstances (e.g., financial hardship, workplace stressors, balancing other familial duties). (See Chapter 4 for more information.) A developmentally appropriate lesson plan along with backup plans make for a successful session, no matter the encountered challenges such as a fussy toddler or a sleeping baby. A strong, working knowledge of all the domains of child development and LSL milestones facilitates diagnostic therapy that views the baby or beginning listener principally by listening age and current level of functioning. LSL practitioners face the huge responsibility of establishing an appropriate rate of progress to close the gap between the child's listening age and CA.

The following is an intervention scenario model for an 8-month-old baby with 7 months listening experience with aided benefit similar to a mild-(30 dB @ 250-500 Hz) to-moderate (50 dB at 1000Hz) to severe-to-profound (85 dB at 2000 and 4000 Hz, 100 dB at 6000 Hz). This baby is a cochlear implant candidate with expected simultaneous implantation at 10 months. This baby can detect /u/, /i/, /a/, /m/ and imitate duration, intensity (conversational level and loud speech, but not quiet speech or whispering), and intermittent pitch changes if modeled with large variations. Speech includes /m/, /ə/, /n/, /d/, /g/, /a/. The focus is on developing this baby's expressive language to vocalize with intent. Before we can expect production, we must input language and facilitate abundant vocalizations.

Intervention Scenario Model:

- Who: mom, practitioner, baby
- Where: home setting in kitchen
- What is happening: getting ready for lunch
- Sample vocabulary for mom and practitioner to use in narrating: highchair, tray, plate, spoon, bib, applesauce, mashed carrots, milk, bottle, wet wipe, chair for mom, sit down, snap the tray, mmmmm, yummy, open your mouth, take bite, eat, drink, wipe, clean, messy, hot, uh-oh, oh no!

Using strategies in this routine involves:

- Repetition, acoustic highlighting, modeling/narrating: *"It's time for lunch! Let's eat, eat, eat. MMMMM that applesauce is sooooooo yummy, yummy yummy. Time to sit down in the highchair. Ooooooopen the tray, sit down, sit down, sit down, snap-snap-snap the tray."*
- Waiting and expectant look: At the end of the utterances, caregiver and/or practitioner would wait and look expectantly at the baby. They have provided rich, redundant input in a familiar routine. Now they need to look at the baby and wait for some type of communication related to wanting to eat or drink. Waiting can be difficult so counting to 15 and looking surprised, expectant or looking at the food may prompt the desired response.
- Serve and return, joint attention, motherese/parentese: After waiting, the baby points to the food and vocalizes *mmmmm*, *məmə*, *dədə* and smiles. Caregiver looks expectantly and replies using parentese, *"You are hungry? Mmmmm that looks sooo good. Mmmmmm."* The baby responds with more vocalizations and excitement about eating. The back and forth or serve and return between baby and caregiver continues throughout the lunch experience. Joint attention is established in this session as everyone is focused on having lunch.

7.10 Summary

Whether a baby or a beginner, learning to listen with the use of hearing technology must always start by laying a strong foundation in receptive language and auditory skills before building up to words. While the ultimate objective is for CHL to have full access to the range of speech frequencies, implementing LSL before cochlear implantation has numerous benefits. Practitioners follow the child and caregivers' leads, meeting them where they are in their hearing loss journey. From conducting appropriate assessment to involving caregivers in crafting goals and home activities that are meaningful to their child and lifestyle, practitioners must possess skills in caregiver coaching, strategies for making the auditory signal most salient, and a keen, working knowledge of development across domains.

7.11 Case Study 1: Early Identification with Early Amplification, LSL Intervention, and Cochlear Implant by Age 1 Year

At 8 months of age: Madeline is an 8-month-old girl with a severe to profound bilateral sensorineural hearing loss. Madeline's hearing loss was identified at birth and confirmed within 1 month of age by auditory brainstem response (ABR). She does not have a family history of hearing loss. Her intake history includes:

- Fitted with hearing aids at 1 month old
- Started early intervention at 3 months old
- Relocated to a different state at 8 months of age
- Neurotypical development, no other complicating conditions
- Cochlear implant candidate with plan to implant one side at 11 months
- Family wants listening and spoken language outcomes

She had minimal auditory benefit with her first set of hearing aids. Changing to more powerful hearing aids improved audibility in the low frequencies and provided access to some speech information before cochlear implantation (**Fig. 7.5**). With new hearing aids and target settings, the child is now able to consistently detect /u/, /i/, /m/, and /a/ at 1–2 feet. At 6 inches from her microphones, the child inconsistently detected /z/, /b/, and /g/ (**Fig. 7.5**). With improved auditory access to speech information, intervention focused on:

- Establishing a listening bubble of a maximum of 2 feet; family to practice determining where sound is most audible for her
- Reducing ambient noise in the household
- Keeping learning opportunities at home within a quiet setting
- Reading aloud daily
- Focusing on LtL sounds (onomatopoeia sounds) that are detectable with aided benefit[22]
  - /m/ mmmm—ice cream (access to 1st formant 250–350 Hz @ 35–40 dB)
  - /a/ ahhhhh—airplane (access to 1st formant 768–1030 Hz @ 55 dB)
  - /e/ hey!—calling out/megaphone (access to 1st formant 536–610 Hz @ 50 dB)
  - /u/ choooo—train (access to 1st formant 430–460 Hz @ 55 dB and 2nd formant 1105–1170 Hz @ 55 dB

At the time of implantation: Madeline, through listening alone, recognized some familiar commands such as "come here," "don't touch," "blow kiss," "wave bye bye." She identified LtL

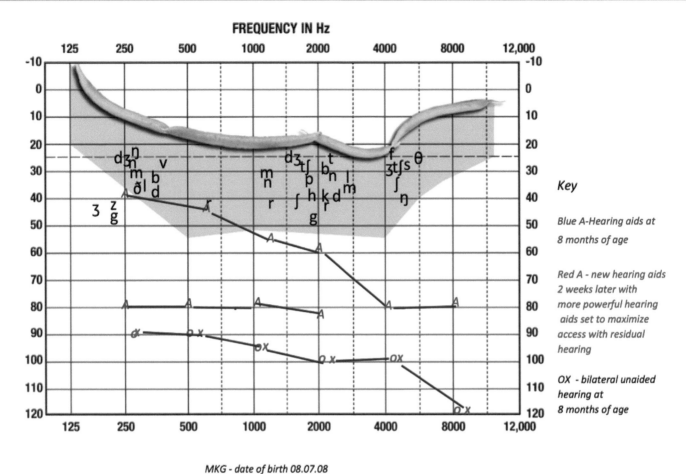

FREQUENCY IN Hz

Key

Blue A-Hearing aids at 8 months of age

Red A - new hearing aids 2 weeks later with more powerful hearing aids set to maximize access with residual hearing

OX - bilateral unaided hearing at 8 months of age

MKG - date of birth 08.07.08

Fig. 7.5 Madeline's pre- and post-cochlear implantation audiograms on the Speech String Bean.[28]

sounds that were just listed plus "quack quack quack quack" for duck. Her speech inventory included:

- Suprasegmentals duration and intensity
- Minimal pitch changes usage and voice quality mildly monotone
- /a/, /u/, /m/ with reduplicated babbling
- One true word "mama" and pointed to mom
- Long and short duration changes, mmmm for ice cream and ah ah ah ah for duck

Post Sequential Cochlear Implantation at 12 and 16 months: She had sequential cochlear implantation with the first CI activation the day before her first birthday and second at 16 months of age. Madeline's mother kept a journal documenting post-cochlear implantation documenting progress.

- 1 week post first implant (12 months chronological age): pointing at objects indicating desire to know what it is
- 10 days post (12 months CA): responding to /ʃ/, imitating *uh oh*, understanding "*brush baby's hair*," imitating *mooooo* for cow, dancing to music, saying "mama" more intentionally and frequently

- During 1–3 months post (13–15 months CA): demonstrates understanding of targeted learning to listen sounds, identifies body parts; points to named pictures in familiar books; says *mo* for *more*; recognizes more Learning to Listen sounds; trying to say *eeek* for a mouse; approximates word *bye-bye*, *um um* for *yum yum*; understands "*get your shoes,*" "*let's go bye-bye,*" "*ring ring where's the phone*"; shows recognition of 2 different songs by doing hand movements; demonstrates auditory closure for familiar songs (examples: attempts "*SNAP*" for crocodile snapping at monkeys in a tree song and "*Oh*" for the Baby Bumblebee song); does movements when hears 4 different songs; uses speech inventory of all previous sounds plus /p/, /b/, /o/, /ə/; makes multiple animal sounds when she hears the animal names
- During 4–6 months post (16–18 months CA): responds to all Ling sounds at 3 feet and attempts imitation of /m/, /a/, /u/ during Ling checks; MacArthur-Bates inventory shows use of 50 expressive true words/word approximations, speech awareness thresholds at 15 dB, understands 15+ familiar commands, puts 2 words together ("get down," "no mama," "more cookie")
- During 7–12 months post (19–24 months CA): has a natural-sounding vocal quality with distinct pitch changes, increases

frequency of 2-word combinations and starting at 8 months post 1st CI has multiple 3-word phrases, using a wide variety of vocabulary (nouns, verbs, adjectives, early pronouns, -ing verb forms, early wh- questions)

- By 16 months post first CI activation (2 y 4 m CA and 16 months CI age): MacArthur-Bates inventory expressive vocabulary of 644 words, uses strings of words and phrases, natural-sounding speech with intelligibility at 90% to unfamiliar listeners

How did this child have exemplary progress within the first 16 months of activation? Her success was multifactorial. In addition to early identification and early hearing aid fitting, the audiologist was not content to accept the initial fitting benefits. By fitting more powerful hearing aids, the child had increased audibility to some low- to mid-frequency information through detection. For children awaiting cochlear implantation, hearing aids programmed so that some speech information is audible increase opportunities to develop auditory brain pathways and reinforce that sound has meaning. Pre-implant auditory intervention stimulates the brain in preparation for future progress post cochlear implant activation. With increased access, the practitioner and family could exploit listening in a salient, functional, and fun manner. As a result, even before the implant, the child demonstrated detection and discrimination, along with emerging identification and auditory comprehension skills.

Another critical part of Madeline's success was her family support and follow through in creating a language-rich environment for her from identification onward. In the first month of therapy sessions, Madeline was not responding to any sounds despite presenting low-frequency noise and speech at 1 inch from her microphone. Not only was she not responding to auditory input; she was continually pulling out her hearing aids. Although she was wearing them all waking hours possible, the lack of auditory response was discouraging. Many parents at this point will question the reason for hearing aids and pre-implant intervention when benefit is not appreciated. Sometimes we see compliance with hearing technology retention and therapy attendance decrease.

Madeline's parents continued to be diligent with technology retention, LSL intervention, and carry-over. After she had new hearing aids fitted and programmed optimally to maximize low- to mid-frequency information, Madeline began responding to her parents' voices, music, and some environmental noises 6–12 feet from her hearing aids. These auditory responses were proof to her parents that she could hear something and attach meaning to sound. That proof motivated and excited them about what was possible then and post cochlear implant activation. While Madeline was awake, they minimized noise, kept her hearing aids on, talked about what they were doing, stayed within her listening bubble, read aloud to her, and worked on developing her auditory function based on her low- and mid-frequency auditory access. As they implemented these activities and strategies, they observed small, definite progress as noted at the beginning of this case study.

Our first session post cochlear implant was the day after activation; her first birthday. At that session, we observed the impact of pre-implant intervention when she:

- imitated suprasegmentals of duration
- imitated a pitch change with *ahhhhhh* for LtL sound for airplane
- moved to music
- turned to knocking on the door
- vocalized back and forth with her parents
- pointed to the airplane when mom said *ahhhhh* and played with the airplane
- attempted *ahhhhh* while playing with the airplane
- pointed to a duck in the picture book when dad repeatedly said, "*quack quack quack quack*"

Madeline's parents recognized the value of hearing aids and LSL intervention before cochlear implantation and during her "1 day post activation" intervention session results.

Pearl

For children awaiting cochlear implantation, hearing aids programmed so that some speech information is audible increase opportunities to develop auditory brain pathways and reinforce that sound has meaning. Pre-implant auditory intervention stimulates the brain in preparation for future progress post cochlear implant activation.

7.12 Case Study 2: Late-Amplified Child

Studying a child referred to here as Connor provides the opportunity for comparing and contrasting the trajectory and outcomes for a child whose hearing loss journey has been far from ideal. Connor is the product of an uncomplicated pregnancy to a family experiencing social and economic hardship in a rural area of their state. They drive three hours round-trip to the clinic where they receive audiological management and LSL/AVT services. Connor's medical history is significant for bilateral tympanostomy tube placement in his first year of life. He did not pass his newborn hearing screening, but his mother reported she and the rest of their family "never thought much of it."

Following sedated ABR testing, Connor was diagnosed at 19 months old with bilateral moderately severe to severe sensorineural hearing loss. He was fitted with hearing aids bilaterally at 20 months old. Subsequently, at age 21 months, he was evaluated by an LSL practitioner and began receiving weekly AVT services consistently. AVT sessions were characterized primarily by behavioral outbursts, including crying, tantrums, and trying to run out of the room. When Connor was interested in and attentive to tasks, he was primarily only repeating central, lax vowels and a few consonant sounds without any clear words. Singing was the most effective tool in sessions. While Connor was not able to imitate changes in vocal pitch or recognizably sing along to the songs, he always immediately began to vocalize along and perform the motions to each "Song of the Week." His auditory skills consisted of imitating duration cues for Learning to Listen Sounds, identifying a few songs, and recognizing some stereotypical phrases, such as "*yay*" by clapping his hands. He could only consistently and accurately detect /u, a, i, m, sh/ of the Ling 6 sounds at about 18 inches. Expressively, Connor was using no more than 3–5 words that were understood by people outside his family (e.g., no, wow). His family reported that Connor used another 10–15 words in familiar contexts around those who knew him best (e.g. "bee-bee" for "drink," "mon" for "come on").

Datalogging revealed poor hearing aid use. For over 1 year, he was wearing his hearing aids for 3–4 hours per day on average. Despite strong commitment by his mother and grandmother to have him wear his hearing aids, Connor would often take them off, throw them and show many accompanying negative behaviors. Aided testing was performed when Connor was 30 months old and revealed aided thresholds in the moderate to severe hearing loss range and detection of the Ling 6 sounds in the moderately severe hearing loss range. Connor was most likely refusing to wear his hearing aids consistently because he was not receiving adequate benefit and meaningful sound from them. The aided speech testing information, along with frequent updates from and concerns voiced by the LSL practitioner, precipitated a cochlear implant evaluation and he was quickly deemed a candidate.

Connor received a cochlear implant on his right side at 36 months old. He maintained a hearing aid in his left ear. Initially, Connor reacted similarly to his cochlear implant speech processor as he did to his hearing aids with many tears shed and tantrums displayed. Within 2–3 weeks following the cochlear implant activation, however, he began bonding with his CI. Connor's mother reported at that time Connor was doing great with wearing his CI processor. She said she noticed that Connor's attention and responsiveness were significantly improving, and the LSL practitioner also observed these changes in behavior during AVT. For the first time in his journey with wearing hearing technology, Connor began requesting, with gestures and vocalizations, for his devices to be put back on when they fell off. He then learned how to put the CI magnet back on himself. He carried this skill over to his hearing aid, as well, by beginning to replace his earmold when needed.

At Connor's third AVT session post-CI activation, Connor was able to imitate, without acoustic highlighting or repetition, all Ling 6 Sounds at 3 feet. These sounds were familiar to Connor from his previous exposure in pre-implantation AVT sessions so that when he had full access to the speech frequencies with the CI, it was not a hard task for him to imitate the sounds. Connor's single word expressive vocabulary was growing by 5 new words per week in the early weeks following activation of the CI.

A month after activation, he began imitating two-word phrases in therapy activities, according to Phase 2 of the Bloom & Lahey Model,[43] but not yet using any phrases spontaneously, as his expressive vocabulary was still taking shape. He demonstrated a growing auditory memory by tracking rote three-word phrases (e.g., "I love you," "where'd it go?"), as evidenced by syllabic marking and intonation. He auditorily attended to stories by pointing to some simple pictures or actions as a book was read. He responded to simple commands without gestural cueing. Connor's speech was characterized by the use of many more vowels (front, central, and back) and the emergence of diphthongs, especially in Learning to Listen activities, through exclamations during play ("OUCH!"), and in songs.

At his second visit to audiology post-activation (approximately 6 weeks later), he progressed up to his loudest mapping program. The family cheered with joy and pride during AVT sessions. They showed understanding of the need to close the 2-year gap between his Current Level of Function age and his CA but were relieved to see him embrace listening as part of his personality and to respond to speech readily in his environment without requiring abundant repetition and a tiny listening bubble. They hoped to have his other side implanted as soon as possible to take advantage of the critical window of LSL development. (For more information on intervention with children with late identified hearing loss, see Chapter 11.

Pearl

Aided testing was performed when Connor was 30 months old and revealed aided thresholds in the moderate to severe hearing loss range and detection of the Ling 6 sounds in the moderately severe hearing loss range. Connor was most likely refusing to wear his hearing aids consistently because he was not receiving adequate benefit and meaningful sound from them.

Discussion Questions

1. Why do we write goals and lesson plans for an infant or child with hearing loss based on their listening age instead of chronological age, bearing in mind the child's current level of functioning and placement along Piaget's stages?

2. What role does optimal access and wear-time with hearing devices play in calculating listening age?

3. When should an LSL practitioner seek the help of additional professionals from other specialties in assisting families of babies with hearing loss?

4. Why is it critically important for LSL practitioners to study and possess a skillful working knowledge of infant and child development across cognitive, play, auditory, speech, and language domains?

5. What are the first steps in developing auditory function with babies with hearing loss or older children who are beginning listeners?

6. How is intervention for babies and beginning listeners similar? How is intervention for babies and beginning listeners different? Give specific examples of development, goals, strategies, and interventions that would be similar and that would be different.

References

[1] Schum R. Psychological assessment of children with multiple handicaps who have hearing loss. *Volta Review* 2004;*104*(4):237–255

[2] Wilson Linder K, Walker B. The Later Years Workshop. Presented at: November 2010; Fort Worth, TX

[3] Flexer C. Start with the Brain and Connect the Dots: White Paper. https://www.hearingfirst.org/m/resources/7179. Published 2017. Accessed October 30, 2021

[4] Ching TYC, Dillon H, Leigh G, Cupples L. Learning from the Longitudinal Outcomes of Children with Hearing Impairment (LOCHI) study: summary of 5-year findings and implications. *Int J Audiol* 2018;*57*(sup2):S105–S111. doi:10.1080/14992027.2017.1385865

[5] Caraway TH. 10 Parent Coaching Strategies. https://www.hearingfirst.org/m/resources/7380 Published 2020. Accessed November 4, 2021

[6] Campbell DR, Goldstein H. Genesis of a new generation of telepractitioners: The COVID-19 Pandemic and pediatric speech-language pathology services. *Am J Speech Lang Pathol* 2021;*30*(5):2143–2154 doi:10.1044/2021_AJSLP-21-00013

[7] Tuohy J, Brown J, Mercer-Moseley C. St. Gabriel's Curriculum for the Development of Audition, Language, Speech, Cognition, Early Communication, Social Interaction, Fine Motor Skills, Gross Motor Skills: A Guide for Professionals Working with Children who are Hearing- Impaired (Birth to Six Years). 2nd ed. Sydney, Australia: St. Gabriel's Auditory-Verbal Early Intervention Centre; 2005

[8] Madell JR, Flexer C. Hearing test protocols for children. In: Madell JR, Flexer C, eds. *Pediatric Audiology*. New York, NY: Thieme Publishing; 2008:60

[9] Rossetti LM. The Rossetti Infant-Toddler Language Scale: Examiner's Manual. East Moline, IL: LinguiSystems; 2006

[10] Lanza JR, Flahive LK. Guide to Communication Milestones: Concepts, Feeding, Morphology, Literacy, Mean Length of Utterance, Phonological Awareness, Pragmatics, Pronouns, Questions, Speech Sound Acquisition, Vocabulary. East Moline, IL: LinguiSystems; 2008

[11] Wilkes EM. Cottage Acquisition Scales for Listening, Language & Speech: User's Guide. San Antonio, TX: Sunshine Cottage School for Deaf Children; 1999

[12] MacArthur-Bates Communicative Development Inventories. https://mb-cdi.stanford.edu/ Published 2007. Accessed November 6, 2021

[13] Caleffe-Schenck N, Dickson CL. Track a listening child. https://www.cochlear.com/0f576aaf-45ce-4256-9b3b-e772663bf661/general_rehabilitationresources_earlyintervention_trackalisteningchild%28tlc%29_en_3.31mb.pdf Published May 2013. Accessed December 31, 2021

[14] Integrated Scales of Development (ISD). https://www.cochlear.com/au/en/home/ongoing-care-and-support/rehabilitation-resources/scales-of-development Published December 2015. Accessed December 31, 2021

[15] Dickson CL. Current Level of Functioning, Pre-Verbal, Verbal. Published 2018

[16] Joint Committee on Infant Hearing; American Academy of Audiology; American Academy of Pediatrics; American Speech-Language-Hearing Association; Directors of Speech and Hearing Programs in State Health and Welfare Agencies. Year 2000 position statement: principles and guidelines for early hearing detection and intervention programs. *Pediatrics* 2000;*106*(4):798–817 doi:10.1542/peds.106.4.798

[17] Chepesiuk R. Decibel hell: the effects of living in a noisy world. *Environ Health Perspect* 2005;*113*(1):A34–A41 10.1289/ehp.113-a34

[18] Cohen S, Glass DC, Singer JS. Apartment noise, auditory discrimination, and reading ability in children. *J Exp Soc Psychol* 1973;*9*:407–422

[19] Keeping Hearing Technology On: Support from Your Child's Caregivers. https://www.hearingfirst.org/m/resources/4226. Published 2018. Accessed December 31, 2021

[20] Anderson KL, Madell JR. Meeting the Challenge: Keeping Hearing Devices on Young Children. https://www.oticon.com/-/media/oticon-us/main/download-center/family-support-materials/professional-all/35537-keeping-hearing-aids-on-young-children.pdf Published 2012. Accessed November 6, 2021

[21] The LMH Test for Monitoring Listening. The Ling-Madell-Hewitt test or the Low-Mid-High frequency test. http://www.janemadell.com/LMH_Discussion.pdf Published 2021. Accessed December 31, 2021

[22] Pollack D, Goldberg DM, Caleffe-Schenck N. Educational Audiology for the Limited-Hearing Infant and Preschooler: An Auditory-Verbal Program. 3rd ed. Springfield, Illinois: Charles C. Thomas; 1997

[23] Graven SN, Browne J. Auditory development in the fetus and infant. *Newborn Infant Nurs Rev* 2008;*8*:187–193 doi:10.1053/j.nainr.2008.10.010

[24] When Can a Fetus Hear: Womb Development Timeline. https://www.healthline.com/health/pregnancy/when-can-a-fetus-hear Published 2018. Accessed December 31, 2021

[25] Law F II, Mahr T, Schneeberg A, Edwards J. Vocabulary size and auditory word recognition in preschool children. *Appl Psycholinguist* 2017;*38*(1):89–125 doi:10.1017/S0142716416000126

[26] Erber N. Auditory Training. Washington DC: Alexander Graham Bell Association; 1982: 92–94

[27] Walker B. Auditory Learning Guide. https://www.hearingfirst.org/m/resources/82 Published 2009. Accessed January 20, 2022

[28] The Shepherd Centre. https://shepherdcentre.org.au/research/functional-listening-index-paediatric/ Published 2013. Accessed December 31, 2021

[29] Estabrooks W. Auditory-Verbal Therapy and Practice. Washington, DC: Alexander Graham Bell Association for the Deaf and Hard of Hearing; 2006

[30] MacIver-Lux K, Perrson AE, Estabrooks W. Is it important to use noisemakers in an auditory-verbal session? In: Estabrooks W, ed. 101 Frequently Asked Questions. Washington, DC: AG Bell; 2012:83–87

[31] Appendix 13-A Learning to Listen Sounds Audiogram and Acoustics of Learning to Listen Sounds Chart. In: Estabrooks W, MacIver-Lux K, Rhoades, E, eds. Auditory-Verbal Therapy for Young Children with Hearing Loss and Their Families, and the Practitioners Who Guide Them. San Diego, CA: Plural Publishing; 2016:466–468

[32] Teacher Tools to Support the Success of Children with Hearing Loss. http://www.janemadell.com/publications/Checking%20For%20Audibility%20in%20School.pdf Published 2015. Accessed December 31, 2021

[33] Flexer C. Familiar Sounds Audiogram eBook. https://www.hearingfirst.org/m/resources/7734 Published 2021. Accessed December 31, 2021

[34] Hart B, Risley T. Meaningful Differences in the Everyday Experience of Young American Children. Baltimore, MD: Paul H. Brookes; 1995

[35] Flexer C. 04 Auditory Brain Development. https://www.youtube.com/watch?v=ArTtXDtNS5A Published 2012. Accessed January 20, 2022

[36] Center on the Developing Child-Harvard University. Serve and return. https://developingchild.harvard.edu/science/key-concepts/serve-and-return/ Published 2019. Accessed December 31, 2021

[37] Carson L. Stages of Early Vocal Development. http://talkingtogether.com.au/wp-content/uploads/2018/08/stages-of-early-vocal-development.pdf Published 2018. Accessed November 6, 2021

[38] NIDCD. Speech and Language Developmental Milestones. https://www.nidcd.nih.gov/health/speech-and-language Accessed November 6, 2021

[39] Your Child's Development. Age-Based Tips From Birth to 36 Months. https://www.zerotothree.org/resources/series/your-child-s-development-age-based-tips-from-birth-to-36-months Published 2008. Accessed November 6, 2021

[40] Ling D. Foundations of Spoken Language for Hearing-Impaired Children. Washington, DC: Alexander Graham Bell Association for the Deaf; 1988

[41] Piaget J. Part 1: Cognitive development in children: Piaget development and learning. *J Res Sci Teach* 1964;*2*(3):176–186

[42] Trelease J. The Read-Aloud Handbook. 7th ed. New York, NY: Penguin Books; 2013

[43] Bloom L, Lahey M. Language Development and Language Disorders. Somerset, NJ: John Wiley & Sons, Inc.; 1978

8 Toddler-Type Language: Putting Words Together and Moving up to Simple Sentences

Darcy L. Stowe

Summary

This chapter dives into the growth and development of toddlers or children in the toddler-type language stage in audition, receptive language, expressive language, speech, play, and more. From learning to follow more complex directions to answering questions and building sentences, a toddler is developing skills in these areas at a rapid rate. This chapter provides a microscopic look into areas of development alongside pearls and pitfalls of intervention for children in the toddler stage with hearing loss and their caregivers.

Keywords

toddler, toddler-type language, receptive language, expressive language, auditory skill development, behavior considerations, caregiver coaching, listening and spoken language intervention, word combinations, sentences, vocabulary, morphemes

Key Points

- Toddlers develop listening, language, and speech at a rapid rate.
- Caregiver coaching is an essential part of listening and spoken language (LSL) intervention with toddlers and older children with toddler-type language because of the time they spend with their caregivers.
- Some important considerations for developing children in this stage are behavior management, cognition, play, and chronological age vs. listening age.
- While this stage may seem simplistic or to some unnecessary (especially for older children), the expansive receptive and expressive vocabulary/language growth that occurs during this time creates the building blocks for the development of flexible and complex language.
- Listening and spoken language strategies are essential for communicating carryover with caregivers during intervention.

The word "toddler" often stirs up several synonyms associated with children of this age—"terrible twos," "threenagers," "temper tantrums," "independence," "meltdowns." Although these stereotypes are often true, the growth and maturity of listening and language in toddlers are immense. From 18 months to 3 years of age, a toddler is still developing neural connections at an astronomical rate—actually faster than they ever will again. If development were a race, children from the ages of birth to 3

years old are running faster than they will for the rest of their lives in the race of brain development. Unfortunately, some children with hearing loss do not have the benefit of early identification and early intervention, which means that this immense growth and maturity of listening and language may be occurring beyond (or even well beyond) the age of 3. Nevertheless, even though the child may be chronologically older, the importance of this stage of language development does not change. This chapter will focus on the unique development, strategies, coaching, and care toddlers and those with toddler-type language need to maximize listening and language learning in this timeframe of their lives.

8.1 How an LSL Provider Knows a Child Is in This Stage

This is an important question to consider before proceeding with content regarding development in the toddler stage. The following are some important factors to consider when determining whether a child with hearing loss is within the toddler stage of development. A child is in this stage if

- The child's chronological age is within 18 months to 3 years and the child demonstrates standard scores within normal limits.
- The child's chronological age is older than 3 years yet their standard scores in speech and language evaluations are greater than one standard deviation below the mean and/or their age equivalents demonstrate language within the 18 months to 3 years range.
- The child has an expressive vocabulary of at least 50 words.
- The child has the ability to follow directions with one or more critical elements through audition only.
- The child is beginning to imitate or combine 2 words into an utterance.
- The child is younger than 18 months of age and is demonstrating any of the previously listed skills.

8.2 Important and Special Factors to Consider with This Stage

Each age and stage of child development comes with unique factors to consider. Toddlerhood is no exception. The following are a few special factors to consider when working with a toddler in LSL intervention.

1. Behavior management: Whether you are a new provider or have many years of experience, you are aware of the possible

challenges with keeping a toddler or an older child with limited language engaged in intervention without too many power struggles. In the early stages of being a one-year-old, toddlers are learning to express their opinion and exert their independence, yet they often don't have the words to do this verbally. Thus, temper tantrums, screeching, flailing, and other less desirable behaviors come into play. Toddlers and older children with delayed language need routine to better predict the beginning, middle, and end of experiences and to help have some sense of control. Independence and control are high priorities for children in this stage. Strategies to support success in LSL intervention sessions related to managing behavior include providing choices (letting the child have control over some aspects of intervention), setting a routine (always starting and ending the session in a predictable way), and expressing empathy in a nonsarcastic manner. For example, if the child throws the green frog off the table in the middle of a play routine, the LSL provider could respond by saying, "Oops! Bummer! I guess the frog is finished," rather than scolding the child for throwing. When working with toddlers and older children with limited language in LSL intervention, keep in mind that behaviors/misbehaviors are always telling us something. Working alongside caregivers to better understand what behaviors are telling us will get to the root of the matter much faster than ignoring or even dwelling too much on misbehaviors. As an LSL interventionist, I want to wonder first whether my goals/activities are too high or too low as compared to the child's skill level. If so, that's an easy answer, and goals/activities can be adjusted immediately to better meet children at their current level.

Pearl

Toddlers and older children with delayed language need routine to better predict the beginning, middle, and end of experiences and to help have some sense of control.

Pearl

When working with toddlers and older children with limited language in LSL intervention, keep in mind that behaviors/misbehaviors are always telling us something.

As with any area, there's a range of challenging behaviors that can come in this age range. Use your keen clinical judgment to help you know when a child is showing developmentally appropriate misbehaviors versus those that are more alarming. Quickly and confidently refer for an outside opinion if you notice behaviors in children that are causing harm to themselves or others in the environment, anger that doesn't calm with relationship, or evidence of any type of abuse or neglect. These could be evidence of trauma and require a skill set outside the scope that can be provided only in LSL intervention.

Toddlers thrive on relationships and experiences. Begin early with a toddler to develop a connection where the toddler can co-regulate with a caregiver, LSL provider, or both when in stressful situations.

2. Motor development: The word "toddler" is derived from the word "toddle," which is a word picture of a child learning to walk and "toddling" around unsteadily as they learn to control their body in space. Toddlers need to stay busy, and play is their "work." Capturing incidental moments to integrate listening and language strategies into motor play is a great tip when working with toddlers. Perhaps the LSL interventionist makes a game out of the walk from the waiting room to the intervention room by narrating "walking walking walking . . . stop!" or whispering "tiptoe, tiptoe, tiptoe down the hall." While in a session, using sensory-stimulating objects in play is a great idea. This could include a weighted ball, sensory tub, or even a slimy spider. For older children in this stage, we must also remember that play is still their "work." Age does not change the fact that actively playing the same walking and tiptoeing games just described will develop more detailed language connections than naming actions on flashcards or worksheets.

Pearl

Capturing incidental moments to integrate listening and language strategies into motor play is a great tip when working with toddlers.

3. Language and cognition: Language guides cognitive development and play. Toddlers and older children with language at this level are seeing many connections in the world around them. They want to explore things on their own and they want to know how things work. They want things when they want them, but they do not yet have the ability to understand all that is said to them or to fully express their thoughts and ideas. The basis for their developing cognition is language, but it is only through the development of rich receptive vocabulary and language in this stage that toddler-type communicators will begin to have the expressive language necessary to share their thoughts and ideas more fully. In the same way, their growth in pragmatics and play is intertwined with the language development. Children who are only beginning to put words together, even if their chronological age is older, do not yet have language and cognitive connections to understand complex relationships. Professionals and parents with reasonable expectations know that toddlers do not fully understand why a parent has to go on a business trip or why the family cannot go to Disneyland today or why a friend wants to play cars instead of dolls. Yet, when a child is older but just beginning to combine words together, professionals and parents may have unrealistic expectations about what the child truly understands; they may expect more based on the child's chronological age. We would not expect a toddler to play interactively with a 5-year-old or participate successfully in a kindergarten classroom. In the same way, we must have realistic expectations for cognitive and pragmatic development of a 5-year-old who is just beginning to combine words.

8.3 Caregiver Involvement in Therapy

Caregivers should be included in all LSL sessions, and this is a crucial part with a toddler or an older child with toddler-type language as well. Children with limited language rely on caregivers to feel safe, comfortable, and at ease. Caregivers' involvement in the session will aid in the toddlers' comfort as well as ensure that the goals and strategies implemented in the intervention are carried over outside of intervention.

8.3.1 Interventionist's and Caregiver's Shares of a Toddler's Time

There are exactly 168 hours in one week. If toddlers or older children with hearing loss and their caregivers attend 1 hr of LSL intervention once a week, they spend merely 0.6% of their week's time in intervention. Yes, LSL intervention is an essential part of maximizing the listening and spoken language potential for a child with hearing loss, yet the momentum behind that development comes from the relationships in the other 99.4% of their time. Equipping and empowering caregivers is an essential component of LSL intervention because, without it, LSL is 0.6% effective (at most). LSL providers should prioritize developing a positive relationship with each caregiver from the very beginning and working to communicate with each caregiver in the way that caregiver most likes to receive and learn new information.[1]

Pearl

LSL intervention is an essential part of maximizing the listening and spoken language potential for a child with hearing loss, yet the momentum behind that development comes from the relationships in the other 99.4% of their time.

8.3.2 What Does Therapy Look Like? The Focus on Caregivers as Equal Players

Caregivers should play an active, participatory role in LSL intervention and not just be observers. LSL intervention is a team with equal players. Caregivers know the child better than anyone else and can speak to daily life as the experts on their child. The LSL provider knows developmental milestones and LSL strategies and can speak as the expert in those areas. Together, the caregiver and LSL provider make a powerful team that is united with one goal—to maximize the listening and spoken language potential of the child with hearing loss.

If this is true of the therapy session, there will be time for feedback and reflection in addition to activities and goals. The LSL provider should aim to start each session with time for feedback from the caregiver. This report could be something to celebrate, a new concern, or a specific story from the family's week. The LSL provider should listen well to this feedback as it may change the course of the intervention plan for the day to maximize what the caregiver is expressing as most pressing for them this week. The LSL provider has a responsibility to clearly explain therapy goals and activities and not assume that observation is sufficient to equip each caregiver to implement goals and activities.

Pitfall

The LSL provider has a responsibility to clearly explain therapy goals and activities and not assume that observation is sufficient to equip each caregiver to implement goals and activities.

Take time to talk and not just "do." Plan play activities (preferably not videos and video games) for toddlers and older children that enable them to remain engaged during times of feedback or reflection between the LSL provider and caregiver. Activities during the LSL session can be discussed as you go or reviewed at the end. Find what works best for you in the relationship you have with individual caregivers and the way they best learn. Don't be shy in asking how the caregiver best likes to give and receive new information, and work to respect that in conversation with the caregiver. Beginning and ending the session with reflection is a great goal for all LSL providers. Keep inquiries open-ended and actively listen in each of these instances to gain insight into the family's greatest concerns or celebrations.[1]

Caregiver coaching can take several forms during an LSL intervention session. Coaching can involve directing an action, giving feedback, or prompting reflection. An LSL interventionist may prompt a parent to action by explaining how the parent can be used as a model before the child has a turn. Also, the LSL interventionist may prompt the parent to take a turn by handing over an activity and providing specific direction on the next steps. Feedback for a caregiver should always include encouragement coupled with specific ideas for improvement. Keep in mind that validating caregivers builds their confidence in growing listening with their child. Caregivers know their child best, and we can reinforce that as LSL interventionists by using validation.

8.4 The Focus of Auditory Development at This Stage

Toddlers are developing auditory skills at a rapid rate. Children with hearing loss in this age range are no exception. For a child with hearing loss who was identified early, fitted with appropriate technology, and enrolled in quality LSL intervention, it is expected that auditory skills would follow a developmental continuum in line with typically hearing peers. For a child who is older chronologically yet has auditory skills similar to those of a toddler due to a shorter duration of listening, these resources are also valuable in setting goals and documenting progress. Erber's Hierarchy (see **Fig. 8.1**),[2] the Auditory Learning Guide,[3] and the Cottage Acquisition Scales for Listening Language & Speech (CASLLS)[4] are three great resources for dissecting auditory skill development in toddlers.

Erber highlights auditory skill development in four categories: detection, discrimination, identification, and comprehension. Those with toddler-type language are typically moving through identification into comprehension at this stage (see **Fig. 8.1**).

Toddlers move from following one-step commands at around 12 months of age to following two-step commands by 24 months of age. Judith Simsers provides great insight into the developmental levels of following commands, which are highlighted in the Auditory Learning Guide. Children begin by understanding familiar commands such as "wave bye-bye." The next step in understanding commands is following one-step commands with one critical element such as "Get the cow." Toddlers and older children at this stage may ease into following one-step commands with one critical element by selecting the desired object from a field of three. As with any task, modeling is key to growing auditory skill development in following commands and moving, from closed set to open set is a

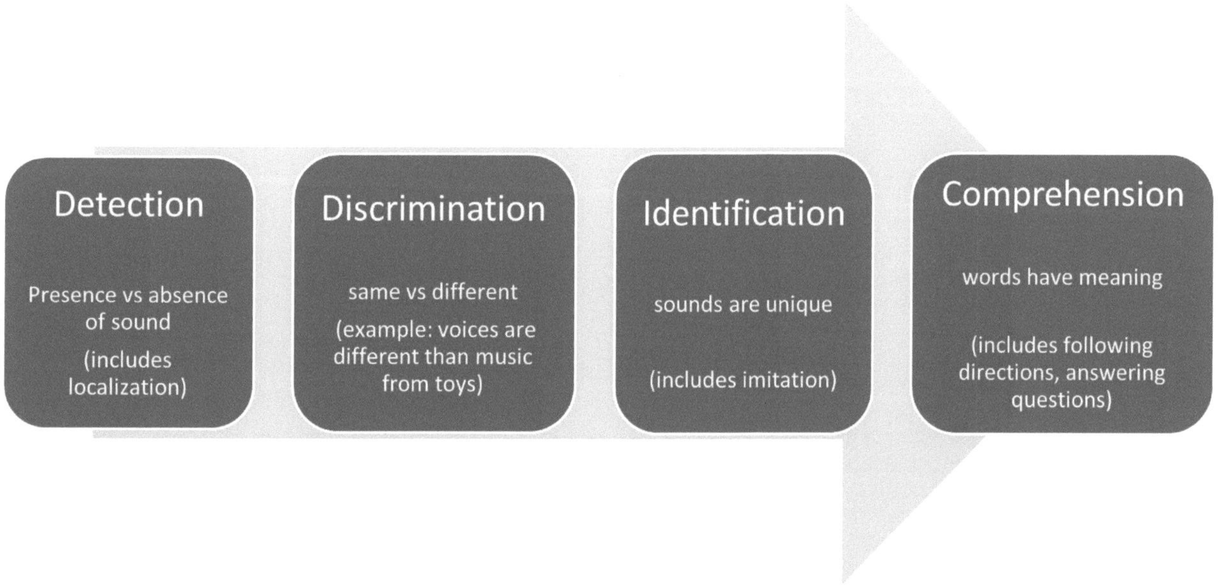

Detection

Presence vs absence of sound

(includes localization)

Discrimination

same vs different

(example: voices are different than music from toys)

Identification

sounds are unique

(includes imitation)

Comprehension

words have meaning

(includes following directions, answering questions)

Fig. 8.1 Erber's four categories of auditory skill development. Adapted from Erber N. Evaluating speech perception ability in hearing impaired children. In: FH, ed. *Childhood Deafness: Causation, Assessment, and Management.* New York, NY: Grune & Stratton; 1977.

natural progression. Simser highlights the intricacies of following commands with two critical elements (see **Table 8.1**).[5]

LSL interventionists should pay careful attention to auditory memory and sequencing development with each child with hearing loss they see in intervention. Moving through goals in auditory memory and sequencing is key to maximizing the potential of children with hearing loss and setting them up for the greatest success in their upcoming academic career. The LSL interventionist must coach caregivers on the intricacies of auditory skill development as well as the "so what" of why this area of development needs attention in the toddler years of development. Growing the ability of a child to follow directions with two or more critical elements can be facilitated in a variety of activities within LSL intervention. For a child in this stage, some of these include:

- Using manipulatives with a book
- Completing a simple craft
- Using two-of-a-kind objects in a barrier game
- Hiding objects in a sensory bin

Table 8.1 Development of comprehension of two-item memory

Type of phrase (in order of development)	Example
Two nouns	Get your <u>shoes</u> and your <u>hat</u>.
Noun & verb	The <u>baby</u> is <u>sleeping</u>.
Verb & object	<u>Wash</u> the <u>car</u>.
Two verbs	<u>Jump</u> and <u>sit down</u>.
Adjective & noun	Go get your <u>blue shirt</u>.
Number & noun	I want <u>three candies</u>.

Source: Adapted from Simser JI. Auditory-verbal intervention: Infants and toddlers. *Volta Review* 1993;95(3):217–229.

- Letting objects go "swimming" in a tub of water
- Inviting passengers on a toy vehicle
- Playing hide and seek with objects in the room

When brainstorming for carryover with caregivers in this area, caregivers might find success targeting auditory memory in the following areas:

- Daily routines: Sorting laundry, picking up toys, sequencing tasks of a morning routine, following a simple recipe
- Play routines: suggesting who wants to play in the dollhouse, cleaning up the playroom, packing a backpack of favorite toys to take on a play date
- Social routines: packing a bag to go visit grandparents, getting items from the grocery list while shopping, reflecting on the child's day at daycare

Several LSL strategies are beneficial when targeting auditory memory and sequencing development in LSL intervention, yet these three are essential:

1. *Audition first:* Letting listeners hear it before they see it. If visual cues (including lip-reading, pointing, gesturing) are used with every presentation of commands, the LSL interventionist cannot conclude that the auditory cortex is solely responsible for the response. Audition first should be utilized naturally and as a way to diagnostically assess whether a child is truly following commands through listening is relying on additional sensory cues to facilitate comprehension. Audition first can be employed simply by establishing joint attention with toys in the session or by using the hand cue if needed in a subtle way (holding a toy or the book from the session in front of the mouth).
2. *Caregiver as a model:* Using the caregiver as a model is critical when teaching any new skill, including auditory memory. Much like

knowing the rules of a game before playing, a child needs modeling to know what is expected with new activities or higher-level goals.

3. *Auditory or listening sandwich*: LSL interventionists and caregivers strive to maintain a high level of expectation for the children with hearing loss, yet there are situations where more supports are needed. In growing auditory memory, the targeted command should be presented through audition first, but what happens if the child doesn't comprehend the message? That's when the auditory or listening sandwich comes into play. Think of audition first as the bottom piece of bread. T he layers of the sandwich on top of that bread are the additional LSL strategies employed to facilitate comprehension. These may include caregiver modeling, acoustic highlighting, a visual cue (such as holding out two hands for two objects), or providing choices. An LSL interventionist may need to employ just one strategy or multiple strategies to facilitate comprehension. Then comes the most crucial part of the listening sandwich: ending with audition first in the repetition of the target. Think of it as a bookend to facilitating comprehension through audition. When the auditory cortex doesn't comprehend the intended message through audition only, LSL interventionists use supports to yield comprehension. But then they must conclude the exchange by putting the command back into audition only, and only then does the auditory cortex have another opportunity for success by connecting a message to comprehension that previously wasn't possible.

8.5 The Focus of Language Development at This Stage

As with audition, language is growing rapidly in the toddler years and should also be growing rapidly for older children in this stage. Language can be sorted into two parts: receptive and expressive. Receptive language is the ability to understand language, and expressive language is using language to express wants and needs. Although this time of life for a child is marked by quantifiable expressive language growth, receptive language is also growing rapidly and deserves equal weight in goals and attention in LSL intervention.

Pearl

Although this time of life for a child is marked by quantifiable expressive language growth, receptive language is also growing rapidly and deserves equal weight in goals and attention in LSL intervention.

8.5.1 Receptive language

A toddler grows from understanding between 3 to 20 words at 15 months to understanding between 250 and 500 words by 24 months.[4] That's a growth of more than 150 times in just one year! Toddlers and those older children who are at this stage of language development must first have an understanding of words before they use them meaningfully. In the toddler stage, receptive vocabulary can be thought of as an empty water tank. When it grows and spills over is when receptive vocabulary begins to become part of expressive vocabulary.

Pearl

In the toddler stage, receptive vocabulary can be thought of as an empty water tank. When it grows and spills over is when receptive vocabulary begins to become part of expressive vocabulary.

Not only are toddlers growing a hefty receptive vocabulary during this time, but they are also growing a very diverse receptive vocabulary. By 24 months of age, a toddler is understanding words in several categories, including toys, foods, clothing, body parts, animals, family, vehicles, household items, verbs, attributes, pronouns, prepositions, and questions. It is important for toddlers to expand beyond nouns alone as they are developing a vocabulary to know and describe the world around them. Also, at this stage, as auditory memory for critical elements and a hefty, diverse vocabulary are developing, so is receptive understanding of an increasing number of critical elements in an utterance. In the Babies and Beginners stage (see Chapter 7), children are understanding one word in an utterance. If a beginning language learner hears, "Grandpa is pouring the milk," "milk" may be the only word that is understood. However, as children enter the emerging word combinations stage, they begin to understand other salient words in the sentence and understand that every change in a critical element can alter the meaning: In our example, Grandpa (not Mommy, not Daddy) is pouring (not drinking, not spilling) the milk (not water, not juice). Understanding an increasing number and variety of critical elements in a sentence is essential to developing complex receptive understanding and flexibility in expressive utterances.

In addition to an increase in vocabulary and understanding of statements, a toddler's receptive language growth is marked by a growing ability to understand questions. **Table 8.2**[6] shows the order of acquisition for understanding questions in the first few years of life. Knowing and considering the hierarchy of developing an understanding of questions are essential in LSL intervention because they guide the selection of goals and activities. Far too often, adults rely on asking yes/no questions with toddlers and children with toddler-type language when children in this stage are capable of much more. Setting the bar high in LSL intervention includes moving forward in modeling next-level questions within an LSL intervention session and relying on yes/no questions only as a rudimentary tool to facilitate understanding rather than a crutch. Guiding and coaching caregivers in the art of questions will provide essential tools for conversational growth in everyday life with children in this stage.

Table 8.2 Development of understanding questions

Age of child	Type of question	Example
< 12 months	Yes/no	*Do you want juice?*
1 to 2 years	What	*What is it?*
	Where	*Where's the ball?*
	Who	*Who is that?*
2 to 3 years	When	*When is your birthday?*
	Why	*Why did it break?*
	How	*How does a bird fly?*

Source: Adapted from Lanza JR. LinguiSystems Guide to Communication Milestones. LinguiSystems, Inc.; 2008.

Pitfall

Far too often, adults rely on asking yes/no questions with toddlers and children with toddler-type language when children in this stage are capable of much more.

For older children who are in this stage of development, the same truths of receptive language development apply. It might seem easier to target expressive language with children who are chronologically older, yet receptive language should receive equal (if not more) attention in writing goals and planning activities. Without comprehensive goals for the development of receptive language and vocabulary, the expressive language development in these older children will remain limited and significantly delayed compared to their typically hearing peers (see Chapter 11).

Pitfall

Without comprehensive goals for the development of receptive language and vocabulary, the expressive language development in these older children will remain limited and significantly delayed compared to their typically hearing peers.

8.5.2 Expressive Language

Expressive language is coming to life in the toddler years, yet expressive vocabulary growth is behind receptive language growth in the race to acquire language—as it should be. **Table 8.3** highlights this difference.[4]

Around the time toddlers have an expressive vocabulary of about 50 words, they will start combining words into two-word utterances, then phrases, and then sentences. Sometimes this

milestone is mistakenly considered to be at 24 months when it should begin occurring around 18 months for typically developing language acquisition. Having an expressive vocabulary that's diverse in both types and intentions of words is essential in learning to combine words into phrases and then sentences.

By 18 months of age, a toddler will demonstrate several language intentions with words. These include labeling, protesting, greeting, requesting, expressing recurrence, and showing possession. Vocabulary mixed with intentions is a recipe for expressing original ideas and being a conversational partner with humans in the environment. For example, a toddler who says "mine" is showing possession. In the same way, a toddler that says "again" is expressing recurrence. These intentions begin in single words and grow to word combinations, then phrases and then sentences as the child grows and develops.

Early expressive phrases include "hi daddy," "more milk," and "no dog." These word combinations mature between the ages of 21 to 24 months to more early sentence structures that can continue to develop. Examples of early two-word sentences include: "Go car!" (action + object), "Bubba stop" (agent + action), and "my ball" (possessive + object). (See **Table 8.4** for a list of expressive two-word combinations by semantic relationship.[4]) To secure the foundation for flexible and varied simple sentences, it is critical that toddlers and older children in this stage develop the ability to combine words in several different patterns.

Morphologic development begins in the toddler stage. Morphemes are a part of language that refer to the smallest unit of meaning. For example, "dog" is one morpheme, but "dogs" is two morphemes (dog + plural *s*). The average length of a toddler's utterances can be measured by calculating a mean length of utterance (MLU). The MLU is calculated by dividing the total number of morphemes in a language sample divided by the total number of utterances. Whether collecting a language sample on your own or thinking about the average length of a toddler's utterances, Brown's stages of language development are helpful in knowing MLU in relation to approximate ages (**Table 8.5**).[7,8]

Morphological development begins around a toddler's second birthday and is marked by simple word endings or prepositions

Table 8.3 Vocabulary acquisition

Age of child	Receptive		Expressive	
	Number of words	Types of words	Number of words	Types of words
15 months	3 to 20	Nouns	1 to 10	Nouns
24 months	250 to 500	Nouns Verbs Attributes Pronouns Prepositions Questions	150 to 300	Nouns Verbs Attributes Pronouns Prepositions Early questions
36 months	1200 to 2000	Nouns Verbs Attributes Pronouns Prepositions Questions (growing in complexity)	800 to 1000	Nouns Verbs Attributes Pronouns Prepositions Questions (growing in complexity)

Source: Adapted from Wilkes EM. Cottage Acquisition Scales for Listening Language & Speech. San Antonio, TX: Sunshine Cottage School for Deaf Children; 1999.

Table 8.4 Development of expressive two-word combinations by semantic relationship

Type of Phrase:	Example:
Agent + Action	*Baby sleep*
Action + Object	*Drink milk*
Action + Recipient	*Hug Daddy*
Entity + Location	*Cup table*
Attribute + Entity	*Little cup*
Possessive + Entity	*Mommy cup*
Negative + X	*No socks*
Introducer + X	*Look car*
What + this / that?	*What this?* OR *What that?*
Question	*Go home?*

Source: Adapted from Wilkes EM. Cottage Acquisition Scales for Listening Language & Speech. San Antonio, TX: Sunshine Cottage School for Deaf Children; 1999.

Table 8.5 Mean length of utterance by age

Stage	MLU	Age (months)	Characteristics
I	1.0–2.0	12–26	Single-word utterances and early word combinations
II	2.0–2.5	27–30	Morphological development begins with: Present progressive verbs (-ing) Prepositions: in, on Regular plural -s Irregular past tense verbs Possessive 's
III	2.5–3.0	31–34	Sentence-form development
IV	3.0–3.75	35–40	Embedding of sentence elements
V	3.75–4.5	41–46	Joining of clauses
V+	4.5+	47+	

Table 8.6 Brown's morphemes

Morpheme	Age of Mastery (in months)
Present Progressive -ing	19–28
In	27–30
On	27–30
Regular plural -s	27–33
Irregular past	25–46
Possessive 's	26–40
Uncontractible copula Example: He is.	27–39
Articles	28–46
Regular past -ed	26–48
Regular third person -s	26–46
Irregular third person	28–50
Uncontractible auxiliary Example: She is.	29–48
Contractible copula Example: He's tall.	29–49
Contractible auxiliary Example: He's drinking coffee.	30–50

Source: Adapted from Owens RE Jr. Language Development: An Introduction. 4th ed. Needham Heights, MA: Allyn and Bacon; 1996.

and moves in complexity to irregular forms of words. Brown[8] compiled data on 14 morphemes that begin around a child's second birthday and continue up to a child's sixth birthday to complete mastery of all 14 (**Table 8.6).**

As with other developmental milestones, it's crucial for LSL interventionists to be very familiar with the order of acquisition of expressive language skills for toddlers and older children with toddler-type language when developing and growing goals for intervention. Toddlers' expressive language can vary from child to child, yet for the most part, it follows a hierarchy that builds on previous development as it grows more complex. For toddlers and older children with hearing loss in this stage learning spoken language, this is no different. First and foremost, LSL interventionists must collaborate with the child's pediatric audiologist to ensure that the child has access to all sounds of speech. Consider the morphemes that are tied to specific high-frequency sounds: plural /s/, possessive /s/, and past tense /ed/ (when it is pronounced as /t/ following an unvoiced consonant as in *hopped*); a child who cannot hear these sounds will not develop the morphemes associated with them.

Finally, with rapidly increasing receptive vocabulary and language, growing flexibility in expressing semantic relationships with two- and then three-word utterances, and expanding morphological development, children are setting the stage to begin using simple sentences rather than telegraphic utterances. At first, these simple sentences will be incomplete or contain child-like errors ("Baby going bed"), but with modeling and practice, they should grow more and more accurate ("Baby going to bed" to "The baby going to bed" to "The baby is going to bed"). Following are some strategies for developing receptive and expressive language in the emerging word combinations to simple sentence stage.

One key LSL strategy to guide and coach families in this stage of expressive language development is expansion. Expansion is modeling the next, more complex concept expressively. Coaching caregivers on the milestones within developing expressive language is a key component to expansion being successful within daily, play, and social routines. For example, if a child says "more" when requesting more crackers at snack time, the caregiver could use expansion and respond with "more crackers." Coaching caregivers in expansion within the LSL intervention session is a great

way to grow the caregiver's comfort level with this strategy for carryover into the child's environment.

On the other hand, commenting is an effective strategy for growing receptive vocabulary in toddlers. Commenting (also known as "self-talk" or "parallel talk") means to add a narrative to a child's world. This can look like commenting as the child plays with toys, commenting as you change the baby's diaper, or adding language to what your child might be feeling or thinking in a situation. Commenting adds spoken language to routines. It provides an opportunity for a child's experiences to have spoken language added to them. Remember that greater than 90% of what children learn, they learn incidentally. Commenting is a great strategy to grow rich vocabularies by giving real-life words to children's interests. With commenting, it's imperative that the caregiver use rich language as much as possible. Consider commenting in the following scenario: the child is playing with a baby doll. Mom can use either these sentences: "Look! You put it there, and now it's here." Or these sentences: "Aww! The baby was sitting in the chair. Now the baby is sleepy. You put him to bed. Shh! Be very quiet." Which of these sets of sentences provides a richer language experience? An LSL interventionist should coach caregivers to use rich language when employing the strategy of commenting because it will provide more mileage growing receptive language than nonspecific language.

Pearl

Remember that greater than 90% of what children learn, they learn incidentally.

Singing is another great LSL strategy to incorporate when focusing on language growth in the toddler years. Singing is a form of acoustic highlighting because it draws attention to sound in a way that differs from regular speech. Think of the classroom setting. Often, early childhood educators will utilize singing in the classroom to get children's attention, define routines, and assist in the transition from one activity to another. Children learn these songs and what they mean quickly. Singing highlights the acoustic signal to get the attention of the listener and also to grow language. Receptively, children will associate gestures with songs before they are able to sing the words of a song. Think of "Pat-a-cake." Children younger than 12 months of age might start clapping when a grown-up starts this familiar routine. Expressively, children will learn to keep a song going by vocalizing and then providing specific words when a grown-up sings a familiar song and then pauses.

8.6 The Focus of Speech Development at This Stage

Speech development in the toddler years is ever-growing and changing. By three years of age, a child consistently produces the following phonemes: /h/, /w/, /m/, /n/, and /p/. By four years of age, a child consistently adds these phonemes: /b/, /d/, /k/, /g/, /f/, and /j/.[9] An LSL interventionist should consider sounds that are emerging as well as routinely produced versus mastered to assess the big picture of a child's speech sounds. See **Table 8.7** for more information.[9]

8.6.1 Milestones and Obstacles in Speech Development

An LSL interventionist should keep in mind that a child with hearing loss must have auditory access to all phonemes of spoken language to produce phonemes clearly. Yet, children with hearing loss are not exempt from articulation or phonological disorders. If LSL interventionists suspect that a child has adequate access to all the sounds of speech and still has speech errors, they should refer the child for a speech evaluation to assess errors and look for patterns of errors that can be targeted in intervention.

As with other developmental milestones, children who are older yet demonstrate speech, language, and listening skills similar to that of a toddler will develop speech sounds sequentially yet possibly at a faster rate than that of a child whose age is within the timeframes previously listed. This is due to the muscle maturity already

established by the articulators in an older child. Keep in mind that "possibly" indicates we should cater goal selection and reasonable expectations based on each child's individual progress and pace.

Pearl

An LSL interventionist should keep in mind that a child with hearing loss must have auditory access to all phonemes of spoken language to produce phonemes clearly.

8.6.2 Strategies for Developing Speech

Acoustic highlighting is the best tool to employ when working on targeted phonemes within a child's speech. Acoustic highlighting gives emphasis to sounds or words to make the targeted phonemes (in this case) more audible. LSL interventionists should keep in mind that acoustic highlighting should be employed as a tool and that caregivers shouldn't always highlight sounds because that's not natural and can distort the message. If children have adequate auditory access to all the sounds of speech, they shouldn't need sounds exaggerated to be able to imitate them correctly.

8.7 The Focus of Cognition and Play at This Stage

Underlying all development at this stage is cognition. Cognition refers to the process of acquiring and understanding knowledge. One way to know about a child's capacity for cognition is a measure of intelligence. A child's potential for development in listening, language, speech, and play all hinges on their cognition. It's important to consider assessing nonverbal intelligence as early as a child is able to know whether the child is reaching his or her potential verbally. The Primary Test of Nonverbal Intelligence (PTONI) can be administered to children as young as 3 years of age. LSL providers should consider assessing nonverbal intelligence at least once in the child's lifetime, and as early as the child's ability and testing measures allow.

Even without a standard score for intelligence, LSL providers should consider the aspect of cognition when planning goals and intervention. Not all children are capable of the same outcomes. It is known that around 40% of children with hearing loss also have one or more additional diagnoses. Some of these affect a child's

Table 8.7 Consonant acquisition

Age (in months)	Consonants emerging (At least 50% correct production)	Consonants routinely produced (At least 75% correct production)	Consonants mastered (At least 90% correct production)
< 18–23	/f/, /k/, /g/, /j/, /ŋ/, /t/	/m/, /b/, /n/, /p/	/h/, /w/
24–29	/l/, /dʒ/, /t/	/f/, /k/, /g/, /j/, /d/, /ŋ/, /t/	/m/, /b/, /n/, /p/
30–35			/f/, /g/, /d/
36–41	/v/, /r/		/k/, /j/, /ŋ/, /t/
42–48	/ɡ/, /ʃ/, /s/		

Source: Adapted from Pena-Brooks A. Assessment & Treatment of Articulation & Phonological Disorders in Children. Austin, TX: Pro-Ed; 2000.

cognition, and thus their potential outcomes in listening, language, and speech. A child with limited cognition will have developmental delays that are not necessarily related to hearing loss. A child with cognition within normal limits should develop listening and spoken language on par with peers (given there are no additional barriers). A child with above-average cognition should develop listening and spoken language above average as compared to peers. Cognition is an imperative consideration in assessing, planning, and executing intervention for children with hearing loss.

Pearl

Cognition is an imperative consideration in assessing, planning, and executing intervention for children with hearing loss.

8.7.1 Considerations for Cognition with Older Children Who Are in This Stage of Development

LSL providers should keep in mind that delays in language development do not mean below-average intelligence. For older children who are late to listening and are in these toddler stages of development, cognition will also be delayed. A child with the ability to follow directions with no more than two critical elements will not have the same critical thinking skills as a child who is capable of six or more critical elements. Consider a group of 6-year-olds listening to a story being read aloud. Will the child with language similar to a 2-year-old understand all the vocabulary, decisions, conflicts, resolutions, and humor that his peers with language skills matching their chronological age? No. Will this same child be able to verbalize a summary of the story in appropriate sentences as well as make predictions from the story? No. Will this same child be able to relate this story to his personal life and verbalize the correlations? No. It's important for LSL providers to consider cognition when choosing play activities to integrate reasonable expectations within intervention and to coach caregivers in carryover.

The development of play skills during toddler years parallels the growth of language during this time period. LSL interventionists should be familiar with the developmental milestones of play in a toddler, as this will guide them in the selection of age-appropriate activities to facilitate language learning. The toddler years are marked by moving from sensorimotor play into the preoperational stage of play (see **Table 8.8**) in Piaget's Stages of Play.[10] The preoperational stage of play includes parallel play

(playing alongside peers but not with peers), pretend play, and acting out of familiar routines in play.

Let's dive deeper into pretend play. As with most developmental skills, pretend play emerges as very basic and becomes more complex over time. Pretend play emerges around a child's first birthday and is shown by the child acting out routines that are encountered in daily life. These can include pretending to sleep, pretending to take a drink, or pretending to leave by getting in the car seat. At the age of 18 months, toddlers begin acting out simple-pretend play routines. These can include pretending to read and engaging caregivers by pretending to give them a drink from an empty cup. See **Table 8.9** for more information about the development of pretend play.

8.7.2 Considerations for Play with Older Children Who Are in This Stage of Development

Unlike several other topics in this chapter, play may be an area where older children who are language-delayed will demonstrate more typical development. Children who are older than 3 years yet have language younger than 3 years can still demonstrate play skills similar to that of their peers of similar chronological age. Yet, the charts provided regarding play in this chapter highlight the development of play skills and can be used a reference for tracking progress and setting goals in order of progression (even without the age information). This is important to consider when planning intervention sessions. Keep in mind the play skills of the child to keep the child engaged in intervention. For example, a child who is 5 years old but demonstrates language and listening skills similar to that of an 18-month-old doesn't necessarily need activities reduced in play to those of an 18-month-old. One of the keys to incorporating listening, language, and speech targets into play routines with older children is to balance the goals within a play framework that is engaging and appealing to the child. The 5-year-old in the previous example might enjoy incorporating monster trucks into a garage/ramp rather than carrying out simple routines with a baby doll.

Pearl

One of the keys to incorporating listening, language, and speech targets into play routines with older children is to balance the goals within a play framework that is engaging and appealing to the child.

Table 8.8 Piaget's stages of play

Ages (years)	Stages of Play	Description
0 to 2	Sensorimotor stage	Includes the five senses, motor play, and exploration
2 to 7	Preoperational stage	Includes parallel play, pretend play, acting out familiar routines in play
7 to 11	Concrete operational stage	Includes logic, problem solving, and turn taking
11+	Formal operational stage	Includes abstract thought, manipulating ideas and hypothetical situations

Source: Adapted from Gallo A. What are the stages of play? Jean Piaget's Theory of Play! Play. Learn. Thrive. https://playlearnthrive.com/stages-of-play-jean-piagets-theory/. Published June 9, 2021. Accessed March 14, 2022.

Table 8.9 Development of pretend play

Ages	Type of pretend play	Description	Example
12–18 months	Self-pretend play	The toddler plays at being herself.	The toddler pretends to fall asleep.
		The toddler performs pretend actions on herself using real-life objects or realistic-looking toys.	The toddler pretends to drink from a cup.
18–24 months	Simple-pretend play	Toddler pretends by performing single actions on people or toys.	Toddler offers adult a toy phone.
		Toddler can substitute a toy object for a real object.	Toddler pretends to eat a toy banana.
		Toddler pretends to do things she sees adults do.	Toddler pretends to read a magazine.
24–30 months	Sequence pretend of familiar events	The toddler performs a sequence of several pretend actions in the appropriate order.	Toddler pretends to prepare and then eat food.
	Beginnings of role play	The toddler plays the role of another person.	Toddler pretends to be a mommy with her baby.
		The toddler can substitute one object for another if it is similar in shape.	Toddler pretends a stacking ring is a donut.
		The toddler gives a doll/animal a more active role in play.	The toddler makes the bear hold a cup and take a drink.
30–36 months	Sequence pretend of less familiar events	The toddler begins to act out less familiar events.	Toddler pretends to be a hairdresser.
		The toddler's pretending is action-based and she may or may not talk during play.	The toddler acts out shopping at a grocery store.
	Substitution of dissimilar objects	The toddler pretends with objects that don't look like the objects for which they stand.	The toddler pretends a block is a car.
		The toddler creates imaginary objects to support her play.	The toddler pets a pretend dog.
3 to 5 years	Sociodramatic Play: *Planned Pretend Themes* (also known as Dramatic Play)	Roleplay	Children will take on make-believe roles.
		Use of make-believe	Children will create imaginary objects for their play: "I am the doctor, and I'm going to cut your bandage" (uses fingers as scissors).
		Use of language to create make-believe actions or situations	Children will use descriptions to engage in play: "Let's pretend that I am the doctor and you came to see me because you broke your arm."
		Extended-play episodes	With no time constraints, children can play for at least 10 minutes in these routines.
		Interaction	At least two children cooperate and interact together in the play episode.
		Verbal communication	The children talk to one another about the play.

Source: Adapted from Weitzman E. Learning Language and Loving It. Toronto, Ontario; Hanen Centre; 1992.

However, we must also recognize that, while the older children with toddler-type language may be physically able to play at a level more consistent with their chronological age, they will lack the receptive and expressive vocabulary and language that accompanies age-appropriate play. Children who have normal hearing have heard the language of familiar routines and activities hundreds of times, so they are able to incorporate this language into play. As indicated in **Table 8.9**, between the ages of 3 and 5, language becomes the basis for play.[11] Older children with hearing loss in this stage have watched and participated in routines and activities hundreds of times but have been hearing the language that accompanies them only for a short time and do not yet understand all the elements in sentences. This makes it difficult for them to follow their peers' dialogue during imaginary play. For example, let's say our five-year-old from the previous example enjoys playing Superheroes. If his peer with typical hearing says, "I'm Spider-Man, and you are Captain America. I put you in a web, so you are stuck and cannot get out until the Hulk breaks the web," our child with hearing loss will have difficulty understanding the rules of play that have been stated and, to the exasperation of his peer, may not participate as directed. Parents and teachers are often concerned because the older child with toddler-like language may play alone or with much younger children. As LSL interventionists, we must educate parents and teachers about the relationship between language and play and create goals that help the child apply learned language to play (**Fig. 8.2**).

8.8 The Focus of Literacy at This Stage

Although they are not yet readers, toddlers are considered emergent readers because they are forming the foundation for critical reading and writing abilities in this timeframe. By the age of 18 months, children take control of reading experiences by pointing to pictures, turning pages one at a time, and asking questions about the story. They label familiar pictures in books but believe all words are labels to the pictures. Toddlers at this age learn that reading gives us information because they watch grown-ups in their world read for information with things like menus, newspapers, and street signs. One-year-olds identify conflict in a story (for example: "uh oh" or "ball gone"). One-year-olds are in the pre-alphabetic stage, which means that any ability they have to recognize words or symbols comes from memorization and not from sound/symbol association with letters from the alphabet. One-year-olds can hold books with proper orientation and turn pages in the correct direction.[12]

As two-year-olds, toddlers continue to grow in their pre-literacy skills. Toddlers in this age group will choose books to "read" independently—meaning they will sit, turn pages, and comment on pictures or even recite a familiar storyline. These older toddlers will begin to have favorites in books and will even choose similar books by their covers (for example, a child who loves Eric Carle's *Brown Bear, Brown Bear* might also select *The Very Hungry Caterpillar* because he notices the similarities on the cover). Toddlers in this age group can fill in missing words in stories, especially those with strong carrier phrases or repeated lines. They will sometimes ask grown-ups what certain words say. They are also beginning to point out letters in their environment, especially those in their own names. Children will also begin commenting on the storyline, characters, conflicts, and beginnings and endings.[12]

Grown-ups engaging with toddlers to grow emergent literacy skills can do so in many ways. First, grown-ups should carve out time daily to read to and with their toddler. This can be at bedtime as a part of a routine or perhaps at a routine time of day that works best for their family. An LSL provider can play an integral role in helping grown-ups identify an ideal time for reading aloud as well as strategies to maximize the time. Reading aloud can include both reading books word-for-word as well as elaborating in a more conversational tone with picture books. Grown-ups should be creative in engaging the toddler as an active participant in reading aloud. Some ideas of how to do this include: provide a snack in the high chair to establish joint attention on books, get toys out to correspond with the story for the toddler to have sensory stimulation, begin to match pictures to objects in place, let the child hold the book and control the page-turning as the grown-up prompts, and stop reading occasionally to have the toddler fill in missing words. Jim Trelease challenges grown-ups to prioritize quality over quantity when it comes to reading aloud—meaning

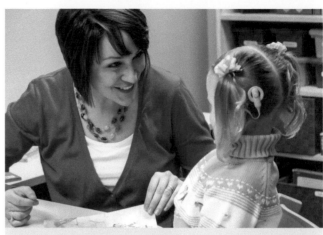

Fig. 8.2 LSL interventionists help children apply learned language to play. Used by permission from family and Hearts for Hearing.

that ten minutes of reading with your child at this language stage can provide a richer experience than 2 hours of sitting in front of a television or playing computer games.[13] Grown-ups should begin using "book language" during the twos, so children develop an awareness of vocabulary related specifically to books. This may include book, cover, page, story, title, beginning, and end. Last but not least, grown-ups can encourage reading by modeling it often in their own lives— with real print books and not just electronics.

Pearl

Prioritize quality over quantity when it comes to reading aloud—meaning that 10 minutes of reading with your child at this language stage can provide a richer experience than 2 hours of sitting in front of a television or playing computer games.[13]

Keep in mind that children who are older yet are within the toddler stage of development must move through reading readiness in a sequential way, just like their younger peers. Children who are 6 years old, for example, and have listening and language similar to a 2-year-old are not equipped for jumping into decoding and reading due to their limited experience with vocabulary, concepts, and language. Literacy should maintain a priority in focus of intervention as LSL providers work on listening, language, and speech goals, but time should be given for those skills that precede reading such as rhyming, book concepts, and reading aloud.

For more information on the development of literacy skills, see Chapter 13. That chapter provides several resources for milestones in literacy, as well as incorporating literacy into LSL intervention (**Fig. 8.3**).

8.9 The Focus of Intervention at This Stage

A listening and spoken language intervention session likely has similar components no matter the child's stage, but there are

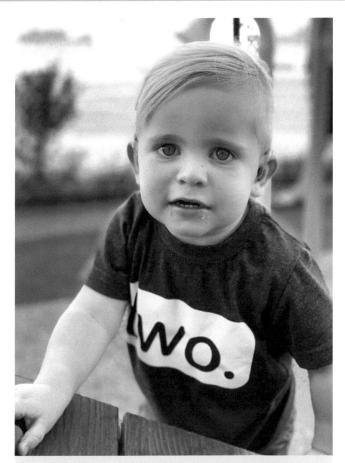

Fig. 8.3 LSL resources for milestones in literacy and incorporating literacy into LSL intervention. Used by permission from family and Hearts for Hearing.

some important things to consider when planning and executing intervention sessions in the toddler-type language stage.

8.9.1 Setting Goals

One of the greatest mistakes in planning intervention sessions is under- or oversetting expectations with goals. An LSL provider should carefully plan session goals based on the next correct step for each child and not just based on the chronological age, listening age, or an item missed on a standardized test. In addition to setting appropriate goals, an LSL provider should be prepared to level up or down as needed during the session, keeping in mind that the goal is not 100% accuracy. If a child is consistently reaching 100% accuracy, the LSL provider should be expecting more and coaching caregivers to push for more. The hallmark of a gifted LSL provider is the ability to adjust midstream to maintain high expectations for the child with hearing loss, yet not overreach expectations. Moreover, if a child is consistently reaching 100% accuracy, then the rate of progress will slow or stop because the intervention lacks a clear roadmap of what the language professionals and parents should be providing to and expecting from the child. An LSL provider should be able to level not only the targets of goals but also the level of modeling, prompting, or assistance needed to achieve the goal, all while

maintaining engagement from the caregiver and child through engaging play routines.

8.9.2 Structure of an Intervention Session

Establishing a Connection

A successful intervention session does not begin in a therapy room but at the moment of connection with the child and caregiver. This may be in the waiting room of a clinic or at the front door or even in the greetings in a teleintervention session. Connecting with a child in this stage is important for setting the context of a pleasant, engaging time. Also, connecting with the caregiver is crucial in setting the tone of the session and allowing the LSL provider to empathize with or celebrate the events of the week. Sometimes a caregiver is eager to share all the celebrations the child and family have experienced in the week. Other times, the caregiver is needing validation in expressing how hard and busy life is outside of the intervention session. Either way, the LSL provider should be sensitive to this from the onset of connecting at each session.

Pearl

A successful intervention session does not begin in a therapy room but at the moment of connection with the child and caregiver.

Again Discussing Caregiver Involvement

As discussed earlier, caregiver coaching is a non-negotiable component of any LSL intervention session. An LSL provider should prioritize caregiver coaching more than any other part of the session because the toddler and the older child with toddler-type language are going to learn listening and spoken language from their caregiver, with whom they spend greater than 99% of their hours! An LSL intervention session without caregiver coaching can be a fun time, but without the depth of a foundation of caregiver coaching, it's weak and lacks influence in a child's development.

Pitfall

An LSL intervention session without caregiver coaching can be a fun time, but without the depth of a foundation of caregiver coaching, it's weak and lacks influence in a child's development.

An LSL provider should plan for caregiver coaching at many times during the session, starting with an open-ended question or statement to gain information from the caregiver since the last session. These opening conversations could start with something as simple as "What's something you celebrated this week?" or "Tell me something good" or "What's your greatest concern?"

Then, coaching continues through each activity. This can take the form of explaining the "so what," turning over the session to the caregiver, or having them watch for certain LSL strategies during an activity. Finally, concluding the session with more time for brainstorming and conversation is key for facilitating carryover (as we will discuss more in this next section).

Equipment Check

Every child with hearing loss who has appropriate amplification maintained by a pediatric audiologist should have adequate access to all sounds of speech if pursuing a spoken language outcome, yet a child with toddler-type language is not yet able to communicate through intricate descriptors if equipment isn't working optimally or there has been a change in hearing. For this reason, an LSL provider or the caregiver should quickly do an equipment check at the beginning of every session. A child in this toddler stage should be able to quickly imitate the Ling-Madell-Hewitt (LMH) 10-Sound Quick Test from increasing distance through audition only. This equipment check should be quick and should not require the LSL provider to take off the technology to troubleshoot unless a change in responses is noted. Ideally, imitation of the LMH 10 sounds should be obtained with each device separately and at increasing distances. If a child consistently imitates all LMH 10 sounds from 3 feet, the LSL provider should double the distance, and thus the volume would decrease by 6 dB. This strategy corresponds with "raising the bar" as discussed earlier in the section on setting goals.[14]

Keep in mind that using a toy with multiple turns may be helpful as a child is learning to imitate all sounds. For example, a ring stacker with multiple rings can be used to elicit imitation by using the parent as a model and each ring mimicking a microphone. When establishing a routine within LSL intervention, using the same toy for the equipment check in each session can provide predictability and aid in carryover.

Literacy Component

Several goals of LSL intervention can be targeted by incorporating a book into each session. For a child in this toddler stage of language development, this is especially true. Integrating literacy provides a springboard for listening, language, and speech growth along with showing how comfortable the child and caregiver are with books. A toddler who has had frequent exposure to books and was read aloud to as a baby will often demonstrate an increased listening attention span compared to a child who hasn't had positive, frequent experiences with books. For children who have not had frequent exposure to books or have not developed the auditory attention needed for listening to them, parents will often report that the child "does not like books and reading." Helping parents learn to choose appropriate books, set appropriate listening expectations, and become engaging readers is often an essential part of LSL coaching.

Pearl

A toddler who has had frequent exposure to books and was read aloud to as a baby will often demonstrate an increased listening attention span compared to a child who hasn't had positive, frequent experiences with books.

Targeting Multiple Goals within One Activity

A toddler's job is play; thus, incorporating targets for listening, language, and speech into play routines is critical for learning. For a toddler whose chronological age is aligned with their listening age, developmental goals should be incorporated into developmentally appropriate play routines. One hallmark of a gifted LSL provider is a session that looks like seamless play routines yet is rich in goals and strategies.

For a child who is older yet is in the toddler stage of language, listening, and speech development, goals can still be incorporated naturally into play routines, yet this can sometimes differ due to the nature of the goals. This intervention is remedial in nature and sometimes requires more structured play-type tasks to facilitate maximizing the potential growth for the child. Assuming a child who is in second grade will do best learning from worksheets is a mistake. Keep in mind that activities lead to carryover and take that seriously when selecting activities within LSL intervention. Perhaps a second grader could be actively involved in choosing the motivating activity to target goals? An LSL provider should be sensitive to the needs of each child and family when choosing goals corresponding with activities within a session and for carryover.

Facilitating Carryover

What good is an LSL intervention session if the goals and strategies cannot be carried over into everyday life for the child with hearing loss and the family? None at all. An LSL provider should make every effort to pause at the conclusion of a session (or jot down notes along the way) to chat with the caregiver about carryover. This conversation will likely take the shape of the learning style of the caregiver, and it should be that way. Some caregivers want to take detailed notes along the way in their notebook that they bring to each session. For this caregiver, carryover accumulates as the session transpires. For other caregivers, they are ready and willing to jump in often during the session for hands-on practice. Then, they can talk through those experiences and narrow down ideas for carryover at the conclusion. The LSL provider can transition into this portion of the session by again using open-ended statements or questions that might include: "What three things are you taking away from today's session?" or "What stood out to you most this week?" or "What are one or two things you want to practice this week?" If a caregiver is focused more on the activities or toys within the session and less on the goals and strategies, this gives the LSL provider a great opportunity to emphasize the importance of the goals and strategies and to devalue any "magic" that might be associated with a certain toy. Teleintervention is a great way to decrease the focus on the toys because the session is using toys and activities from the child's home and enhancing those with new goals and strategies.

Pearl

If a caregiver is focused more on the activities or toys within the session and less on the goals and strategies, this gives the LSL provider a great opportunity to emphasize the importance of the goals and strategies and to devalue any "magic" that might be associated with a certain toy.

8.10 Summary

Toddler-type development is robust and rich, as seen throughout this chapter. The toddler stages of listening, speech, and receptive and expressive language development are crucial for developing more rich language, literacy, and academic skills beyond the toddler years. Both children who are within the toddler stage of development at the same time that they are toddlers and those children who are in this stage at an older age due to acquiring listening later in life can each demonstrate progress and success with the help of enlightened caregivers and intentional pediatric audiologists and LSL providers. LSL providers should strive to grow knowledge in developmental milestones at this age, raise the bar for each child and prioritize caregiver coaching as the key to optimizing listening, speech, and language for the toddler with hearing loss.

8.11 Case Study 1: Child Chronologically Appropriate for This Stage

Evie, age 2 years, 2 weeks, has been diagnosed with a moderate sensorineural hearing loss bilaterally. She was diagnosed at less than 1 month of age via auditory brainstem response (ABR) after referring three times to her newborn hearing screening. Evie has a family history of hearing loss, including her older sister and father having sensorineural hearing loss and utilizing hearing aids, yet Evie's father and sister were not diagnosed with hearing loss until after Evie was diagnosed with hearing loss. She was fitted with digital hearing aids at 1 month of age. Evie also uses a personal remote microphone system at home. She has been seen for weekly auditory-verbal therapy sessions since 1 month of age and attends a parent-toddler group weekly with her mother.

Currently, Evie demonstrates an emerging skill of following commands with two critical elements. She can more easily follow two familiar commands together with high context such as "put it in the bucket and wave bye bye" or "throw it away and wash your hands." Expressively, Evie requests more often with one word rather than two such as "more" or "cookie" rather than "more cookie." When following a model, she will use two words to request in therapy and also at home. Evie's speech is typical for her age, yet is not adult-like yet. She consistently substitutes /k/ for /t/, /d/ for /g/, and /p/ for /f/. She also sometimes leaves off the last sounds of words. Lastly, Evie is full of strong opinions. She remains more engaged in therapy when choices on activities are given.

Of note, Evie's speech and language scores are within normal limits, yet this does not negate her need for intervention. Keep in mind that hearing loss is a risk factor for delays in listening, speech, and language development. Developmental intervention is no less important than remedial intervention for children with hearing loss within the first three years of life—when the most learning is occurring.[15] A toddler cannot adequately verbalize a shift in hearing or a change in hearing technology; thus it is imperative to continue with early intervention at least until the age of 3 to closely monitor listening, speech, and language growth over time.

See **Table 8.10** for scores from Evie's most recent language evaluation. She was 2 years, 2 weeks old at the time of this assessment.

8.12 Case Study 2: Older Child in This Stage

Justin, age 4 years, 7 months, has been diagnosed with a profound sensorineural hearing loss bilaterally. His birth history includes being born full-term and passing his newborn hearing screening (NBHS). Pertinent medical history (PMH) includes the following: At one week of age, Justin was diagnosed with hypoplastic left heart syndrome. He was immediately hospitalized and received a heart transplant at 8.5 months of age at a children's hospital out of state. At 11 months of age, he acquired bacterial meningitis and was hospitalized for 2 months due to complications. He did not pass the hearing screening before being discharged from the hospital. Justin received his first cochlear implant at 16 months of age with activation of that device at 17 months of age. Justin has not yet received a second cochlear implant due to chronic health issues with his ears. He originally only received one cochlear implant because it was the surgeon's preference at the time. Justin also uses a personal remote microphone system at home and at school. He has been seen for weekly LSL intervention sessions since 17 months of age. Justin also currently attends a public school where he is in a mainstream pre-kindergarten class for most of the day. Justin is on an individual education plan (IEP) through the school and receives speech therapy, physical therapy, and occupational therapy.

Currently, Justin wears his cochlear implant during all waking hours. His mother is actively involved in each therapy session. Justin is making slow but steady progress. Some considerations for Justin's delays include limited language input during hospitalizations, limited exposure to peers until being enrolled in school due to health issues, and likely cognition greater than one standard deviation below the mean. (Assessment at the age of 5 years, 7 months demonstrated Justin has a nonverbal IQ of 84.) Despite his delays in development, Justin is very social. He loves engaging with staff and other adults at the clinic every time he comes in for therapy. His strength expressively is with social phrases such as "How's it going?" or "What's your name?" Yet, he struggles with appropriate syntax when generating sentences and questions that are not memorized. For example, he can clearly say "What's up?" but when prompted to find out mom's favorite color, he will say "Mom favorite color?" (with question inflection but not worded as a question). He is not yet using appropriate verb tenses (such as adding "s" for present tense or "ed" for past tense when appropriate). He also consistently leaves off plural and possessive "s" and omits helping verbs. Receptively, Justin can consistently follow directions with two critical elements when presented through audition only, but he struggles with three or more. He not only

Table 8.10 Evie's Preschool Language Scale, Fifth Edition (PLS-5)

	Standard Score	Percentile	Age Equivalent
Auditory comprehension	103	58	1 yr, 10 months
Expressive Communication	105	64	1 yr, 9 months
Total Language	104	61	1 yr, 9 months

Table 8.11 Justin's speech and language evaluation (chronological age: 4 yr, 7 mo)

	Scaled score	Standard score	Percentile	Age equivalent
Clinical Evaluation of Language Fundamentals, Preschool, 2nd Edition (CELF-P 2)				
Sentence structure	1		0.1	< 3 yr, 0 months
Word structure	1		0.1	< 3 yr, 0 months
Expressive vocabulary	1		0.1	< 3 yr, 0 months
Concepts and following directions	1		0.1	< 3 yr, 0 months
Recalling sentences	1		0.1	< 3 yr, 0 months
Basic concepts	1		0.1	< 3 yr, 0 months
Core Language		45	<0.1	
Receptive Language Index		45	<0.1	
Expressive Language Index		48	<0.1	
Language Content Index		45	<0.1	
Language Structure Index		48	<0.1	
Peabody Picture Vocabulary Test, Fourth Edition (PPVT-4)		70	2	2 yr, 8 months
Expressive Vocabulary Test, Second Edition (EVT-2)		70	2	2 yr, 8 months

struggles to remember three or more items but often confuses the order of presentation. For example, when playing a barrier game with toys, mom may ask Justin to "put the baby under the chair." Justin would likely understand baby and chair but then put the baby "in" the chair as a guess. Another example during a barrier game: mom may ask Justin to "put the cat and dog in the cup," and Justin would likely put the cat in the cup and not select the dog. Justin's intelligibility of speech is good even with unfamiliar listeners. He uses most age-appropriate phonemes with the exception of /l/ and /r/. He even uses most consonant clusters spontaneously and correctly. Lastly, when tasks become too challenging, he has been observed to attempt to divert attention or change the subject to something familiar and comfortable.

See **Table 8.11** for scores from Justin's most recent language evaluation. He was 4 years, 7 months old at the time of this assessment.

Discussion Questions

1. Given each child's current age and level of functioning, what would you expect their play skills to be?
2. Given each child's current age and level of functioning, what would you predict some goals for LSL intervention to be? Provide goals for audition, receptive language, expressive language, and speech.
3. Given each child's current age and level of functioning, what would you predict could be challenging in an LSL intervention session?
4. Given the description of the caregiver and child relationship, what caregiver coaching techniques do you feel would be effective in intervention with this child?

References

[1] Estabrooks W, Morrison H, MacIver-Lux K. Auditory-Verbal Therapy: Science, Research and Practice. San Diego, CA: Plural Publishing; 2020
[2] Erber N. Evaluating speech perception ability in hearing impaired children. In: Bess H, ed. Childhood Deafness: Causation, Assessment, and Management. New York, NY: Grune & Stratton; 1977
[3] Walker B. Auditory Learning Guide. Pennsylvania Speech-Language-Hearing Association. https://www.psha.org/member-center/pdfs/auditory-learning-guide.pdf Updated April 3, 2009. Accessed March 14, 2022
[4] Wilkes EM. Cottage Acquisition Scales for Listening Language & Speech. San Antonio, TX: Sunshine Cottage School for Deaf Children; 1999
[5] Simser JI. Auditory-verbal intervention: infants and toddlers. *Volta Review* 1993;95(3):217–229
[6] Lanza JR. LinguiSystems Guide to Communication Milestones. East Moline, IL: LinguiSystems, Inc.; 2008
[7] Brown R. A First Language: The Early Stages. Cambridge, MA: Harvard U. Press; 1973
[8] Owens RE Jr. Language Development: An Introduction. 4th ed. Needham Heights, MA: Allyn and Bacon; 1996
[9] Pena-Brooks A. Assessment & Treatment of Articulation & Phonological Disorders in Children. Austin, TX: Pro-Ed; 2000
[10] Gallo A. What are the stages of play? Jean Piaget's Theory of Play! Play. Learn. Thrive. https://playlearnthrive.com/stages-of-play-jean-piagets-theory/. Published June 9, 2021. Accessed March 14, 2022
[11] Weitzman E. Learning Language and Loving It. Toronto, Ontario: Hanen Centre; 1992
[12] Phillips L. A Canadian Language and Literacy Research Network Handbook. http://www.theroadmap.ualberta.ca/home. Accessed March 30, 2012
[13] Trelease J. *The Read-Aloud Handbook*. 6th ed. New York, NY: Penguin Books; 2006
[14] Madell JR, Hewitt JG. The LMH Test Protocol. https://hearinghealthmatters.org/hearingandkids/2021/3245/
[15] Cole E, Flexer C. Children with Hearing Loss Developing Listening and Talking. 4th ed. San Diego, CA: Plural Publishing; 2020

9 Preschoolers and More Proficient Communicators: Using Complex Language to Communicate and Think

Elizabeth Tyszkiewicz and Lyndsey Allen

Summary

This chapter covers key points related to deaf or hard of hearing (DHH) children's transition from simple, factual language to the kind of talk that encodes thinking and is crucial in educational and social settings for the rest of their lives. Readers are invited to reflect on the different aspects of spoken language that characterize this process and to develop an informed, intentional plan for each of the children in their care. The crucial role of the family is stressed, and the challenges of accessing classroom education are discussed.

Keywords

complex language, thinking, communication, auditory development, auditory memory, grammar, vocabulary, intervention planning

Key Points

- Therapy and education planning needs to take into account the child's whole developmental profile, as well as allow for individual variation.
- Family life, school life, and other authentic experiences are the richest material for language learning, and caregivers are the main agents of change.
- The quality of a child's access to sound is a crucial determinant of success, and there must be close adult supervision of hearing technology use, as the child becomes independent in a variety of other ways.
- Progress in vocabulary, syntax, and speech production is necessary but not sufficient. The child needs to develop and consolidate pragmatic and social knowledge, as well as engage in using language for complex thinking.
- When DHH children come late to intervention, careful attention needs to be paid to individual adaptation of the support program, enabling them to "catch up."
- Physical and social environments have a powerful effect on a child's ability to participate in collective learning, and when appropriate adaptations are made, these enhance interaction and access to information.

9.1 Characteristics of This Stage

Children who are following a typical developmental trajectory enter this stage with mastery of functional communication, allowing them to use spoken language to have their needs met

(*I want some juice*), to control their environment (*go away dog*), gain information (*where's daddy?*), and enjoy noticing and labeling an increasing number of things of interest to them in the world. The next big developmental leap is the one that takes them into language that supports thinking and refers to processes in our minds that are not visible in the concrete environment.

Early word combinations and "telegraphic" utterances evolve into simple sentences with more complete morphological markers. As language and vocabulary grow, children begin combining simple sentences and move to using more and more complex utterances. By the end of this stage, at approximately 5 years of age, typically hearing children talk constantly, have extensive, descriptive vocabularies, and use compound and complex sentences with generally correct grammar. They ask innumerable questions and can sometimes correct their own errors. Their language approximates adult-like language, which is the foundation they need to become competent learners in an academic (preschool or school) setting.

Pearl

By the end of this stage, at approximately 5 years of age, children's language approximates adult-like language, which is the foundation they need to become competent learners in an academic (preschool or school) setting.

Many of the learning processes that stimulate this development occur through communicative experience and cannot be directly taught. Compare the level of language and thinking required, for example, in the following questions asked during play with toy vehicles:

Simple, concrete level: *Where's that truck driving to?*

Thinking/reasoning/projecting: *What do you think the driver will say when your truck meets that big dumper truck coming over the bridge?*

We examine the stage beyond toddlerhood, when language is "exploding" in the context of a complex and rapidly evolving developmental picture. Children expand their social circle and begin to use language within increasingly complex interactions with a variety of communicative partners. We discuss the close link between a range of emerging skills and the spoken language abilities for which they provide the scaffold.

As Jenny Willan states, "Development is a holistic process of interaction between body and brain, involving reciprocal physical, social, emotional and intellectual responses. It is dependent on the interplay of heredity, character, family, neighborhood and culture, and no two children will develop in exactly the same way."[1]

9.2 Special Considerations for This Stage

Children are not only moving into this next stage of language—they have an array of emerging skills in many domains. When chronological and language age are aligned, or at least not more than a year out of synch, rapid consolidation of both gross and fine motor skills makes children increasingly autonomous, able to explore and act on the environment. They develop awareness of the different thoughts and ideas of others and begin to show "helping" behaviors (e.g., bringing someone their shoes without being asked as the family prepares to go out). Fine motor skills enable real participation in care routines and other activities of daily life, and tasks such as drawing become of increasing interest.

When a child is older in years, but has severely delayed language, this is a crucial consideration for planning intervention. Children may have limited receptive and expressive language skills, and yet be acutely aware of what is socially and cognitively appropriate for their age group. An easy trap to fall into is that of presenting a child with activities matched to their "language age," which they will consider an affront to their dignity and self-perception. We need to offer them tasks, activities, and games that match their age group, while setting listening, speech, and language targets at an appropriate level of attainment. For example, a seven-year old who has come late to listening needs to build auditory discrimination/identification and basic auditory feedback (the ability to reproduce vocally what has been heard) by working on sound-object associations. This child is too mature to find playing with toy objects very engaging but will be stimulated by and interested in a modified version of a competitive card game that incorporates the same auditory targets.

Pearl

Communication development is inseparable from all other aspects of the child's developmental profile.

Pitfall

Where language is delayed, don't offer babyish activities, but match what you offer to the child's chronological age and interests while setting early communication goals.

9.3 Family Involvement in Learning: Crucial for Academic Success

Dathan Rush writes, "When we focus on weaving communication intervention into daily routines and activities, we no longer need to tote a toy bag, or even a tablet, to early-intervention sessions. The focus has shifted to the family's activities and keeping the parent or other primary caregiver in the lead."[2]

It is unfortunate that the moment when the big push from simple to complex language with all its associated cognitive and social development occurs often coincides with the child's move away from the family circle into group settings. This can create the understandable belief that the next stage is the responsibility of the preschool and school professionals, with the family taking more of a supportive role. In addition, support services, such as specialist educators and therapists, may move to the school setting, leaving the family with only occasional contacts or updates. In fact, this process can mask the crucial realization that a child doesn't enter school to learn the language of school; they need to enter with much of the language in place. This language, and its associated thinking skills, is one key to academic success. You cannot learn the history of your family and community without a concept of time and the language to talk about past and future (for example, a standard preschool activity is to look at simple timelines and place pictures of the children as babies on them). You cannot take part in classroom discussion without understanding and knowing how to ask and answer questions beyond the immediately concrete, such as *why do you think that will happen? how do you know? what if...?* You cannot understand stories and begin to navigate social relationships without a grasp of emerging theory of mind and a growing repertoire of "mind minded" terms (*think, want, know; feel, hope, jealous, excited, disappointed*). This language is not an explicit part of the school curriculum because it is assumed that the children will be in the process of developing it and will use it to access curriculum content. A useful distinction is drawn in the field of second language acquisition by children between Basic Interpersonal Communication Skills (BICS) and Cognitive Academic Language Proficiency (CALP), reminding us that, as Jim Cummins explains, "Academic language is characterized by being abstract, context reduced, and specialized. In addition to acquiring the language, learners need to develop skills such as comparing, classifying, synthesizing, evaluating, and inferring when developing academic competence."[3]

While this example does not exactly mirror the situation of DHH children, the practical implications for support services are clear: families need support, resources, training, and encouragement to maintain the learning and input their child requires to be successful in education. Close home-school-therapy service collaboration is crucial, and ideally, therapy services to the family need to continue with a strong emphasis on enabling caregivers to raise their expectations and push the child to the next, less concrete stage of language.

Pitfall

The child's move to formal education settings can create the understandable belief that the next stage is the responsibility of the preschool and school professionals, with the family taking more of a supportive role. In addition, support services, such as specialist educators and therapists, may move to the school setting, leaving the family with only occasional contacts or updates. In fact, this process can mask the crucial realization that a child doesn't enter school to learn the language of school; they need to enter with much of the language in place.

If there are other, typically hearing children in the family, the adult caregivers may well be providing them with good-quality input in response to their questions and curiosities. A good starting point, in this case, is to identify the helpful elements and support the adults in providing the same learning to the DHH child. For their child with hearing loss, they may be unconsciously limiting their language or focusing exclusively on "academic" skills such as learning letters and numbers. The job of the support professional is not to point out these limitations, but to enable caregivers to broaden their view of the next stage to be reached, providing them with the tools to bring about progress. Much of the necessary language input can take place in everyday contexts and through home routines. A therapist can help a parent to upgrade language in a way that promotes dialogue, thinking, and discussion. For example, *put the lid on the toothpaste tube* is a simple, concrete command, but *what do you think will happen if you leave the lid off the toothpaste tube all night?* is a preschool science question. The more adventurous will, in fact, leave the lid off and make some follow-up observations in the morning. They will move into some speculative theory of mind-based questioning: *what do you think Dad will say when he wants to clean his teeth and the toothpaste has become dry and hard?*

To move to this level of language, parents and caregivers are likely to need support and explicit information to enable them to understand how it develops the skills their child needs for school learning. Teachers need similar information to enable them to enrich the conversation in their classrooms and to raise their awareness of the needs of the DHH student.

If we can convince families that home is not just for the child's leisure time but a unique incubator for thinking and brain-building, they can tackle the next stage of their child's language learning with enthusiastic optimism, rather than just hoping that school can do the job. Even when the first stage of language acquisition has gone well, the family is likely to need further intervention to move out of their "comfort zone" and push on to more demanding conversations with their child.

Pearl

If we can convince families that home is not just for the child's leisure time but a unique incubator for thinking and brain-building, they can tackle the next stage of their child's language learning with enthusiastic optimism, rather than just hoping that school can do the job.

9.4 The Focus of Auditory Development at This Stage

Typically hearing children learn from direct interaction and also overhear language used in a range of different situations, trying out expressions or constructions to test their mastery and explore the meaning of what they are learning, sometimes to the amusement of the adults around them.

Clearly, all this is more challenging when a child has impaired hearing. Overall listening time is reduced, the available auditory speech information can be degraded by many different factors, and children's lower level of language attainment may mean that they have fewer problem-solving and meaning-making strategies than children with a wider vocabulary. This means that there is a need for great vigilance and a concerted effort by all those who support the child to bring the child into this next stage of language development. If the child does not progress into the next stage, it is not fair or realistic to expect them to comprehend academic learning and to function as equals among their typically hearing peers. The role of the support professional, as children enter preschool and early education settings, is to keep this goal at the forefront of everybody's mind. Families need to know how they can help the child progress at home, and school staff need training and input to raise their awareness of what needs to be in place for the child to excel academically. Sadly, it is possible for a child with severely delayed language ability to "pass" in a mainstream classroom, apparently accomplishing academic tasks, but with no understanding of the language, thinking, and learning they contain.

Pitfall

When a child has impaired hearing, overall listening time is reduced, the available auditory speech information can be degraded by many different factors, and children's lower level of language attainment may mean that they have fewer problem-solving and meaning-making strategies than children with a wider vocabulary.

Of course, it is a joyful moment for the adults who care for a DHH child when they observe that auditory learning has become integrated into everyday life and that language is developing as a result of listening experiences. Sometimes, the relief and delight can lead to a relaxation of vigilance and to reduced insistence on rigorous use of the hearing technology, especially in busy family life and childcare settings. At this stage, children are still very adaptive and may not have a strong ability to notice and comment if their listening experience has decreased in quality. Four-year-olds who can happily spend a morning at preschool with their shoes worn on the wrong feet are unlikely to have a sophisticated ability to let adults know their hearing technology is malfunctioning. We need to promote independence and self-care, but also remain quite fanatically aware of the need for the technology-dependent child to have hearing devices that are working optimally at all times. We also need to keep training the listening brain to tackle increasingly complex information in ever more challenging listening environments.

This means that we:

1. Make sure, as practitioners, that we have checked with the family what their thoughts, perceptions, assumptions, and experiences are in relation to the child's hearing loss.

This is the feedback from the family of a 4-year-old named Chen, when asked about achievements so far and concerns: "We can't imagine Chen without his hearing aids. He has a moderate-to-severe hearing loss. They really are a part of him, and when, occasionally, he gets some middle ear congestion after a cold, it is immediately noticeable how it makes his hearing less sharp. Chen needs adult supervision when he has to change his clothes for swimming because he can easily knock out and lose a hearing aid. We have to prepare him ahead of time for swimming lessons and use visual strategies because he cannot swim with the hearing aids on. We are working towards him taking responsibility for putting in his earmold, changing his battery, and other basic tasks. We need to make sure that his teachers and other caregivers know how to use his personal assistive technology, and that they are vigilant both about that and his access to sound. With his therapist, we continue to work on 'brain level' auditory skills, such as fine discrimination, auditory recall, and distinguishing signal from noise.

We also have recently realized that Chen does not know many adults who use hearing aids and believes he will not need them when he grows up. We are not sure what is best to do about this."

From this direct inquiry with the child's caregivers, we learn that:

- He is a consistent and committed hearing aid user, but the adults around him may need support and guidance in continuing to optimize his access to sound.
- While he hears well, Chen may not have developed the advanced auditory skills that are necessary for him to flourish socially and fulfill his academic potential.
- This child has not yet had access to DHH peers and role models and may not have a clear idea of himself as an adult who uses hearing technology in the future.

2. Observe the child himself and take into account his level of understanding, as well as his competence in managing his own equipment and listening situation.

"I am Chen and I am five years old. I use two hearing aids and I wear them all the time I am awake. Actually, I like to fall asleep with them on because I don't like the lonely feeling when I'm in bed at night and I can't hear clearly. My favorite things to do are playing with Legos, swimming, and having adventures outside with my brother Eddie. Sometimes I forget that I have my hearing aids on. Once I was jumping in the autumn leaves in the garden and I lost one. It took my parents ages to find it, and they were a bit worried it was gone forever. My Grandad has just got a hearing aid, but none of the other adults I know use them. Probably when I am grown up, I won't need my hearing aids any more."

Observation of and conversation with the child tell us that he loves to hear, but we need to inquire more closely to find his baseline auditory abilities.

- Does he learn from overhearing and incidental conversation? Adults should be noticing the child's use of words and expressions not directly taught. It can be a shock the first time a taboo word is uttered by the child, which family or teachers are quite sure they have never used, but it is an encouraging indicator of incidental language learning.
- Does he accurately process the finer elements of grammar and vocabulary in the utterances he hears? For example, *the baby kissed grandma* has a different meaning from *the baby was kissed by grandma*. A listener who relies on key words and guesswork will not be able to discriminate between the two.
- What level of spoken memory load can he manage, and with what kind of information? A child at this stage should be able to listen to and attempt to retell a simple story. He should be able to follow standard multipart classroom instructions such as *change your shoes, get your reading books, and sit on the carpet.*

- Is there evidence of "listening ahead"? This is a crucial element of the brain-level processing we bring to our perception of connected speech. From early in their development, children can display the skill of "auditory closure" in which they can fill in the possible next words of an interrupted utterance. This starts with easy, rote-learned items such as *ready…get set…_____*, but continues throughout our listening life. We listen to what is said and can narrow down the range of semantic, syntactic, and logical possibilities for what is going to come next, as in *the girl was very tired, so she____* or *we mustn't eat too much candy because _____*. A listener who is unable to do this faces the exhausting task of determining the meaning of each element from an enormous set of possibilities and will not be able to keep up with the flow of information in a classroom interaction or a conversation.

3. Plan intervention using our knowledge of the entire developmental profile of the child, as this is important in determining what learning experiences best support the language and communication progress we are working to attain.

As Weisberg and coworkers state, "When children are in environments where learning is occurring in a meaningful context, where they have choices, and where they are encouraged to follow their interests, learning takes place best."[4]

When the baseline for auditory skills has been established, therapy and teaching can be planned to enhance the child's capabilities and move on to the next stage.

At any specific point, each child has a unique profile in relation to these areas of development. Close observation enables therapy and daily goals to be tailored to the individual's learning needs.

9.5 Auditory Development Considerations for Children Who Come Late to Intervention

Unfortunately, it is not unusual to encounter children whose chronological age is much greater than their listening experience and skills. This can be the result of factors such as late identification of hearing loss, illness, inconsistent use of hearing technology, or, as in the case of some children who arrive from overseas, belated access to appropriate equipment and services. These children need to work through the initial steps covered by their age peers in a more timely fashion. A baseline needs to be established (using the information from previous chapters in this book), and the challenge for practitioners is to devise activities that satisfy age-appropriate physical, cognitive, and social needs, while providing auditory learning opportunities at a "younger" level.

Pearl

Intentional building of "brain level" auditory skills is paramount at this stage.

Pitfall

Do not relax vigilance when providing optimal auditory access through technology, even though the child may be becoming more independent.

9.6 The Focus of Spoken Language Development at This Stage

It is crucial that language goals and the activities planned for implementing them are based on a firm grasp of typical development. Speech and language therapists (pathologists), teachers, and all other support workers need to refer frequently to texts such as Fahey, Hulit. and Howard's *Born to Talk,*[5] research articles, and other information sources, to ensure they are up to date with the latest findings. Our goal in this chapter is not to provide a comprehensive account of everything a child needs to learn at this stage, but rather to lay out guidance for the reader in thinking about what needs to be provided and how to enable the child's transition from talk about what is concrete and visible to talk about what is going on in our minds as we think. Typically developing children drive this transition themselves through their comments and questions. Children with impaired hearing, although they may have plenty of cognitive potential, are at risk of stalling in their learning and of entering the school system without adequate language to take advantage of what is offered or to truly participate in the life of their peer group. The following is an outline of some of the language skills that characterize this stage of development, and then a reflection on how these goals can be implemented by families, teachers, and therapists.

Pitfall

Children with impaired hearing, although they may have plenty of cognitive potential, are at risk of stalling in their learning and of entering the school system without adequate language to take advantage of what is offered or to truly participate in the life of their peer group.

Norm-referenced language assessments that are commonly used to evaluate language ability provide, at best, a crude guide to the child's attainment in relation to age peers by sampling a representative set of test items and providing a score that can be compared to the expected standard. When this score falls significantly below chronological age, children are usually considered eligible for support and therapy services. However, these assessments do not, and cannot, measure the complex thinking abilities for which advanced language is used. This means that children who score at or above average on standardized assessments are most at risk of being considered ineligible for further therapy input; in some educational systems, even children with hearing loss whose scores fall in the low average range do not qualify for services. While these children may have acquired the basic "tools" needed, they are expected to manage the intricate and difficult transition

to complex thinking with minimal support. Without continued intervention, academics and peer relationships become more and more challenging for these children because the language and cognitive demands increase. On the other hand, if intensive, coordinated intervention programms are in place, the child can establish and consolidate the next stage of learning and become well equipped to progress through the education system. This has resourcing implications that can and should be addressed.

Pitfall

Norm-referenced language assessments that are commonly used to evaluate language ability provide at best a crude guide to the child's attainment in relation to age peers. However, these assessments do not, and cannot, measure the complex thinking abilities for which advanced language is used.

9.7 Receptive Language

To access the higher order of thinking that complex language makes possible, a child needs to have the verbal memory capacity to retain and review a string of spoken information that includes content words, but also the semantic and grammatical structures that enable reasoning and theorizing to be encoded. To function in an environment where learning ability is challenged and stretched, a child must learn to listen purposefully, ignore redundant or intrusive information, identify items that need clarification, overhear indirect talk, and make and test informed guesses (which means taking risks and accepting that errors also help us learn). In a classroom, children may be challenged to comprehend speech while engaged in an activity or to participate in discussions with multiple talkers. They must understand and respond to a range of questions, including those that require a speculative, unverifiable answer. They must become aware of the social impact of what is said and the contexts that alter the prosodic features and the language used. This emerging awareness of communication style is apparent when parents at home observe the child's toys being told off in "teacher style" or see the child adopt voices and attitudes when role-playing.

Pearl

To function in an environment where learning ability is challenged and stretched, children must learn to listen purposefully, ignore redundant or intrusive information, identify items that need clarification, overhear indirect talk, and make and test informed guesses (which means taking risks and accepting that errors also help us learn).

Family, teachers, and therapists must bear in mind that language experience needs to be both wide and deep. There is more to knowing a concept than simply being able to label an example of it, such as when the child can say *dog* or *rectangle* or *rain* when presented with a picture. To be really confident to participate in classroom discourse and conversation, a child needs experience of semantic networks,[6] verbal reasoning (*How does Mother Bear know somebody has been eating her porridge?*), causal-explanatory talk (*Baby Bear is very upset because....*), and the finer points of syntax (*Father Bear has the <u>biggest</u> bowl because he eats <u>the most</u> porridge*). Consolidation at this level of detail provides children with a sound foundation on which to rest their own thinking and problem-solving. Adults may sometimes withhold information about more complex concepts because of a (possibly unconscious) belief that children with hearing loss find them too challenging, thus inadvertently depriving them of the rich experience that enables age-appropriate learning to occur.

Pitfall

Adults may sometimes withhold information about more complex concepts because of a (possibly unconscious) belief that children with hearing loss find them too challenging, thus inadvertently depriving them of the rich experience that enables age-appropriate learning to occur.

9.8 Expressive Language

At the stage of language we are describing, a child needs to formulate answers to questions that are beyond the immediate and concrete. *What, who,* and *where* questions are mastered in the previous stage of language use (see Chapter 8), but *how, why, what if, what happened* require responses that are expressed in a more complex form. (See the Cognitive Skills Chart and other resources in Chapter 22 for open-ended, complex question forms.) Clauses need to be linked, reflecting the development of thinking and reasoning. This means mastering the use of *because, but, so that, or,* and *then,* to express connected thinking. Narration and stories require expression of a series of events, which must be held in the mind, formulated as spoken sentences, and conveyed to the listener in an organized fashion. In this stage, the child begins exploring falsehoods, simple jokes, and language play; uses language to imagine and create alternative realities by speaking in a role; and develops emerging awareness of register and socially appropriate conversation.

9.9 Vocabulary

By age 5, children typically have an expressive vocabulary of approximately 2,000 words and a receptive vocabulary that is at least twice as large. Vocabulary size is positively correlated with a range of important skills for language and literacy,[7] and this clearly presents a challenge for children with hearing impairment, for whom the all-important incidental opportunities to learn are likely to be compromised. Every adult around the child needs to be aware of the importance of broadening and increasing vocabulary and presenting the child with multiple opportunities to encounter new words in a meaningful context. Parents and professionals alike may unconsciously "adjust" their vocabulary to an easier word because they think the child will

not know the more challenging one, thereby losing an opportunity to help the child grow receptive and expressive vocabulary. A child who knows *big* is at the starting point, but one who has the opportunity to learn *huge, gigantic, large, enormous,* and *massive* is on the way to being a successful reader and an engaged student. It's clearly hard to learn pronouns from adults who only ever say *would you like grandma to do it?* or *hold daddy's hand,* when talking about themselves.

9.10 Strategies for Facilitating Language Development

Children who are moving into complex language use cannot simply be "taught." They need input from adults who are prepared to wonder and question with them, following their interests and curiosity, as well as using these as a scaffold to support a level of language that goes beyond the concrete. At this stage, knowing a concept is far beyond simply being able to say *dog* when shown a picture of one or pointing one out from a selection of items. Because the first stage of spoken language learning has been effortful and highly specific, the adults around the child sometimes feel overwhelmed by the task of moving into a "higher gear," and, as discussed above, they may also have an unconscious reluctance to challenge the child for fear of exposing everybody involved to failure. It remains easier to ask a closed question (one that has a specific, single answer, usually known by the questioner) such as *what do we need now?* than an open one (that seeks new information, unknown to the questioner, generated by the person who answers) such as *what do you think should happen next?*

The role of the coach, teacher, or therapist is to support the adults around the child in stretching, enriching, and challenging listening and spoken language to promote brain growth and enable the transition to complex thinking. This is only possible to a limited extent in a therapy room or a formal learning situation. It needs to permeate the whole life of the child and family.

Language embedded in a purposeful, real-life context provides optimum opportunities for genuine understanding and consolidation across different environments. Put simply, a sorting task with plenty of associated complex talk, such as putting away the laundry, is a more solid basis for abstract preschool math tasks (e.g., creating sets of colors or shapes) than a boxed game in the therapy room.

Another area of learning that takes on importance at this stage is the language used among peers and the exposure the child has to unfamiliar environments and people through moving away from the family circle for part of the day. As Dr Stephen Briers says:

Other relationships are much less tolerant, much less forgiving than the one that exists between parent and child. You are ideally placed to provide the sensitive coaching, feedback and support that your child will need as she gets to grips with the difficult business of getting along with others.[8]

Emerging research findings[9] are uncovering some disturbing evidence of subtle social exclusion in the free play of children who experience a range of communication differences. These observations hold true even when the children concerned have average or above average scores on standard measures of language, speech, and educational attainment. The researchers hypothesize that the influence of the environment on behavior has a major bearing on their findings and encourage work with architects and designers to make modifications that enhance social interaction.

Pitfall

Emerging research findings are uncovering some disturbing evidence of subtle social exclusion in the free play of children who experience a range of communication differences. These observations hold true even when the children concerned have average or above average scores on standard measures of language, speech, and educational attainment.

Adults cannot and should not follow the children into their peer group but should nevertheless be vigilant in their observation of successes and challenges, as well as creative in coming up with modifications that enhance learning. This could be as simple as controlling noise in a free play environment to give each child the best chance of hearing and communicating effectively with peers, as well as reducing stress and conflict.

Formal, standardized assessment provides a necessary, but not sufficient starting point. It can enable us to identify gaps in the child's knowledge or weaknesses that need to be remediated for the academic curriculum to be learned. If we simply "teach to the test" and try to fill in what we view as the missing content, the child will be no further along in acquiring the competencies previously described as characterizing the true complex language user. As is often the case, the changes we need to bring about relate to the attitudes, expectations, and skills of the adults who support the child's learning.

So how is intervention to be planned and delivered as a child makes the transition from simple to complex language?

We have to both raise expectations and provide the support that will allow everyone to enter a new, rewarding but challenging stage of learning. It means enabling children to strive, problem-solve, seek clarification, and make errors that are rich in learning opportunity, and generally to move beyond what they already know. We have to present them with new information and help them tackle it. A specific example concerns a classroom helper allocated to the DHH child to enable the child's participation in mainstream education. The class teacher gives a 3-part instruction such as *finish your paintings, wash your hands, and then get your lunchboxes.* The helper can and often does facilitate the child's success at the task, by breaking it down into a series of one-element commands and supplying the next one only when the child has completed a single task. Although this assistance may be well-intentioned and effective on the surface, it maintains the child at a lower level of language and processing than typically hearing classroom peers. Alternatively, we can intervene with the helper, coaching them in ways to build a listening and language brain by having the child develop strategies for rehearsing verbally (saying back to oneself the information to be memorized), asking for clarification or repetition from the teacher, counting off the elements on one's fingers, or questioning a peer about the information.

The child. of course, needs information, but also strategies for accessing it independently, memorizing it, and using it effectively in a variety of situations.

Pearl

Transitioning to complex language means enabling children to strive, problem-solve, seek clarification, make errors that are rich in learning opportunity, and generally to move beyond what they already know.

9.11 Language Considerations for Children Who Come Late to Intervention

As outlined in the Audition section, some children come into the preschool/school program without having benefited from early access to hearing technology and language input. Each of these children will have an individual profile, and it is crucial that their language ability is carefully evaluated to provide a baseline for therapy planning. A general "rule of thumb" suggests that where such children have a discrepancy of 24 months or more between their chronological age and their age-equivalent language scores, it is not realistic to expect them to access the curriculum in an entirely mainstream setting. It is crucial that all those involved (family, school, and therapy team) co-ordinate closely, to provide intensive remediation, and enable the child to begin "closing the gap" For more information, see Chapter 11.

Pitfall

A general "rule of thumb" suggests that where such children have a discrepancy of 24 months or more between their chronological age and their age-equivalent language scores, it is not realistic to expect them to access the curriculum in an entirely mainstream setting.

Children who have missed the developmental "window" for specific skills may find it particularly challenging to make the leap to more abstract language and concepts, needing extensive support through stories, roleplays, and repeated experience to begin to develop Theory of Mind[10] and to move away from exclusively literal interpretations.

9.11.1 The Focus of Speech Development at This Stage

Speech sound development is highly individual, even within families.[11,12] There is also extensive documentation on a variety of associated developmental difficulties in children with hearing impairment. For additional information, see Chapter 15. As with typically hearing children, such difficulties may include oral motor weakness or apraxia, and where these are suspected despite optimal auditory access through technology and optimal intervention, individualized, specialist assessment and advice must be sought. However, that is beyond the scope of this chapter, in which we assume that early amplification fitting, appropriate intervention, and underlying typical development have occurred when we discuss general guidelines for incorporating speech goals in planning for the 3- to 6-year-old age group.

Speech accuracy is often a concern for caregivers and other adults around the child. It is the most noticeable indicator of progress toward age-appropriate skills and can cause a good deal of anxiety if it appears to be falling behind.

Even in cases where hearing technology is fitted and optimized in the first year of life, children with hearing impairment are likely to have had a listening and speech trajectory that differs from that of their typically hearing peers. Time in the auditory world is reduced because of care needs and the difficulties of managing amplification in very small children. Babbling, which incorporates both auditory feedback and motor rehearsal of speech sounds, may be reduced or absent,[14] and there may be a mismatch between language ability and speech production skills. None of this needs to be a matter for concern because continuing, good-quality auditory and communication experience usually allow speech production to come into line with other skills. Thoughtful observation and a "light touch" approach to intervention often yield the best results.

Pearl

A mismatch between language ability and speech production skills does not necessarily need to be a matter for concern because continuing, good-quality auditory and communication experience usually allow speech production to come into line with other skills. Thoughtful observation and a "light touch" approach to intervention often yield the best results.

It is helpful to remind ourselves of some basic principles when evaluating speech production skills and errors in this age group:

1. Consider auditory experience.

What is the hearing age of this child? How much time has the child had with optimal access to the sounds of speech? Time without technology, malfunctioning or inappropriately fitted technology, unfavorable listening environments, and middle ear congestion slow progress in all areas, and speech sound development is no exception. If technology was not fitted until 12 months of age or older, the child may have skipped the "babble" phase and be trying for words and sentences with a history of reduced non-communicative speech practice.

2. Is the child's speech sound system developing and changing?

Where the speech sound system is immature, developmental changes can have a powerful effect on production with an associated temporary deterioration of accuracy. Villiers and Villiers,[15] documenting these processes in detail, give this example:

… amid the fragmented early words there may be the isolated words that the child pronounces flawlessly. At fifteen months, our son Nicholas produced a perfect turtle for the various toy turtles that swam in his bathtub. Later on, when the child begins to form systematic strategies or rules for the pronunciation of words, these "progressive idioms" are brought into line with the new patterns of pronunciation. So at eighteen months, Nicholas's turtle became kurka. (p. 30)

3. Is the child attempting longer and more complex utterances?

As the child moves from short, simple utterances to more complex formulations, the cognitive load associated with this can lead to a reduced capacity to monitor and self-correct speech errors. Thinking about the vocabulary and grammar for the message you want to put across, together with attending to the communicative interaction, can leave very few resources for attempting challenging speech sounds and their combinations. A good general rule is to focus on accurate speech production when using familiar, well-known vocabulary and communicative situations and to allow for a temporary deterioration in intelligibility when the subject matter, sentence structure, or vocabulary is more challenging. For example, repeated practice of /n/ is likely to be more successful in a game or story that allows frequent repetition of *no no no,* and harder when a child is trying to share a newfound enthusiasm for *Ninja Turtles.*

4. Do the child's errors fit into the sequence of typical development?

For English-speaking children, there is a wealth of documentation about typical speech sound development,[11] and the equivalent information, if available, should aid evaluation in any other language.[16] Processes such as fronting, reduplication, or final consonant deletion[11] may be in line with the child's hearing age and spoken language experience. Substituting a non-speech sound, such as throat-clearing for certain fricatives, does not fit into the expected developmental pattern and should prompt further investigation, starting with verification of the child's auditory access to accurate speech information through hearing technology.

Speech development is "a marathon, not a sprint," and norms for typically developing children show a wide age range for the acquisition of specific sounds.[17] In the preschool age group, we need to make careful observations of the individual child and not be too hasty in our recourse to intensive intervention. We are often able to support the evolution of the system, rather than providing immediate specific remediation. In typical development, the following is a useful rough guideline:

General principles to be gleaned from the current study are that most of the world's consonant phonemes are acquired (on average) by the time children are 5 years old, and, by this time, over 90% of consonants within words are produced correctly.[12]

However, when a hearing loss affects the duration and quality of a child's access to sound, we need to allow for discrepancies in relation to the expected rate of development.

Let's consider the following example:

9.11.2 Ashley

I am Ashley and I am 3 years old. I know lots of words, and I love to tell people about things that I am interested in, and I am excited that I can make longer sentences now. I told my grandpa that I have a tent in the garden, but he didn't understand. I had to take him there and show him. He said "Oh! You mean a tent in the garden," but that's what I had told him.

Ashley's Adults

Ashley is a lively, friendly, sociable boy who loves to chat. He started out with hearing aids following newborn hearing screening and made slow but steady progress in his listening and speaking. At 14 months, he was fitted with bilateral cochlear implants, and we were amazed at the improvement to both the rate and quality of his spoken language progress after he had access to the whole range of speech frequencies. Recently, he has been trying to say more and more, but we have noticed that he has become harder to understand, sometimes even for those who know him well. We are wondering if we should be working with him on specific speech sounds.

Strategies for Facilitating Speech Development

Ashley's Listening and Spoken Language Specialist (LSLS), together with his parents, listens carefully to his speech in the therapy setting, and the LSLS listens to the parents' comments on the changes they have observed. They agree that Ashley's speech sound system is evolving and that the loss of intelligibility may be temporary and caused by a number of linked factors that affect his production. They will support him in a range of ways and enlist all of those who care for him in providing enjoyable, developmentally appropriate experiences to move him through this phase.

They know that Ashley's audiologist must be recruited as a crucial participant, ensuring that he can hear and discriminate the sounds he is expected to produce through his cochlear implants.

Rather than using a specific activity as an example, this last section lists the strategies to be used throughout Ashley's participation in home and preschool life:

1. Provide opportunities for relaxed, extended vocalization with adequate breath support. Children who have had limited opportunities for pre-verbal practice sometimes try for words and phrases when they have not yet firmly established some of the underlying skills. Everyday, low-verbal exclamations and onomatopoeia provide enjoyable ways to compensate for this: *oooooh, wheeeee, wow, mmmmmm* etc

2. Build stamina for syllable repetition and alternation, while using relaxed breath. Many sound-object associations, stories, songs and rhymes can be incorporated into play allow for this: singing *aye aye yippee yippee aye* ("She'll be Coming Round the Mountain"); *ee aye ee aye oh* ("Old Macdonald Had a Farm") ; *fee fie fo fum* (Jack and the Beanstalk); *I'll huff and puff and huff and puff* (The Three Little Pigs) ; *trip trap trip trap* (The Three Billy Goats Gruff). Give the child plenty of chances to produce utterances in imitation of a model, in motivating contexts such as story-telling.

3. Provide intensive experience, in context, of particular target sounds. See Chapter 22 for materials that provide vocabulary, phrases, activities, songs, and stories for each English consonant. For example, a mother aware that her child needs to practice plosives comments as he is playing *you're blowing in the bottle, blow blow blow!* as he puts a toy ketchup bottle to his mouth, rather than, for example, *you're having some ketchup.*

4. Rather than arbitrarily picking missing sounds to target, make a careful tally of those the child can produce and use these to facilitate new skills. Listen for successful productions and note the words and positions that the child can manage competently—we are always aiming for communicative success. For example, a child who has mastered initial /m/ and can combine it with a vowel is in a position to make meaningful, rewarding use of this skill when saying *mine, me, more, messy, Big Mac, Mom.* If the sound has been acquired in initial position in words, there is the potential to move it to final (*Mom*) and medial (*yummy*) positions and to try longer sequences with variations of vowels (*more for me Mommy, it's yummy*) etc. The take-home message here is that even speech production learning is contingent on real situations and meanings. It requires nimble thinking and creativity on the part of parents and therapists.

5. Model prosodic variations while telling stories and offer the child opportunities to imitate and to come up with his own variations: *how do we speak when we're sad? telling a secret? annoyed? Who in the story or game has high pitch and who speaks in a low voice? Who speaks fast and who slowly?*

6. Support the child in organizing his words and slowing down. Using an "introducer" such as *guess what?,* and telling the story in a more organized way gives the listener time to tune in and scaffolds the child's speech effort, especially if there has been some rehearsal such as *when we see Grandpa, tell him "Look, I've got new shoes."*

7. Support success by using what our late colleague Jacqueline Stokes called the "Tell the man" technique, where, in more challenging situations, the child is provided with a model of the words he needs to say, but in the presence of the person he needs to speak to, so that he is successful even if his production is not perfect, e.g., *Tell the man: "I want pizza please."*

This cannot, of course, be an exhaustive account of every speech development difficulty and its remedy. We have given an example of a typical case and some guidelines for thinking developmentally about a particular child's situation. In this age group of DHH children, who all have different histories, the speech sound system is likely to be evolving and developing. The basic guidelines are: never lose sight of the importance of audition, make careful observations, and provide positive, communicative opportunities for practice. Bear in mind that more cognitively demanding communication uses capacity that cannot then be allocated to working on speech.

Pearl

The basic guidelines are: never lose sight of the importance of audition, make careful observations, and provide positive, communicative opportunities for practice. Bear in mind that more cognitively demanding communication uses capacity that cannot then be allocated to working on speech.

9.12 Speech Considerations for Children Who Come Late to Intervention

The child's "hearing age" (or time with effective hearing technology) affects every aspect of development including speech. After children have access to auditory information, they are able to begin building auditory feedback, breath support, and stamina (the ability to repeat, alternate or combine syllables rapidly as in connected speech), and then to begin developing a phonological repertoire. This may need to be supported through some specific intervention, and as always, the challenge is to devise age-appropriate activities that address learning need from an earlier stage. Rhymes, songs, stories with a repeated theme, and games with catch phrases (e.g., *go fish!*) are all part of the toolbox to be used at home, at school, and in therapy. Repeated practice in a meaningful context is, as always, the basis for goal-setting and intervention.

9.13 The Focus of Communicative Pragmatics and Play at This Stage

At this developmental stage, language learning is embedded in widening social experience and an increasingly complex context. Communication takes place in different circumstances, including with other children who may not have the skills that adults bring to helping the conversation go smoothly. There are unfamiliar environments and the need to address strangers, such as teachers and other day-care or school staff. Register change begins to become relevant: can you speak to an unfamiliar adult as you can to your sibling at home? Some topics or words are taboo, or transgressive, and we have to make judgments about when they can be used and for what purpose. It is a tremendous challenge for the adults who support children with hearing impairment to find the balance between directly providing the knowledge the child needs and, at the same time, ensuring that the child can do the crucial learning that takes place during independent experience away from the family or therapy room. The growing body of research in pragmatics supports this broad view of language development:

> During conversation, children are not only learning vocabulary and syntax, but they are also acquiring the tools they need to become full members of their culture…In that sense, culture organizes and gives meaning to interactions between caregivers and children, and this is especially the case in parent-child discourse. Narrative practices such as reminiscing constitute the arena in which children learn and practice the necessary linguistic skills for narrative development; at the same time, reminiscing is a context in which children acquire the cultural knowledge necessary to become competent members of their community.[18]

The family provides essential experiences that equip children to hold their own in the wider social circle they will encounter as they enter preschool and primary education.

Pearl

It is a tremendous challenge for the adults who support children with hearing impairment to find the balance between directly providing the knowledge the child needs and, at the same time, ensuring the child can do the crucial learning that takes place during independent experience away from the family or therapy room.

Play becomes both more social and more verbal as children discover the power of language for co-creating alternative realities. We can both be other people, as when playing "house" and taking on roles within an imaginary setting, and also speak and act for characters within a game with miniature objects (such as Playmobil™ or Lego™). Typically developing children spontaneously display these play behaviors, whereas DHH children, especially those who come late to intervention, may need prompts and modeling from adult play partners to move into this next play stage.

Therapists need to be aware that this can be a perplexing and difficult role for parents, and some feel genuinely defeated by being asked to engage in "pretending," confessing that they don't know what to say and don't have "imagination." If there are typically developing children in the family, they will usually have moved through the stages of play development themselves, enlisting adult help and participation as needed, but without specific input. As they reach approximately 5 years of age, children become able to create socially interactive scenarios and play within them, acting out roles based on what they have learned from a range of sources. How do people speak to one another in an office? What do people do in a bike shop? What did the princess say when the unicorn came out of the forest? For children with hearing impairment, the quantity and quality of knowledge and experience that allow this development may be significantly reduced. If they cannot participate effectively in group play, they will not have the opportunity to learn how to be a part of it. Small children also have variable abilities in producing clear speech, organizing their spoken messages, and displaying appropriate pragmatic skills such as avoiding vocal clash (everyone speaking at the same time) and checking that the listener has understood. This is why adults sometimes need to support the development of pretending and role play for a DHH child by participating in it themselves, however odd this may feel to some people. Therapists will provide the most effective support if they take time to find out what is most comfortable for the particular family. People who cannot imagine a conversation with a unicorn may feel more at ease within a structure such as playing "shops" or "school." A child can be prepared for new experiences such as a visit to the dentist by participating in a guided pretend play sequence about it, which is likely to feel more purposeful for a parent. Acting out a story from a book or from a favorite film can provide a scaffold to more inventive activities. In some cultural contexts, it is very unusual for adults to take part in play directly, and the support team may need to look to older siblings as the models.

Successful social interaction requires the development of Theory of Mind (TOM), the ability to take into account the thoughts, feelings, and preferences of others, as well as awareness of our own mental processes. Two crucial sources of learning in this domain are pretend play and stories.[19] The adults around the child at this stage have a responsibility to ensure there is rich and plentiful access to this type of learning opportunity as the child tackles the complexities of the world beyond home and family.

The skill set covered by pragmatics is wide and complex. It is sometimes poorly understood, even by practitioners in the field of early communication, as the relevant research and literature are of relatively recent vintage. Communicative pragmatics includes basic abilities such as taking and handing over conversational turns, introducing and maintaining a topic, and determining what type of response is required by a conversational partner. In addition, we acquire social knowledge, such as how and when to interrupt, how to join in, how to respond to remarks such as compliments, and how to adapt our communication to the situation. We need to start determining what is actually meant by formulating an idea of what the speaker may intend, as in the following dialogue:

Q: Would you like some ice cream?
A: I've already eaten some jelly.

Pragmatic knowledge allows us to make a guess as to whether this respondent does or does not want ice cream, or isn't sure, based on our understanding of their apparently unconnected statement. It is intricately linked to TOM and to the need for awareness of the thoughts and intentions of others.

The previous information should drive home the point yet again: the learning of complex language takes place through interactions. It is situational and experiential. It cannot be "taught" directly, so the interventionist needs to have input into every aspect of the child's life to bring on board the adult caregivers who are the true agents of change.

The drive to increase language skills and knowledge can sometimes lead us to lose sight of the crucial role played by pragmatics and the need to empower children to use words for a range of purposes with people around them. As so eloquently expressed by experts in early communication, we are "building a brain"[10] and need to provide children with direct experience of using verbal communication to forge their identity, express their thoughts, exchange or negotiate with others, and grow to occupy their own place within the community.

9.14 Communicative Pragmatics and Play Considerations for Children Who Come Late to Intervention

Research indicates that TOM begins to build very early in life and is founded on a range of experiences including witnessing and overhearing interactions between others.[20] Even capable children, who rapidly acquire factual knowledge and "pure" academic skills such as calculation, may struggle with TOM and need specific, intensive intervention and experience to grasp the concepts involved. As with other types of learning, this is most effective when offered as a collaborative program across all the settings in which the child is learning. Not offering grandpa tea because you know he prefers coffee and understanding why your school friend won't play the game you have chosen are all part of the complex web of knowledge we need to interact successfully with the people around us. When a child comes late to this learning, explicit, intensive intervention is likely to be needed, based on mind-minded talk, play, experience, stories, and real-life situations.

9.15 The Focus of Cognition at This Stage: Home and School in Tandem

Cognitive development, as children prepare to enter the education system, is intricately intertwined with language because they need to become able to understand and manipulate linguistically encoded ideas in addition to making empirical observations of the world. An example to illustrate this is the progression from putting your finger in a candle flame and noticing that it is painful, to being able to answer *what would happen if you put your finger in a candle flame* without any candle being there. Clearly, the move to complex thinking cannot occur unless language keeps pace with it. Most of the learning, thinking, and reasoning that occurs beyond the early exploratory stage of activity is inseparable from the increasingly complex language system that encodes and communicates it.

9.16 The Focus of Literacy at This Stage

In her excellent summary of issues related to reading for DHH children, Carol Flexer reminds us that:

High levels of literacy are needed to do well in school and in a job, and to have choices and flexibility in career success. The bottom line is that literacy is tied to knowledge. This includes knowledge of the words, sounds, and infrastructure of our language, as well as knowledge of what's going on in the world.[21]

The foundations for literacy are laid in the first stages of a child's development through the sharing of story books that provide great enjoyment, but also build brain capacity for a range of reading-related skills: remembering characters and sequences of events; understanding motivations and feelings within a story; becoming aware of rhyme, alliteration, and the prosodic characteristics of different voices; developing an understanding that written information can be decoded, and acquiring some early skills for this (e.g., recognizing initial letters). Young children also respond to familiar graphic information long before they can formally read (as many parents know from driving past McDonald's).

At the transition to complex language, the child will build on these early skills to begin acquiring the diverse set of abilities needed to use the many forms of written information that surround all our day-to-day activities. We don't just enjoy stories; we read instructions, web pages, recipes, subtitles, road signs, greeting cards. Stories also become more challenging, needing both social understanding (theory of mind, awareness of rules and conventions, humor) and advanced language processing for both vocabulary and syntax. This can be illustrated by opening almost any story-based picture book. Consider, for example, the first few lines of "The Digging-est Dog" by Al Perkins and Eric Gurney:[22]

I was the saddest dog you could ever see
Sad because no one wanted me
The pet shop window was my jail
The sign behind me said "for sale."

Some of the questions a reader needs to be able to answer to fully understand this passage are: *why does nobody want this dog? what does "for sale" mean? is the dog in a shop or in jail? what is a sign, and why does the dog have one behind him? who wrote it, and why did they put it there? what is a pet shop?* The text does not yield these answers. The reader has to bring some prior knowledge and some interpretation ability to the text, and we cannot take for granted a DHH child's capacity to simply "pick these things up" as they develop.

A verbally skilled child still benefits from intentional, sustained, attentive shared reading support with adults who are willing to take the time to explore everything that the text has to offer. *Jim Trelease's Read-Aloud Handbook*[23] has clear indications for how to go about this and many suggestions for relevant resources.

In practical terms, there is no shortcut. Families, if it is not their habit to read regularly with their children, need coaching and specific input to make it part of their daily routines. Classroom practice and staffing arrangements must accommodate this essential activity. Therapists, and others who provide advice, must be prepared to spend time and effort ensuring that children acquire the necessary skills. These include phonological awareness, the decoding of text with all its attendant subskills, and then the all-important linguistic competence that enables them to understand the meaning of what they read and query the parts they are not clear about. Like all other complex learning, this is experiential, but also needs "bottom-up," skills-based instruction. Children who do not have age-appropriate literacy cannot access the curriculum or fulfill their cognitive potential. All school subjects require the understanding of written information, whether this is the rubric for a math problem, directions for a science experiment, or a class newsletter. Daily, purposeful shared reading needs to be a non-negotiable component of every child's program, and all those who care for the child must be encouraged to participate. In cases where the family finds it harder to contribute because of challenges such as not being fluent in the majority language, having poor literacy themselves, or experiencing family stresses, it is vital that these needs are addressed within the support program by seeking additional resources and putting facilitative structures in place. This might be by identifying and involving other reading partners in the family circle, such as older siblings or grandparents, and ensuring they are provided with information and skills. Because this learning is interactive and based on dialogue, it cannot occur through exposure to video or audio versions of stories. As always, there must be purposeful talk.

Pearl

Daily, purposeful shared reading needs to be a non-negotiable component of every child's program, and all those who care for the child must be encouraged to participate. Families, if it is not their habit to read regularly with their children, need coaching and specific input to make it part of their daily routines.

9.17 Literacy Considerations for Children Who Come Late to Intervention

Auditory and language skills need to be in place for written language to be meaningfully learned. Sometimes, basic abilities such as knowing the alphabet or recognizing some familiar written words are mistaken for encouraging signs of progress in literacy for children who have not had the opportunity to acquire the necessary foundation skills in listening and language. We cannot expect reading development to fill in all the holes in delayed spoken language, vocabulary, and academics for these children. The therapist or education support professional needs to address the language and learning needs of each child in response to the individual profile and ensure intensive remediation is provided; otherwise the child is at risk of functioning superficially within the classroom without access to genuine learning

Pitfall

Decoding words on the page is not the same as really understanding the meaning of the text.

9.18 The Focus of Planning and Intervention at This Stage

As seen throughout this chapter, the move into complex language learning is thrilling, multifaceted, and highly dependent on rich interactive experiences. For DHH children, there are challenges to this process that their hearing peers do not experience, but with enhanced input and appropriate intervention, they have the opportunity to fulfill their potential. There is no "cookbook" for planning and goal-setting, but interventionists need a thorough knowledge of typical spoken communication development in all its aspects and can work to the following guidelines:

- Build a team, including family, school, and therapists, and ensure that all members are committed to providing the child with a rich, focused experience.
- Build a comprehensive profile of the individual child, including physical, cognitive, social, language, and speech abilities, to establish the baseline for goal-setting.
- Create goals that address any identified, underlying auditory, language, speech, and pragmatic learning needs, and ensure that all team members are aware that academic and social goals will be fully attained only with age-appropriate, complex language skills.
- Enlist all those around the child by providing them with knowledge, confidence, modeling, coaching, and feedback so that they can intervene effectively.
- Make sure the child's views, tastes, and preferences are taken into account in the activities offered, with particular regard to using age-appropriate materials, even when the listening/language level is at an earlier stage.

This stage of language is the gateway to full social and educational participation, but without the intentional extra "push" to get them started, children are at risk of appearing to manage, when in fact their learning continues to be superficial. With appropriate, coordinated intervention, though, the sky really is the limit for DHH who have access to appropriate technology and whose family and team have high expectations.

9.19 Summary

The move from simple to complex language is not a simple linear progression but a colossal step in brain development, social knowledge, and language. For children whose access to information is compromised by hearing impairment, it behooves us to be extremely vigilant as they embark on this essential stage of their learning. Standard test scores are not sufficient to indicate progress. All concerned adults need to be informed and enabled to provide optimal input, and close attention must be paid to progress in auditory skills, speech, language, pragmatics, and social participation. Complex language development is crucial for participation in education, for literacy, and for subsequent participation in employment, and it starts at this stage. There are great interest and enjoyment to be found, both for the child and the adult caregivers, in embarking on this next stage.

9.20 Case Study 1: Child Chronologically Appropriate for This Stage

Ismail

Ismail has just turned 4 and loves sea creatures. He has a big collection of them and can tell you their names and characteristics, for example, "Octopus eight legs." He was born with a mild to moderate sensorineural hearing loss, for which he uses bilateral hearing aids.

Ismail lives at home with his mom, dad, grandma, and older brother. His cousins live next door. His family mostly speaks English, but his grandma is more comfortable speaking Urdu, so she uses both languages with him.

As he's due to start his first year of formal schooling, in 3 months, Ismail's family is worried he'll struggle, because at home he enjoys being the "baby" in the family and is not very independent.

Audition

Ismail Can:

- Imitate the Ling sounds *mm, oo, ah, ee, shh, sss* from approximately 6.5 feet.
- Follow instructions that have three to four key pieces of information such as *give me the big red fish.*
- Follow two-step instructions in sequence, e.g., *first we stir and then pour*
- Predict language and fill in a gap left by someone else (a task described as auditory or linguistic closure); e.g., *this is Daddy's chair, this is….* (mummy's chair)

Language

As Ismail is growing up in a bilingual home, scores from assessments normed on monolingual populations must be interpreted with caution. Measured in English only, a recent assessment scored Ismail's language as delayed by 12 months (overall language score) and a delay of 6 months for vocabulary knowledge.

Ismail can:

- Name 30 sea creatures and describe their characteristics
- Use phrases with 3-4 key words such as *I want two biscuits or Give mummy big octopus*
- Consistently use negatives *no, not*
- Sometimes use pronouns *me, my, I, you, your* (often he uses the person's name)
- Answer *what, who, and where* questions
- List a sequence of nouns with "and", e.g., *apple and banana*
- Talk about things happening in the present, e.g., *Mummy eats chocolate* and use *-ing* endings, e.g., *I'm running!*

Speech

When saying single words or short phrases, Ismail is mostly intelligible to the listener. With longer sentences, as the language processing demands increase, the accuracy of his speech decreases. He continues to use some substitutions such as /t/ for /k/ and reduces clusters such as *poon* for *spoon*.

Six-Month Language Goals

1. Develop understanding of indirect information and inference.

Goal—In well-known and familiar contexts, Ismail will demonstrate understanding of questions and comments where information must be inferred on ten occasions.
   Examples

- *The little dog's all wet, I wonder what happened to him?*
- *I know daddy's home because his car is here.*
- *I was really hungry, so I went into the kitchen and…..*

2. Develop understanding of mental states and language of emotion to support TOM.

Goal—Ismail will use 10 new words or phrases relating to mental states or emotions on 5 occasions.
   Examples

- *Granny **likes** those biscuits*
- *What do you **think** is in this box?*
- *I **know** it's under your bed, I saw it there!*
- *The boy's very sad, he's **upset** his toy broke.*

3. Develop aspects of "thinking" and provide opportunities for "auditory or linguistic closure."

Goal—Ismail will draw on different aspects of thinking to take a contingent response and complete sentences on 10 occasions.
   Examples

- Retelling stories from memory: *Once upon a time there were three bears, and they...*
- Reasoning: *We'd better take our rain boots, because...*
- Planning: *We're making a sandwich, so we need bread, and butter and ....*
- Making up stories: *The shark said I'll eat you up, and the little fish said....*

Reflective Questions

1. Ismail's parents are worried about his speech and keep asking you to include speech activities in your session. Is this appropriate? If not, why not? What would your plan of action be?
2. You talk with Ismail's family about developing TOM, but they seem confused.
   a. Describe 3 activities that would be appropriate for goal 2.
   b. Write down how you would explain theory of mind to Ismail's family.
3. On your last home visit, you saw Ismail's grandmother interacting with him as if he were a much younger child. She feeds him, wipes his mouth with a cloth, and pre-empts all his needs without opportunity for communication.
   a. What are two reasons Ismail's grandmother may behave in this way?
   b. How would you approach this with the family?
4. Ismail will start formal schooling in 3 months' time. Write down three language goals that would work toward his being "school ready."

9.21 Case Study 2: Older Child in This Stage

Poppy

Poppy is 7 years old, and she loves Disney princesses. She enjoys dressing up and likes to listen to stories. Shortly after her birth, Poppy's parents were told that, during pregnancy, Poppy had been infected by cytomegalovirus (CMV). Because of CMV, Poppy is profoundly deaf in both ears, her motor milestones are delayed (she walked at 2 years), and spoken language has been slow to develop. Poppy finds it hard to regulate her emotions and sensory systems, so she is supported by an Occupational Therapist who specializes in sensory integration.

At age 2, Poppy received bilateral cochlear implants and began developing spoken language. She lives at home with her mom and older sister, Emily; both girls attend their local mainstream school.

At school in the mornings, Poppy has 1:1 support from a teaching assistant, and once a week a Teacher of the Deaf (TOD) visits to provide support and advice.

Audition

Poppy can:

- Imitate the Ling sounds *mm, oo, ah, ee, shh, sss* from approximately 6.5 feet.

- Listen to simple stories and answer simple questions about them
- Fill in words and phrases to familiar stories

Language

Standardized Assessment

At 7 years 3 months, Poppy is slightly older than the normed age range for the Preschool Language Assessment PLS4-UK, but age equivalent scores can be useful as a means of tracking progress.

PLS4-UK Results: Chronological Age (CA) 7.3
Age Equivalent (Total Language Score) 4.6

Poppy Can:

- Use sentences with 4 to 5 words and include small words such as *a, the, is*
- Change verb tenses to show when events happened in time, e.g., *she jumps, she jumped*
- Use words to describe mental states, e.g., *I think, I know, I forgot*, and emotions such as *angry, happy, excited, sad, disappointed*
- Ask *why* and *what happened* questions
- Explain cause and effect reasons using *"because,"* e.g., *I cried because it broke*

Phonics

Poppy Can:

- Read the first 100 high-frequency words
- Read CVCC words (*jump, nest, belt*)
- Write the common grapheme for most given sounds (e.g., *e, ee, ie, ea*).

Speech

Poppy's speech is highly accurate and intelligible to all listeners. As she's easy to understand, adults often over overestimate her language capabilities and presume Poppy understands when she doesn't.

Poppy at School

Poppy can be cheerful in nature and attempts to build and maintain peer relationships by being a bit of a "clown" to make people laugh. Although Poppy interacts with others, she doesn't belong to any of the social groups, and her delayed language makes it difficult for her to access the increasingly complex social interactions going on around her. She takes home feelings of sadness and becomes angry or withdrawn. Easily distracted and without the necessary linguistic skills, Poppy finds it hard to work independently and therefore requires a high level of support to access the curriculum. School can fund 1:1 support only in the mornings, so in the afternoon Poppy is exhausted and prone to emotional meltdowns, which often result in her being withdrawn from class.

Six-Month Language Goals

1. Develop understanding of more complex questions that require thinking past the information that is given.

Goal—Given a story, Poppy will give contingent answers to three questions that move beyond the concrete information with 60% accuracy in four out of five opportunities.

Questions to start with are *how, why, what if, what happened, what might happen next?*

2. Develop the ability to tell a short narrative.

   a. Goal—Given a picture scene, Poppy will RE-TELL a short narrative and include the elements in the following list (with 80% accuracy on 4 out of 5 opportunities).

   b. Goal—Given a picture scene, Poppy will GENERATE a short narrative and include the elements in the following list (with 80% accuracy on 4 out of 5 opportunities).

   c. Goal—Poppy will GENERATE a personal narrative (talking about her own experience) and include the elements in the following list (with 80% accuracy on 4 out of 5 opportunities)

   Elements to be included:

   • Who was there?
   • What happened?
   • How did they fix it?
   • How did they feel?

3. Develop perspective taking and theory of mind by recognizing emotions and intentions of others, and be able to use causal explanatory talk.

Goal—Given a short story, Poppy will give contingent responses (with 80% accuracy in 4 out of 5 opportunities) to the following questions:

• How did they feel?
• Why did they feel like that?
• Why did they do that?
• Why did they want that?'

Discussion Questions

1. Consider the Strategies for Facilitating Language Development previously discussed. How do you envision the teaching assistant supporting academics and teacher-directed instruction? How do you envision the assistant supporting classroom instructions and independent work? What role does Poppy's teaching assistant have in supporting her to access the social aspects of school? Consider what training she might need and what support could look like?

2. A meeting of family and professionals is called to discuss Poppy's afternoon emotional meltdowns. What factors may be contributing to the emotional meltdowns? Based on each personal or professional view, what might each of the following people suggest as an appropriate plan of action?
   a. Parent
   b. Speech and language pathologist
   c. Teacher of the deaf
   d. Audiologist
   e. Occupational therapist (specialist in sensory integration)

3. While working on goal 2, Poppy generates a short narrative from a picture prompt. She says: *The boy's painting a picture. Then, he knocks over the paint. His mom says, "Get a cloth and wipe it up."* Poppy needs to expand this narrative to include more elements. Describe activities and language strategies you would use to help her.

References

[1] Willan J. Early Childhood Studies, a Multidisciplinary Approach. London, UK: Palgrave; 2017

[2] Rush D. From couching to coaching: How do we get families engaged in early intervention? It starts with us communicating their enormous influence on their children's development. *ASHA Lead* 2018;23(10):46. doi: 10.1044/leader.FTR1.23102018.46

[3] ¡Colorín Colorado! What are BICS and CALP? WETA Public Broadcasting. https://www.colorincolorado.org/faq/what-are-bics-and-calp Published 2019. Accessed March 20, 2022

[4] Weisberg D, Hirsh-Pasek K, Golinkoff R, Kittredge A, Klahr D. Guided play: principles and practices. *Curr Dir Psychol Sci* 2016;25:177–182

[5] Fahey K, Hulit L, Howard M. Born to Talk: an Introduction to Speech and Language Development. 7th ed. Pearson; 2018

[6] Talbot P. Topics in Auditory Verbal Therapy. 2nd ed. Language Launchers Inc.; 2016:49

[7] Currie NK, Cain K. Children's inference generation: the role of vocabulary and working memory. *J Exp Child Psychol* 2015;137:57–75

[8] Briers S. Superpowers for Parents, the Psychology of Great Parenting and Happy Children. Edinburgh, UK: Pearson Prentice Hall Life; 2008

[9] Rieffe C. Social inclusion: creating an inclusive schoolyard. Focus on Emotions: Developmental & Educational Psychology. https://www.focusonemotions.nl/play/social-inclusion Accessed March 20, 2022

[10] Westby C, Robinson L. A developmental perspective for promoting theory of mind. *Top Lang Disord* 214;34(4):362–382

[11] SLT for Kids. Phonological milestones. https://www.sltforkids.co.uk/ages-and-stages-developmental-milestones/phonological-milestones/ Published 2022. Accessed March 21, 2022

[12] McLeod S, Crowe K. Children's consonant acquisition in 27 languages:a cross-linguistic review. *American Journal of Speech-Language Pathology* 2018;27:1546–1571 doi:10.1044/2018_AJSLP-17-0100. https://ajslp.pubs.asha.org/article.aspx?articleid=2701897

[13] Wiley S, Moeller MP. Red flags for disabilities in children who are deaf/hard of hearing. *ASHA Lead* 2007;12(1):8–29 https://leader.pubs.asha.org/doi/10.1044/leader.FTR3.12012007.8

[14] Kishon-Rabin L, Taitelbaum Swead R, Ezrati Vinacour R, Kronnenberg J, Hildesheimer M. Pre-first word vocalizations of infants with normal hearing and cochlear implants using the PRISE. Elsevier International Congress Series. Vol. 1273; 2004:360–363

[15] Villiers A, Villiers J. da-da – Early Language. London, UK: Fontana Open Books; 1979

[16] Hua Z, Dodd B., eds Phonological Development and Disorders in Children: a Multilingual Perspective. Bristol, UK: Multilingual Matters; 2006

[17] McLeod S. Summary of 250 cross-linguistic studies of speech acquisition. Bathurst, NSW, Australia: Charles Stuart University. https://www.csu.edu.au/research/multilingual-speech/speech-acquisition Published 2012. Accessed March 21, 2022

[18] Carmiol AM, Sparks A. Narrative development across cultural contexts. In: Matthews D, ed. Pragmatic Development in First Language Acquisition. Amsterdam/Philadelphia: John Benjamins Publishing Company; 2014:281

[19] Fivush R, Habermas T, Waters TEA, Zaman W. The making of autobiographical memory: intersections of culture, narratives and identity. *Int J Psychol* 2011;46(5):321–345

[20] Morgan G, Meristo M, Mann W, Hjelmquist E, Surian L, Siegal M. Mental state language and quality of conversational experience in deaf and hearing children. Cogn Devel 2014;29:41–49 https://openaccess.city.ac.uk/id/eprint/5058/ Accessed March 21, 2022

[21] Flexer C. How to grow a young child's reading brain. Continued Early Childhood Education. https://www.continued.com/early-childhood-education/articles/to-grow-young-child-s-22759 Published April 17, 2018. Accessed March 21, 2022

[22] Perkins A, Gurney E. The Diggingest Dog. London, UK: Harper Collins Children's Books; 2006

[23] Trelease J. Jim Trelease's Read-Aloud Handbook. 8th ed. New York, NY: Penguin USA; 2019

10 Auditory-Verbal Strategies to Build Listening and Spoken Language Skills

Sherri J. Fickenscher

Summary

The goal of auditory-verbal practice is to equip children who are deaf or hard of hearing with the necessary listening and spoken language skills to develop sufficient auditory skills to achieve good communicative competence and meet their full potential educationally and beyond. This chapter discusses the listening and spoken language (LSL) strategies that are critical to accomplishing this goal.

Keywords

joint attention, take turns, parentese (infant-directed speech), increased auditory experience, optimal positioning, auditory sandwich, model language, wait time, acoustic highlighting, repetition, prompt, expansion, whisper, asking open-ended questions, sabotage

Key Points

- Listening and spoken language (LSL) strategies are critical tools for children who are deaf or hard of hearing to achieve conversational competence, succeed in school, and meet their full potential.
- LSL strategies are chosen based on goals and desired outcomes for children.
- LSL clinicians learn strategies to focus on making speech more audible, to encourage the proper production of specific speech sounds, to increase access to receptive language and to encourage and expand expressive language skill of the children they serve.
- LSL clinicians are uniquely poised to impact the life-long learning of infants and toddlers by coaching and guiding caregivers not only in strategies that foster the growth of listening and spoken language skills, but in interactive strategies to encourage strong brain architecture.
- LSL clinicians ensure that strategies are decided on with parent input and work to coach and guide parents on the use of strategies in the child's everyday routines and experiences.

10.1 Introduction

The goal of auditory-verbal practice is to equip children who are deaf or hard of hearing with the necessary listening and spoken language skills to develop sufficient auditory skills to achieve good communicative competence and meet their full potential educationally and beyond. Listening and spoken language (LSL)

strategies are critical to accomplishing this goal. LSL strategies are often categorized by skill development, for instance: auditory skills, receptive language skills, and expressive language skills. This chapter will categorize, define, and discuss LSL strategies according to the developmental stages identified in other chapters of this book:

- Babies and Beginners: Starting with Nothing and Building up to Words (see Chapter 7)
- Toddler-Type Language: Putting Words Together and Moving up to Simple Sentences (see Chapter 8)
- Preschoolers and More Proficient Communicators: Using Complex Language to Communicate and Think (see Chapter 9)

In addition, LSL strategies for the following settings will be included:

- Caregivers/infants in daycare settings
- Providers in mainstream settings

While the LSL strategies discussed are categorized by developmental stages, LSL clinicians are expected to use their own professional knowledge and judgment to employ all strategies that move children closer to their goals. The strategy chosen must be appropriate for the developmental stage of the child. Each child and family is unique and will follow their own unique trajectory, and it is up to the discretion of the LSL clinician to decide when to use various strategies. Strategies are categorized here by stages for ease of learning, and as a way to consider teaching and coaching LSL strategies as a child grows and develops. Each section will list potential goals that could be considered when choosing a particular strategy. The LSL strategies defined and discussed in this chapter are by no means exhaustive.

Many strategies are considered best practice across the field of child development (joint attention, child-directed speech, repetition, and expansion, to name a few) and many are used almost exclusively in the field of LSL (auditory sandwich, acoustic highlighting when used for audibility purposes, auditory closure, expectant look, to name a few).

Additional resources to further learning on LSL strategies are included in the Resources for Clinicians chapter of this book. The reader is strongly encouraged to explore these resources for a deeper knowledge and understanding of LSL strategies.

10.2 Rationale for Learning LSL Strategies

LSL strategies are employed to foster rich, varied, and robust linguistic input in a manner that increases the likelihood of children gaining the necessary skills to be successful in educational environments and in all future life endeavors. LSL clinicians utilize these strategies because children who are deaf or hard of hearing are at a greater risk for language delays as hearing loss hinders the level of input these children receive.[1]

Professionals interested in providing Listening and Spoken Language services must be knowledgeable about the Nine Domains of Knowledge outlined by the AGBell Academy for Listening and Spoken Language.[2] These nine domains, or core competencies, are:

- Hearing and Hearing Technology
- Auditory Functioning
- Spoken Language Communication
- Child Development
- Parent Guidance/Coaching, Education, and Support
- Strategies for Listening and Spoken Language Development
- History, Philosophy, and Professional Issues
- Education
- Emergent Literacy

Strategies for listening and spoken language development account for 14.9% of the LSLS (Language and Spoken Language Specialist) certification examination; therefore, the importance of knowing, coaching, and applying LSL strategies cannot be understated.[2] Additional information regarding certification can be found in the Resources for Clinicians chapter.

LSL strategies are critical to the success of children who are deaf or hard of hearing learning to communicate effectively in a hearing world. A clinician learns strategies to focus on making speech more audible, to encourage the accurate production of specific speech sounds, to increase access to receptive language, and to encourage and expand expressive language skills of the children they serve.

LSLSs are not only knowledgeable about what strategy to use when, but can explain, model, and coach parents, caregivers, and other professionals in the use of strategies and the "why" behind the use. Over time, clinicians move from being consciously competent in these skills to unconsciously competent in these skills, always learning and always growing alongside the children in their practices.

Pearl

LSL strategies are employed to foster rich, varied, and robust linguistic input in a manner that increases the likelihood of these children gaining the necessary skills to be successful in educational environments and in all future life endeavors.

10.3 Brain Builders: First Things First

Strategies are meant to encourage the development of listening and speaking skills, but that focus alone is not enough. Strategies

are meant to contribute to the overall development of children. Before discussions on strategies that build listening and spoken language can take place, discussions on strategies and practices that build strong brains must take place.

- The Center on the Developing Child at Harvard University takes the complicated topic of how brains develop down to relatable and understandable terms. Brains are shaped by genes and experiences. [3] LSL clinicians must be knowledgeable about the genetic links and causes of hearing loss and must also be knowledgeable about how experiences are the building blocks of strong brain architecture. LSL clinicians must be uniquely poised to impact the life-long learning of infants and toddlers by coaching and guiding caregivers not only in strategies that foster the growth of listening and spoken language skills, but in interactive strategies to encourage strong brain architecture. While there is nothing clinicians can do about the genetic makeup children are born with, they can have a tremendous influence on the experiences of children. It is the relationship with caring and responsive adults that fosters strong brain architecture, which LSL clinicians have been doing for decades and decades through focusing on parent coaching and engagement. Two key points to consider are:

- Strong brain architecture is built by interactive relationships. Some of the LSL strategies that foster interactive relationships are *joint attention, taking turns, and asking open-ended questions.*
- Interactive relationships build resilience. Resilience supports children in overcoming challenges and adversity and encourages a "stick to it" attitude!

Strong brain architecture and resilience will lead to the best outcomes for all children. Linking the use of LSL strategies to brain building concepts contributes to strong listening and speaking skills, strong brains, and increased resilience in children. These are exactly the skills all children need to thrive!

Pearl

It is the relationship with caring and responsive adults that fosters strong brain architecture, which LSL clinicians have been doing for decades and decades through focusing on parent coaching and engagement.

10.4 Choosing the Appropriate LSL Strategy

Strategies are chosen based on desired outcomes for children and in careful consideration of the family's culture, dynamics, needs, and abilities. For appropriate goals and outcomes to be determined, a professional must evaluate a child's current levels of functioning (CLF) in all areas of development. CLF are determined through formal and informal assessments, observations of the child, and discussion with parents and other members of a child's Individualized Family Service Plan (IFSP) team or Individualized Education Program (IEP) team. The reader is referred to Chapter 6 for further learning on this topic.

After a child's CLF is determined, then goals are determined and discussed with caregivers. Some questions that drive strategy selection and use are:

- What is the goal?
- What strategy will assist in meeting that goal and why?
- Was the strategy effective?
- What is the next step?

When the goal is the focus (vs. the strategy), the clinician has a way to evaluate the effectiveness of the LSL strategy. LSL clinicians are diagnosticians and are continually collecting the data necessary to move a child and their caregivers to the next level of learning.

The selection of the appropriate LSL strategy is driven by the stage of listening and talking the child is currently moving through. LSL strategies must be thoughtfully chosen to advance children through these levels of listening and speaking. To choose appropriate goals, the LSL practitioner must have a thorough understanding of the stages of listening and talking, as well as how the children's current levels of functioning fall into these stages.[4]

Pearl

When the goal is the focus (vs. the strategy), the clinician has a way to evaluate the effectiveness of the LSL strategy.

Pearl

What strategy could be used to advance a child through each of the stages of listening and talking? It is the LSL clinician's responsibility to know this! (**Table 10.1**)

It is often surprising to some to realize that the skills listed in the stages of listening and talking are usually attained by children with typical hearing during the first year of life and are considered the foundation for all future listening and spoken language skills! Between the ages of 1–6 years of age, the child then develops higher level listening skills and by 6 years of age has acquired nearly perfect grammar.[5]

If a clinician is unaware of the various stages of listening and talking, then the likelihood of underestimating a child's ability is high, which decreases the likelihood of closing the language gap that can exist for children who are deaf or hard of hearing.

Early identification, amplification, and enrollment in a program with an LSL focus increase the likelihood that the gap between chronological age and language equivalencies remains as small as possible until the gap no longer exists. This is completely possible for children born with hearing loss today who are identified early, fitted with appropriately set technology, and receive proper use of LSL strategies to aid the development of these foundational skills.

Pitfall

If a clinician is unaware of the various stages of listening and talking, then the likelihood of underestimating a child's ability is high, which decreases the likelihood of closing the language gap that can exist for children who are deaf or hard of hearing.

Many LSL strategies hold many different names while essentially describing the same action. For instance, the strategy *"auditory sandwich"* can also be referred to as *"listening sandwich."* Other possible names of LSL strategies are listed in this chapter as each strategy is defined.

10.5 Babies and Beginners: Starting with Nothing and Building up to Words

Just as newborn hearing screening, early amplification, and technology have changed, research on early brain development has influenced the use of various LSL strategies. But where do practitioners begin? LSL clinicians begin with the understanding that a newly diagnosed baby often leaves parents feeling ill-equipped. Once concerned with managing the hectic, but typical life with a newborn which includes diaper changes and feedings as well as managing the rest of their lives, parents of a child with hearing loss are now faced with audiology appointments, new terminology, as well as feelings of doubt, grief, anxiety, guilt, and sadness.[6] While the importance of establishing full-time use of technology is critical, so is reminding parents that they *do* know how to communicate with their newborn! LSL clinicians must balance the sense of urgency about technology use with the parents' capability to take in the information about navigating this new world. Parents are concerned mostly that they will not know how to communicate with their new infant; this is a thought that creates roadblocks for developing foundational skills. The strategies listed in this section are not listed in order of importance. How these strategies are introduced and discussed with families

Table 10.1 Stages of listening and talking

Stages of listening	Stages of talking
auditory awareness	crying
attention	cooing
localization	smiling
discrimination	laughing
auditory feedback	vocalizing
sequencing	babbling
auditory memory	imitating
auditory processing	blowing
	jargon
	first words

will vary greatly depending on the needs of the caregivers and goals the LSL clinician creates together with the caregivers.

A discussion that is critical prior to introducing LSL strategies with families is: *What is your baby communicating to you?* By asking this question, the LSL clinician reminds the parents that they are the expert on their child and that they have intuitive skills that will begin their child's communication journey. Parents often do not see their caregiving as communication and the LSL clinician can aid tremendously in this effort. It helps to remind parents that when their baby cries, the baby is communicating and their response to their child (picking the baby up, changing the diaper, feeding) helps build neural connections in the brain of their newborn. LSL clinicians guide and coach caregivers to notice and respond to all communication attempts. For more in-depth learning of this stage, the reader is referred to Chapter 7.

Pearl

LSL practitioners ask: What is your baby communicating to you? This reminds the parents that they are the expert on their child and that they have intuitive skills that will begin their child's communication journey.

Pitfall

The LSL practitioner is mindful that parents may believe they have to learn a special way (i.e. the use of LSL strategies) to communicate with their child. This misconception often creates roadblocks to communication.

The strategies discussed in this section are also the place to start with beginning listeners who are older but have not developed early listening skills. LSL strategies to consider during this stage of development are discussed later in this chapter.

10.5.1 Joint Attention

Joint attention is the intentional sharing of focus between two people and is recognized as a building block for social competence. Joint attention can be classified as a form of communication[7] and in a primitive form begins at birth as babies are able to share eye gaze. Human faces tend to hold the most interest for newborns, so this joint attention is one of the earliest signs of communicative and social behavior. This is an important skill to recognize and encourage when working with babies and children as communication is most successful when people share a common focus or topic of discussion.[8] Joint attention, however, is not defined by just sharing eye gaze, but must include intentional sharing of attention and the acknowledgment that two people are sharing attention with the same objects, people, or events. This begins between 6 and 9 months of age and is firmly established by 18 months of age.

Joint attention allows caregivers to provide language to hopefully match the child's thoughts and to bathe the child in language. When caregivers encourage joint attention and label what a child focuses on, the child's vocabulary increases at a faster rate.[9] Joint

attention is most effective when words are provided based on the child's interest and the label is given at the moment when joint attention is naturally established, rather than if the adult attempts to constantly redirect the child's attention.[10] Joint attention is often accomplished when adults in a child's environment act as keen observers and acknowledge what seems to be of most interest to the child and then follows the child's lead. A child's preferred activities can act as springboards for learning.

Joint attention with a child who is deaf or hard of hearing helps to establish context to ensure the message is clear. When a child and adult share visual focus on a particular object, the child is also in an "auditory only" position and the adult has the opportunity to build both auditory and language skills at the same time.

An example of both joint attention and following the child's lead would be when a child receives a gift and is way more interested in the bow or wrapping paper than the gift! Typically, the adult tries to change the child's focus to the gift, but what if the child were allowed to explore the bow or the wrapping paper that really interests them and the adult layered on the language (following the child's lead) while sharing joint attention? It might look something like this:

Child: (rips paper)
Adult (pointing to their own ear or the child's ear): Oh, I hear that paper ripping. That is fun, isn't it?
Child: (puts paper in mouth)
Adult: You put the wrapping paper in your mouth. Does that taste yummy? Paper is for ripping, Let's take it out of your mouth. Let's rip some more (taking the interaction back to what the child was previously interested in, so acknowledging what the child showed attention to, but attempting a shift). Ripping paper is fun!
Child: (rips paper again and excitedly waves hands with paper in it)
Adult: Wow! You are holding tight on that paper. Let's listen to it again as we rip the paper. That is noisy, isn't it?

One of the important aspects of following the child's lead is that this can occur during daily routines as a caregiver, parent, or teacher notices and notes activities or toys that are of particular interest to a child.

Goals of joint attention could be to:

- increase attention to auditory input (when child & caregiver are both looking at an object, they are naturally in the listening only state, not speechreading)
- build social cognition[11]
- develop theory of mind[7]
- increase caregiver contingent talk

Other names for joint attention include shared focus and joint reference.

10.5.2 Take Turns

Communicative competence is a two-way street. Encouraging caregivers, colleagues, and children to *take turns* models the reciprocal interactions that are expected from communication partners. Research is abundantly clear: turn taking between children and their caregivers builds stronger brains! One such study focuses on the neural mechanisms found by neuroimaging that revealed greater activation in Broca's area (left inferior frontal regions) for children experiencing more conversational turn taking with caregivers. More conversational turn taking also resulted in increased verbal abilities.[12] The Center on the Developing Child at Harvard University refers to turn taking as "serve & return" interactions and houses a library of multimedia research focusing key findings in the field of child development (See links provided in the Resources for Clinicians chapter of this book.)[3]

Communication exchanges are most effective when caregivers learn to wait for a nonverbal or verbal response from a child before they take another turn in the communication exchange. Infants may coo or kick their feet as a conversational turn, while a three-year-old child is expected to give an appropriate verbal response. The goal when adults take turns is to elicit participation from the infant or child. With infants this can also involve imitation. When a baby coos at the caregiver, the caregiver can *take a turn* by cooing back in imitation of the baby, or by pretending to have a conversation with the baby even though there are no true words. For instance:

> Baby coos
> Adult coos back imitating baby
> Baby coos
> Adult: "Wow! Tell me more about that!"
> Baby smiles
> Adult: "Oh... your smile tells me you are happy."

One concept to consider when focusing on taking turns is the "equal time pie."[13] The amount of time the practitioner, caregiver, and child talk should be equal. This is difficult to do without focusing on the use of LSL strategies such as turn taking and wait time.

The content of the *turn taking* will eventually become more complex, so this LSL strategy should always be in use even when children become established conversationalists. Turn taking builds social development.

Pearl

Turn taking builds social development as well as language development.

Pitfall

Talk time by the clinician and the child should be about the same, but the clinician is often the one doing the most talking. Watching videos of sessions can help to reveal if this is the case!

Recent research by Donnellan found infants' vocalizations that were paired with eye gaze and were met with a timely response from caregivers were one of the best predictors of expressive language development at 2 years of age.

Goals of taking turns could be to:
- increase auditory attention to speaker
- increase neural connections in the brain
- encourage expressive language
- build conversational competence
- build relationships

Another name for turn taking is serve & return.

10.5.3 Parentese (Infant-Directed Speech)

Parentese is a form of acoustic highlighting that is characterized by abundant variation in the suprasegmentals of speech. The adult makes changes to their vocalization in duration (elongation of vowels and consonants), pitch (sometimes as much as an octave higher), and intensity (often decreasing their intensity). It is when an adult naturally changes pitch and prosody (stress and intonation patterns) when talking with a child. Sentences are typically shorter and often repeated and reduplication patterns are utilized (referring to a bottle as a "baba"). Adults produce sounds more clearly when they are practicing parentese, and babies pay attention longer. This phenomenon is not taught to anyone, and yet, it occurs across genders, socioeconomic status, and age.[14] This is one of the great wonders of language learning: parentese is used naturally and unconsciously by most adults.

Research on parentese indicates that it helps babies with typical hearing to "crack the code" of language.[14,15] The well-formed and elongated vowels and consonants parents employ during parentese make it easier for a child to map the sounds of their native language.[14] Adults intuitively change not only their acoustic patterns of speech as the infant ages, but the content of what they say. In the first 3 months of life, the caregiver tends to talk about what the child is experiencing or feeling and tends to use one-word utterances. By 7 months of age, the caregiver includes more labeling of objects and people with action words being used more between 11 and 24 months of age.[8]

Some research reports parents of children who are deaf or hard of hearing often use less parentese than parents of children with typical hearing.[15] This may mean children who are deaf or hard of hearing and who already receive less auditory experience, may not have exposure to the richness in the language provided by parentese. This may not be because the child does not have auditory access, but because the parent may be hesitant to use this type of speech.

The use of parentese naturally decreases by the time of the child's second birthday, which is, again, unfortunate for a child who is deaf or hard of hearing, as parentese so naturally utilizes the suprasegmentals of speech. Thus, decreased use means that some deaf or hard of hearing infants and toddlers may miss out on the many benefits of parentese. Parentese is often referred to as infant-directed speech, especially in research, and these terms are often used interchangeably. Parentese should be encouraged for every child, regardless of the child's auditory access.[16]

Parents often feel silly being encouraged to use parentese. One technique that can be encouraged by LSL clinicians that taps into the benefits of parentese is singing. Singing is considered a technique; a way of doing something with a goal in mind but no specific way of doing it (a strategy is specific in how it is carried out). Singing is natural for most parents until the diagnosis of hearing loss is confirmed and suddenly parents find themselves quiet at a time when their child desperately needs exposure to speech and language. Singing gives children the benefits of parentese when it might seem difficult or unnatural to parents. Singing exposures children to natural vocal rhythms and has a way of capturing attention. Singing and listening to music is a tremendous activity to tap into the listening brain while having fun, too.

Goals of parentese could be to:

- increase attention to speaker
- enhance auditory perception of speech[17]
- expose child to increased vowel repertoire
- "crack the code" of language[14,15]
- encourage vocal turn-taking such as cooing
- encourage social-emotional development

Other names for parentese are infant directed speech, motherese, caretakerese, and child-directed speech/language.

10.5.4 Increased Auditory Experiences (Listen, Listen, Listen)

Increased auditory experiences, sometimes referred to as "auditory bombardment," involve the conscious planning of exposure to meaningful auditory input. In the beginning stages of listening, this is primarily based on pointing out sounds in a child's environment and connecting those sounds with words. Children who are deaf or hard of hearing need extra practice linking sound to meaningful events. This is often accomplished through listening walks around the house or outside and pointing out sounds in the environment. Sounds that may appear ordinary can be linked in fun ways to babies and beginning listeners. When a sound (perhaps it is the clothes dryer indicating the completion of a cycle) is presented, the caregiver calls attention to the sound, points to their ear and excitedly proclaims "OOOOOO! I think I heard something! What is that beeping sound? Let's listen! There it is again. I heard *beep-beep*. Let's go find out what made that beeping noise." This simple daily activity is increased auditory experience.

Pointing to the ear is a visual signal that can aid understanding that listening is interesting, important, and expected. The fun then continues as the caregiver and child explore together until the source of the sound is found. In this manner, sound has been acknowledged, attended to, and linked with meaning again increasing auditory experience.

Careful attention, however, must also be given to monitoring the acoustic environment of children who are deaf or hard of hearing. Increased auditory experience is not the same thing as noise. Multiple speakers, televisions, music playing in the background, and even the hum of refrigerators or heating and cooling systems create a tremendous amount of background noise. Background noise makes listening more difficult. This occurs in the home, in daycares, and in classroom settings, and the LSL clinician works to raise awareness to the acoustic roadblocks to learning. When

attention is paid to the reduction of noise in the child's environment, the ease of learning is increased .[4]

Increased auditory experience encourages a child to use hearing as the primary sensory modality and creates multiple meaningful opportunities for the child to be exposed to environmental sounds, individual speech sounds, words, and as the child grows in listening experience, to grammatical structures. The end goal of providing increased auditory experience is that the child will link the targeted sound, word, or grammatical structure to meaning and eventually this translates into increased language opportunities.

Goals of increased auditory experience could be to:

- increase auditory awareness/attention to sound
- create a listening environment[17]
- increase comprehension through listening[18]
- highlight proper articulation of speech sounds as the child ages

Other names for *increased auditory experience* are auditory bombardment, focused auditory stimulation, or bathing the child in sound.

10.5.5 Optimal Positioning

Optimal positioning involves the awareness of the distance that exists between the sound source, typically a human voice, and the intended audience, in this case a baby or new listener. Distance, background noise, and reverberation are three factors that dramatically impact the quality of the signal for those with hearing loss; even when they are fit with appropriate technology. Children with typical hearing learn language incidentally, that is, from overhearing others around them.[8] This is often not the case for children with hearing loss, so positioning becomes critical for auditory skill development and exposure to speech and language. Speech perception capabilities can be improved by decreasing the distance between a speaker and listener. LSL practitioners are greedy for every single decibel of sound so that the best possible auditory signal arrives to the brain. The closer the child is to the sound source, the greater the intensity of sound which then allows for a more precise signal. (See information on the speech bubble in Chapter 3.)

Pearl

LSL practitioners use positioning as a strategy because they are greedy for every single decibel of sound and work to provide the best possible auditory signal to the brain.

If a child has one ear that hears better that the other, optimal positioning means the LSL clinician is aware of the asymmetrical loss and coaches and guides those in the child's life to be on the side of child's better hearing ear.

The goal of optimal positioning is to give the best possible auditory signal to the brain. As the child ages, experiences with distance listening are explored, but for the beginning listener closer is better. Remote microphone (RM) technology assists in ameliorating the detrimental effects of distance. The reader is encouraged to read about the critical importance of RM technology in Chapter 2.

Goals of optimal positioning could be to:

- increase auditory awareness/attention to sound
- create a listening environment[17]
- facilitate auditory processing[17]
- increase access to subtle conversational cues[16]

10.5.6 Auditory Sandwich

When a child is not getting a message using audition alone, the auditory sandwich is useful. With this strategy, auditory information is presented alone, then auditory information is presented with visual information and finally, information is presented again using audition alone. (Listen, listen and look, listen.) The analogy of the "sandwich" assists in coaching purposes.

Bread: Presentation through audition alone ("I think I hear a cow! Listen…. mooooooo. Yes, that's a cow. Let's see!")

Meat: Audition paired with visual support (pull out toy cow and talk while child is looking at object: "Wow! It's a cow. The cow says moooooooo.")

Bread: Presentation through audition alone again when the child's focus is off of the cow but not looking directly at the clinician. ("Moooooo says the cow.")

The science behind the auditory sandwich begins with the understanding of auditory neural development and brain plasticity. If the auditory cortex of the brain is not exercised, it will be reorganized for the processing of other information such as visual information.[19] The LSL clinician encourages listening first to stimulate the auditory centers of the brain prior to activating the visual centers of the brain.

The auditory sandwich can also be used as a teaching tool to link known vocabulary to new vocabulary. For instance, when a child understands the word "big," it is time to learn another word! Perhaps it is "huge" or "gigantic." The LSL clinician could say "The elephant is a *huge* (new word said with acoustic highlighting; audition alone) animal. It is really, really big (linking "huge" to a word they do know, "big"). The elephant is a huge animal." This provides multiple opportunities to hear a new word and to link the new word to an already known word.

Goals of the auditory sandwich could be to:

- increase attention to auditory input and to the speaker
- encourage caregiver belief that the child is able to gain meaning through listening alone
- stimulate the auditory centers of the brain
- increase ability to process language through listening

Other names for auditory sandwich are listening sandwich, prompting for listening first and last, and auditory/audition first.

10.6 Toddler-Type Language: Putting Two Words Together and Moving up to Simple Sentences

Early exposure to talk and interaction, especially during the critical age period of 18–24 months, has been linked to levels of school-age language and cognitive outcomes.[20] By two years of age, typically developing children have approximately 150–300 expressive words and are putting two words together in utterances. LSL strategies used during this period encourage utterances such as "Daddy up" to become "Daddy, pick me up" and stress the importance of continually moving a child along the language continuum. The reader is encouraged to explore Chapter 8, which goes in depth about this developmental stage.

The LSL strategies listed for this developmental stage should also include the strategies listed in the previous section ("Babies and Beginners"). As the knowledge of professionals, caregivers, and parents grows, their capability to use multiple strategies in multiple situations grows as well. Practitioners continually reflect and evaluate their practice and are cognizant of when a strategy isn't working, why it may not have worked, and what other strategy they can employ.

The LSL strategies to consider during this development period are listed a little later in this chapter, but clinicians are not limited to these strategies alone.

10.6.1 Model Language

For all children to communicate through spoken language, they must have language modeled for them. Children who hear language that is meaningful and appropriate have a higher likelihood of using spoken language.[21] The goal of modeling language is to expose children to a rich and abundant language system and to speak in a way that ensures the message is received and understood. Some areas to consider when modeling language include:

- Rate of speech: Children between the ages of 3 to 5 years of age process between 120 and 124 words per minute. Most adults speak at a rate of 160–180 words per minute.[22] This can create a disconnect especially for children who are not hearing optimally. Speaking too quickly also makes unstressed words (pronouns, articles, etc.) more difficult to hear and learn.
- Volume: Adults often speak too loudly to children who wear technology. This does not aid in audibility and often gives more power to sounds that don't need more power (like vowels) and less power to sounds that do need it (like consonants). Caregivers who are naturally soft spoken may need to be encouraged to speak with a bit more intensity or to be more aware of how far they are from the child.
- Articulation: Adults often drop word endings when their rate of speech is too fast. This makes it harder for children to learn word endings.
- Word choice: LSL clinicians encourage the use of rich and varied vocabulary, taking care not to limit word choice for children. Modeling involves exposing children to new words

all the time. Labeling nouns often seems intuitive for most caregivers. The LSL practitioner encourages the use of verbs, attributes, and relations such as positional, locational, and size words. These basic concepts have been linked to later academic success, so it is critical to encourage caregivers to use them frequently.[17]

- Length and complexity of message: To keep children moving towards longer and more complex sentences, LSL clinicians model and coach caregivers to speak in sentences that are grammatically correct and are one step ahead of where the child is speaking. For instance, when a child is putting two words together, the caregiver speaks in sentences of 4–6 words to stretch the child.

Additional forms of modeling language can be:

- narrating (adult offers a "play-by-play" of what is naturally occurring)
- self-talk (adult talks about what they are seeing, doing, feeling, or thinking)
- parallel talk (adult talks about what the child is seeing, doing, feeling, or thinking)

Goals of modeling could be to:
- increase likelihood message is received and understood
- increase receptive language skills
- increase use of appropriate grammatical structures
- build neural connections in the brain[21]
- promote knowledge of language[17]

Modeling can also be referred to as narrating, self-talk, parallel talk, play-by-play, rephrase, scaffold or recast.

10.6.2 Wait Time

Wait time is the pause used between an adult's interaction with a child and the child's expected response, which allows adequate time for the child to process the auditory information and formulate a response.[23] This pause signals to children that some response is expected from them; therefore, this LSL strategy focuses on pragmatic skills as well as listening and spoken language skills. Wait time is a form of acoustic highlighting. The response the child gives can be verbal or nonverbal, but it is critical that the LSL clinician model wait time and discuss with families the importance of a child having the necessary time to respond. For older children *without* auditory and language deficits in typical classrooms, it is recommended that teachers give 3 to 5 seconds of wait time before answering a question.[24] For many adults, 5 seconds of wait time can feel uncomfortable, causing them to jump in quickly to repeat or rephrase. Yet, if typically developing children may need 5 seconds of wait time, how much longer might a child with auditory and language delays need? Children with hearing loss may need 5 to 10 seconds of wait time to process information and formulate their response. Adults must learn to wait quietly and expectantly despite their discomfort to allow the child time to respond. However, it is important to keep wait time natural. If a child loses interest after a few seconds and has moved on to something new, then the child is not using that wait time to formulate a response and the strategy is ineffective.

Pitfall

It is important to keep wait time natural. If the child loses interest after a few seconds and has moved on to something new, then the child is not using that wait time to formulate a response and the strategy is ineffective.

Seminal work by educator Mary Budd Rowe described the efficacy of wait time in research that spanned 20 years.[25] Rowe's findings have implications for the LSL clinician as she found when school-aged children were given 3 or more seconds of undisturbed wait time not only the students' responses, but future interactions of the teachers, were positively impacted. A few of the findings relevant to LSL clinicians were: the length and correctness of responses of students increased, the number of students who gave "I don't know" responses decreased, the number of teacher follow-up questions that required higher-level thinking increased, and the variety of teacher questions increased.

To utilize wait time, the LSL practitioner:

- maintains eye contact
- raises their eyebrows to indicate interest and expectation of a response
- leans their body toward the child
- counts to 8–10 seconds (or an appropriate amount of time individualized to the child's needs). Parents can be encouraged to count on their fingers as they wait.

Goals of wait time could be to:
- increase length of a response
- increase likelihood of a response from a child
- build communicative intent
- build turn-taking skills[8]
- facilitate spoken language skills[17]
- allow time for auditory processing

Wait time may also be referred to as think time or pausing.

10.6.3 Acoustic Highlighting

Acoustic highlighting is an umbrella term, of sorts that includes many LSL strategies under this one general term. Most often acoustic highlighting is referred to as adding vocal emphasis on specific sounds, words, parts of phrases, or grammatical structures. This is done by either pausing before or after a targeted word, sound, or grammatical structure or by increasing the intensity or duration of the target. Perhaps the most primitive form of acoustic highlighting is parentese. Other forms of acoustic highlighting covered and discussed in other sections of this chapter are: positioning, whispering, singing, repetition, and wait time. Acoustic highlighting is used to increase audibility, processing time, and comprehension of the spoken word.[17,26]

Acoustic highlighting is based on speech acoustics and is used to make sound more audible for a beginning listener and progresses to less highlighting for a child who listens well. The goal of acoustic highlighting is to focus a child's attention on the intended target and then to drop the use of the strategy as soon as the child meets with success. Acoustic highlighting is achieved by adjusting pitch, intensity, stress, or timing.

Examples

1. While cleaning up toys before lunchtime

    Caregiver: "Let's have a race. Please get the yellow ball and the horse."

    Child: returns with blue ball and horse.

    Caregiver: "Wow, that was fast. You brought the blue ball and the horse. Listen again! Please get the (slight pause) *yellow* (said with a touch more intensity) ball and the horse."

2. During a language lesson, a classroom teacher notices a student is improperly using the pronoun she.

    Teacher: "I heard you say *he*, but Aubree is a girl. So, you could say: (slight pause) *She* (increased intensity) is picking up the doll."

The goal ultimately is for the child to use the proper pronoun, but if the child is not yet able to do this successfully, the teacher is giving the student ample opportunity to hear the proper use of the pronoun.

Goals of acoustic highlighting could be to:

- increase attention to auditory signal or speaker
- increase audibility of certain sounds, words, or phrases
- encourage response from the child
- facilitate auditory processing[17]
- enhance auditory perception of speech[17]

10.6.4 Repetition

Repetition is the frequent and varied use of rich vocabularies, grammatical structures, phrases, or sentences that adults use to expose children to spoken language.

Language input has been determined to be a major contributor to overall language development. The seminal work of Hart and Risley confirms the validity of the LSL strategy of repetition as this work revealed the number of words a child heard early in life correlated to language scores later in life.[27] Repetition is a form of modeling language and is based on the theory that the more often a word is heard, the earlier it should be learned.[28]

Children who are deaf or hard of hearing are at an increased risk for language delays, so the LSL clinician utilizes models and coaches the strategy of repetition to expose children to as much spoken language as possible.

LSL clinicians are mindful that it is not just the quantity of words, but the quality of words, including word classes, that

adults expose children to through the use of repetition. Typically, the earliest words children learn are nouns along with some personal-social words (*yes/no*; *want*; *hi/bye-bye*; *night-night*) followed by verbs and adjectives. Adults educate themselves about typical language development to monitor the growth and complexity of language development of the children they support.

Pearl

Children who are deaf or hard of hearing are at an increased risk for language delays, so the LSL clinician utilizes models and coaches the strategy of repetition to expose children to as much spoken language as is possible.

Pitfall

Repetition without linking to meaningful input is unsuccessful. LSL clinicians are mindful that it is not just the quantity of words, but the quality of words, including word classes, that adults expose children to through the use of repetition.

Goals of repetition could be to:

- develop auditory feedback loop
- increase receptive and expressive language
- increase knowledge of proper grammatical structures

10.6.5 Using Prompts

Prompts are a broad category of strategies that are used as a stimulus to support or encourage expressive language. Prompting is typically used in conjunction with other LSL strategies and is the use of a verbal, visual, or physical indicator to encourage responsiveness from a child. Prompting can be used when a child has said nothing, when a child has said something that includes an error such as an incorrect word choice or grammatical error, when the adult wants to expand the child's language, or when a message is incomplete or inaccurate.[29]

Verbal prompts	Physical or visual prompts
Modeling expected language "you could say '*help me please*'"	Leaning in towards child
Use of auditory closure	Expectant look
Use of sabotage	Use of sabotage
Adult prompts with "Tell me more about that" or "Tell me in a whole sentence"	Use of picture or print

A skilled LSL clinician uses prompting to encourage turn-taking and expand and extend conversational competency. The more practice a child has at talking, the better the child becomes at talking. Prompting is used for exactly this reason: to encourage more talking.

Goals of prompting could be to:
- increase verbal working memory[30]
- increase auditory attention
- increase expressive language skills
- increase use of proper grammatical structures

10.7 Preschoolers and More Proficient Speakers: Using Complex Language and Using Language to Think

In the United States, many children enter preschool around 3 years of age with the capability to use language to meet their emotional, physical, academic, and social needs. Preschoolers use anywhere from 5–8-word phrases to request politely, recount events of the past, talk about future events, and even have the social constructs to "promise" and tell lies to others.[31] Most 3-year-olds have developed large receptive and expressive vocabularies. While preschoolers continue to experience vocabulary growth, the primary task now is to refine their grammar (syntax) and pragmatics and to increase their capability to use language efficiently and effectively. In short, to become good conversationalists!

Auditory skills continue to be a critical component as preschoolers must listen to gain information and meaning and to build conceptual vocabularies.[32] Preschoolers listen not only to obtain meaning, but to gain proficiency in the grammatical structures of their language, so during this time, syntax acquisition occurs rapidly. These complex syntactic abilities are a predictor of reading comprehension in elementary school.[33]

Studies consistently show that when compared to their typically hearing peers, children with hearing loss have weaknesses in the use of verb tense, *wh*-clauses,[1] length of their utterances, and demarcation of plurals.[33] For more in depth learning on this stage of learning, see Chapter 9.

Many of the LSL strategies already discussed in this chapter continue to be crucial for the overall development of the preschooler and more proficient speaker. In particular, taking turns, modeling, acoustic highlighting and prompting aid in increasing awareness of the syntactical structures of language. In addition, the following LSL strategies are offered for consideration to continue to build the necessary skills to be successful conversationalists and to succeed in mainstream school settings.

10.7.1 Expansion/Extension

Expansion occurs when an adult repeats a child's utterance providing a more grammatically complete language model without changing the child's intended meaning.[34] The terms expansion and extension are often used interchangeably in literature; however their meanings are slightly different. An expansion is when an adult repeats back what a child has said in a grammatically correct fashion without adding anything new. An extension is when the adult provides the correct syntax and adds additional information.[8] For example:

Child: "I knowed Henry name"
Adult using expansion: "Oh. You knew (slight acoustic highlighting) Henry's (elongate /s/ sound) name."
Adult using extension: "Oh. You knew Henry's name because you heard the teacher say it?"

The length and complexity of language input from caregivers have been shown to contribute to overall language development,[35] so the use of expansions and extensions can provide this enriched exposure.

Expansions and extensions can be used in the naturally occurring context of conversation, which enables this strategy to be used effectively by parents at home, teachers in the classroom, and clinicians in auditory verbal sessions.

Because expansions are based directly on the child's utterance and improve or correct what the child said, they therefore hold deep and inherent interest to the child.[16] When some previous information is used to deliver the new information and capture the child's attention, expansions can lead to increases in utterance length and grammatical development.[8] Expansion also provides a corrected language model without the negative aspect of correcting a child.[21]

Goals of expansion/extension could be to:
- increase length of utterance[8]
- encourage complexity of responses from a child[16]
- increase receptive language skills
- increase expressive language skills

Expansion may also be referred to as recast, extension, adding something new, elaborate, or expatiation.

10.7.2 Whisper

A whisper is accomplished when the speaker turns off their voice and reduces the suprasegmental of intensity. Whispering is a form of acoustic highlighting and is used to give less audible high-frequency phonemes more saliency. These are typically the voiceless phonemes of /h/, /s/, /t/, /k/, /p/, /sh/, /ch/, /f/, and /th/. Vowel sounds carry the power or increased energy of speech while consonants carry the intelligibility of speech.[27] Whispering, when close to the child's technology, can make sounds easier to hear by decreasing voiced sounds which can make voiceless phonemes more audible. *Whispering* is also used to capture a child's attention by adding an element of surprise or by calling attention to the speaker.

Goals of whispering could be to:
- increase auditory attention to speech sounds
- increase auditory accessibility of high-frequency sounds
- enhance auditory perception of speech[18]

10.7.3 Asking Open-Ended Questions

Open-ended questions are questions that require more than a one-word or targeted "correct" response from a child. Asking open-ended questions keeps the conversational volley going while yes/no questions or questions that only require one-word or a "correct" answer to respond, tend to stop conversation. Asking open-ended questions offers adults the opportunity to gain insight into what a child is thinking, feeling, or curious about and encourages the child to use language to express themselves effectively.

Open-ended questions begin with the words: *why, why not, how, what do you see/hear, what happened, what do you think,* or *what happened when or next,* as well as statement words that encourage expanded responses such as *describe, explain,* or *tell me about.* Yes/no questions often begin with the words *are, do, will,* or *would.*[36] Closed-ended questions often begin with *who, what, what color, how many, where,* and *when* and are easy to answer with a short phrase. Open-ended questions cause a child to think and reflect before responding.

The habit of asking open-ended questions takes some practice for all adults. Parents who are well versed at asking open-ended questions find conversations with their teenagers more robust. Here are a few examples of changing closed-ended questions into open-ended questions:

Did you have a good day? becomes *What was something good that happened today?* or *Tell me about your day.*

Was Roberto sick today? becomes *Why do you think Roberto was not at school today?*

Did that make you happy? becomes *How did that make you feel?*

Did you play outside today? becomes *What did you do outside today?*

Pearl

Parents who have mastered the art of asking open-ended questions when their child is young, may find conversations with their teenagers a bit easier!

Pitfall

Asking too many questions or asking questions that the adult already has an answer to can discourage conversation. The goal of asking any question is not to quiz a child, but to engage them in meaningful dialogue.

Goals of asking open-ended questions could be to:

- encourage critical thinking
- facilitate spoken language and cognition[17]
- increase the number of conversational turns a child takes
- engage a child in discussion and increase topic maintenance

10.7.4 Asking "What Did You Hear?"

There are bound to be times when a child who is deaf or hard of hearing is unsure of what was said or asked of them. When a child gives an incorrect or inappropriate response, fails to respond, or experiences a communication breakdown, the adult can ask, *"What did you hear?"* or "What do you think I said?" to prompt the child to give back the part of the message that was heard and attempt to repair the communication breakdown. Asking "what did you hear?" or "what do you think I said?" also holds the child accountable for listening. Clinicians, parents, teachers, and even siblings should consider using this strategy prior to automatically repeating a question, comment, or sentence to a child. Sometimes children have heard the message clearly but lack confidence in their listening capabilities. Sometimes they have heard part of the message, but not the entirety and are seeking clarification. The LSL clinician recognizes the value of knowing what part of the message the child heard and uses this knowledge to advance listening skills. It should be noted that, if the child has consistent difficulty hearing some sounds (such as /s/, /z/, etc.) or hearing in specific settings, the clinician should let the audiologist know because it may be possible to modify technology settings to help the child hear the missing sounds.

Moreover, this strategy is much more effective than teaching the child to say, "Can you repeat that?" as it forces the child to think about what was heard and attempt to fill in the blanks of missing information.[34] Questions to consider could be: What part of the message did the child misunderstand? Was it the beginning, middle, or end of the sentence? Is this linked to the child's auditory memory? Did the child just mishear one word, perhaps acoustically similar words like *dish/fish* or *boat/bat,* and was unable to use the context clues of the sentences to take a guess? Did the child hear correctly, but not know the meaning of a new vocabulary word? Is the child's confidence lacking or is their personality such that they don't want to risk being wrong?

All of these questions, and many more, contribute to an LSL clinician being a diagnostician. Everything a child does, doesn't do, says, or doesn't say gives clues to their current levels of functioning.

Pearl

Asking "what did you hear?" or "what do you think I said?" also holds the child accountable for listening. Clinicians, parents, teachers, and even siblings should consider using this strategy prior to automatically repeating a question, comment, or sentence to a child.

Example of Identifying What Child Did Not Hear

Parent: After soccer practice today, we need to stop at the store to pick up groceries.

Child: What?

Parent: *What did you hear?*
Child: After soccer practice, we need to stop . . . where?
Parent: Oh, at the store to pick up groceries.

Example of Identifying Communication Breakdown

Parent: I bought orange marmalade at the store.
Child: What?
Parent: *What do you think I said?*
Child: You bought an orange microwave at the store???

Parent recognizes that the child is not familiar with the word "marmalade" but has matched syllables and beginning sound of the word.

Goals of asking "What did you hear?" could be to:
- increase attention to the auditory signal or speaker[17]
- increase confidence in listening skills
- increase repair strategies for communication breakdowns
- facilitate auditory processing[18]
- assist LSL clinician in determining cause of communication breakdown

10.7.5 Sabotage

Sabotage creates an unusual or unexpected situation with familiar items or routines that is contrary to the child's expectation or understanding.[17]

One way to use sabotage is for the adult to create an element of surprise with a purposeful mistake or contrived situation.[38] This starts a "cause and effect" cycle of intentional communication. The adult can elicit language from the child if they place materials just out of reach, provide fewer materials than the child needs, or "forget" materials or parts of a routine. For example, the child's chair may be broken, parts of the game may be missing, or the clinician may have a wrench rather than a can opener for a cooking activity. It is then up to the child to bring the need to the adult's attention, and the dialogue continues until a resolution occurs. These contrived situations are helpful to practice certain words, phrases, or skills and to create opportunities for the child to use problem-solving skills.[27] The key to the effective use of sabotage is awareness of the child's listening and language capabilities. Sabotage is ineffective if the adult uses language or concepts that are not yet mastered by the child. For example, if a teacher says while holding two dinosaurs: "I have one triceratop" hoping the child will correct the utterance, but the child does not yet have the word *triceratops* as part of their expressive vocabulary, then the sabotage will tend to add confusion for the child, instead of eliciting an expressive response. Sabotage is used only when the situation can be easily repaired or solved, so this is more like a game than a trick.

Sabotage can also be used to teach self-advocacy skills in relation to the child's hearing equipment. After a listening check, the teacher can hand the student's equipment back but leave it powered off. The goal is to see if the child notices something is wrong and asks for assistance. The teacher may then need to prompt

the child with a question such as "Can you hear me?" "What did I say?" or "Is your hearing aid/CI working?"

Goals of sabotage could be to:
- create opportunities to practice spoken language
- facilitate spoken language and cognition[18]
- encourage expressive language and thinking skills

Sabotage may also be referred to as creating the unexpected.

10.7.6 Strategies for Caregivers of Children in Daycare

For many professionals in daycare environments, working with a child who wears technology is new and intimidating. Without the LSL clinician explaining and stressing the importance of amplification, the child's technology may not be understood and valued as the key to accessing the brain. Caregivers in daycare settings are responsible for caring for multiple infants, toddlers, and young children all at the same time, all day long. Sometimes the responsibility of maintaining use of the child's technology is not a priority, so it is the LSL clinician's role to ensure there is an understanding of the importance of technology and its impact on the developing brain. Often inviting the professional in the daycare to listen to the hearing aids through a stethoset and to actually hear how the child's remote microphone technology works can be a game changer! The LSL clinician is sure to coach the family on stressing the importance of wearing the technology as well so that before a child enters a daycare environment, the parent is prepared to explain that the use of the child's technology is non-negotiable. Parents can be encouraged to make short little videos on how to change batteries, which they can send to the caregivers to have on hand when needed. Parents are expected to check their child's technology every morning before drop-off, to be sure to have back-up equipment in the child's belongings, and to impress on the caregivers in daycare that a phone call should be made immediately to the parent if the child's technology doesn't appear to be working. Parents are coached, sometimes in role-playing with the LSL clinician, what to say and how to respond if they show up to pick up their child and the technology is in the backpack, in the cubby, on the child incorrectly, or not working.

One topic of conversation that can have a huge impact on daycare providers is when the LSL clinician links the LSL strategies they are introducing to the benefits all children in their care will receive when these strategies are embraced and employed. Most LSL clinicians have a short window and limited amount of time to interact with the daycare provider, so keeping the message short, memorable, and meaningful is critical. This can be done by the Three Ts messaging provided in Dana Suskind's book *Thirty*

Million Words: Building a Child's Brain.[21] The Three Ts stand for: *Tune In, Talk More, Take Turns*. This messaging applies to all children and keeps the complicated theory and terminology simple and practical, thereby avoiding roadblocks to action.

Tune In involves the conscious effort of observing a child and talking about what they find interesting. This involves the LSL strategies of joint attention, positioning (often daycare providers are down on the child's physical level, which is helpful, so the benefits of this should be pointed out), and following the child's lead. To *Tune In*, the caregiver notices and acknowledges how a baby or child is communicating to them and what they are communicating. *Tuning In* increases the likelihood of meaningful interactions between caregivers and children.

Talk More is fairly self-explanatory and can be linked to the LSL strategies of modeling language, parentese (which may very well be in use in the infant rooms), acoustic highlighting, expansion, and repetition.

Take Turns is an LSL strategy that clinicians are quite familiar with! Caregivers might need a bit of coaching on the LSL strategies of wait time, expectant look, asking open-ended questions, and prompting.

The biggest message to send caregivers in daycares is using these three strategies; *Tune In, Talk More and Take Turns* creates language rich environments that will grow the brains of all of the children in their care. Add a fourth "T": *Technology* for the child who is deaf or hard of hearing.

For Spanish-speaking providers, Suskind offers the Three C's: *Conéctese (Tune In), Converse Más (Talk More), and Comparta Turnos (Take Turns).*

Pearl

Daycare providers may be more willing and likely to use LSL strategies when the LSL clinician makes the case that the LSL strategies they are introducing will benefit all children in their care.

10.8 Strategies for Practitioners in Mainstream Educational Settings

Many children who are deaf or hard of hearing are educated alongside their hearing peers (typically referred to as mainstream settings) for their whole educational experience. Some children may begin in schools or programs that are specifically designed for children with hearing loss and eventually move to educational settings with hearing peers. Either way, the individual child's success is based on many factors, and the purpose of this section is to highlight just a few of the strategies that are beneficial to children in mainstream educational settings. The reader is referred to Chapter 16 for more in-depth learning on this topic.

Many teachers of the deaf (TOD) push in during a child's regularly scheduled classes for the purpose of observing how the child interacts in the classroom as well as taking the opportunity to model, coach, and guide mainstream teachers in effective LSL

strategies. When direct services to the child are offered, these are to be outside of the classroom environment and should be expressly outlined in the child's IEP whether services are consultative, direct, or for coaching purposes. The TOD is not providing push-in services to act as an aid to the child.

Accommodations that professionals in the mainstream need to be aware of should be written in the child's IEP. However, if there is not someone present at the IEP meeting who understands the needs of children with hearing loss who use audition to communicate, some critical accommodations can be missing. Many of these factors are considered prior to placement in a specific classroom and can include: acoustics of the environment and modifications that may be necessary, the child's use of technology (including remote microphone technology), class size, the teacher's knowledge of children with hearing loss, and their use of strategies that support children's access to the curriculum.[37]

Any of the LSL strategies discussed in this chapter can support children in the mainstream. Many of the strategies are considered best-practice for *all* students and may already be in use in mainstream settings. Several key strategies and questions to consider are listed in the following sections.

10.8.1 Positioning

Where is the child seated in the classroom? Where is the classroom positioned in the school? Classrooms that are in high-traffic areas or near noisy areas (playgrounds, gymnasiums) are difficult listening environments for children with hearing loss. Positioning also refers to where the teacher is within the classroom during instruction. Some important questions to consider are:

How is audibility impacted if the teacher walks around the room during instruction?

Does the teacher talk about important information while turning away and writing on a black, white, or smart board?

Of equal importance is how the student is positioned in relation to the peers. LSL clinicians are aware of the child's hearing loss and whether one ear may have greater auditory access than another, so they can educate the other professionals in the child's environment to be aware of the importance of positioning.

10.8.2 Wait Time

Teachers in the mainstream are encouraged to be especially mindful of allowing the child who is deaf or hard of hearing the appropriate wait time to listen, process, and respond to questions, comments, or directions. Sharing resources with teachers on the seminal work by Mary Budd Rowe,[25] discussed earlier in this chapter, and the effects of wait time on all students may prove beneficial.

10.8.3 Open-Ended Questions

Open-ended questions can be utilized as a great tool for comprehension checks for all students in the class. The classroom teacher is coached to be mindful of not singling out the child with hearing loss and impacting their social and emotional health. Asking guided questions at the end of class to sum up or review is an effective way to check all students' comprehension.

Frequent comprehension checks provide repetition of important information to the child with hearing loss as well as all the children in the classroom creating an enriched learning environment for all.

10.9 Summary

Children who are deaf or hard of hearing have limitless possibilities today, regardless of the severity of their hearing loss. The use of appropriately programmed technology and access to trained professionals are keys to their success. LSL professionals who are competent in their practice can describe why strategies are chosen, how strategies are carried out, and what the expected outcome is, and then coach caregivers or other professionals on the effective use of strategies.

LSL clinicians employ a wide range and variety of strategies and move fluidly through the use of multiple strategies in any given interaction with a child who is deaf or hard of hearing. Strategies that are incorporated into daily routines and daily living are most effective.

LSL strategies are a key component to children meeting their full potential, mastering communicative competence, and meeting with success in all life endeavors. LSL clinicians have an obligation, therefore, to become proficient in their knowledge and implementation of LSL strategies.

Discussion Questions

1. Why do LSL clinicians need to be knowledgeable about LSL strategies?
2. Which LSL strategies also encourage strong brain architecture by encouraging interactive relationships?
3. What aspects of speech and language are taken into account when modeling language?
4. How does an LSL clinician choose which LSL strategy to focus on?

References

[1] Donnellan E, Bannard C, McGillion ML, Slocombe KE, Matthews D. Infants' intentionally communicative vocalizations elicit responses from caregivers and are the best predictors of the transition to language: A longitudinal investigation of infants' vocalizations, gestures and word production. Dev Sci 2020;23(1):e12843 doi: 10.1111/desc.12843

[2] AG Bell Academy. The AG Bell Academy for Listening and Spoken Language. https://agbellacademy.org/certification/lsls-domains-of-knowledge/ Accessed November 27, 2021

[3] Center on the Developing Child at Harvard University. Serve and return. https://developingchild.harvard.edu/science/key-concepts/serve-and-return/ November 21, 2021

[4] Estabrooks W, MacIver-Lux K, Rhoades EA. Auditory-Verbal Therapy for Young Children with Hearing Loss and Their Families and the Practitioners Who Guide Them. San Diego, CA: Plural Publishing, Inc; 2016

[5] Pollack D, Goldberg DM, Caleffe-Schenck N. Educational Audiology for the Limited-Hearing Infant and Preschooler: An Auditory-Verbal Program. Springfield, IL: C.C. Thomas; 1997

[6] Luterman D. Counseling Persons with Communication Disorders and Their Families. Austin, TX: PRO-ED; 2017

[7] Gavrilov Y, Rotem S, Ofek R, Geva R. Socio-cultural effects on children's initiation of joint attention. Front Hum Neurosci 2012;6(286):286 doi: 10.3389/fnhum.2012.00286

[8] Cole EA, Flexcer C. Children with Hearing Loss Developing Listening and Talking Birth to Six. San Diego, CA: Plural Publishing, Inc; 2020

[9] Gleason J. The Development of Language. Pearson Education; 2005

[10] Tomasello M, Carpenter M, Call J, Behne T, Moll H. Understanding and sharing intentions: the origins of cultural cognition. Behav Brain Sci 2005;28(5):675–691, discussion 691–735 doi: 10.1017/s0140525x05000129

[11] Mundy P, Newell L. Attention, joint attention, and social cognition. Curr Dir Psychol Sci 2007;16(5):269–274 10.1111/j.1467-8721.2007.00518.x

[12] Romeo RR, Leonard JA, Robinson ST, et al. Beyond the 30-million-word gap: children's conversational exposure is associated with language-related brain function. Psychol Sci 2018;29(5):700–710 doi: 10.1177/0956797617742725

[13] Sindrey D. Listening Games for Littles. London, Ontario, Canada: Word Play Publications; 1997

[14] Gopnik A, Meltzoff A, Kuhl P. The Scientist in the Crib. New York, NY: Harper Collins Publishing; 1999

[15] Bergeson-Dana T. Spoken language development in infants who aer deaf or hard of hearing: the role of maternal infant-directed speech. Volta Rev 2012;112(2):171–180

[16] Fickenscher S, Gaffney E. Auditory-verbal strategies to build listening and spoken language skills. 2016. http://www.clarkeschools.org/AVstrategiesBoo

[17] MacIver-Lux K, Rosenzweig E, Estabrooks W. Strategies for Developing Listening, Talking, and Thinking in Auditory-Verbal Therapy. In: Smolen E, ed. Auditory-Verbal Therapy Science, Research, and Practice. San Diego, CA: Plural Publishing; 2020:521–561

[18] Simser JI. Auditory-verbal intervention: infants and toddlers. Volta Rev 1993;95(3):217–229

[19] Kral A, Lenarz T. How the brain learns to listen: Deafness and the bionic ear. Neuroforum 2015;21(1) doi:10.1515/s13295-015-0004-0

[20] Gilkerson J, Richards JA, Warren SF, Oller DK, Russo R, Vohr B. Language experience in the second year of life and language outcomes in late childhood. Pediatrics 2018;142(4):e20174276 doi: 10.1542/peds.2017-4276

[21] Suskind D, Suskind B. Thirty Million Words: Building a Child's Brain. New York, NY: Dutton; 2015

[22] Madell J. Can children understand fast speech? Hearing And Kids. https://hearinghealthmatters.org/hearingandkids/2013/can-children-understand-fast-speech/ Published April 24, 2013. Accessed September 27, 2021

[23] Dickson CL. Sound Foundation for Babies. Cochlear. https://www.cochlear.com/au/en/home/ongoing-care-and-support/rehabilitation-resources/sound-foundation-for-babies Published July 1 2021. Accessed September 27, 2021

[24] Stahl RJ. Using "think-time" and "wait-time" skillfully in the classroom. https://files.eric.ed.gov/fulltext/ED370885.pdf. Accessed August 14, 2021

[25] Rowe MB. Wait time: slowing down may be a way of speeding up! J Teach Educ 1986;37(1):43–50 doi: 10.1177/002248718603700110

[26] Ling D. Foundations of Spoken Language for Hearing-Impaired Children. Washington, DC: Alexander Graham Bell Association for the Deaf; 1989

[27] Hart B, Risley TR. Meaningful Differences in the Everyday Experience of Young American Children. Baltimore, MD: Brookes Publishing Company, Inc.; 1995

[28] Goodman JC, Dale PS, Li P. Does frequency count? Parental input and the acquisition of vocabulary. J Child Lang 2008;35(3):515–531 doi: 10.1017/s0305000907008641

[29] White E. Listening & spoken language preschool programs. In: Preparing to Teach, Committing to Learn: An Introduction to the Education of Children Who Are Deaf/Hard of Hearing. http://www.infanthearing.org/ebook-educating-children-dhh/index.html Accessed August 15, 2021

[30] Newbury J, Klee T, Stokes SF, Moran C. Exploring expressive vocabulary variability in two-year-olds: the role of working memory. J Speech Lang Hear Res 2015;58(6):1761–1772 doi: 10.1044/2015_jslhr-l-15-0018

[31] Mclean JE, McLean LK. How Children Learn Language. San Diego, CA: Singular Pub. Group; 1999

[32] Morrison HP. Development of listening in auditory-verbal therapy. In: Auditory-Verbal Therapy: Science Research and Practice. San Diego, CA: Plural Publishing; 2020:303–338

[33] Werfel KL, Reynolds G, Hudgins S, Castaldo M, Lund EA. The production of complex syntx in spontaneous language by 4-year-old children with hearing loss. AJSPL 2021;30(2):609–621 doi: 10.1044/2020_ajslp-20-00178

[34] Cruz I, Quittner AL, Marker C, DesJardin JL. Identification of effective strategies to promote language in deaf childrenwith cochlear implants. Child Dev 2012;84(2):543–559 doi: 10.1111/j.1467-8624.2012.01863.x

[35] Hoff E. The specificity of environmental influence: socioeconomic status affects early vocabulary development via maternal speech. Child Dev 2003;74(5):1368–1378 doi: 10.1111/1467-8624.00612

[36] wikiHow. How to ask open ended questions. wikiHow. https://www.wikihow.com/Ask-Open-Ended-Questions Published October 21, 2021. Accessed September 27, 2021

[37] Sexton J. Preparing for more deaf or hard of hearing children in mainstream schools. District Administration. https://districtadministration.com/preparing-for-more-deaf-or-hard-of-hearing-children-in-mainstream-schools/ Published July 9, 2021. Accessed August 14, 2021

Resources

The reader is referred to the following resources for additional learning on LSL Strategies:

AGBell Academy for Listening and Spoken Language Exam Blueprint: https://agbellacademy.org/wp-content/uploads/2018/12/LSLS-Certification-Exam-Blueprint_FINAL.pdf

AGBell Academy for Listening and Spoken Language Certification: https://agbellacademy.org/certification/

Auditory Verbal Strategies to Build Listening and Spoken Language Skills by Sherri Fickenscher and Elizabeth Gaffney. Retrievable from www.clarkeschools.org/AVstrategiesBook

Auditory-Verbal Therapy: Science, Research, and Practice by Estabrooks, Morrison, & MacIver-Lux (2020),[3] Chapter 15: "Strategies for Developing Listening, Talking, and Thinking in Auditory-Verbal Therapy."

Hearing First offers Learning Experiences specifically on LSL strategies: https://www.hearingfirst.org/learning-experiences/ The catalog of Learning Experiences can be viewed here. Parent friendly handouts of LSL strategies can be found here: https://www.hearingfirst.org/m/resources/7380

Preparing to Teach, Committing to Learn: An Introduction to Educating Children Who Are Deaf/Hard of Hearing by Lenihan (2020). Chapter 7: "Listening and Spoken Language Strategies." Retrievable here: https://www.infanthearing.org/ebook-educating-children-dhh/chapters/7%20Chapter%207%202020.pdf

Video examples of strategies can be viewed at the following websites: https://www.jtc.org/ideas-advice/video-tips/; https://www.jtc.org/es/ideas-y-consejos/consejos-en-video/

Welcome To Rehab At Home | The MED-EL Blog: https://blog.medel.com/rehab-at-home/

11 Late to the Party: When Children Come Late to Listening and Spoken Language Therapy

Joan G. Hewitt

Summary

Despite concerted efforts to identify hearing loss at birth, a significant number of children are late identified. This chapter considers reasons why hearing loss may be late diagnosed and the effects this can have on listening, language, cognitive, and academic development. This chapter also helps practitioners determine the appropriate developmental stage for beginning intervention with children whose hearing loss was late identified and discusses best practices for ensuring that this population develops the language skills necessary to be successful in the education system and beyond.

Keywords

Late identification, late diagnosis, newborn hearing screening, misdiagnosis, developmental stage, grief process, developmental sequence, developmentally appropriate, splinter skills, annual growth, catch-up growth, functional language, receptive language, expressive language

Key Points

- Even with well-established universal newborn hearing screening programs an estimated 15% to 40% of children with hearing loss are still late diagnosed.[1]
- Late diagnosis may be the result of an error in newborn hearing screening, failure to follow up on a newborn hearing referral, no availability of newborn screening in the place a child is born, or progressive hearing loss.
- Parents of children with late diagnosed hearing loss need the same emotional, educational, and coaching support as parents whose children are enrolled in early intervention. Depending on the age of the child, this may mean adopting a novel approach to therapy so that parents can be participants in intervention, especially in the educational setting.
- Children who are late diagnosed can have varying degrees of hearing loss and language delay.
- Detailed assessment and observation of all areas of language development—listening, speech, receptive language, expressive language, and pragmatics—are essential to determining the starting point for intervention because these children may have "splinter skills" with development in some areas and significant delays in others.
- For these children to develop rich, flexible language commensurate with their hearing peers, intervention must follow the typical developmental sequence. This process cannot be circumvented by providing simple "functional" language.
- Language level, not chronological age or grade level, is the determining factor of where to begin intervention (e.g.,

Chapter 8, "Babies and Beginners"; Chapter 9, "Toddler-type Language" or Chapter 10, "More Proficient Communicators").
- To catch up, children who are late diagnosed will need to make more than 1 year's progress in 1 year's time. Practitioners working with these children need to be committed to partnering with parents to ensure this intensity of intervention throughout the child's day.

11.1 Introduction

With the advent of newborn hearing screening, early diagnosis, early hearing aid fitting, and early cochlear implantation, it is easy to assume that all children with hearing loss will receive early intervention and quickly close the gap between their language development and that of their hearing peers. Unfortunately, far too often this is not the case. It is estimated that 15% to 40% of children with hearing loss are late identified, so practitioners need to be well-versed in how to develop language in those children who are late to the party.[1]

11.2 Why Are Children Late to Listening, Speech, and Language Intervention?

11.2.1 False Negative Results

First, newborn hearing screening, like other tests, can have false negative results in which the infant appears to pass but actually has hearing loss.[2]

False negative results can occur because of equipment malfunctions, lack of technician training, or failure to follow appropriate testing protocols, including administering the test too many times to obtain a "pass." Also, depending on the sensitivity of the screening equipment, infants with minimal or mild hearing loss may pass their newborn hearing screening. Finally, if an infant has auditory neuropathy spectrum disorder (ANSD) and otoacoustic emissions (OAEs) are administered, the baby can pass the screening, which is why auditory brainstem response (ABR) testing is the test of choice for newborn hearing screening.

11.2.2 No Newborn Hearing Screening

In the United States, in 2019, 2.1% of infants, which is more than 75,000 infants, did not receive newborn hearing screening.[3] This can occur because the parents declined the screening in the hospital, did not follow up with a medical facility to have the testing, or because the baby was born at home, so the parents did not receive information about hearing screening. It is also important to remember that not all countries have universal newborn hearing screening. Thus, children who were born in another country may not have had access to early diagnosis and intervention.

11.2.3 Lost to Follow-Up

Unfortunately, many babies who do not pass their newborn hearing screening do not receive all necessary follow-up care. In 2019, 27.5% of infants (over 16,000 infants) who did not pass their newborn hearing screening were lost to follow-up.[4] A major factor in families' failure to pursue needed follow up is the lack of understanding of the effects of hearing loss and the importance of diagnosis and treatment.[5] Too often parents are told by technicians, nurses, or even pediatricians that their child's failed screening was "just an equipment problem or some fluid in their ears." This failure to educate parents about the importance of further testing can interfere with their motivation to follow up during those stressful early days with an infant. A lack of education or significant parent grief, especially denial and depression, can also lead to parents' rejecting intervention after permanent hearing loss is diagnosed. When babies have a mild or moderate hearing loss, they do respond to sound, so some parents have a difficult time accepting that the child has a hearing loss which will affect language learning and that the child will need hearing aids. In some cases, lack of health insurance coverage may interfere with obtaining follow-up services. A final reason that many children do not receive follow-up services is because many families are transitory. A county or a state may be trying to contact a family for follow-up testing or intervention, but if that family has moved, reaching them and connecting them to a different area's screening system can be challenging.

11.2.4 Other Health Issues at Birth

Diagnosis and intervention of hearing loss in babies with serious health issues or other challenges may be delayed because other medical procedures and treatments need to take precedence over hearing testing. In addition, parents may be overwhelmed by the sheer number of medical appointments, so adding additional appointments to test hearing can seem like a low priority. While medical procedures, treatments, and appointments do need to be prioritized for these babies, it is important that their parents be educated about the need to follow up with hearing testing or intervention as soon as reasonably possible.

11.2.5 Poor Quality Follow-Up

Although it is painful to admit, there are still places in which babies do not receive diagnostic testing and follow-up with audiologists specifically trained to assess infants and pediatric patients. All clinicians working with this part of the population should be well-trained and highly experienced or they should refer to others. Poor quality follow-up can lead to delayed diagnosis, incorrect diagnosis, delayed intervention, or inappropriate intervention.

11.2.6 Progressive Hearing Loss

In addition to poor quality follow-up, the failure to recognize the progressive nature of a hearing loss can lead to significant delays in appropriate diagnosis and intervention. Failure to provide audiological testing at regular intervals (every 3 months for newly identified children) and to cross-verify electrophysiological results with behavioral results and parent/clinician observations can lead to delays in identifying hearing changes and making necessary technology adjustments. Failure to identify disorders such as Enlarged Vestibular Aqueduct (EVA) or cytomegalovirus (CMV) can also lead to assumptions that hearing loss is stable when it is not.

11.2.7 Hearing Loss Onset after Birth

As we know, hearing loss can develop after birth. Infants can accurately pass their newborn hearing screening but develop hearing loss at some point after birth. The parents of these children may be unaware of the signs of hearing loss, or they may have a false sense of security because their child passed newborn hearing screening. They may also have a difficult time navigating the medical system to obtain testing because their child is no longer within the newborn screening system.

11.2.8 Misinformation/Poor Advice

Unfortunately, even with universal newborn hearing screening for more than 20 years, much of the public and some medical practitioners are still misinformed or uneducated about the capability to accurately assess hearing in infants and young children and the effects of hearing loss on listening, speech, and language development. If parents suspect a child's hearing loss after the child passed newborn hearing screening, they may discuss their concerns with extended family members or friends. All too often well-meaning family members or friends share advice like "There's no need to worry. Your brother did not talk until he was 3, and he's fine." Even more alarming is that, when families discuss their concerns with their physicians, there are still some pediatricians who minimize the parents' concerns and even some who counsel parents that hearing cannot be accurately tested in infants and young children.

Parents can also receive misinformation or poor advice about types of technology, technology wearing schedules, and appropriate therapeutic intervention. If a child is utilizing hearing aids but needs cochlear implants, significant delays will occur. If the family was counseled that it is fine to take breaks from hearing aids or cochlear implants, then wearing time may not be sufficient for developing audition. If the parents want to develop spoken language but were counseled that any therapy approach is fine, inappropriate intervention may result in further delays rather than progress.

11.2.9 Poor Follow-Through

Some children can be considered late to the party even though they had very early diagnosis and excellent intervention. If parents do not follow through with hearing technology all the child's waking hours, do not act as language facilitators at home, or if other family stresses (poverty, illness, employment, neglect, etc) interfere with follow-through, the child may begin school with significant delays.

11.2.10 Misdiagnosis

Children with undiagnosed hearing loss can appear to have attention, speech/language, social, cognitive, or behavioral issues. While hearing testing should always be completed *first* before assessing for any of these other issues which rely on hearing, there are children who have been diagnosed with attention deficit disorder (ADHD), speech-language delay, apraxia, autism spectrum disorder (ASD), cognitive delay, auditory processing disorder, or oppositional defiant disorder (ODD) when undiagnosed hearing loss was present. Unfortunately for these children, not only were their diagnosis and intervention delayed, but they may also have received inappropriate intervention in the form of medication, speech/language therapy practices, or behavioral therapeutic interventions for a disorder they did not have.

11.3 Where Do We Begin Our Intervention?

We must start at the beginning and make use of the same early interventions and strategies we have discussed thus far in this textbook!! As practitioners, we know that time is of the essence for all children with hearing loss but even more so with these children whose listening, speech, and language development has been significantly delayed. Our goals may be to obtain hearing technology and begin auditory-verbal therapy to develop language as quickly as possible. Moreover, parents may be happy to relinquish responsibility and decision making to us. However, this push to move forward does not change our collective responsibility to educate these parents and partner with them so that they can become their child's primary language facilitators.

Pearl

As practitioners, the push to move forward does not change our collective responsibility to educate these parents and partner with them so that they can become their child's primary language facilitators.

Educating and partnering with parents of late identified children takes skill, consideration, and empathy. While we know it is essential to move forward with obtaining an accurate diagnosis, fitting technology, and beginning auditory-verbal therapy, we must remember that these parents are most likely in shock; many feel that the child they thought they were raising has been replaced by a completely different child. They are trying to deal with emotions of loss as they are being pushed to make decisions, accept unfamiliar technology, and begin changing the way they are interacting with their child. It is often overwhelming for them. In addition, if the diagnosis has been delayed for several years, the

professionals working with the parents may no longer be early intervention specialists who are used to walking through the grief process with parents. Practitioners must slow down, recognize the parents' emotional and mental state, and tailor intervention appropriately. In the long run, overwhelming parents with information they cannot yet comprehend or allowing them to relinquish all responsibility to clinicians is detrimental to the parents' growth and their child's progress. (See Chapter 4, "Empathy: Changing the Culture of Communication.")

Pitfall

In the long run, overwhelming parents with information they cannot yet comprehend or allowing them to relinquish all responsibility to the clinicians is detrimental to the parents' growth and their child's progress.

In addition, if the hearing loss was not diagnosed or intervention was not started until preschool or school-age, the practitioners and education system may not be set up to assist parents, but everyone must recognize that the child will need significant language input outside the academic day. Thus, it is essential to these children's progress that their parents receive the training to become their child's primary language facilitator. This may mean being creative in how to include and coach parents in all therapy sessions. Some possibilities are scheduling sessions with the DHH early intervention specialist, setting up individual therapy before or after school so parents can attend, scheduling remote sessions when the child and parents are at home, using a "flipped" therapy model where the parents attend through an online platform, or providing private individual auditory-verbal therapy for the child and parents. As discussed in Chapter 5, school systems may be unfamiliar with the model of parent inclusion and coaching, but after professionals see the benefits, they should be highly supportive of it.

Pearl

If the hearing loss was not diagnosed or intervention was not started until preschool or school-age, the practitioners and education system may not be set up to assist parents, but everyone must recognize that the child will need significant language input outside the academic day. Thus, it is essential to these children's progress that their parents receive the training to become their child's primary language facilitator.

Finally, we must also recognize that older children diagnosed with hearing loss may go through a grieving process. Their world is changing, and they are struggling, but until their hearing loss is identified or changes in their hearing are documented, they do not know why. After the hearing loss is identified, they must attend a number of appointments, accept technology, and begin therapy. Some children may express anger, anxiety, or sadness about the hearing loss and all it entails, but often children's emotions are reflected in their behaviors. Practitioners and parents must recognize the signs of grief in children and provide the necessary support and resources for children to express and work through their emotions.

11.4 Where Do We Start Our Speech and Language Intervention with Children Who Are Late to the Party? The Beginning!

Children who are late to the listening, speech, and language party do not fit neatly into one developmental category, so the beginning is specific to each individual child. For example, the child might be a 4-year-old with a mild to moderate hearing loss that was diagnosed at birth, but the parents chose not to proceed with amplification. At preschool, concern was expressed that articulation was somewhat unintelligible and language seemed immature. Or the child might be a 3-year-old who received hearing aids for a mild to moderate hearing loss at 2 months of age but did not have regular follow-up with a pediatric audiologist, has not made good progress despite intensive auditory-verbal therapy, and is now found to have a moderate to profound hearing loss from EVA. Another example might be a non-verbal 2-year-old who passed newborn hearing screening because of technician error, was diagnosed with a profound hearing loss related to Connexin 26 at 18 months, and was required by the implant team to complete 6 months of hearing aid use before implantation. Another possibility is a 5-year-old child who was diagnosed with ASD at 16 months of age because spoken language was not developing. Because newborn hearing screening was passed, hearing was considered normal without further assessment. Recent testing for kindergarten revealed no markers for ASD, so hearing was tested, and a profound hearing loss was diagnosed. Finally, the child might be an 8-year-old who has a moderate hearing loss that has never been aided and who has moved from another country with poor language development in his native tongue and no language development in English.

Despite the fact these children are different ages with different hearing losses and different amounts of listening and language experience, we need to start at the same place with each: the beginning! As we discussed, listening is the foundation for the development of spoken language. Each of these children, to a greater or lesser degree, has missed important listening time. If the parents' goal is to maximize spoken language development, we must insist on full-time use of appropriate hearing technology to access listening and full-time input of language in all environments, and then we must begin intervention at the appropriate starting point.

When the appropriate hearing technology is in place, we must assess the children's listening, speech, and language to determine where they are developmentally and begin there. Even though the children may be older, following a developmental model will ensure that important skills are not missed and that rich, flexible, not atypical, language develops. This means that our assessments

will direct us to the appropriate stage or stages of language development. Moreover, with these children, it is essential that we complete detailed assessments and observations as their skills may be splintered with progress in some areas but significant deficits in others. Failure to assess all areas of listening, speech, language, and pragmatics can lead to intervention that neglects important skills and leaves the child with continued delays.

Pearl

Even though the children may be older, following a developmental model will ensure that important skills are not missed and that rich, flexible, not atypical, language develops.

Pitfall

Failure to assess all areas of listening, speech, language, and pragmatics can lead to intervention that neglects important skills and leaves the child with continued delays.

From the previous examples, neither the late diagnosed 2-year-old nor the misdiagnosed 5-year-old would be expected to have any receptive or expressive language. Thus, it is essential that we begin intervention with the expectations and goals detailed in Chapter 8 ("Babies and Beginners"). Age does not change the fact that these children have not developed the auditory foundation of listening and receptive language necessary for spoken language. Yes, activities will need to be modified to be interesting and appropriate to the child's age, but the goals of therapy will be consistent with those for beginning language learners.

For the 4-year-old with inconsistent hearing aid use, the 3-year-old with unrecognized progressive hearing loss, and the 8-year-old English language learner, detailed assessments and observations will be the key to determining the starting point. If the child has a limited receptive vocabulary and is only using single words, then you will turn to Chapter 9 ("Toddler-type Language"). Again, the activities you use to coach the parents will need to be modified for the child's age and level of cognitive development, but the basic expectations and goals will be consistent with ensuring good auditory attention, building a greater receptive language base, and encouraging word combinations and sentences. If the child has a listening and receptive language foundation such that they are using simple sentences, then you would refer to Chapter 10 ("More Proficient Communicators").

We must remember that it is not possible to skip steps or jump ahead in language development. If we want children with hearing loss to develop rich, flexible language and the thinking skills that accompany that language, they must build the skills of each developmental level. Obviously, our goal is to accelerate the time it takes the child to move through lower developmental levels, but we must clearly understand that it is **always** the child's developmental listening and language level, not the child's chronological age or grade in school, that determines our starting point for intervention.

Obviously, our goal is to accelerate the time it takes the child to move through lower developmental levels, but we must clearly understand that it is *always* the child's developmental listening and language level, not the child's chronological age or grade in school, that determines our starting point for intervention.

11.5 But Wait, Don't Children Need "Functional Language" to Express Themselves?

All too often, when children are late to intervention, the authors have seen a list of goals encouraging expressive language development without goals for building a foundation of listening or receptive language development. Consider for yourself the pitfalls of this approach. Imagine you arrive in a foreign country where they speak a language you have never encountered before. Although you do not know the language at all, everyone you meet is speaking to you in that language and expecting you to respond in that language. When you do not respond because you do not understand what is being said, everyone appears to be coaching you to say something, but you have no idea what you are saying or agreeing to. If you are truly imagining this scenario, you should have that anxious feeling that comes with being lost and overwhelmed and you should be thinking to yourself right now, "Help! This is ridiculous! I have never heard this language! I have no idea what they are saying or what they are asking me to say! I need time to listen so I can begin to understand the language before I start saying words and sentences!" Exactly! If you cannot begin speaking an unfamiliar foreign language without building a receptive language base (when you already have a well-developed primary language), why are we thinking that children with hearing loss can do that? As we discussed in Chapter 1, we are building language and need a strong foundation of listening and receptive language before we can expect expressive language regardless of our age.

Pearl

If you cannot begin speaking an unfamiliar foreign language without building a receptive language base (when you already have a well-developed primary language), why are we thinking that children with hearing loss can do that?

Moreover, within these expressive language goals, the authors often see an emphasis on the development of "functional" language such as: *more, I want, help me, please, and thank you.* While the idea to provide non-verbal children with functional language seems appropriate on the surface, the focus on expressive language without a receptive foundation and the focus on these specific words and phrases can be quite problematic. Imagine that I walked up to you on the street and said, "More." What are you going to do for me? As you try to decide what I want and what you are going to do

for me, I will continue to say, "*More, more, more.*" Did that clarify my request for you? Were you able to give me what I wanted? I am guessing that you still did not understand what I wanted, so now I will say, "*Please, please, please.*" Did that clarify my request for you? Again, I am guessing not, so now I will say, "*Help me, help me, help me.*" If you are correctly imagining this exchange, you should see that these "functional" words are not functional unless there is a detailed context. Moreover, even within a detailed context, these words are often not functional. To give you an example, in a recent visit, a patient became increasingly agitated at the beginning of an appointment and kept saying, "*More*" which was the targeted expressive language goal from his therapist. The audiologist offered him every toy available while his father offered him all the snacks he had brought. Nothing offered was what the child wanted, so he became increasingly upset. In the end, the audiologist and parent figured out that the child wanted his mother in the appointment, not his father. This exchange clearly illustrates how "more" was *not* functional communication. "More" means an additional amount of something you already have, but in this case, the child had nothing and actually wanted something that was not present. In other words, the child was using "more" to mean "give me something or someone different" which is not appropriate to the meaning of "more" and ineffective for communication of his true desire. "More" in no way provided a functional representation of what he wanted.

In addition, we must realize that initially focusing on these "functional" words and phrases to elicit communication is not developmentally appropriate. In typical language development, as receptive vocabulary builds, early language learners are beginning to understand that certain objects have specific names. Thus, the majority of children's first words are nouns.[6] In the previous example, the child wanted "mama" which is one of the first words children generally acquire. However, this child was late to the language party, so the well-meaning, but misguided professional had targeted "functional" language over developmentally appropriate language. Bypassing the typical developmental order meant this child lacked the specific (and very basic) word which would have expressed what he wanted (mama!) and left him with an inappropriate, generic word which had no meaning in the context he used it. Thus, while functional words are an integral part of communication, we must ensure we are teaching them at a developmentally appropriate time and using them in a way that enhances communication development.

Pitfall

We must realize that initially focusing on these "functional" words and phrases (e.g., *more, I want, help me, please, thank you*) to elicit communication is not developmentally appropriate.

According to the Cottage Acquisition Scales for Listening, Language, and Speech (CASLLS) Pre-Sentence Level,[7] typically developing children begin using "more" to express recurrence ("do it again") at 15 to 18 months of age when they have a receptive vocabulary of at least 50 words and an expressive vocabulary of 10 to 20 words. They begin using "more + a noun" at 21 to 24 months of age when they have a receptive vocabulary of 250 to 500 words and an expressive vocabulary of 150 to 300 words. Along the same lines, "please" and "thank you," which are merely polite requests with little linguistic meaning, are not used by typically hearing children until 21 to 24 months of age. According to the CASLLS Simple Sentence Level, typically developing children begin using "I want + a noun" between 24 and 30 months of age when they have extensive receptive and expressive vocabularies. From this data on typically developing children, it should be evident that targeting these utterances as first words for functional language is not developmentally appropriate. By targeting these words and phrases as "functional" language instead of building the appropriate listening and receptive foundations, professionals must realize that they are circumventing typical development, fostering atypical development, and leaving children with ineffective communication. Instead of teaching a child to say "more" or "please" or "I want" to obtain a desired item, think of the significantly increased depth and breadth of language we are inputting if we ask, "Do you want juice or milk?" "Your red pants or your green shorts?" or in the case of our example, "Your mommy or your daddy?" (Note that none of those examples are yes / no questions, but instead choice questions which provide exposure to necessary vocabulary.) By building a rich receptive foundation with developmentally appropriate language, we are encouraging the development of a truly functional expressive repertoire that enables children to state their wants and needs.

Pitfall

By targeting these words and phrases (*more, I want, help me, please, thank you*) as "functional" language instead of building the appropriate listening and receptive foundations, professionals must realize that they are circumventing typical development, fostering atypical development, and leaving children with ineffective communication.

Pearl

By building a rich receptive foundation with developmentally appropriate language, we are encouraging the development of a truly functional expressive repertoire that allows children to state their wants and needs.

In the same way, focusing on learning colors, numbers, letters, and even prepositions because a child is of preschool age does not develop meaningful and developmentally appropriate communication. According to the CASLLS Simple Sentence, typically developing children begin using "color + a noun," "number + a noun," or "preposition + a noun" when they are 24 to 30 months old. At that age, they have extensive receptive and expressive vocabularies and are combining words into meaningful phrases. Colors, numbers, and prepositions only become meaningful when they are put together into telegraphic utterances or simple sentences with a rich collection of nouns. If the child is not yet putting words together, then their chronological age and academic skills are secondary to the need to build the listening and receptive language skills necessary to move from single word utterances to combined words.

So, yes, children who are late to the party need "functional" language, but we must remember that language that develops typically and naturally is the most functional language of all. Only by identifying a child's development in each area of listening, speech, language, and pragmatics can we identify where the late-to-the-party child's intervention should begin: Chapter 8 (developing listening, receptive language, and first words), Chapter 9 (putting words together and beginning to use simple sentences), or Chapter 10 (moving to more complex language).

11.6 What if a Child Has Skills at Different Levels?

It is highly possible that a child who is late to intervention will have "splinter skills" with more progress in some areas and less progress in others. For instance, the 3-year-old with progressive hearing loss may have developed a good collection of nouns, some adjectives, and a few rote phrases during early language development but then started to lose hearing and did not develop verbs or word endings. The child may be able to combine familiar nouns, adjectives, and stereotypic phrases into coherent utterances, but otherwise, language is limited. It may be tempting to begin with Chapter 9 because the child can combine words, but before working with this child on longer expressive utterances and simple sentences, the practitioner will need to return to more basic listening and receptive language skills from Chapter 8 to develop the missing listening, receptive, and expressive skills. In other words, for children with skills at differing levels, it is essential that practitioners recognize that strong, well developed language is dependent on mastering all listening, speech, language, and pragmatic skills at each developmental level.

Pearl

For children with skills at differing levels, it is essential that practitioners recognize that strong, well-developed language is dependent on mastering all listening, speech, language, and pragmatic skills at each developmental level.

11.7 How Long Will It Take Late-to-the-Party Children to Catch up to Their Hearing Peers?

As we have discussed throughout this chapter, there is no one description for children who are late to language intervention. From our earlier examples, the 4-year-old with inconsistent hearing aid use may have language which is 1 year delayed while the child who was misdiagnosed as being on the autism spectrum may be 5 years delayed. While some practitioners, especially school personnel, may want to focus on academic development, progress in academics is dependent on spoken language development; thus, language development should be prioritized over academics.[8]

It is critical that, not only clinicians, but also teachers and administrators recognize that the cognitive development needed for academics is intertwined with language development. All children entering kindergarten need to be approaching adult-like language and vocabulary so that they can now apply to their knowledge of language to literacy and learning.[9] They will use their knowledge of language to begin learning abstract concepts and problem-solving complex issues. Research has clearly demonstrated that language deficits in school-aged children are closely tied to lower cognitive and executive function scores[10,11] and poorer academic performance.[12] In other words, well-developed language drives strong cognitive and academic development, but poor language development can easily lead to poor cognitive and academic development.

Many professionals and parents think that teaching a child to read will solve the language deficit problems, but we cannot read what we do not understand. Consider what happens when, while visiting a foreign country, you come upon a sign, directions, or museum description written in a language you do not know. Without a foundation in that language, you will not know what you are reading. You may have developed the skills to decode the words but have no receptive language to understand and derive meaning from what you are reading. This lack of sufficient language development is one of the reasons children with hearing loss traditionally struggled to develop reading skills above a 3rd grade level; they learned to decode but lacked the breadth of language necessary to read for meaning.[13]

In addition, children with delayed language struggle to understand abstract concepts and complex issues. Consider our late diagnosed 2-year-old and 5-year-old. If these children enter school without having developed the receptive understanding of past tense verbs and their markers, how will they understand the time continuum of historical events? If any of our examples have not developed complex vocabulary and language, how will they compare and contrast life in the US with life in Japan or understand the complex relationship between the two countries?

Moreover, we must recognize that, without language that is within 1 to 2 years of their hearing peers, children with hearing loss are virtually cut off from the language of the classroom and their fellow students.[9] In other words, academic subjects are taught through age appropriate language; thus, until children with hearing loss have age appropriate language, they cannot fully participate in and benefit from academic learning.

Children who are late to listening and spoken language need to make accelerated progress every year until they catch up. Typically developing children should make 1 year of language growth each year, which is called annual growth. Annual growth is the typical developmental changes and learning which occur from one year to the next. For instance, annual growth includes all the developmental changes which make a two-year-old more advanced than a one-year-old or a five-year-old more advanced than a four-year-old. Children who are behind are those who have failed to make appropriate annual growth. This places these children in a position where they must, not only make annual growth, but also catch-up growth to reach the same level of skills and learning as their peers. Thus, children who are significantly behind in spoken language development must make 1 year of annual growth plus at least 1 year of catch-up growth each year if they are to narrow the gap between their language and that of their peers.[10] In the previous examples, the 4-year-old who is 1 year behind would need to make 1 year of annual growth **and** 1 year of catch-up growth which is **2 years of growth in 1 year** to enter kindergarten

at the same language level as the hearing peers. In contrast, if the 5-year-old who was misdiagnosed makes 1 year's annual growth *and* 1 year's catch-up growth **every year for 5 years,** then that child will reach the language level of the hearing peers at age 10. Practitioners working with children with hearing loss who have significantly delayed language need to clearly understand that targeting 1 year's progress in 1 year's time will maintain the same delay year-to-year and will never allow the child to catch up. Moreover, those professionals who are committed to and skilled with intervention that creates a minimum of 2 years' growth in 1 year's time should be the ones in charge of care for this special population of children who need this intensity of service.[10] In all cases, professionals and parents need to clearly understand that focusing on intensive language intervention is the key to setting the foundation for cognitive and academic development.

Pitfall

Practitioners working with children with hearing loss who have significantly delayed language need to clearly understand that targeting 1 year's progress in 1 year's time will maintain the same delay year-to-year and will never allow the child to catch up.

Pearl

Those professionals who are committed to and skilled with intervention that creates a minimum of 2 years' growth in 1 year's time should be the ones in charge of care for this special population of children who need this intensity of service.

11.8 Summary

Practitioners who work with children with hearing loss are going to see children who are late to the listening, speech, and language party. Because of the many reasons for late diagnosis that can lead to inappropriate intervention or even misdiagnosis, our late-to-the-party children can have any degree of hearing loss and any amount of exposure or lack of exposure to speech and language development. Moreover, their parents can arrive in various stages of the grief cycle without a full understanding of hearing loss and the necessary intervention. Thus, it is the responsibility of all practitioners to understand that, although time is of the essence, the children must receive the necessary support to move through the stages of language in a developmentally appropriate sequence. At the same time, practitioners need to clearly recognize that the children's parents must receive the support to move through the stages of grief, the education to understand the hearing loss, and the coaching to become their child's primary language facilitators. (For more information, see Chapter 4, "Empathy: Changing the Culture of Communication" and Chapter 5, "Parents as Partners.")

To ensure appropriate listening and language development, practitioners must adhere to the sequence of typical development. To do this, they must thoroughly assess the child's skills; identify the child's level of functioning in each area: listening, speech, language, and pragmatics; and then select the appropriate developmental level (Chapter 8, "Babies and Beginners; Chapter 9, "Toddler-type Language"; or Chapter 10, "More Proficient Communicators") regardless of the child's chronological age or grade level. Practitioners must remember that coaching parents and children to develop rich, flexible language is a long-term goal that passes through many stages and cannot be achieved by simply targeting "functional" language. Moreover, practitioners must be committed to ensuring that these children receive an intensity of intervention that enables them to make more than 2 years' progress in 1 year's time so they can close the gap and develop language commensurate with their hearing peers. It is critical that parents and professionals alike clearly recognize that age-appropriate language development is the key to strong cognitive development and future academic success.

Discussion Questions

1. You are an SLP or TOD on the school district's preschool team. On your caseload, you have a newly diagnosed 3-year-old with a mild to moderately severe sloping hearing loss. This child did not pass newborn hearing screening but was lost to follow up. Consider the following questions:
    a. What might the parents be experiencing? What support and coaching might they need? How will you accommodate that support and coaching in your setting?
    b. What might the child be experiencing? What specific deficits do you think assessments in listening, articulation, receptive language, expressive language, and pragmatics will show? At what language level (beginner, toddler-type, more proficient) do you think intervention will begin? Why?

2. You are an SLP or TOD on the school district's DHH team. On your caseload, you have a 3-year-old with a profound hearing loss whose parents declined newborn hearing screening, so the loss was not diagnosed until 17 months of age. Initially, the parents chose to use manual communication, but found it difficult to learn so they decided to pursue bilateral implantation when the child was 26 months old. For the first year of implantation, device use was less than 3 hours per day. The child has now entered the DHH classroom in your program. Consider the following questions:
    a. What might the parents be experiencing? What support and coaching might they need? How will you accommodate that support and coaching in your setting?
    b. What might the child be experiencing? What specific deficits do you think assessments in listening, articulation, receptive language, expressive language, and pragmatics will show? At what language level (beginner, toddler-type, more proficient) do you think intervention will begin? Why?
    c. Based on your assessment, how many years delayed do you think the child's language development is? How much language growth in 1 year will you target? Based on the growth you are targeting, when will this child's language catch up to the hearing peers?

3. You are an SLP or TOD in an elementary school. On your caseload, you have a newly diagnosed first-grader with a mild to moderate hearing loss. The previous year the kindergarten teacher had raised concerns about a possible

learning disability or ADHD because the child did not attend well and was not developing any reading skills. Through a full developmental evaluation, it was learned that the child had been diagnosed with this hearing loss at birth, but the parents declined amplification and intervention because their child "could hear." Moreover, it was also learned that, since birth, the child's caregivers during the day do not speak English. Consider the following:
    a. What might the parents be experiencing? What support and coaching might they need? How will you accommodate that support and coaching in your setting?
    b. Will you include the caregivers in your intervention? If so, how will you include them?
    c. What might the child be experiencing? What specific deficits do you think assessments in listening, articulation, receptive language, expressive language, and pragmatics will show? How do you think exposure to a second language has affected the child? At what language level (beginner, toddler-type, more proficient) do you think intervention will begin? Why?
    d. Because there is concern that the child is not developing reading skills, how will you balance academics with speech and language intervention?

References

[1] Fitzpatrick EM, Ham J, Whittingham J. Pediatric cochlear implantation: Why do children receive implants late? Ear Hear 2015;36(6):688–694

[2] Hidenobu T, Morimoto N, Minami S. False negative error in newborn hearing screening. Pediatric Otorhinolaryngology Japan 2009;30(1):47–53. https://doi.org/10.11374/shonijibi.30.47

[3] CDC EHDI. (2021). (rep.). 2019 Summary of Hearing Screening Among Total Occurrent Births. Retrieved from https://www.cdc.gov/ncbddd/hearin-gloss/2019-data/02-screen.html

[4] CDC EDHI. (2021). (rep.). 2019 CDC EHDI Hearing Screening & Follow-up Survey (HSFS)

[5] Pynnonen MA, Handelsman JA, King EF, Singer DC, Davis MM, Lesperance MM. Parent perception of newborn hearing screening. JAMA Otolaryngol Head Neck Surg 2016;142(6):538–543 10.1001/jamaoto.2015.3948

[6] Waxman S, Fu X, Arunachalam S, Leddon E, Geraghty K, Song HJ. Are nouns learned before verbs? Infants provide insight into a longstanding debate. Child Dev Perspect 2013;7(3). https://doi.org/10.1111/cdep.12032

[7] Wilkes EM. Cottage Acquisition Scales for Listening, Language & Speech: User's Guide. San Antonio, TX: Sunshine Cottage School for Deaf Children; 2001

[8] Ling D. Foundations of Spoken Language for Hearing-Impaired Children. Washington, DC: Alexander Graham Bell Association for the Deaf; 1989

[9] Early childhood literacy: the National Early Literacy Panel and beyond. Choice Reviews Online. 2013;50(12):50-688650-6886. doi:10.5860/choice.50-6886

[10] Noble KG, Norman MF, Farah MJ. Neurocognitive correlates of socioeconomic status in kindergarten children. Developmental Science. 2005;8(1):74-87. doi:10.1111/j.1467-7687.2005.00394.x

[11] Hart B, Risley TR. American parenting of language-learning children: Persisting differences in family-child interactions observed in natural home environments. Dev Psychol. 1992;28(6):1096-1105. doi:10.1037/0012-1649.28.6.1096

[12] Shanahan T, Lonigan CJ. The National Early Literacy Panel: A summary of the process and the report. Educ Res. 2010;39(4):279-285. doi:10.3102/0013189x10369172

[13] Qi S, Mitchell RE. Large-scale academic achievement testing of deaf and hard-of-hearing students: past, present, and future. J Deaf Stud Deaf Educ. 2012;17(1):1-18.doi:10.1093/deafed/enr028

[14] McConkey Robbins A, Koch DB, Osberger MJ, Zimmerman-Phillips S, Kishon-Rabin L. Effect of age at cochlear implantation on auditory skill development in infants and toddlers. Arch Otolaryngol Head Neck Surg 2004;130(5):570–574 10.1001/archotol.130.5.570

[15] Fielding L, Kerr N, Rosier P. Annual Growth for All Students: Catch-Up Growth for Those Who Are Behind. Kennewick, WA: New Foundation Press; 2007

IV
Adding the Second Floor

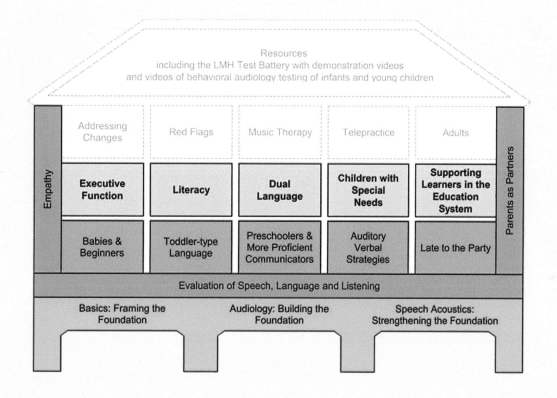

12 Executive Function Therapy Integrated into Auditory-Verbal Practice

Amy McConkey Robbins

"If the brain is a symphony then executive function is the conductor." Thomas E. Brown

Summary

This chapter covers the topic of executive functioning (EF) interventions in children with hearing loss. Executive functioning encompasses a set of brain-based processes that are important for virtually everything children need to do in their childhood years. EFs are responsible for the active management and control of cognitive resources, emotions, and behaviors to plan, organize, and achieve goals. Children with hearing loss are at much higher risk for EF delays, due in part to reduced exposure to and development of spoken language, and reduced exposure to auditory experience (resulting both from deafness and from degraded auditory signals transmitted by current hearing technologies). Children's executive functions can be improved following targeted therapy, and are most efficiently addressed by integrating EF goals into speech-language or LSL interventions. The chapter presents numerous goals and activities, supported by research findings and clinical experience, for practitioners to employ as they help to improve EF in children with hearing loss. For all suggested techniques, EF skills are targeted through activities that also address a child's needs within communication domains such as listening, spoken language, conversational competence and literacy. It is no longer enough to help children who are deaf or hard of hearing achieve speech and language skills at age- and grade-level. They must also be on a path to become well-adjusted, emotionally healthy, respectful, tax-paying citizens. In other words, they must compete with other children in the realm of EF. This chapter is a step in that direction.

Keywords

executive functioning in children who are deaf or hard of hearing; executive functioning intervention; executive functioning therapy and hearing loss; LSL intervention; auditory-verbal therapy; pediatric cochlear implant intervention

Key Points

This chapter will cover the following:

- Case study of an LSL child struggling with executive function (EF) weaknesses
- A definition of EF and its components
- The relationship between EF and language in young children
- The unique EF challenges faced by children with hearing loss

- Rationales for incorporating EF into LSL activities for children with hearing loss
- 10 principles for integrating EF into intervention for children with hearing loss
- Suggested teaching activities to address each of the 10 principles
- Emphasis on home and school carry-over as essential components of success
- Pearl and pitfalls to guide the LSL practitioner

12.1 Introduction: Drake

Drake, a six-year old boy with bilateral cochlear implants (CIs), is sulking and teary during our session because his mother won't let him bring a fast-food plastic puppy with him from the car. Though he has age-appropriate scores on speech and language tests, Drake's parents and I are concerned about other deficits in his communication and behavior. He often lets small problems escalate into crying scenes because he can't put them behind him. He has few close friendships with classmates because he is poor at social negotiation on the playground. If given a turn in conversation, he'll dominate until other children walk away. When the class self-divides into duos for a cooperative learning activity, no one wants to be paired with Drake. His mother is exasperated with him in the mornings when she must drag him through the steps of his routine so he is ready for the school bus. This is in spite of her having awakened him in plenty of time and having used multiple reminders that worked well for his older sister. On afternoons when he has a short homework assignment, he sprawls across the study table, whines, uses poor effort and sloppy handwriting on his spelling words and addition facts, even though they are easy for him. His language and math tests scores are at or above grade level. His case conference committee argues that Drake no longer qualifies for speech/language services because his test scores are all within normal limits. Yet we see a profile that suggests significant struggles. Why? Testing at a large cochlear implant center reveals that Drake has significant deficits in multiple domains of executive functioning.

12.2 What Is Executive Functioning (EF)?

Executive functioning (EF) encompasses a set of neurocognitive or brain-based processes responsible for the active management and control of cognitive resources, emotions, and behaviors to plan, organize, and achieve goals.[1] Because of the complexity of processing involved in self-regulation and goal-attainment,

EF comprises multiple domains, including controlled attention (active regulation of the direction and content of mental processing), inhibition (delay in behavior to consider situations and goals), working memory (active maintenance of information in immediate memory during other mental processing), and flexibility/shifting (switching strategies based on feedback). Due to its role in recruiting and regulating other psychological processes, EF is critical for multiple domains of functioning in daily life such as self-control, focus, learning, language development, memory, and goal-attainment. *In other words, EF is important for virtually everything children need to do in their childhood years.* In fact, EFs are more important for school readiness than is IQ and they continue to predict math and reading competence throughout all school years.[2] The risk of EF delays begin at preschool ages, and, without intervention, delays can persist into childhood and young adulthood.[3,4] To understand the components of EF, an organizing scheme is helpful that groups EF skills into two categories based on how each skill functions: whether it contributes to how a child *thinks* (cognition) or to how a child *does* things (behavior).[5] (See **Table 12.1**.)

With Drake's diagnosis of EF deficits and the skillful explanation of test results by the psychologist examiner, Drake's profile of learning, behavior, and daily living came into sharp focus for his parents. EF deficits were disrupting Drake's ability to do almost everything that makes up a six-year-old's life: stick to a schedule, manage feelings, work on a task until completion, get along with peers, tolerate a reasonable level of frustration, work toward a goal before receiving a reward, react to an emotional situation in a way that is proportional to its severity, and so forth. For the first time, they could understand how he demonstrated excellent speech understanding and articulation, a strong vocabulary, and age-appropriate spoken language skills (which were primary goals when they chose bilateral cochlear implantation for him as an infant) yet also struggled in the many ways they had observed. They were curious to know if Drake's congenital hearing loss or his cochlear implants had caused his delays in EF and whether there was any way to improve them.

Pearl

Executive functioning is more important for school readiness than is IQ, and it predicts math and reading competence throughout the school years.

EFs are brain-based skills that develop as a result of two main contributors: biology and experience. EFs depend on a neural circuit in which prefrontal cortex is central. The potential for EF is hard-wired, ready to develop from birth, much as symbolic language is. But that innate ability or biological "equipment" may be altered by a host of other factors, including damage to the brain, especially to the frontal lobe, or a genetic, familial predisposition for attention deficit or organizational challenges. On the experience front, if the environment a child grows in is hostile, toxic or otherwise unhospitable, EF development is at risk of suffering. And, if the child's environment has never modeled or expected good EF, the likelihood of delays in EF is high.

Table 12.1 Components of EF organized by thinking vs. doing

COGNITION: Thinking skills	BEHAVIOR: Doing skills*
Working memory	Response inhibition (Impulse control)
Planning/Prioritization	Emotional control (regulation)
Organization	Sustained attention (controlled attention)
Time management	Task initiation
Metacognition	Goal-directed persistence
	Flexibility/Shifting

*Words in parentheses are alternate terms.

Reprinted with permission from Dawson P, Guare R. Identifying your child's strengths and weaknesses. In: *Smart but Scattered: The Revolutionary "Executive Skills" Approach to Helping Kids Reach Their Potential*. New York, NY: The Guildford Press; 2009.

12.3 Relationship between Executive Functioning, Hearing Loss, and Cochlear Implants

A growing body of literature has documented that there is a correlation between hearing loss and EF. Importantly, research confirms that CIs do not contribute to EF risk and may actually ameliorate EF delays. For example, very young deaf children who receive CIs show rapid development of EF skills at a rate similar to their normally hearing (NH) peers after implantation.[6] At the same time, individuals with hearing loss are at a higher risk of EF deficits than those with NH. About 25-40% of children with CIs show EF deficits depending on age and EF domain.[7] Multiple factors contribute to the risk of EF delays in children with hearing loss, including reduced exposure to (and delayed development of) spoken language and reduced exposure to auditory experience (resulting both from deafness and from degraded auditory signals transmitted by current hearing technologies).[8] Language is important for EF development because children use language as a tool to represent goals (e.g., labeling goals), to regulate attention and behavior (e.g., with self-directed speech), and to manage and organize the contents of thinking. Auditory experience provides valuable practice with focus, resisting distraction, holding information in memory, and controlled sequential attention and processing, all of which are EF components. Furthermore, although children with CIs are at 2 to 5 times greater risk of having clinically significant EF deficits compared to children with NH, at least half of children with CIs do not show clinically significant EF delays.[3,7] Thus, while children with CIs are at elevated risk for EF delays compared to NH peers, many children with CIs show considerable resilience and positive development of EF skills. The factors that cause this variability in EF in children with CIs may be targets for interventions to improve outcomes in at-risk children.

Pitfall

Research confirms that cochlear implants themselves do not contribute to the risk of executive functioning (EF) weakness and may actually ameliorate EF delays.

12.4 Can EF Be Improved through Intervention?

The short answer to this question is "yes." Evidence-based interventions have been rigorously studied and have shown that children's executive functions can be boosted following structured therapeutic, educational, neuropsychological, and socioemotional programs.[2,9] Consider that executive function development can be substantially promoted or hindered by environmental factors including early childhood stress, family structure, and educational opportunities. Fortunately, this means these skills are extremely malleable and amenable to improvement.[10]

Pearl

EF can be affected by factors such as early childhood stress, family structure, and education. Fortunately, this means EF skills are extremely malleable and amenable to improvement.

12.5 Why Are EF Interventions Effective within LSL Practice?

The listening and spoken language (LSL) approach to developing oral communication in children who are deaf or hard of hearing (DHH) is an effective platform for incorporating EF targets, because it emphasizes audition as the foundation of symbolic language. Techniques to foster language growth, enrichment, and mastery are at the core of LSL practice and these serve to support EF development, as well. Furthermore, LSL uses a diagnostic-teaching approach[11,12] where the clinician is teaching *and* evaluating the child in the same session to assess what techniques work and don't work, which modifications accelerate progress, and whether supports that scaffold a child's learning are still necessary or may be removed. Each of these features is also appropriate in interventions that address EF. Furthermore, parent-child relationships are key to the development of EF. It is the parents' and the family's constant support, shared experiences, and time spent together enjoying everyday activities like reading books, cooking, or dancing that help scaffold children's self-regulatory skills. These are, undoubtedly, the most effective and lasting EF foundations.[10] Recall that, because LSL practice views the parent as the primary "teacher" for the child[13] and helps clinicians become skilled at coaching parents,[14] this approach promotes one of the most important components of successful EF intervention, that of carry-over of skills from therapy to home.

There is a mutually beneficial relationship between EF therapies and LSL practice in that improved EF allows a child to progress more easily within LSL sessions, and participation in LSL strengthens the foundations of listening, language, and learning that are known to support EF maturity.[15] Given that most children who are DHH are already involved in ongoing speech-language or LSL sessions, and that EF is best addressed when bundled with other meaningful activities, blending the two makes great sense. When I meet with families about using this integrated approach, I make clear what my goal is for doing so. I emphasize that the ultimate

goal is not to have the child use the strategies and behaviors we teach there in our sessions. Rather, the goal is for the child to generalize those strategies and behaviors outside the intervention setting, spontaneously putting them to good use in the everyday events that make up the child's life. That is the true measure of effectiveness of our integrated intervention plan.

Pitfall

The ultimate goal is not for a child to use EF behaviors in our sessions, but to generalize them, using them spontaneously in everyday life at home, school, and in social situations.

12.6 Planning and Implementing EF Goals and Activities

In this section, I review ways to integrate EF goals into existing LSL or SLP practice. In doing so, we double our efficiency because activities address both LSL and EF goals. For clinicians new to this process, knowing where to begin may be challenging. Dawson and Gaure[5] outline useful principles for improving EF to get us started. Two of these are especially relevant to LSL practice: (1) Consider both EF developmental expectations and the child's current EF skills; and (2) Support external-to-internal transition of EF skills. An explanation of these is found later in this chapter.

Consider both EF developmental expectations and the child's current EF skills. As practitioners who have studied child development, we are accustomed to choosing activities based on the developmental level of the child's cognitive, language, and/or hearing age. But in the realm of EF, we may not be as familiar with what children are expected to do at different ages within the domains that make up EF. It is helpful, therefore, for clinicians to review some expectations for everyday EF developmental tasks in typical children. **Table 12.2** shows broad guidelines for expected behaviors across a number of the domains within EF.

Knowing what EF behavior is expected at a certain chronological age, however, is not the whole story. The clinician also must identify what the child's actual EF functioning is at the present time. (This is analogous to describing the gap between chronological age and language age in children who are DHH.) These two sets of data, EF developmental expectations and current EF skills, combine to steer us toward (1) the goals we will set for the child and (2) the techniques and strategies we will use to achieve them.[5] Many students with hearing loss are not functioning at age level in EF skills. Consider, for example, that typical children are expected to do a 20-minute homework assignment independently, with some redirection, by the end of second grade, at about age eight-and-a-half. For some children with hearing loss and EF delays, they have never completed their homework independently. Thus, the structures and strategies that work with most 8-year olds will probably not work for them. We need to match the task demands to the child's actual developmental level *for that EF skill,* break down the demands into smaller steps and provide support and reinforcement.

Another example will be familiar to LSL practitioners. Typically developing children are expected to demonstrate the EF maturity of inhibiting certain speech behaviors, such as blurting,

Table 12.2 Developmental tasks requiring executive skills

Age range	Developmental task
Preschool	Run simple errands (for example, "Get your shoes from the bedroom")
	Tidy bedroom or playroom with assistance
	Perform simple chores and self-help tasks with reminders (for example, clear dishes from table, brush teeth, get dressed)
	Inhibit behaviors: don't touch a hot stove, run into the street, grab a toy from another child, hit, bite, push, etc.
Kindergarten to grade 2	Run errands (two- to three-step directions)
	Tidy bedroom or playroom
	Perform simple chores, self-help tasks; may need reminders (for example, make bed)
	Bring papers to and from school
	Complete homework assignments (20-minute maximum)
	Decide how to spend money (allowance)
	Inhibit behaviors: follow safety rules, don't swear, raise hand before speaking in class, keep hands to self
Grades 3–5	Run errands (may involve time delay or greater distance, such as going to a nearby store or remembering to do something after school)
	Tidy bedroom or playroom (may include vacuuming, dusting, etc.) Perform chores that take 15-30 minutes (for example, clean up after dinner, rake leaves)
	Bring books, papers, assignments home and take them back to school
	Keep track of belongings when away from home
	Complete homework assignments (1-hour maximum)
	Plan simple school project such as book reports (select book, read book, write report)
	Keep track of changing daily schedule (for example, different activities after school)
	Save money for desired objects, plan how to earn money
	Inhibit/self-regulate: behave when teacher is out of the classroom; refrain from rude comments, temper tantrums, bad manners
Grades 6–8	Help out with chores around the home, including daily responsibilities and occasional tasks (for example, emptying dishwasher, raking leaves, shoveling snow); tasks may take 60-90 minutes to complete
	Babysit younger siblings or other kids for pay
	Use system for organizing schoolwork, including assignment book, notebooks, etc. Follow complex school schedule involving changing teachers and changing schedules
	Plan and carry out long-term projects, including tasks to be accomplished and reasonable timeline to follow; may require planning multiple large projects simultaneously
	Plan time, including after-school activities, homework, family responsibilities; estimate how long it takes to complete individual tasks and adjust schedule to fit
	Inhibit rule breaking in the absence of visible authority

Reprinted with permission from Dawson P, Guare R. Identifying your child's strengths and weaknesses. In: *Smart but Scattered: The Revolutionary "Executive Skills" Approach to Helping Kids Reach Their Potential.* New York, NY: The Guildford Press; 2009.

interrupting or speaking without raising their hand in class, by early elementary school age. Many children who are DHH are delayed in these inhibition skills and speak whenever a thought comes into their mind. This means they interrupt, talk over others and are poor conversational partners. Such children (and adults, for that matter), suffer negative social consequences for this EF immaturity because others do not tolerate someone who dominates conversations. Parents of children who are DHH may accept this behavior at home, and even may have encouraged it in the early stages of a child's spoken language development. At that age, clinicians and parents are delighted whenever the child expresses himself. But as the child ages, the lack of developmental expectations within the environment is actually holding the child back, from both maturity and social standpoints.

Support external-to-internal transition of EF skills. This is one of the most fundamental EF principles and central to our work. As mentioned, executive functions are brain-based—primarily frontal lobe—skills that increase with age and maturity. When children are young, parents largely act as their child's frontal lobe. As caring adults, we structure, alter and organize a child's environment to compensate for the child's EF skills that are yet to develop.[5] Very young children, for example, cannot handle being near water unattended. Adults provide external structures, install safety gates, supervise children at all times, and set rules about wearing a life vest. Gradually, because adults have repeated rules, such as, "Always have an adult with you when near the water," a child internalizes the rules and practices good water safety. In other words, we first modify the external environment to essentially substitute for immature EF, gradually expecting children to do this on their own. This is the "external-to-internal transition" that is the mark of maturing EF skills. Whenever we set a goal for a child to develop more effective EF, we should always begin by changing things outside the child (the external) before advancing to strategies where the child is required to change (the internal).[5] Consider Billy, a child whose parents encouraged him to speak, anytime, anywhere, when he was first learning to listen and talk. They altered the external environment (their behavior) to support his participation. As he ages, the family must set boundaries and model behaviors that require Billy gradually to internalize the rules of social discourse and control his own blurting and interrupting. LSL practice abounds with techniques that incorporate this fundamental external-to-internal transition. For example:

1. When young children are first learning to say "thank you," adults initially prompt them with "What do you say?" when they're given a treat. Over time, adults provide less direct external prompting. Rather, the parents model "thank you" when they are given a treat, use expectant eye gaze or hold onto the treat, expecting the child to internalize the behavior and eventually say, "thank you" without any prompt.

2. We initially repeat instructions for very young children, even when they have not requested it, to help them follow the instruction. We might say, "Get the bunny. Go get it. Give me the bunny. Where is the bunny?" We are modifying the external environment so the child achieves success. As the child ages, we reduce the number of repetitions given, use pause time, and wait for the child to express his needs. Through modeling, he develops a repertoire of queries, from "What?" at the earliest stage, to "Please repeat" to "Did you say to get the buggy?" indicating he is internalizing the skill of requesting clarification.

3. We initially read a young child's mind when he appears not to have understood a question. Parents sense when their child hasn't understood and jump in to help. They modify the external environment by offering unsolicited prompts and multiple choice options. Gradually, we teach the child that it's okay not to know an answer, but he must tell us that and actively seek the information he needs. If our expectations do not increase, we find older children who, when unsure of an answer, shrug their shoulders and passively make eye contact with their parent, who answers for the child. If the child says, "I don't know" to a question, we further facilitate the external-to-internal transition by replying, "Someone here knows," encouraging him to turn to his parent and ask, "Do you know the answer, Mom?"

As we integrate EF activities into LSL intervention, we should keep in mind that our long-term goal is not for the child to demonstrate better EF skills *in our sessions.* That is just a means to an end. Rather, it is for the child to internalize and spontaneously use these skills *in the real world*, in everyday life, at home, at school and beyond.

Pearl

Whenever we set a goal for a child to develop more effective EF, we should always begin by changing things outside the child (the external) before advancing to strategies where the child is required to change (the internal).

12.7 Ten Principles of EF Interventions for Children with HL

Robbins and Kronenberger[15] outlined 10 principles for integrating EF techniques into existing LSL or SLP sessions (see **Table 12.3**). In this section, I discuss and make suggestions about activities to address each of these principles. Keep in mind that, though activities are listed under a specific heading, many are cross-over activities that organically focus on more than one EF. For example, barrier games target Theory of Mind (ToM), perspective-taking, language organization, and more.

Principle 1: Prior to initiating intervention, assess the child's EF and identify at-risk domains.

EF involves multiple abilities and varies considerably across children who are DHH; some children show broad delays across multiple EF domains, while other children show delays in only a few EF domains, and still others show no delays at all.[7] As a result, before launching an intervention, it is critical to understand whether a problem with EF exists, and if so, which domains are affected. Several parent- or teacher-report behavior checklist measures of EF are available for clinicians to conduct an initial survey. These include:

The Behavior Rating Inventory of Executive Function (BRIEF).[16] As a questionnaire developed for parents and teachers of school-age children, the BRIEF assesses executive function behaviors in the

Table 12.3 Ten principles of EF interventions for children who are deaf or hard of hearing

Principle 1: Prior to initiating intervention, assess the child's EF and identify at-risk domains

Principle 2: Integrate EF strategies into existing LSL and SLP treatments

Principle 3: Utilize specific language that structures and supports EF behavior

Principle 4: Teach time awareness, such as planning, predicting, and time management, to children who have EF delays

Principle 5: Focus on organization skills as a component of EF training

Principle 6: Target inhibition and impulse control in EF/AVT practice

Principle 7: Teach and encourage self-regulation, including emotional control, through modeling, practice, and imaginative play

Principle 8: Strengthen WM and metacognition with Boss-Your-Brain strategies and scaffolding

Principle 9: Provide accommodation and extra help using the "Magic R's" with children who have EF delays:
  1. Reduce memory or work load
  2. Regularly provide templates for child to fall back on
  3. Rehearse extra times; repeat, and repeat again
  4. Reinforce auditory material with visual cues
  5. Rhythm/rhymes make information stick (because musical elements are "memory magnets")
  6. Re-expose the child to the learning [? Or skill?] in different contexts
  7. Rewind to encourage emotional self-regulation
  8. Review with child as active participant

Principle 10: Embed EF interventions into the day-to-day home and school experiences of the child.

school and home environments. A Spanish version of the BRIEF is also available, adding to the usefulness of this measurement tool.

The Behavior Rating Inventory of Executive Function–Preschool (BRIEF-P). [17] The BRIEF-P measures behavioral manifestations of executive function in preschoolers and may be administered to parents of children 5 months to 2 years of age.

The Learning, Executive and Attention Functioning Scale (LEAF). [18] This behavior checklist has been used widely across the world. It is easy to administer, score, and interpret, and is valid in identifying specific EF delays in children with CIs. Data from the LEAF have been reported in published studies of children with cochlear implants, giving this measure special relevance to LSL clinicians. The LEAF has four versions: LEAF Parent-Report/Teacher-Report Scale; LEAF Self-Report Scale for adolescents and adults; LEAF language-revised self-report version for adolescents and adults, with content modified to improve readability and meaning; and LEAF Preschool Scale for children aged 3-6 years (prior to first grade). Getting permission to use the LEAF, free-of-charge, is available through this website: https://drk.sitehost.iu.edu/LEAFinfo.html which explains the process of getting access to the LEAF. The requesting clinicians must download from the site the "LEAF Permissions and Use" document, which includes the required language to request LEAF use, as well as the authors' email address. Users request permission via email and are sent a password. This ensures that the LEAF is distributed to qualified providers and that its use is tracked.

Informal EF questionnaires. Clinically useful questionnaires are available in the book, *Smart but Scattered.* [5] There are separate questionnaires for children at the following levels: Preschool/Kindergarten, Grades 1–3, Grades 4–5, and Grades 6–8. A teen version of the questionnaire is also available (Guare, Dawson, Guare). [19] Parents score the results and are able to see a profile of EF strengths and weaknesses for their child. Another useful tool by these authors is the EF questionnaire for parents to take, yielding their own profile of EF strengths and weaknesses. Understanding both the child's and parent's EF profiles serves as a useful counseling tool and can make selected goals more realistic. For example, if the child's primary weaknesses are organizing and initiating (homework, school projects and so forth) but one parent is weak in time management, it is likely this will not be a good fit. Because the time-challenged parent often may be late in helping the child get organized and started on projects, the clinician could suggest that the other parent or another adult take this role. Likewise, if a child and parent are both weak at emotional regulation, the parent may need to recruit another adult for support and guidance and to develop creative approaches to help the child who cries when challenged. There is little to be accomplished if both parent and child dissolve into tears or engage in heated argument.

Principle 2: Integrate EF strategies into existing LSL and SLP treatments. It is acknowledged that to improve EF, focusing narrowly on them is not as effective as a holistic approach that encompasses emotional and social development (as does LSL practice) and physical development (shown by the positive effects of aerobics, martial arts, and yoga). [9] A large body of research has demonstrated that language and EF are strongly associated in children with hearing loss, in many cases stronger than in NH peers. [20] Not only does language provide support to improve self-regulation and WM, but EF provides controlled, focused

mental effort to enhance language processing. [21] Integrating EF training into LSL or SLP practice allows for both sets of abilities to be used to support and improve each other. Furthermore, because children who are DHH routinely attend SLP and/or LSL sessions, integration of EF training with that practice allows convenient access to EF skills training. LSL practice is highly compatible with incorporating EF targets, because it emphasizes audition as the foundation of symbolic language. [15] Finally, because LSL practice views the parent as the primary "teacher" for the child, [13] it promotes an essential component of successful EF intervention, that of carry-over of skills from therapy to home. **Table 12.4** lists some intervention targets appropriate for integrated EF, speech-language, and LSL therapies, with corresponding activities and purposes shown. Note that auditory standards for LSL practice apply to sessions where EF goals are integrated, including the use of well-fitted hearing technologies, a quiet learning environment with limited background noise, use of a remote microphone to enhance the speech signal, and close monitoring of the child's listening abilities (see Chapter 2).

Principle 3: Utilize specific language that structures and supports EF behavior. The close association between EF and language during childhood, and certainly after cochlear implantation [7] suggests that language-based interventions may improve EF. LSL practice is a language-rich method and the coaching and guidance of parents is focused heavily on language enrichment within every session, including carry-over at home. Some suggested ways to utilize specific language in LSL activities that structures and supports EF include:

- Designated words or phrases, known as verbal prompts. When used repeatedly by adults, these verbal prompts are important cues for children as they move from external to internal EF control. They function as a mini version of a rehearsal, reminding the child of a previous discussion about strategies or rules. Consider the prompt, "Let's rewind." If I tell a child, "In this game, I want you to pick the thing that is thinnest," a child with poor emotional control may respond impulsively in a loud and exasperated tone, "It's going to be too hard!" My response is to say, "Let's rewind." (Pause, imitating the rewinding of a video.) "Billy, in this game, I want you to pick the thing that is thinnest." This strategy allows the child a do-over to respond with better emotional control than his initial response. Perhaps after the rewind, Billy says, "Okay, I'll try" or perhaps, "I don't know what 'thinnest' means." In the latter case I clarify, "I'm glad you used self-control and told me that, Billy. Thinnest means skinniest. Thin and skinny are synonyms." Another verbal prompt, "Hold that thought" is used when the child interrupts to say something. It indicates that though the adult is interested, the child's idea will have to wait for an appropriate time in the conversation when the child may add his comment. "Instruction!" is a one-word rehearsal cue from the clinician who is about to deliver a command. Rather than an instruction coming out of thin air, which some children fail to follow the first time it is presented, this cue helps to prime the child by indicating that the next thing said will be an instruction. This allows time for the child to focus attention and prepare for what is coming next, which will be a command. This is especially

Table 12.4 Intervention targets that integrate EF and speech-language goals with corresponding activities and purposes

Intervention Target	Activity/Purpose
Time awareness/management	Daily schedules at therapy, home, school; Support auditory schedule with visual input, as appropriate; Multi-color timer to manage steps within a larger task; YTT discussions at home
Model and encourage imaginative play	Language stories that encourage self-regulation (Tarshis et al, 2016);[23] Figures/dolls/animals that "talk" to each other and support roleplaying; Storybook game builds emotion into play*
Facilitate transfer of child's behavioral control from external (adult) to internal (self)	Plus/Zero chart* for immediate, focused feedback; Gradually fade feedback, ask child to self-rate
"Invisible" mental states made tangible and explicit	Use thought bubbles; Form & test hypotheses in 20 Questions game; Boss-Your-Brain strategies* (Visualization; Act-it-Out)
Impulse control: Child "thinks before doing"	"Mother, May I?", "Simon Says", "Slap the Jack" games; Preparation Is Everything (PIE) techniques
Enhance comprehension using categories, address class inclusion/exclusion concepts	Utilize algorithms for categorizing & sub-categorizing; Surprise Table: ("Is it a vehicle? Does the vehicle have wheels? Does it use gasoline?")
Maturity of Self-regulation/impulse control	Teach alternatives to interrupting: "Hold that thought" and "Excuse me!"*. Child's conversational and social skills benefit; Play What are You Wearing Today? Game;*
Take advantage of language to mediate thought and action	Encourage re-auditorization because "when you do that, your brain can hear yourself think."*
Working memory (WM) improvement	Tasks requiring a "mental sticky-note" while doing another task (e.g., "Keep your score in your mind while you roll the dice, then add them up"); Employ motor rehearsal (Act-it-out) and re-auditorization (Say-it-aloud) strategies; Visualization + corresponding language to support WM (e.g. "I can see that in my mind"; "Your words make me picture...")* Teach chunking, mnemonics, e.g., "I write with my right, so this is my left."
Emotional regulation	Use rewinds* to practice a better response (e.g. Child responds in a whiney voice, adult says, "Let's rewind and do that again."); Size of the Problem technique (Garcia Winner)
Use musical elements of rhythm and melody for pacing and entrainment to help routines and long-term memory storage	Boss Your Brain* with finger cues, melody, rhythm, e.g., learn phonics or board game rules with rhythmic chants
Support expressive language retrieval and organization	Templates; Thinking in Threes* (e.g., "Tell 3 things about the movie you saw"); 3 Rules to every game: How you win, how you move/play, and something else*
Encourage reflection vs. impulsivity; model language that describes these	"You took your time before answering. I'm proud of you for being reflective and not impulsive." Teach child to ask: "May I have a moment to think, please?"; Respect silence as another person in the room*
Maximize auditory access provided via the CIs; provision of clear, disambiguated auditory input	Remote mic technology; quiet workspace; background noise reduced; Use of AV techniques e.g., acoustic highlighting*
Silent breaks with non-verbal tasks to decrease listening fatigue and provide an end point to cognitively demanding lessons	Use Transition Tasks*: Mindfulness techniques that "wipe our mental whiteboard clean"
Foster flexibility of thought and action; encourage use of a range of solutions for problem solving.	Superflex Social Thinking (Madrigal & Garcia Winner, 2008) concepts e.g., "Rock Brain" is not a good problem-solver
Use of language that supports and scaffolds EFs	Designate specific words and phrases as verbal prompts, e.g., "Instruction!"* to prime child's attention and performance
Higher Order Thinking Skills (HOTS); advanced vocabulary; multiple word meanings	Pyramid game; Surprise Action Table; Three for Me and Tribond games
Develop empathy, ability to understand others' perspectives	Take an OPV (Other Person's Viewpoint) (DeBono, 1998); Assume another's opinion: "Speaking as an optimist....", "Speaking as Alexander Hamilton..."
Organization of thoughts and surroundings; Completing tasks	Teach child to FACE (Finish and Check Everything); Take photo of finished task, e.g., his organized and cleaned room
Interpret thoughts and feelings of others using their words, tone of voice, facial expressions/body language and what we already know about them	Poetry "Packs a punch" with dense meaning. Comic strips are short but full of inference and have speech and thought bubbles + facial expressions/body language

*See Robbins for descriptions and select video clips.[11]

effective when accompanied by an index finger flicking up near the temple (like a lightbulb coming on), drawing visual as well as auditory attention to the upcoming instruction. As with all strategies, we fade its use when the child no longer requires it.

- Thinking in Threes.[11] Many things in the real world can be itemized or condensed into a set of three. This is an important skill for children who speak before organizing their thoughts, produce run-on sentences or use difficult-to-follow stream of consciousness output. I use the prompt, "Let's think in threes" as a reminder that expressive language is not just the words that come out of our mouth, but also should be a reflection of what we think. Condensing to three ideas also suggests that we prioritize what we say and do so concisely. Not every thought in our head is worthy of expression. Adults should provide frequent models to help a child become accustomed to listing three things across a variety of topics, including: three rules to every board game; three events from the past day; three highlights of a vacation; three ideas that summarize the plot to a movie; three comments in a conversational turn. This may be more or less than a child would typically say, but either way, it is practice with prioritization and self-regulation.

- Language and concepts from "We Thinkers!"[22] social stories. These stories employ distinct language that captures a targeted executive function. These are highlighted in engaging books that tell a story about the EF and use repeated vocabulary and phrases that become highly familiar to the child and adults. Some examples of these include: "Think with your eyes" is a reminder to extract visual cues from other people in your surroundings; "Are you on my plan?"[23] prompts the child to remember he is not operating alone but is in a group that has a unified plan, set by the adult in charge; "Body in the group" (or "BIG") reminds us that when we maintain an appropriate physical presence—not too close, not too far away—others feel comfortable and the group plan keeps going; The adult comment, "You're having a thought about me," draws attention to the internal state of thinking that children may not be aware of; "Show me you're thinking about me" suggests that eye contact and visual attention are not just physical behaviors but represent internal, mental states. Each concept in the social stories is paired with a catchy song. After children are familiar with them, we act out the stories, as noted, and use the supplemental teaching suggestions for each concept.

Pitfall

When our teaching focus includes EF, skills such as eye contact and visual attention are not just physical behaviors but represent internal, mental states, with language that represents those states.

The appendix lists recommended resources for integrating LSL/SLP and EF goals.

- Language that reflects ToM. Even at the earliest stages of a child's language development, we are conscious of utilizing mental state words as we speak. Repeated exposure to words such as: *think, remember, forget, wonder, imagine, believe, process,* has been shown to facilitate a child's ability to grasp these mental state concepts. It is important to model and discuss this with parents, as they may have received the message that language to their child should reflect only the concrete, here-and-now. I point out that the here-and-now includes comments such as, "I *wonder* what is inside that box," "I *think* Daddy just got home," and "I don't *remember* her name."

- Doing Includes Thinking. In EF-embedded LSL practice, clinicians are in the habit of modeling and asking parents to share their *thought processes*, not just a factual account of events. For example, if a child talks about what they saw at the school carnival, I ask two consecutive questions, "Mom, is that how you *remember* it? Is that what *happened*?" I pair these two questions together—one reflecting a mental state, the other an action—so that the child hears the cohesiveness between them. Likewise, when I encourage a child to re-auditorize what she has heard, I am not just suggesting a behavior but also a mental action. I explain that, "when you say things out loud, your brain can hear yourself think."

Principle 4: Teach time awareness, such as planning, predicting, and time management, to children who have EF delays. Problems with time management and time awareness are common causes and characteristics of EF disorders in children with normal hearing,[24] and are also delayed in children and adolescents with CIs.[3] Suggested activities include:

- "News of the Day" activity.[11] This is another example of an EF-infused LSL activity. On the way to our therapy space, I do a pitch-matching activity using a clinician-created song. I descend the stairs with the child one step behind, making this a listening-only activity. In the song, I review the date and tell something noteworthy about my day as the child echoes me. Each line is sung one half-step lower than the previous line, covering about one full octave of descending notes. Adults may observe the child's pitch matching and open-set understanding. A sample "News of the Day" song is: "Today (Today) is (is) Wednesday (Wednesday) May First (May First) and this morning (and this morning) something happened (something happened) that made me (that made you) feel worried (feel worried)." A conversational hook is added to the auditory aspects of this song, as evidenced by the last sung comment. At the bottom of the steps, the child may ask, "What happened that worried you?" with genuine concern. Parents and children take their turns as leader as soon as appropriate. For very young children, we may only sing today's date and day of the week. I suggest parents start the day at home with this information, too, as it helps children orient to their schedule, which is often anchored by specific events on certain days.

- Visual Schedules. Begin each session by reviewing a visual schedule of the session activities to support predictability and time sense. The child can see a beginning and, importantly, an ending point. These time anchors often improve compliance and self-regulation for the entire session for children with poor time sense. Imagine being summoned to a meeting but not knowing what the agenda was or whether it would last 10 minutes or 2 days. Your attention would be reduced throughout the meeting, concerned for what came next and how long it would take. Schedules alleviate that concern. I have a rubric for the printed schedule to make it more challenging over time, eventually fading it to an auditory-only schedule, if appropriate for an individual child.

- Child-friendly clocks, timers, and other devices give children a way to segment and measure time. A timer with green, yellow, and red lights indicates time allotments for the steps required to complete a task, which reduces anxiety in children who cannot yet tell time or who are anxious and struggle with emotional regulation. Smart technologies, such as a Hatch monitor, have functions that set programs to cue a child for tricky transitions, including nap time, clean-up time and bedtime, using colored lights and auditory signals.

- "Yesterday, Today, Tomorrow" (YTT) discussions. At home, YTT dinnertime discussions of the child's past day's activities and next day plans, are a helpful summary and a way to prepare for tomorrow. Use of these may improve awareness and monitoring of time-based behavior and planning. Knowing that we have prepared a plan helps to alleviate anxiety, which is desirable in both children and adults. Morning routines are typically stressful for families of children with time management deficits. When the family makes a plan to address this, getting teacher support of the plan is important, particularly in the event the child is late for school.

Principle 5: Focus on organization skills as a component of EF training. Studies of concept formation have found that children with CIs may have more difficulty with complex categorization skills than normal-hearing peers, even when the groups do not differ in nonverbal intelligence.[25] Additionally, delays in organizing and processing complex information are found in some children with CIs.[3,7] As a result, children benefit from learning strategies to organize their environment as well as their thinking. Suggestions include:

- Category-based concept formation. The ability to group items based on similar characteristics can be taught with language categories and category exemplars (e.g., playing "I Spy" and focusing on categories to look for in the environment, such as vehicles, animals, etc.). We play "Three for Me," a game requiring participants to select three pictured tiles that are all related in some way. As a child progresses, we emphasize the flexibility of categories and the notion that one item can belong in many different categories. We group and then regroup one tile with new tiles that now form a different category. Tribond Jr. or Tribond are even more challenging and abstract, because participants must tell what three things have in common (a "Threezer"), without any visual cues.

- Surprise Table. This activity combines work on categorization, WM, use of mental state words and metacognition. The clinician covers a common object and encourages the child and parent to discover the identity of the object by posing questions based on categories and sub-categories (e.g., "Is it a food? Does it fall in the vegetable category? Can you eat it raw or does it need to be cooked?"). As a central principle of a "dialogue" rather than "tutorial" therapy style,[26] the participants switch roles frequently so that sometimes the child knows the identity of the object and the parent and clinician pose the questions. Different skills are required as sender vs. receiver of information, so both roles are important. If children get stuck, we recruit the strategy, "Review what we know," using re-auditorization and finger cues to list aloud the information already given. Players must remember the clues that have been said (WM) and form an idea of what the object is. If a player thinks he knows the answer, he says, "I have a hypothesis," and asks a question that will confirm or deny his idea. If the answer denies his idea, the player says, "I withdraw my hypothesis" and play continues. To further support categorical organization and visual support when needed, I post a chart that lists common categories.

- Surprise Action Table. This game follows the format of the Surprise Table, but the target is an action (verb) rather than a noun. As such, it tends to be challenging for children so we progress to this level after they have been successful guessing nouns. The corpus of questions is different for verbs than nouns (e.g., "Is this an action you can see?" "Do you need to be taught to do this?" "Do only humans do this action?"). Initially, I may supply a chart with possible questions a child and parent may ask. This provides visual support as needed and helps children organize the information they ask about and receive.

- Algorithms for organization. Some children are intrinsically organized, whereas children with EF organizational weakness often don't even "see" messes nor tidying-up solutions. Therefore, strategies for organizing toys, games or clothing, and keeping track of important school papers must be directly modeled and taught. I plan specific activities where we clean up materials we have been using in our session, using verbal labels to sort and organize. I find we make more progress over time if I take a picture of the area *when it is in an organized state.* For example, I'll take a photo of the child standing beside a bookshelf in my therapy room where I've organized our materials and games, before we use any of them. Near the end of the session, I plan for enough time that the child returns the materials to the bookshelf, using the organized picture as a visual guide. Verbal mnemonic devices or adult-created songs that the child says or sings while organizing are valuable (e.g., "Legos go in a bin that's blue, blocks do too, and my tools; Board games go in a bin that's green, and that is how I keep things clean" to the tune of "Here We Go 'Round the Mulberry Bush"). I call music a "memory magnet"[27] because things we learn in musical form, such as T.V. theme songs and commercial jingles, stick with us almost involuntarily. I help children recruit music for remembering facts, rules, or other rote information. I use piggyback tunes (Chapter 19: "Music Therapy for Children with Hearing Loss," Barton and Robbins) to teach children their address and phone number because these are important for a child's safety. Home carry-over of these strategies is highly encouraged.

Pearl

For children with organizational challenges, keep a photo of the finished "product," such as a clean room or an organized backpack. As they organize, they'll have a visual image of their goal.

- Finish and Check Everything (FACE). We emphasize that "a job isn't done until you've finished and checked everything or FACE'd." Many children with EF delays don't know what a finished task looks like.[5] To teach this rule, we use a three-step process. First, we look together at a "finished" task. I show a backpack that is organized with school supplies in a pouch, papers requiring a parent signature in one folder and homework in another. Second, the child describes what he sees in the organized backpack to ensure he recognizes the steps and components that make up a "finished" task. Third, we write a list of the steps and components that the child and I reviewed. We send this home to be posted so that there is a visual reminder each time the child gets his backpack ready for school. Parents may rehearse at home by prompting, "Have you FACE'd your backpack?"

- Graphic organizers. These are visual and graphic displays that organize ideas and demonstrate relationships between different concepts and facts. They are especially helpful to students who struggle with organizing and arranging information, including both receptive mastery of ideas and expressive skills needed in written language activities. Some of those I use frequently are: *T-charts*, where information is divided into two columns; *Main Idea (or Semantic) Maps*, used for brainstorming and generating ideas for planning or writing tasks; *Venn diagrams* to compare and contrast two groups; *Sequence Charts* that display a series of steps or events in order, including timelines. These help clarify the sequence of events in a story or history lesson; *Multiple Outcomes diagrams*, which encourage prediction about possible outcomes, support a child's imagination in proposing different endings for a story, and prompt children to problem-solve with multiple solutions, an important EF skill of cognitive flexibility.

- Pyramid game. This is a challenge-level game for older children and teens. Modelled after the gameshow "100,000-Dollar Pyramid," I say successive items from an unnamed category. The task is for child and parent to call out the category, using successive clues to narrow down the correct answer. If I give the clues "the ring" and "the gloves" the parent calls out, "Things at a wedding," which is incorrect. If I add "the referee" the child guesses, "Things at a boxing match," which is correct. Real-world and experiential knowledge, multiple word meanings, and advanced vocabulary all enter into this game. We switch roles so that each person gets to "host" and read the clues.

Principle 6: Target inhibition and impulse control in EF/LSL practice. Impulse control is the capacity to think before you act, to resist a sudden response until you've assessed the situation. Impulsive behavior is one of the most common concerns of parents of children with CIs, and evidence suggests that impulsivity is elevated in children with CIs even when language delays are accounted for.[8] Furthermore, impulse control is a central component of EF[28] that, when delayed, can lead to significant behavioral and learning problems[24] and negative social consequences. Because parent involvement is important in interventions that address impulsive behavior in children,[29] parents attending LSL sessions should be taught strategies to improve impulsivity in children with EF delays, beginning at very young ages. Suggested activities include:

- Games requiring impulse control. These are games that emphasize a time delay and thinking before acting. For example, the rule in "Simon Says" is that players should only carry out an instruction if the leader has prefaced it with "Simon says." Children must delay their impulse to act out the instruction immediately, and instead think back on whether those key words were said. The game, "Mother May I?" requires self-control and impulse control since, before carrying out the leader's (or "Mother's") direction, players must always ask, "Mother, may I?" The latter activity also taxes WM because players must retain the direction given, pause to ask permission from Mother, then return to carry out the direction. As with all EF behaviors, our goal over time is to transfer external regulation (provided by the adult) to internal, child-controlled behavior regulation. Games such as "Slap the Jack" or "Hands Down" are won when a player recognizes a specific visual target and acts on it but controls the impulse to act when a non-target appears.

- The Plus/Zero chart.[15] This simple technique gives a child immediate feedback when we are targeting an explicit, impulsive behavior. Say the child impulsively guesses at unknown words when reading aloud rather than sounding them out. We review the reminder: "If you guess at a word, you'll probably be wrong, but if you use a rule [to decode it], you'll probably be right." If this isn't successful, I make a chart with two columns labeled "+" and "0." We don't use a minus because the chart isn't a punishment, but a reminder to help the child do better. We target only one behavior at a time and keep the chart within the child's view. If he sees the word "hesitate" and rushes through it, guessing, "headache," I reach over and write a "0" on his chart. On the next page, he takes time to sound out a word, so I write a "+" on the chart. I don't interrupt what we're doing, but the chart gives feedback to the child that he has been impulsive. As children are motivated by rewards, the child will get one if he has more "+" than "0" marks at the end of the activity. Some children with poor impulse control have requested that I make a +/0 chart to help regulate their behavior and be less impulsive.

- "Hold that thought," a prompt described earlier, is another impulse control technique. I say it when children have interrupted a discussion without using an appropriate conversational structure, such as "excuse me." I accompany the verbal prompt with as a visual reminder that the thought should stay in the child's brain until it is his turn to speak.

- What Are You Wearing Today.[11] Activities that provide practice for a child to engage in authentic dialogue and meaningful conversation, rather than rote drill work, best foster EF development. For example, a game such as "What Are You Wearing Today?" marks clothing as the conversational topic, with parent and clinician posing questions regarding the child's attire. Roles within language interactions, and the rules that govern them (e.g., we don't start talking about a new bicycle when the topic is clothing), address the EF skill of impulse control, and children must resist the temptation to answer questions asked of others or to blurt out an unrelated comment. Sustained attention, another EF skill, also is addressed in this activity, because children must follow a dialogue thread with multiple contributors, over a course of many exchanges, all components of conversational competence.

- Preparation Is Everything (PIE) for impulse control. Preparing or priming a child just before engaging in an activity that requires impulse control can make all the difference. Before we play "Mother May I?" I ask, "What will you do after you hear Mother's instruction?" And I ask the same question of the parent to reinforce the response: "I'll ask 'Mother, may I?' before I move!" Initially, I prime a child on each turn, but gradually see external-to-internal control wherein the child needs less priming. It is equally important for parents to prepare a child during real-life situations as a rehearsal of impulse control. Before they go to a neighborhood carnival, the parent asks, "What will you do if there's a long line to buy tickets?" They discuss what behavior would be acceptable if they must wait their turn.

Pearl

To address impulsivity, practice PIE. or Preparation is Everything. Prime the child just before going into a situation where impulsivity is likely. Rehearse beforehand what a reflective response could be.

- Respect silence as if it's another person in the room.[11] Adult modeling of behavior is critical when dealing with impulse control. When children struggle with inhibition, it is critical that adults show them what it means to think before doing, including to give oneself moments to be quiet and re-group. Though parents have sometimes been taught to fill the space with spoken language, I suggest we "respect silence as if it's another person in the room." Quiet, language-free moments are important for a host of reasons. A planned period of silence, with no spoken language, is an important mental break between activities. In every session, we do a motor imitation game, the Transition Task,[11] between activities and say that "It wipes our mental chalkboard clean so we can concentrate on the next activity." This notion that silence should be respected, almost as if it's another person in the room, was suggested in a workshop by Dr. Parker J. Palmer.

Principle 7: Teach and encourage self-regulation, including emotional control, through modeling, practice, and imaginative play. Children learn not just through didactic teaching, but also through experiential modalities such as imitation/modeling, repeated practice, and imaginative play. In fact, because didactic teaching relies heavily on language skills and self-control (both of which are at risk for delays in children with CIs), modeling, practice, and imaginative play are likely to be more effective in engaging and teaching EFs. Examples include:

- Encourage dialogue between figures, dolls or animals that "talk" to each other, while including targeted EF concepts. The figures pretend to "boss their brain" as an image of self-control. For example, suppose a child has poor self-control when frustrated and does not work well in a group. We set up a role-playing scenario where three action figures are trying to solve a problem. We model with two figures each proposing a solution, trying theirs, and finding that neither works. While

staying calm, they ask the third figure for a solution, which is successful. Adults interject EF vocabulary such as, "I'm not being impulsive, I am being reflective" or "We stayed on the group plan and found a solution."[22]

- Books focused on EF. After reading a book with the child that targets self-regulation and impulse control, engage in roleplaying with dolls, puppets, or yourselves, re-telling the book, such as *Waiting Isn't Easy*[30] or *I Can Handle It*,[31] using acting, a medium that involves motor rehearsal. After acting out the story, we all switch roles. This is a key step because characters vary from one another in books; some ask more questions, some repeat a refrain, others supply a key word or a rhyme. Experiencing each role is enriching for the child and encourages flexibility and understanding multiple points of view, both important EF skills, and offers the chance to act out goal behaviors multiple times.

- "Size of the problem" concept.[32] When a child's reaction to a problem is larger than the original problem, it creates new problems and causes peers to be uncomfortable. This overreaction is often seen in children with delayed EF. "Size of the Problem" is a social skills concept used to help students identify the severity of their problems which then allows them to choose an appropriate reaction. Small problems warrant small reactions or none at all, but this requires emotional regulation. When students have a common language to describe their problems and reactions, they can identify solutions. A catchy song, "Size of the Problem" sung by Tom Chapin, reviews the steps needed to discern how big a problem really is. The Social Thinking materials include a thermometer-like gauge for children to judge their problems and their reactions.

- Preparation is Everything (PIE) for emotional regulation. Preparing, also called priming or rehearsing, for situations where emotional regulation will be challenged is critical. Doing so allows rehearsal for the child to practice self-regulation. If the family has chosen a movie to see, the parent asks beforehand, "What will we do if that movie is sold out?" As a child is preparing to attend a birthday party, the parent queries, "What will you do if it gets too noisy at the party?" Rehearsing and problem-solving with the child can avoid meltdowns. Some parents resist this preparation with the concern that just discussing the possibility of an imperfect outcome will trigger their child to have a meltdown. This is all the more reason those families need to implement PIE at home.

Principle 8: Strengthen WM and metacognition with Boss-Your-Brain strategies[33] *and scaffolding.* These EF skills are grouped together because we boss our brain both to remember things (WM) and to practice new ways of problem-solving and thinking about other people and situations (metacognition.) These terms are further described below:

1. WM is like a ***temporary sticky note*** in the brain that keeps track of short-term information. It lets us work with information without losing track of what we're doing. It holds new information in place so the brain can work with it briefly and connect it with other information. For example, a child doing three-column subtraction must suspend subtracting temporarily to borrow from the next higher column, then resume subtracting.

If a child is reading a chapter book, she is engaged in understanding the text, then encounters an unfamiliar word. She temporarily goes into decoding mode, "sounds out" the word, recognizes its meaning, then returns to the comprehension task without losing what she's already understood about the story. Like impulse control, WM (particularly verbal WM) is an EF component that has consistently been shown to be delayed in children with CIs.[7] Keep in mind that language provides structure to hold memory in the face of distraction. This means children benefit by using language to consolidate short-term memory information so that it is more resistant to interference from distractions.

Pitfall

Verbal working memory and impulse control are EF components consistently delayed in children with CIs. Goals to address these should be regularly integrated into LSL and home activities.

2. Metacognition is a multifaceted brain-based process that allows individuals to stand back and take a bird's-eye view of themselves, including to observe how they problem-solve. Metacognition allows awareness and insight into one's own learning. It also involves the ability to evaluate social situations, both an individual's own reactions and the behavior and reactions of others. Metacognition is considered an essential step toward mature thinking. Suggested activities:

- Teach Boss Your Brain (BYB) strategies.[32] I incorporate Boss Your Brain strategies to help children learn ways of remembering, organizing and retrieving what they have heard and understood. For example, the reauditorization or "say it aloud to yourself" strategy aids memory by hearing one's own voice repeat information. The "finger cue" strategy is useful for information in a list or series of steps because each finger marks a single item as it is spoken, aiding both memory of the items and their sequence. I tell children this is the world's best memory aid because you'll never forget your fingers at home or leave them in your backpack. They are always with you. A "visualization" strategy is used frequently because it is known that adept listeners and readers form visual images in their mind. The parents and I make this process explicit by describing our images and using vocabulary such as *picture, image,* and *visualize.* I might say, "Mom, I'm visualizing a girl with Little Orphan Annie hair." The parent replies, "I saw her hair differently in my mind." I add, "The words made me picture a girl with short, red, curly hair," and so forth. These strategies set the stage for important EF and ToM skills. I use BYB techniques with children as young as age two to model selected strategies and teach them to the parents. Young children are not required to use the strategies themselves, but often begin to do so spontaneously, after repeated exposure. Over time, this incorporates the important EF skills of metacognition and cognitive flexibility, since the child must evaluate his performance on a task (e.g., "Did I use the most effective BYB strategy? Would another strategy be more successful?"), then make changes based on self-evaluation.

Pearl

Incorporating Boss Your Brain (BYB) strategies into LSL teaching helps children learn ways to better remember, organize, and retrieve what they have heard, read, and understood.

- Auditory-only schedules. Remembering the sequence of activities in a schedule is an auditory memory task used with children who do not require a visual schedule. At the beginning of each session, I say the schedule of activities—usually seven total—and encourage children to pick one or more Boss Your Brain strategies that will help them remember. They quickly learn how helpful it is to use finger cues to mark each item, re-auditorization ("so my brain will hear and remember"), and sometimes visualization ("I see the activity in my mind.") After each activity, I prompt the child to say his schedule and determine what comes next. I don't insist that children use the BYB strategies because I want them to see for themselves how much easier remembering is when they do use them. It is more powerful if children decide on their own that they are helpful.

- Attribute Ranking. This game has multiple goals and involves the classic WM feature of holding information in short-term storage while solving another task. I tell the child how to rank the words I say. For example, "Rank these from fastest to slowest" and the child names the dimension involved. This reinforces the concept of dimensions such as *speed, depth, width, time, age,* and so on. I then say four words on that dimension, such as "bicycle, car, trike, airplane." The child uses BYB cues (usually re-auditorization and finger cues) to remember the four words then shuffles their order mentally before responding, "airplane, car, bicycle, trike."

- Remember and Classify. These games integrate WM, classification/organization and auditory memory. The child hears me say several words, repeats them, and says which of two categories each word belongs in. To double efficiency, I use categories from the child's academic content. If the classroom science focus is on living things, I say four words, the child repeats them and tells if each is living or non-living. For geography, I list four countries, the child repeats and tells if each is in the northern or southern hemisphere. For English support, I say four words, the child repeats and tells if each word is an adjective or adverb. To increase familiarity with classifying, I ask children to make categories based on their academic work and bring them to our next session.

- Add One Each. I say a random series of three numbers, such as "Eight, two, five." The child repeats back the series after adding one to each number, so the correct response is: "Nine, three, six." I model and encourage the use of the strategy "Invisible Blackboard,"[34] where we write information with our finger in a space in front of us, our invisible blackboard. We can add or subtract from the invisible numbers we've written. This is also helpful for writing alternatives to tricky spelling words or writing a phone number we need to remember short-term. I make the game more challenging by increasing the length of the series, using higher numbers, or proposing "Multiply by four each" or "Divide by three each."

- Read the Word I Spell. To target WM, I spell aloud a familiar word to the child, who must "read" and identify it without writing it down. I begin with short, easy words but progress to longer ones where the child must chunk letters into syllables, in sequence, to identify the word. The invisible blackboard, a motor rehearsal strategy, has high pay-off. We switch roles often, so children see that I succeed when I use my invisible blackboard to write letters as they are said, chunk them into syllables, and "read" the word.

- Card games such as "Crazy Eights," "Uno," and "Go Fish." These activities improve WM in two ways. First, by requiring the child to remember the rules of the game, which we review each time we play, supported by the BYB strategy of finger cues. For young children, I also solidify the rules by putting them to rhythm or melody. Second, by establishing motivation for players to remember when cards they and others have played. Players who do so are likely to win, which is a strong motivator for most children.

- Additional WM strategies. Other examples of strategies to address WM include making associations of memory information with other well-known information (e.g., rhymes or songs, such as singing the days of the week to the tune of "The Addams Family" theme song), chunking multiple memory units into fewer/larger/meaningful wholes (e.g., remembering the phone number 531-8642 as three decreasing odd numbers and four decreasing even numbers), and using mnemonics to cue information in memory storage (e.g., "Roy G. Biv" to help to remember the first letters of the colors in the rainbow: red, orange, yellow, green, blue, indigo, violet). "Top-down" comprehension strategies, such as cuing memory for details of a language passage by remembering the overarching theme or meaning of the passage, are supported visually by an umbrella outline.[33] This helps with memory by putting meaning (e.g., comprehension) on to language material that might otherwise have to be stored by rote rehearsal. Top-down strategies include previewing information so that it is meaningful when held in memory or reviewing information so that it is meaningful when retrieved.

- Barrier Games: Two players, separated by a barrier, must arrange identical sets of materials in exactly the same configuration, using verbal exchanges without visual access across the barrier. Barrier games are ToM in action because they demonstrate how clear language has to be for another person to understand your perspective. There are multiple goals embedded in these games, including the use of specific, rather than vague, language. For example, if I can't see a child's board and he tells me to "Put the dog right over here" I am not able to complete the direction. This ties into another goal, which is the taking of another's viewpoint. Barrier games are ideal for addressing ToM because they demonstrate that we communicate from our viewpoint, whereas others only see their viewpoint. In other words, different people have different perceptual experiences.

Pearl

Barrier games are ideal for addressing Theory of Mind (ToM) in young children because they demonstrate that we communicate from our viewpoint, whereas others only see their viewpoint.

- Tell and Show.[11] This game addresses EF and LSL goals. The child brings an object (e.g., a stuffed dog) from home, keeps it hidden from me, and describes it without showing it. I must create a picture of it in my brain, based on the features mentioned. After I have a mental picture, I am shown the object and I use rich, descriptive language to contrast how I saw it in my mind vs. how it actually looks. I might say, "I was picturing a long, bushy tail, because you didn't mention how his tail looked, but now I see the dog has a short, stubby tail." We switch roles and I become the sender, so that the child experiences both aspects of the activity. As one child said, "You will be the listener and I will be the teen-ener." We build visualization skills by making mental images based on the words we hear, a critical skill for reading comprehension and auditory memory.

- Cartoons and thought bubbles. With school aged children, I show a cartoon strip which we interpret, frame-by-frame, using both the speech and the thoughts of the characters, as both are represented in bubbles. I ask, "What did Jeremy's mother mean when she wrote him the note? And what did Jeremy think his mother meant?" Cartoons typically have multiple cues to meaning, including the words and thoughts written in bubbles, facial expressions, and even the font style and size, which can indicate emotional intensity. Single-panel cartoons are often an advanced level, with the reader required to make one or more inferential leaps to see the humor. I sometimes write things I am thinking in our session on a thought-bubble white board as an extension of this concept. Children may be taken aback and moved when they become aware of the internal thoughts others write (e.g., "I wish Billy would be more respectful of his mother.") I have observed that this technique enhances a child's self-regulation and improves awareness of others' feelings.

- Doing an OPV (Other Person's Viewpoint).[35] Many thinking situations involve other people. What these other people think is just as much a part of the situation as the facts. Though in the same situation, these people may have a very different viewpoint. It is an important part of thinking to be able to tell how other people are thinking, a skill that is often delayed in children with EF challenges. Poetry is a vehicle to appreciate that two people may have divergent understandings in the same situation. I use the poem "Skating"[36]: "They said come skating;/ They said it's so nice./ They said come skating;/ I'd done it twice./ They said come skating;/ It sounded nice..../ I wore roller-/ They meant ice." Another resource to develop this concept is the program "Thinking for Action"[35]. This teaches how to see things from another person's viewpoint by doing an OPV. A beginning step is an exercise that demonstrates what happens to our view when a child and I are face to face. I can't see what they're seeing behind me, and vice versa. With that simple, observable foundation, the program develops into higher-level understanding of how others think and feel differently from us and the importance of appreciating that.

Principle 9: Provide accommodation and extra help using the "Magic R's" with children who have EF delays. In addition to teaching EF skills to children with CIs, the environment should also endeavor to help the child by offering accommodations so that EF skills are not overwhelmed. Examples of these accommodations include the "Magic R's"[15]: *reduce* memory or work load, *regularly* provide preview and verbal prompts for developing skills, *rehearse* desired behaviors extra times then repeat and repeat again, *reinforce* auditory material with visual cues, *rhythm/ rhymes* make information memorable, *re-expose* the child to the skill in different contexts, *rewind* to encourage self-regulation and *review* with the child as an active participant. Integration of EF accommodations into educational and therapy plans makes all the difference so I offer teachers a poster of the Magic R's. Carry-over into classrooms reinforces target behaviors and provides predictability and repeated practice to children. Teachers report that modeling and teaching the Magic R principles help all the children in the class, not just those who are DHH.

Principle 10: Embed EF interventions into the day-to-day home and school experiences of the child. Formal didactic teaching alone is unlikely to result in significant behavioral change without the opportunity to practice, apply, and generalize EF skills.[8] Children learn much better when they are exposed to target information repeatedly, over long periods of time, in real-world contexts, with behavioral examples, and with logical consequences. Therefore, embedding the child in home and school environments that use, demonstrate, and encourage EFs will produce the most dramatic and durable outcomes. Modeling of EF skills by parents and teachers, repeated reinforcement of target EF behaviors by the child in daily life, and discussion of EF goals integrated into daily interactions are examples of embedding a child into an EF-rich environment.[15] With many of the suggested activities in this chapter, I have included a home and parent component to maximize carry-over. Programs with specific suggestions for environmental components that surround the child with positive EF models and examples can be found in books and learning curricula describing ways to improve EF.[37] An LSL technique for assessing a parent's understanding of intervention goals is to query, "Tell me how you will explain our EF techniques, and why we use them, to another person (e.g., spouse or grandparent)". This allows the clinician to provide additional information to a parent who may need it and to tailor it to a specific family situation. Parents often will raise their expectations and change the rules for their child if a clinician approaches this as an issue of increased competence. The clinician might say to a parent whose seven-year old child blurts and interrupts, "When Billy was younger, you encouraged any of his spoken communication attempts and even stopped talking to let him speak. That showed your sensitivity to his communication level and was the right strategy to use. Now, Billy has advanced and this strategy no longer serves him. Because I know you want him to thrive in social and school settings, let's talk about some new rules we will set for him that I'll utilize in our sessions and you'll utilize at home. I'm confident that Billy will be able to rise to these new expectations."

Pearl

An LSL technique to assess parents' understanding of EF intervention goals is to ask, "Tell me how you will explain our EF techniques, and why we use them, to another person, e.g., spouse."

12.8 Summary and Conclusions

Helping children who are DHH achieve speech and language skills at age- and grade-level is no longer enough. They must also be on a path to become well-adjusted, emotionally healthy, respectful, tax-paying citizens. In other words, they must compete with other children in the realm of EF. In laying out principles and techniques for EF interventions in this chapter, I acknowledge they are illustrative, not exhaustive. Supported by research findings, each principle points us in clinical directions that target relevant at-risk domains of EF in children in LSL practice. The specific techniques proposed are based on suggestions from EF intervention programs for NH children and by experiences in my own clinical practice. The children and parents have been my teachers and have tolerated trial-and-error attempts and numerous mistakes I've made in the pursuit of integrating LSL and EF intervention into one service provision. Parents, in fact, have been the real catalysts for my mission to blend EF into LSL practice. For numerous families, including Drake's, whose story began this chapter, parents were delighted with their child's LSL progress but frustrated by the other weaknesses in behavior and thinking that reflected EF delays. Improving EF in these situations has helped the child, which has helped the family. This is in line with the tenants of LSL practice, which pledge a strong commitment to family centered principles. It is my goal that improving EF along with communication skills in children who are DHH brings us a step closer to a full flourishing across all developmental domains in the children whose care is entrusted to us.

Pearl

Helping children achieve speech and language skills at age- and grade-level is no longer enough. They also must be on a path to become well-adjusted, emotionally healthy, respectful, tax-paying citizens. In other words, they must compete with their peers in the realm of EF.

12.9 Resources

Appendix 1 is a list of recommended resources for integrating LSL/SLP and EF goals.

Discussion Questions

1. The transition of EF control from external-to-internal is a pivotal tenet of intervention. In addition to the examples given in the text, what are some ways that this transition manifests itself in therapy?

2. EF intervention is more effective when bundled with LSL/SLP sessions. Describe some LSL techniques that are well-suited to incorporating EF goals (e.g., impulse control games.)

3. Well-meaning parents can, unintentionally, work against EF maturity in their child. What are some conversational conventions and rules that the practitioner may need to address with the family?

4. Explain two teaching activities that focus on improving working memory.

5. How can Boss your Brain strategies improve Theory of Mind and metacognition?

6. List several resources that enable families and practitioners to incorporate EF goals into therapy and daily life.

References

[1] Barkley RA. Executive Functions: What They Are, How They Work, and Why They Evolved. New York, NY: Guilford Press; 2012

[2] Diamond A, Lee K. Interventions shown to aid executive function development in children 4 to 12 years old. *Science* 2011;*333*(6045):959–964 10.1126/science.1204529

[3] Kronenberger WG, Beer J, Castellanos I, Pisoni DB, Miyamoto RT. Neurocognitive risk in children with cochlear implants. *JAMA Otolaryngol Head Neck Surg* 2014;*140*(7):608–615 10.1001/jamaoto.2014.757

[4] Beer J, Kronenberger WG, Castellanos I, Colson BG, Henning SC, Pisoni DB. Executive functioning skills in preschool-age children with cochlear implants. *J Speech Lang Hear Res* 2014;*57*(4):1521–1534 10.1044/2014_JSLHR-H-13-0054

[5] Dawson P, Guare R. Smart but Scattered. New York: Guilford; 2009

[6] Kronenberger WG, Xu H, Pisoni DB. Longitudinal development of executive functioning and spoken language skills in preschool-aged children with cochlear implants. *J Speech Lang Hear Res* 2020;*63*(4):1128–1147 doi: 10.1044/2019_JSLHR-19-00247

[7] [Kronenberger WG, Pisoni DB. Neurocognitive functioning in deaf children with cochlear implants. In: Knoors H, Marschark M, eds. Evidence-Based Practices in Deaf Education. London: Oxford; 2018

[8] Kronenberger WG, Pisoni DB. Why are children with cochlear implants at risk for executive functioning delays: Language only or something more? In: Marschark M, Knoors H, eds. Oxford Handbook of Deaf Studies in Learning and Cognition. New York: Oxford; 2020

[9] Diamond A. Activities and programs that improve children's executive functions. *Curr Dir Psychol* Sci 2012;*21*(5):335–341 10.1177/0963721412453722

[10] Calderon J. https://www.health.harvard.edu/blog/executive-functionin- children-why-it-matters-and-how-to-help-2020121621583. Published December 16, 2020. Accessed September 1, 2021

[11] Robbins AM. Auditory-verbal practice: A conversational competence approach. In: Moeller MP, Ertmer D, Stoel-Gammon C, eds. Promoting Language and Literacy in Children Who Are Deaf or Hard of Hearing. Baltimore, MD: Brooks Publishing; 2016

[12] Estabrooks, W. (2012). 101 FAQs for AVTs

[13] Simser J, Estabrooks W. Why are parents required to participate in auditory- verbal therapy and education? In: Estabrooks W, ed. *101 Frequently Asked Questions about Auditory-Verbal Practice*. Washington, DC: AG Bell; 2012

[14] Talbot P, Estabrooks W. What are the characteristics of an effective parent-practitioner relationship in auditory-verbal therapy and education. In: Estabrooks W, ed. *101 Frequently Asked Questions about Auditory-Verbal Practice*. Washington, DC: AG Bell; 2012

[15] Robbins AM, Kronenberger WK. *Principles of Executive Functioning Interventions for Children with Cochlear Implants: Guidance from Research Findings and Clinical Experience*. Otol Neurotol 2021;*42*(1):174–179

[16] Gioia GA, Isquith PK, Guy SC, Kenworthy L. *Behavior Rating Inventory of Executive Function-2 Manual*. Lutz, FL: Psychological Assessment Resources; 2015

[17] Gioia GA, Espy KA, Isquith PK. *Behavior Rating Inventory of Executive Function – Preschool Manual*. Lutz, FL: Psychological Assessment Resources; 2003

[18] Castellanos I, Kronenberger WG, Pisoni DB. Questionnaire-based assessment of executive functioning: Psychometrics. *Appl Neuropsychol Child* 2018;*7*(2):93–109 10.1080/21622965.2016.1248557

[19] Guare R, Dawson P, Guare C. Smart but Scattered Teens. New York: Guilford; 2012

[20] Kronenberger WG, Colson BG, Henning SC, Pisoni DB. Executive functioning and speech-language skills following long-term use of cochlear implants. *J Deaf Stud Deaf Educ* 2014;*19*(4):456–470 10.1093/deafed/enu011

[21] Kronenberger WG, Henning SC, Ditmars AM, Pisoni DB. Language processing fluency and verbal working memory in prelingually deaf long-term cochlear implant users: A pilot study. *Cochlear Implants Int* 2018;*19*(6):312–323 10.1080/14670100.2018.1493970

[22] Palmer KW, Tarshis N. We Thinkers! Santa Clara, CA: Think Social Publishing; 2013

[23] Tarshis N, Hendrix R, Palmer KW, Garcia Winner M. Social Explorers Curriculum. Santa Clara, CA: Think Social Publishing; 2016

[24] Barkley RA. Attention-Deficit Hyperactivity Disorder. 4th ed. A Handbook for Diagnosis and Treatment. New York, NY: Guilford; 2014

[25] Castellanos I, Kronenberger WG, Beer J, Colson BG, Henning SC, Ditmar A, Pisoni DB. Concept formation skills in long-term cochlear implant users. *Deaf Studies Deaf Edu*, 20(1), 27–40. https:// doi.org/10.1093/deafed/enu039

[26] Robbins AM. Rehabilitation after cochlear implantation. In: Niparko J, ed. Cochlear Implants: Principles and Practices (2nd ed). Philadelphia, PA: Lippincott, Williams, & Wilkins; 2009:269–312

[27] Robbins AM. Music and singing in auditory-verbal therapy. In: Estabrooks W, MacIver-Lux K, Morrison HM, eds. Auditory-Verbal Therapy: Science, Research, and Practice. San Diego, CA: Plural Publishing; 2020

[28] Miyake A, Friedman NP, Emerson MJ, Witzki AH, Howerter A, Wager TD. The unity and diversity of executive functions and their contributions to complex "Frontal Lobe" tasks: a latent variable analysis. *Cognit Psychol* 2000;*41*(1):49–100 doi: 10.1006/cogp.1999.0734

[29] Barkley RA. ADHD and the Nature of Self-Control. New York, NY: Guilford Press; 1997

[30] Williams M. Waiting Isn't Easy. New York, NY: Hyperion Books for children; 2014

[31] Wright L. Mindful Mantras: I Can Handle It. Laurie Wright Publishing; 2017

[32] Palmer KZ, Tashis N, Hendrix R, Garcia Winner M. We Thinkers! Vol. 2. Santa Clara, CA: Think Social Publishing; 2016

[33] Robbins AM. (2005). Bossing your brain: A history lesson with a middle school student who is hard of hearing. *Volta Voices*, July/August, 38–40

[34] Bell N. Visualizing and Verbalizing. San Luis Obispo, CA: Gander Publications; 1991

[35] De Bono E. Thinking for Action: Learn How to Focus Your Mind and Get Things Done. Hong Kong: DK Publishing; 1998

[36] Silverstein S. Come Skating. A Light in the Attic. New York, NY: HarperCollins; 2009

[37] Dawson P, Guare R. Coaching Students with Executive Skills Deficits. New York: Guilford; 2012

Appendix

Suggested Materials for Use in Integrated Executive Function, Speech-Language and Auditory-Verbal Intervention Activities

Games and Toys

Blurt (www.educationalinsights.com)

Bubble Talk: The Crazy Caption Boardgame (www.technosourceusa.com)

Buzz Word and Buzz Word, Jr. (www.patchproducts.com)

Chess (www.wikihow.com/Play-Chess)

Concept (Repos Production)

Dinkee Linkee for Kids (bananagrams.com)

Fast 5 (www.educaborras.com)

Headbanz for Kids (www.patchproducts.com)

Learning Well board games: *Predicting Outcomes, Getting the Main Idea, Inference, Cause and Effect, Reading for Detail, Following Directions* (www.eaieducation.com)

Line Up: The Memory Game of Quick Looks and Tricky Crooks (www.mindware.com)

Simon electronic toys (www.hasbrogaming.hasbro.com)

Sloth in a Hurry: An Improv Game (www.eeboo.com)

Sort it Out!, Jr. (www.universitygames.com)

Super Mind Pack: Negotiation Game, Word Planning Game and others (de Bono, 1998, DK books)

Taboo (www.hasbrogaming.hasbro.com)

Three for Me (www.patchproducts.com)

Tribond and *Tribond Kids* (www.patchproducts.com)

Watch This Face: An Emotional Literacy Activity (www.eeboo.com)

Books

Coaching Students with Executive Skills Deficits (Dawson & Guare, 2012)

See Time Fly: Visualizing and Verbalizing History Stories (Bell, 2001)

Smart but Scattered (Dawson & Guare, 2009)

Smart but Scattered for Teens (Guare, Dawson & Guare, 2013)

Social Explorers Curriculum (Tarshis et al, 2016.)*Superflex: A Superhero Social Thinking Curriculum* (Madrigal & Garcia Winner, 2008)

Thinking about You Thinking about Me (Garcia Winner, 2007)

Thinking for Action games (de Bono, 1998; www.dk.com)

Visualizing and Verbalizing for Language Comprehension and Thinking (Bell, 1991)

Other

642 Things to Write About: Young Writer's Edition (www.chroniclebooks.com)

Graphic Organizers, downloadable online or found in *Graphic Organizers* (www.teacgercreated.com)

Joke books, including knock-knock jokes, puns, play on words, double meanings

Six-Way Paragraphs (Pauk, 2000)

Specific Skill Series, including *Main Idea, Drawing Conclusions, Using the Context* and others

The Expressionary: The Ultimate Dictionary Companion for Idioms, Everyday Phrases and Proverbs (Schmidek, 2003) (www.acadcom.com)

Time Tracker visual timer and clock (www.learningresources.com)

13 The Auditory-Verbal Approach and Literacy

Lyn Robertson

Summary

This chapter argues that the Auditory-Verbal approach provides excellent preparation for literacy development in children with hearing loss and offers specific thoughts about building this preparation into therapy. Learning to listen and speak in a language-rich environment enables children to develop language comprehension and word recognition capacities necessary for productive listening, speaking, reading, writing, and thinking. The larger the child's spoken language and experiential repertoire, the better prepared she or he is prepared for becoming a literate individual who can think critically and participate in all aspects of society.

Keywords

literacy, listening, speaking, reading, writing, thinking, interacting cueing systems, language comprehension, background knowledge, vocabulary, language structures, verbal reasoning, literacy knowledge, word recognition, phonological awareness, decoding, sight recognition, read-alouds, language experience books, critical thinking

Key Points

- Listening, speaking reading, writing, and thinking are interacting language capabilities that mature with practice in the company of people who do them well.
- Auditory-Verbal practice prepares children with hearing loss to use spoken language as preparation for becoming literate members of society.
- Children learn to read and write by reading and writing with others in meaningful ways.

13.1 Introduction

As described throughout this book, professionals who work with children with hearing loss are vitally important in setting them on the path to participating in all aspects of life. Learning to listen and speak underlies their social, emotional, and intellectual functioning, all of which influence the extent to which they attain literacy. Much of this comes in the form of equipping parents and others who have daily contact with each child with the knowledge and skills they need to ensure the child is immersed in a language-rich environment that stimulates the person-to-person interactions that enable the child to acquire well-formed spoken language abilities.

This chapter focuses on reading and writing and makes the case that Auditory-Verbal therapy *is* preparation for literacy. The

mantra "Talk, talk, talk!" can translate into "Language, language, language!" It cannot be stressed enough that knowing and being able to use the spoken language encoded in print is a necessary prerequisite to learning to read and write that language. The more such knowledge the reader has, the more likely she or he is to become a proficient reader.

Pearl

Auditory-Verbal practice teaches parents how to listen to, speak, read, and write with their children.

Had the pioneers of the Auditory-Verbal approach begun with the intent of making literacy possible for children with hearing loss, they would not have needed to proceed differently. Learning spoken language through listening and speaking about daily activities and things in one's environment builds the requisite comprehension, word knowledge, and reasoning processes necessary for the increasingly complex thinking required for higher level literacy. Children with hearing loss who are not immersed in spoken language made accessible through technology are in the unfortunate situation of the children in the well-known Hart and Risley study[1] who experienced an estimated 30 million fewer words spoken with and around them between ages 2 and 4 compared to the children who fared better at school, and learned to read well when they were of school age. In analyzing the results of their investigation into the amounts and kinds of words used with very young children, Hart and Risley concluded: "The extra talk of parents in the professional families and that of the most talkative parents in the working-class families contained more of the varied vocabulary, complex ideas, subtle guidance, and positive feedback thought to be important to cognitive development."[2]

Suskind[3,4] wisely seized on this information when she realized that some of her patients, recipients of cochlear implants, learned spoken language far better than others. In response, she has proactively set up the Thirty Million Word Center for Early Learning and Public Health that serves children both with and without hearing loss.[5] It is precisely the attention that Auditory-Verbal practice gives the linguistic sounds, words, ideas, and communication that prevents a debilitating lack of linguistic input and prepares children for literacy.

13.2 The Importance of Literacy

Let us begin here with a "thought experiment." Imagine what it would be like not to be able to read and write. Make a list of all that would be closed to you and consider the opportunities you would not be aware of in your life. It has been well known and well documented[6,7,8,9,10,11] that children who do not develop a good working knowledge of the spoken language they are to read, achieve well below their peers with typical hearing on standardized reading tests. As recently as forty years ago, parents of children diagnosed anywhere along the continuum of moderate to profound hearing loss were advised that their children would need to attend special schools or programs and that their educational attainment would be severely limited. A lesser emphasis on spoken language and diminished access to people speaking in well-formed language hindered their ability to communicate and build the foundations for literacy. As technology has enabled both audition and ever-finer discrimination between and among the sounds in words, children presented with an Auditory-Verbal approach have increasingly thrived in the mainstream in schools where most of their peers enjoy typical hearing.[12,13,14,15,16,17,18,19,20,21] Indeed, we now know of many young adults with significant hearing loss who use cochlear implants and/or hearing aids who have advanced degrees and serve in professional roles, alongside their colleagues with typical hearing.[22,23]

Reading and writing at high levels across multiple genres is essential to the many modes of communication needed for living an independent life in which a person can seek, evaluate, and express information and opinion, think critically, and move easily in social and professional circles. Add to these the emotional benefits of pleasure reading, recognized as "bookjoy" by the National Council of Teachers of English,[24] and it is clear that high-level literacy contributes greatly to the living of a full life.

13.3 Multiple Literacies

While the focus in this chapter is reading, writing, and thinking, it is necessary to realize there are other literacies, all of which require basic reading and writing capabilities. Twenty-first century literacies take into account the digital, the global, and the diversity accessible in the burgeoning networks that make up our world. The literate person is actively involved in consuming and constructing meanings and in keeping up with a rapidly changing world. In the words of the National Council of Teachers of English[25]: "Literacy has always been a collection of communicative and sociocultural practices shared among communities. As society and technology change, so does literacy. The world demands that a literate person possess and intentionally apply a wide range of skills, competencies, and dispositions. These literacies are interconnected, dynamic, and malleable. As in the past, they are inextricably linked with histories, narratives, life possibilities, and social trajectories of all individuals and groups."

The speed of change in the ways we communicate using ever-changing language forms and modes of transmission demands far more than the basics. Everyone is struggling to keep up in this exciting time, and professionals dealing with hearing loss must heed the call to work with children and their families with this in mind. The reader is urged to read the entirety of the NCTE statement (https://ncte.org/statement/nctes-definition-literacy-digital-age/).

13.4 Academic Disciplines and the Study of Reading and Writing

Various ways of investigating reading and writing have developed over the years, and they continue to develop. There is no one, correct, way to conceptualize the processes, and it is more productive to understand them as building on one another in kaleidoscopic fashion. *Behaviorists* think in terms of word identification: one sees the letters, and sounds them out or sees a whole word, hears the word and connects it to a meaning.[26] *Linguists* and *psycholinguists* think about the language being read in terms of its structure and how the structure informs prediction of words and their meanings.[27] Co*gnitive psychologists* pay close attention to the role of background/previous knowledge and how the brain organizes, retrieves, and analyzes it in constructing meaning.[28,29] *Sociolinguists* consider the role of social location of the reader and how language(s) are used and regarded.[30] *Literary theorists* regard each episode of reading as one in which the reader makes a new meaning in the presence of text.[31] *Critical theorists* pay attention to the access the writer and reader have to societal power.[32] A basic difference between and among these disciplinary views involves the question of where meaning resides. Is the reader identifying a meaning the writer intended? Or, is the reader creating a meaning based on knowledge and experience the reader brings to the text? Can some of both be happening simultaneously?

It serves us well to use all of these ways of explaining reading and writing, particularly in an ever-changing world. Interestingly, we can go as far back as the early twentieth century to Thorndike's rather comprehensive definition of reading comprehension that anticipated at least some of what has followed in literacy research and that can still serve us well in our work: "Understanding a paragraph is like solving a problem in mathematics. It consists in selecting the right elements of the situation and putting them together in the right relations, and also with the right amount of weight or influence or force for each. The mind is assailed as it were by every word in the paragraph. It must select, repress, soften, emphasize, correlate and organize, all under the influence of the right mental set or purpose or demand."[33]

In general, literacy is thought to involve an interaction of all the capabilities the individual has amassed up to the point of doing a particular reading or writing task, and continued experience with reading for meaning and writing with purpose hones these capacities further. The abilities involved in all of these conceptualizations of various aspects of literacy comprise the goals that can be realized using an Auditory-Verbal approach.

13.5 Interacting Cueing Systems Involved in Reading and Writing

A useful construction of the reading process has been offered by Scarborough.[34] Scarborough's discussion rests on research and assumptions based on the hearing world, the world that children with hearing loss enter through technology use, instruction, and experience in listening and speaking. Many researchers are concerned with children with typical hearing who struggle with reading and writing because they exhibit gaps in one or several of these components, and professionals who deal with hearing loss will recognize these categories. Note that writing is often described as the "flip side" of reading, and the writer makes use of the same components while composing a message.

Scarborough divides the intertwining, overlapping processes of language comprehension and word recognition and represents them visually as accumulated strands that form a braid or rope. Language comprehension comprises background knowledge, vocabulary, language structures, verbal reasoning, and literacy knowledge. Word recognition involves phonological awareness, decoding, and sight recognition. Language comprehension becomes "increasingly strategic" and word recognition becomes "increasingly automatic" as the reader moves through practice toward skilled reading, defined as "fluent execution and coordination of word recognition and text comprehension."[34]

Strands of Early Literacy Development

Language Comprehension
1. Background knowledge
2. Vocabulary
3. Language structures
4. Verbal reasoning
5. Literacy knowledge

Word Recognition
1. Phonological awareness
2. Decoding (includes spelling and predictions)
3. Sight recognition

All are necessary to the overall reading process, yet not every category is elicited during every instance of reading. Adams[35] posits that during every decision point during a given reading, all the cueing systems are poised to contribute to a suitable reading that produces a "click" of understanding. The systems that win the race at that split second are the ones triggered in the reader to create meaning. As soon as that happens, the systems reset themselves and the race begins anew. Good readers have developed strengths in all of the systems and can create meaningful readings through active engagement with the text using the systems in quick succession until satisfied. For example, the comprehension process of language structure might suggest that the next word in a sentence should be a noun, so the reader's focus is on "nounness." The vocabulary process might suggest an array of suitable meanings for the word. And, the decoding process helps the reader decide exactly what the word is. For example,

She went to see the brown _____. [many things—nouns—are brown]

She went to see the brown ho_____. [what is this story about? a house? a horse?]

She went to see the brown horse. [the "r" makes it a horse, not a house!]

When the process is working well, all of this goes on without the reader's awareness. An expert reader can make meaning of this sentence in one glance, without reading it word by word, or letter by letter, unless an ambiguity within the sentence trips him or her up, causing a closer examination of the letters on the page.

Pitfall

Parents may approach reading as only a mechanical process of sounding out words. The Auditory-Verbal practitioner should discuss with parents why reading involves more than sounding out words.

Children learning to read must have a well-developed comprehension of the language they are learning to read; word recognition skills are important, but they cannot be employed in the absence of established knowledge of the words on the page, sign, screen, or anywhere print can reside.

The next pages lay out the eight processes involved in Language Comprehension and Word Recognition, linking each in turn to Auditory-Verbal practice.

13.5.1 Language Comprehension: Background Knowledge

The building of background knowledge begins well before birth, evidenced by the observation that newborns with typical hearing recognize their mother's voices.[36] And then, every experience contributes to a growing understanding of the world. Cognitive psychologists have developed schema theory to account for how people organize, store, retrieve, and use the content and process knowledge gained through experience. Simultaneously, language plays an important role in these processes by enabling communication and enhancing thought. A schema is a unit of information, understanding, or idea stored in memory. A person's take on the world is made up of numerous schemas (alternate plural: schemata) connected within an ever-growing, dynamic memory network. As discussed in Anderson,[28] schemas serve a variety of functions in interpreting experiences, information, and texts. They:

1. provide slots that foster assimilation.
2. help one know what is most important and where to put one's attention.
3. help one make inferences.
4. help one search memory to reconstruct the events in the text.
5. help a reader decide what to keep and what to leave out in a retelling.
6. help with figuring out what must have happened.

Consider that a small child is learning about the world and the language and concepts that people use to explain it. As that child attends preschool for the first time, much is unknown, and the child "learns the ropes," i.e., develops a schema, by figuring out over the first few weeks how his/her preschool works. Perhaps there has been an orientation to introduce the child to what to expect. This sets up the basic slots for a day at school (mommy takes you to the room where your class is; the teacher greets you and says your name; there are other children to play with; there's circle time, play time, naptime, and snack time; and—finally—daddy comes to take you home). As the days at preschool unfold, each of the slots begins to contain its own set of slots. Playing with other children begins to have certain expectations, such as taking turns with valued toys. Mommy packs the snack because of a food allergy. And, so on. New information that fits easily into existing slots will be easily understood and remembered; learning the words for each bit of information aids in building and relying on a solid schema for preschool. The child isn't surprised when it's naptime, because it happens every day.

After a while, when asked what happened at preschool, the child knows to choose the event that was unusual in the day, because it stands out as different. Putting attention there signals knowing that mommy or daddy generally know what to expect and want to know about something new and interesting. Based on this, the child learns to make inferences when an episodic memory is not a strong one. When asked about snack time, the child might say: "I guess I ate crackers today" (because Mommy often packs crackers). Or, if the memory is vivid: "Lila sat next to me" (because she always does). Knowing the schema for preschool helps the child do a memory search in order to anticipate and then reconstruct the events of a day; the schema guides the child in transitioning to each activity and then in telling about it later. The schema helps the child know what to keep and what to leave out in talking about the day and allows for figuring out what must have happened. In the preschool schema, there is almost always a naptime.

An idea can be retrieved from memory in a variety of ways, both linguistic and non-linguistic. Schemas are strengthened when words are attached to them, though, because the addition of language to other retrieval cues (images, for example) expands the memory. Words help in linking related aspects of knowledge to each other by labeling stored categories of over-arching and subordinate ideas that carry other labels. When language is used, the idea, or referent, is represented by language tags stored in memory. These tags enable the person to use that knowledge in some way in listening, speaking, reading, and writing, all of which are ways of thinking. The more experiences a person has and the more connections that person makes, both consciously and unconsciously, between and among them, the more options the person can bring to bear in making sense of the world and of text and in communicating about them. This is helpful in understanding how sociocultural forces influence the meanings readers bring to words. "Even a simple word like *dog* is interpreted through the lens of personal experience which, in turn, is filtered through cultural representations of dogs and other animals.[25]"

Auditory-Verbal Practice and Background Knowledge

A strength of Auditory-Verbal practice is that parents can learn during sessions how to introduce their child to many, many experiences in the world they might not have considered necessary in a very young child's life. Visits to friends and family, the zoo, the arboretum, the beach, the mountains, the playground—even the grocery store and the restaurant, and so on, are vital to building the background knowledge necessary to operate in the world. The same is true for learning to bake bread and cookies, use a vacuum cleaner, and do other household tasks. Meeting and talking with the mail carrier, the fire fighter, the trash collector, and the pilot also count. When an activity cannot happen in person, it can happen using toys, books, make believe, and pretend play. In short, the goal is to introduce the child to as much as possible that goes on in the world. Making a Language Experience Book entry and talking about such outings and play help the child consolidate and store concepts in memory networks.[23] Steps in making and using this practical technique are discussed later in this chapter, as well as in the therapy chapter (Chapter 3, "Speech Acoustics: Strengthening the Foundation").

Pearl

The Auditory-Verbal practitioner is in a good position to help the family understand the critical importance of employing literacy-building practices and experiences with their child on a daily basis.

13.5.2 Language Comprehension: Vocabulary

Vocabulary growth is fostered within rich experiential context. Children learn new words by hearing them used in meaningful context and having opportunities to try them out and receive feedback in the form of a meaningful response when they use them.[27] I once observed a mother reading a book with her son, a child learning through auditory-verbal means. The story involved a flood, and the word "flood" was used several times. The boy stopped his mother and asked, "What *happened?!*" and his mother replied: "There was a flood!" She went on reading, and her son interrupted her again with "What *happened?!*" and she replied again, using the word "flood." This went back and forth a few more times, and suddenly the mother realized that "flood" wasn't in her child's experience or in his vocabulary. Then, she explained using words she knew he understood, that it had rained for a long time, and there was so much water around the house that it floated. They looked at the pictures together and talked, and "flood" began to be a concept for him, grounded in words he already knew and pictures he could see. Instruction that attempts to build memory for isolated words is often less than successful, as it is less likely to be linked to background knowledge already stored in the schematic network.

The reason for reading is always to make meaning in the presence of print; therefore, on its own, the ability to pronounce words in text is insufficient for stimulating comprehension. Pronouncing a word one does not know is simply not helpful, and dwelling on that aspect of reading without attention to reading's other attributes creates a damaging message for the child that reading is a meaningless process. A large, well-understood vocabulary of related words encompassing multiple synonyms, antonyms, and word parts prepares a child for learning to read in that it makes possible the bringing of meaning to print. As the child moves through school, the demands of texts become more challenging. At this point, the child needs to learn to make sense of new words by using known context and consulting words and word parts. At the beginning, though, the child needs to know and be able to use in speech most of the words in the text and to have access to good illustrations and explanations of new words.

Auditory-Verbal Practice and Vocabulary Development

The Auditory-Verbal (A-V) practitioner needs to demonstrate to parents ways of using spoken language to help the child build more spoken language. This can take many forms well-known to Listening and Spoken Language Specialists (LSLS). For example, parents need to learn how to:

1. Carry on conversations based on experiences, real objects, pictures, and relationships.
2. Wait for responses from the child and then follow up with language that provides useful feedback.
3. Speak in expansive sentences that provide synonyms and antonyms that the child needs to learn. ("Your *dog*, Beau, is a good *pet* who keeps you *company* by *playing with you* in the backyard." "Your preschool *field trip* to the *arboretum* was a fun *excursion.* You got to see many *kinds of trees* you hadn't seen before.")
4. Read aloud and write with the child on a daily basis.
5. Play games that both require and supply new language and vocabulary. (I Spy with My Little Eye, 20 Questions, and so forth)

13.5.3 Language Comprehension: Language Structures

By the age of three, children with typical hearing have internalized and are able to use the basic structures of the language(s) spoken around them,[37] and children with hearing loss who are learning to listen can achieve this milestone, as well. Fry[38] observed similar attainment by the age of 6 or 7 in children with hearing loss who were learning to listen. They do this by being immersed in language, through hearing people talking and trying out their growing understanding of how speech and language work, and then modifying their own speech on the basis of feedback they receive from the mature speakers of the language(s) in their midst. This includes parts of speech (nouns, verbs, adjectives, adverbs, pronouns, prepositions, conjunctions, and interjections), prefixes and suffixes that can be added to words to change their meaning in some way, and markers for number (singularity and plurality), tense, and degree (for example, strong, stronger, strongest). Clauses and phrases contribute additional information in conventional ways. After these structures are established, the person spends a lifetime adding content words to them. The complexity of "wrapping" a present for someone to "*un*wrap" at the party involves a core word modified by tense and negation, as well as movement from the present to the future, all expressed with subtle structural linguistic changes. Children learn these subtleties by honing their listening and speaking without knowing what these structures are called. As they learn to think about language, they may say they speak the way they do because it "sounds right."

Language structures matter in reading because the internalized sense of what kind of word usually comes next in a well-formed sentence helps the reader predict the next word without even looking at it, and the many rapid series of predictions and confirmations (or disconfirmations) create the same meaningful flow in reading that fosters making sense while listening. Predictions rest on interactions between and among the schemas, the vocabulary,

and the structural cues associated with meaning making. Return to the example previously given:

> She went to see the brown horse.

Conventional English syntax rules out a sentence such as "She went to see the horse brown," unless "brown" suddenly becomes a verb, as in "She went to see the horse run."

Auditory-Verbal Practice and Language Structures

Auditory-Verbal practitioners use well-formed, sentence-length spoken language with children with hearing loss well before the children can understand the language, and the children store it away and try it out bit-by-bit, just as children with typical hearing do. Practitioners should explain this process, encourage parents to speak in these ways at home with their children, and emphasize that doing so lays the foundation for literacy development. "Baby talk," while cute and fun, serves other purposes and should not be the primary way parents and young children converse.

13.5.4 Language Comprehension: Verbal Reasoning

Words in English are fraught with ambiguity,[39] and many of the seemingly simple words that children encounter in early reading experiences carry multiple meanings. For example, can, light, and run can all be used as nouns, as well as verbs. In a study of ambiguity detection skill, Cairns, Waltzman, and Schlisselberg[40] followed children from preschool through 3rd grade, tracking their ability to recognize multiple meanings in words and testing their reading comprehension. They gave children sentences such as "The man's nails were very sharp" (lexical ambiguity) and "The child talked about the problem with the teacher" (structural ambiguity), constructions that can represent at least two different meanings. The study's results indicate that ambiguity detection skill is associated with readiness for reading instruction in first grade and progress in reading achievement in second and third grade.

Learning how to think using language involves content and structural knowledge that extends from the concrete "here and now" and becomes increasingly complex with experience. Even simple language is replete with figures of speech that include metaphors, similes, and analogies, all of which stimulate meaning making by comparing and contrasting words and ideas. "I'm as quick as a cricket," "I'm as slow as a snail," and "I'm as small as an ant" make up the first several pages of *Quick as a Cricket,*[41] a book of similes for children. Rich illustrations introduce the child to basic comparisons people make between themselves and animals. Knowing basic comparisons facilitates making inferences, a necessary part of interpreting both the world of experience and the meaning of text. Being able to do simple verbal reasoning in listening and speaking ought to precede applying such reasoning during reading.

Pearl

Parents need models, practice, and feedback from the Auditory-Verbal practitioner while learning to talk with children in ways that expand their language and thinking.

Auditory-Verbal Practice and Verbal Reasoning

Riddles are particularly fun for children and can be offered and laughed about during A-V sessions. Zipke[39] offers multiple examples such as:

- What has an ear but cannot hear? Corn!
- Will you join me in a bowl of soup? Do you think there's room for both of us?
- Why did the bear tiptoe through the campground? He didn't want to wake the sleeping bags!

These well-worn jokes rely on extensive background knowledge that needs to be explained to children as they catch on to multiple meanings and the ways riddles work. Zipke suggests making explanations using words the child already knows, drawing pictures to illustrate meanings, and poring over books of riddles designed for children.

Other kinds of word play using nursery rhymes, fill-in-the-blanks, following directions, treasure hunts, and nonsense words can be emphasized during A-V sessions and then employed by parents at home. Such practice is foundational to promoting a love of words and the many ways of using them.

13.5.5 Language Comprehension: Literacy Knowledge

Teaching children about books, letters, words, and sentences is probably what most people think about when they consider helping a child learn to read. Children learn about these concrete, practical aspects of the ways spoken words are represented in books during frequent read-alouds that introduce them to the conventions of text while conveying a story. Some conventions are deduced as the child sees and hears what the adult does with a book, and some are learned as the adult makes explanations and applies terms to them. Direct instruction, whether at home or in preschool, usually begins with letters and the sounds they represent. Over time, children learn what a spoken and printed word is and how to determine where to demarcate the beginnings and endings of words. They need to be introduced to ways of talking about language and the contents of books, known as Concepts About Print.[42] For English, the language of Clay's focus, these include: front of the book; back of the book; title; author; where to begin reading; left to right [right to left in Hebrew or Arabic]; top to bottom; first word on a page; last word on a page; first letter in a word; last letter in a word; capital and lower-case letters; and punctuation marks.

Auditory-Verbal Practice and Literacy Knowledge

The Auditory-Verbal practitioner can include read-alouds and create experience-book entries during sessions with a child to prepare the parent and child for doing these activities together at home. Parents can be asked to talk about what is happening as they read and write with their child, so the practitioner can assist in making these experiences go well. Practical steps recommended for reading and writing with a child are discussed toward the end of this chapter.

13.5.6 Word Recognition: Phonological Awareness

Difficulty with phonological awareness has often been associated with hearing loss, as one cannot identify, store, and retrieve from memory what cannot be heard. Facility with the phonology of the language to be read is understood as causal in learning to read and write.[43] Interestingly, some children with typical hearing have difficulty with phonological awareness that is deemed to be the cause of their reading delay,[44] and the recommended remedies for them are similar to Auditory-Verbal practices that help children discriminate between and among target sounds. A highly developed auditory awareness of the individual sounds and segments that make up words, then, is a necessary precursor to instruction in translating print to the spoken sounds and words it represents. As a child's vocabulary grows, she or he must learn to assign words and word parts in memory to specific linguistic compartments so as to access and remember them with efficiency when listening; otherwise the memory load becomes too large to handle.

In Goswami's explanation, "There is considerable developmental pressure to represent these [new vocabulary] words in the brain in a way that will distinguish them from other words and allow the child to recognize them accurately and quickly during speech comprehension. For example, a 2-year-old probably knows the words 'cot,' 'cat' and 'cut,' 'hot,' 'not,' and 'lot,' and 'cough.' All these words differ from 'cot' by a single phoneme. To distinguish between these similar-sounding words both quickly and accurately, child linguists argue that children must begin to represent the sequences of sounds that constitute each known word in their brains. They must represent the 'segmental phonology' of the words they know."[43]

In typical development, children learn how words differ from one another through listening and speaking experiences while immersed in the pronunciations of one or more dialects of the language(s) used in their environment, thus, Goswami's examples do not work for all ways of pronouncing English words. Learning these differences spurs the growth of phonemic awareness, the finer-grained auditory skill necessary for discovering and understanding the alphabetic principle, the concept that the smallest linguistic sounds match up with the specific letters and letter blends that represent them.[45] For this reason, helping children learn to differentiate between and among the sounds of their language is an essential part of preparing them for reading and writing.

Pearl

Teaching children about letters and the sounds they represent is more likely to be successful after phonemic awareness has been established.

Traditionally, early childhood is a time for word play. The rhymes, repetitive songs, word games, and riddles referred to in the last section build various kinds of knowledge, including phonological and phonemic awareness. Another kind of phonological awareness that predicts learning how to read is the ability to tap out and count syllables in spoken words.[45] Learning music helps children learn about syllables, phonemes, sight identification, orthography, and patterns, all of which assist them in reading fluently.[46] All of these help children map the sounds onto the letters and syllabic letter combinations.

Consider the nursery rhyme, "Twinkle, Twinkle, Little Star," which has the same tune and rhythm as "The Alphabet Song":

Twinkle, twinkle, little star
How I wonder what you are
Up above the world so high
Like a diamond in the sky
Twinkle, twinkle little star
How I wonder what you are

This song has repetition ("twinkle, twinkle"), alliteration ("twinkle, little"; "wonder what"), rhyme ("star," "are"; "high," "sky"), and a pace that is easy to clap out. It provides a bit of information about the world and how we want to know more about it, and it's fun to learn and sing over and over again, providing many opportunities for important discoveries to develop.

Auditory-Verbal Practice and Phonological Awareness

The Auditory-Verbal approach addresses this aspect of literacy head-on by helping children discriminate between and among sounds in the language in both listening and speaking, and the practitioner can coach parents in using the various forms of word play on a daily basis. Suggesting specific nursery rhymes, songs, word games, and riddles to use at home during a given week helps parents know they are using good materials with their children. Many of these are found in children's books.

13.5.7 Word Recognition: Decoding

The sounding out of words is the usual way of referring to decoding, and many words can be spoken from print by putting sounds to the letters in left-to-right fashion. But, this works in making meaning only if the reader already has the words in his or her working vocabulary, and it is only helpful in writing words spelled in conventional ways. That said, automaticity in decoding is helpful in informing the numerous predictions taking place during a given reading.

Auditory-Verbal Practice and Decoding

During the preschool and early elementary years, the Auditory-Verbal practitioner should employ informal play with sounds as one way of establishing the listening skill necessary for phonemic awareness. Working with children who are not yet of school age does not need to dwell on helping a child learn letters and their sounds, though children who show interest in connecting sounds and letters should be accommodated. The practitioner's role is that of making sure that children are developing knowledge of all facets of language through listening and speaking as preparation for formal literacy instruction in school.

13.5.8 Word Recognition: Sight Recognition

Many words do not conform to decoding rules and, instead, need to be identified as whole or sight words, for example: could, have, and what. As with decoded words, such recognition is useful only when the word is already part of the child's meaningful vocabulary, so recognizing such words in the context of a phrase, sentence, or story is a good way to lodge them in long-term memory.

Auditory-Verbal Practice and Sight Recognition

The Auditory-Verbal practitioner should focus on all facets of language and its auditory components and need not work formally on sight word recognition, though if a child shows interest, informal word play and the incorporation of written whole words into tasks during therapy sessions can be helpful. The practice of mounting written words on objects and furniture in a room (for example, "table" taped onto the table; "toys" taped onto the toy box) is a subtle way to match the written word with its referent without directly teaching about it.

13.5.9 A Note about Decoding and Sight Recognition

Many people have an awareness of a debate between teaching reading through a decoding (phonics) approach vs. teaching through a whole word/sight word approach. There is no need for such debate, as mature readers use both cueing systems and all the processes attendant to them. They are both pathways to word recognition, also called word identification, and both serve important purposes that complement each other. Further, there is no perfect system for teaching reading. Children learn what is salient to them at a particular moment, and they do not always learn what someone is trying to teach them. It is more productive to see the learner as an active constructor than as a vessel to be filled.[47,48] Blaming or praising a particular reading curriculum for a child's reading achievement misses the point that listening, speaking, reading, writing, and thinking are interacting language capabilities that mature with practice in the company of people who do them well. Indeed, children who learn to read early have usually had extensive experience in daily shared reading with an adult.[49] These shared reading sessions strengthen the child's abilities to master the components described, often without formal instruction in reading.

Pearl

Children learn language and become ready for literacy by interacting with role models who talk, listen, read, write, and think (figure things out) *with* them.

13.6 Theory of Mind

Theory of mind (ToM) is an important concept bearing on comprehension, in general, and on reading comprehension as it pertains to this chapter. Children developing typically experience a growing understanding that others have knowledge, feelings, intentions, and beliefs apart from their own, and their emerging ToM readies them for social interaction and social reasoning. Lags in ToM interfere with friendship, likeability, leadership, and persuasion and are associated with loneliness and deception. In short, a well-developed ToM is essential for mental health throughout life.[50] Numerous studies have documented difficulty in ToM development in children with hearing loss, particularly in signers with parents who have typical hearing, and attribute this to language delay and lack of conversational experience, particularly the dearth of talk about mental states.[51] One study of children with cochlear implants described as "oral deaf" found significantly lower ToM performance in them[52]; another study found no delay in children using cochlear implants.[53] The interested reader can delve deeply into these findings by reading these studies and those reviewed in the work of Wellman and Peterson.[50,51] This writer could find no studies that address the development of children with whom the Auditory-Verbal approach has been or is being used. The hypothesis that children with hearing loss who learn to listen and speak will progress more typically in developing ToM needs to be studied, and close attention should be given to the listening and spoken language status of the subjects involved.

The connection between ToM and reading comprehension of narratives involves the reader's ability to identify with the mental states of the characters in a story. Dore[54] proposed that the "age at which children [with typical hearing] reach important developmental ToM milestones is notably similar to the ages at which they seem to master significant narrative processing abilities" (p. 1072). Dore et al. cite milestones that begin around age 3 with the child understanding the spatial perspective of a main character. By age 4 or 5, the child begins to understand what a character might be thinking, and by age 7, the child can usually identify mixed emotions in a character. The assumption is that ToM typically develops apace with spoken language facility. The ability to infer, monitor, and talk about a mental state in one or more characters in a story makes for richer comprehension. In general, children apply what they know in their own interpersonal lives with others to what they encounter in a story read to them and then to stories they read themselves, so the need to cultivate ToM in children with hearing loss becomes obvious. In addition, listening to stories and then talking about the characters' feelings and intentions may spur on ToM development.

Auditory-Verbal Practice and Theory of Mind

The Auditory-Verbal practitioner can contribute to children's development of ToM by bringing mental states into therapy sessions and demonstrating for parents ways they can do so on a daily basis. Discussing with parents the need for social interaction and healthy friendships, as well as how age-appropriate ToM assists with literacy development contributes to their motivation to add this to their daily interactions with their children. Practical

ideas include teaching labels for emotions, and asking questions about causal factors, feelings, and perspectives. For example:

- Ask questions such as: Why did Goldilocks go into the bears' house? Was she curious? Did she know the bears wouldn't want her in their house? Why did Goldilocks run out of the bears' house? How did she feel? Scared? Embarrassed? Sorry? Was she smiling? No. Show me how her face looked.
- Using toy figures, act out a story with the child, with each player taking different roles and switching roles when possible (This time, you be Goldilocks, and I'll be Papa Bear). Give the child opportunities to talk from each character's point of view.
- Seek out and use books that present different points of view. *Brown Bear, Brown Bear, What do you See?*[55] and *A Weekend with Wendell*[56] are classic books that invite seeing from another's perspective.

Pearl

During therapy sessions, the parent can both observe the practitioner carrying out a literacy practice and then try out the practice with the child to get feedback and guidance from the practitioner

13.7 Listening and Spoken Language Specialist (LSLS) Domain 9: Emergent Literacy

The subcategories of Domain 9 incorporate Scarborough's categories discussed previously, as well as the five categories determined important to reading by the National Reading Panel: phonemic awareness, phonics, fluency, vocabulary, and comprehension.[57] **Table 13.1** lists the many targeted listening and experiential practices used by practitioners and taught to parents by practitioners to use frequently with their children. These make intentional the practices and experiences that typical hearing makes available to children without hearing loss.

The Auditory-Verbal practitioner's role is to foster age-appropriate speech, language, and comprehension and to watch for difficulty in one or more of the Domain 9 categories, all in the service of enabling the child to enter mainstream schooling prepared for instruction in literacy and in content across the curriculum; for appropriate adjustment to schooling; and for meaningful social interactions.

13.8 Literacy-Building Practices

The Auditory-Verbal practitioner is in a good position to help the family understand the critical importance of employing literacy-building practices with their child on a daily basis. These can be built into therapy sessions during which the parent can both observe the practitioner carrying out a practice and try out the practice with the child to get some feedback and guidance. Many practices listed in **Table 13.1** can be incorporated into the

Table 13.1 Linking LSLS domain 9 and literacy theory with auditory-verbal therapy

LSLS Domain 9	Literacy Theory: National Reading Panel Category	Auditory-Verbal Therapy: Practices
a. Reciting finger plays and nursery rhymes	Phonemic awareness Phonics Fluency Vocabulary Comprehension	Targeted listening practice • Example: Discriminating between 1 and 2-syllable words whose phonemes differ by one (ex: mat-bat, bat-bam, batter-matter, batter-badger) • Exposing child to melody, expression, rhythm, rhyme, intonation • Using repetition
b. Telling and/or retelling stories	Vocabulary Comprehension	Targeted listening practice • Responding with spoken language • Waiting for and requiring child to use spoken language • Daily interactive read-alouds with the child • Positioning close to the microphone • Using acoustic highlighting • Pausing, waiting (providing thinking time for the child) • Changing voices for characters • Asking and answering questions in a conversational manner • Using classic literature, songs, nursery rhymes
c. Activity and story sequencing	Vocabulary Comprehension	Targeted listening practice • Responding with spoken language • Waiting for and requiring child to use spoken language
d. Singing songs and engaging in musical activities	Phonemic awareness Phonics Fluency Vocabulary Comprehension	Targeted listening practice • Exposing child to melody, pitch, expression, rhythm, rhyme, intonation • Using repetition
e. Creating experience stories/experience books	Vocabulary Comprehension	Targeted listening practice • Developing conversations using natural interactions • Highlighting vocabulary • Paying attention to word order • Changing words by adding prefixes and suffixes
f. Organization of books (e.g., cover; back; title; author page)	Vocabulary Comprehension	Incorporating book-reading vocabulary during read-alouds
g. Directionality and orientation of print	Vocabulary Comprehension	Incorporating book-reading vocabulary during read-alouds

h. Distinguishing letters, words, sentences, spaces, and punctuation	Phonemic awareness
	Phonics
		Targeted listening practice
		• Acoustic highlighting
		  o Suprasegmental
		  o Segmental
		• Asking, "What did you hear?"
		Pointing out and talking about letters, words, sentences, spaces, and punctuation

i. Phonics (e.g., sound-symbol correspondences and letter-sound correspondences)	Phonemic awareness Phonics	Targeted listening practice • Preparing a child who listens for formal instruction that leads to understanding the alphabetic principle
j. Phonemic awareness (e.g., sound matching; isolating; substituting; adding; blending; segmenting; deleting)	Phonemic awareness Phonics	Targeted listening practice • To one's own speech • Six-sound Test • Nursery rhymes • Music and singing
k. Sight word recognition	Fluency	Allowing sight word identification to develop naturally during read-alouds without focusing directly on this aspect of reading during the emergent reading period

l. Strategies for the development of listening, speaking, vocabulary, reading and writing	Phonemic awareness
	Phonics
	Fluency
	Vocabulary
	Comprehension
		Targeted listening practice
		• Focus on building
		  o auditory memory
		  o receptive and expressive spoken language
		Providing the child with mature models of spoken and written language structure and function
		Playtime alone, with parent, and with other children

Continued on page 190

Table 13.1 *(Continued from page 189)* Linking LSLS domain 9 and literacy theory with auditory-verbal therapy

LSLS Domain 9	Literacy Theory: National Reading Panel Category	Auditory-Verbal Therapy: Practices
m. Contextual clues to decode meaning	Vocabulary Comprehension	Having frequent conversations with the child in the course of daily activities fosters meaning making
n. Oral reading fluency development	Fluency	Having frequent conversations with the child in the course of daily activities fosters fluency in spoken language and reading
o. Text comprehension strategies (e.g., direct explanation; modeling; guided practice; and application)	Vocabulary Comprehension	Narrating life as it happens Bringing sounds to life through meaningful experiences Having frequent conversations Learning through exposure • Semantics • Morphology • Syntax Learning to • Turn statements into questions, exclamations, etc. • Apply words to objects, actions, relationships modifiers, and ideas • Use pragmatic aspects of language • Apply memories of experiences to text
p. Abstract and figurative language (e.g., similes; metaphors)	Vocabulary Comprehension	Focusing on abstract and figurative language with the child during • Frequent conversations • Daily read-alouds
q. Divergent question comprehension (e.g., inferential questions; predictions)	Vocabulary Comprehension	Asking divergent questions of the child during • Frequent conversations • Daily read-alouds

From Chapter 9 (Robertson & Wray), *Auditory-Verbal Therapy: For Young Children with Hearing Loss and their Families and the Practitioners Who Guide Them* (pp. 270-273) by Estabrooks, W., MacIver- Lux, K., & Rhoades, E.A. Copyright © 2016 Plural Publishing, Inc. All rights reserved. Used with permission.

two main literacy-building practices of Daily Read-Alouds (also called Shared Reading) with the child and creating and using a Language Experience Book (LEB) with the child. Both should be conducted with the intent of interacting with the child using meaningful language with as much frequency as possible. And, both should be regarded as great fun for both the adult and the child. Meaning must always be the emphasis; too much focus on letters, words, and sounds can cause the child to conclude that reading and writing are just complicated guessing games, and he or she can come to misunderstand the purposes of sitting down with a book or trying to write something on paper.[58]

Pearl

The Auditory-Verbal practitioner should help parents learn why reading and writing with very young children who are learning to listen is necessary to their language development and their later academic achievement and social adjustment.

13.8.1 Read-Alouds

Reading with a child should be great fun. In the words of Mem Fox, "When we get involved in reading aloud to our babies and other children, we often forget entirely that we *should* be reading aloud. We have such a rollicking good time, and we relate so warmly to our kids as we read together, that it becomes a delicious "chocolate" kind of experience.[59]

Children need the emotional closeness and the word and language play that can emerge during interactions about a book, whether it is a story or informational. We want them to love and look forward to reading with mom, dad, or another adult. It is never too early to begin, and many parents read with their infants during the first few days at home. It may seem pointless to read with an infant who does not know much about the world, words, and language yet, but reading aloud and interacting with the baby begins to build that very foundation in much the same way that narrating daily experience helps the child build essential knowledge. It is also never too early or too late to begin, and it need never stop. Children, especially children with hearing loss, need to learn how to listen and to use listening to learn. In the exchanges over the content of a book, the child can begin to approximate how to use language, create meaning with it, and modify it according to the responses she or he receives from the adult. Children's books offer the rhyme, rhythm, and repetition described in this chapter as essential to learning about language and reading, and the adult can make this fun by emphasizing them with voice changes, hand motions, expressive faces, and requests to join in saying and singing them. Props can be used to represent characters and objects in acting out the story in a concrete way. Reading with a child can involve both indirect and direct teaching of language and literacy, and the importance of helping the child be an active participant in either case cannot be overstated. The adult involved needs to be aware of the child and his or her interests and background knowledge in relation to the material at hand. This is not a time to "fill up the child" with words or knowledge, but, instead, to involve the child in actively constructing meaning together in the presence of the words and pictures in the book.

Indirect Teaching During Read-Alouds

Indirect teaching while reading with a child provides multiple opportunities to practice conversational language; make explanations in terms of the child's life experiences; use new words and phrases in context; present new combinations of sounds, syllables, and environmental sounds; explore longer sentences, items in a series, and story structures; map descriptions onto pictures; and talk about what might happen next and how to solve a problem. Reading together builds attunement between the child and adult and creates opportunities to talk about feelings and emotions: How does this character feel? Why? How would you feel if you were the kid in this book?

It is important to regard the book as a guideline for these kinds of interactions. There will be times when the child shows more interest in a particular picture than in the words read aloud, and it is fine for the adult to ignore the words and just talk with the child, giving the child ample time to respond and bring up whatever he or she is thinking about. This gives the adult good clues about where and how the child is functioning in thinking and in language. By following the child's lead, the adult demonstrates deep regard for the child's thoughts and feelings, emotional bonds are created, and both will look forward to and engage in more reading sessions and, thus, more reading and language practice.

Direct Teaching During Read-Alouds

Children are ready for direct teaching about reading when they start showing interest in the mechanics of reading. This can involve actions such as trying to turn the page, pointing to a letter or word and saying it, running a finger along under the words being read, and so on. Such direct teaching can take the form of questions, explanations, and directions: Do you know this letter? This word? Can you find an m on this page? Can you find the letter your name starts with? How many b's can you find? This word is star. Show me which way we go here. Here is the title of this book. Show me how to turn the page. Where do I start?[60] All of this should be done in fun and without coercion. If the child enjoys it and wants to know more, that is fine. If not, the adult can save it for another time.

Reading Aloud with a Child with Hearing Loss

When preparing for a read-aloud, the first step is to make sure the child's technology is working and that the child is getting the clearest sound possible from it. The pair should sit comfortably next to each other with the book visible to both and conversation about it enhanced by good listening conditions.

Just as in reading with a child with typical hearing, two worthy goals include: (1) reading for a total of 45 minutes a day, split into two or more sessions,[61] and (2) reading three stories during each session: a favorite, a familiar, and a new one.[59] Fox calculates this adds up to more than one thousand stories a year and a huge number of stories and words that can be accumulated before the child begins school and formal reading instruction.

The adult should concentrate on clear, simple steps, beginning with a welcome or a description (Let's read this book together. I think you'll like this book. It is about trains.). Reading should be enthusiastic, and the adult's voice should vary in pitch and tempo according to the story and the characters involved so as

to help the child create meanings that connect the words heard to the pictures seen. Practicing reading the book aloud before the reading session is recommended.[62] The best readings by adults are readings for meaning and for excitement; if the meaning is not being processed by the adult, it will not show up in the auditory signal, and it will be harder for the child to connect it to what he or she knows. Stopping to look at pictures, make explanations using words the child already knows, and to exchange questions and answers promotes thinking and learning. These steps are the same for children of all ages with appropriate increases in vocabulary level as the child grows older. Parents and children can read together well into upper elementary and high school.[62] If this seems extreme, consider that adults enjoy going to readings presented by the authors of books that interest them.

Language Experience Book

Writing with a child should also begin at a very young age so the child learns that the words people say can be written down and that speech is segmented into words with spaces between them. Ideally, this takes place mainly between the parent(s) and the child, because they are usually together on a daily basis. The practitioner, teacher, and other adults can participate as circumstances allow. It is important for the child to see the adult writing and drawing pictures and then to enjoy listening to the adult read the words, followed by looking at and talking about the pages together. This provides listening, vocabulary, usage, and conversational practice. The LEB, especially for the younger child, narrates that child's life, recording the accumulating day-to-day experiences of the child in a simple notebook or in single booklets, each about a particular experience. At first, the adult supplies the language and the image (a drawing, a photo, a souvenir), using words already being used with and by the child. The goal is to make daily entries or books and to use these special books during read-alouds. In these first "readers," the child has the advantage of encountering words in print that he or she knows in speech, thus facilitating both reading comprehension and word identification.

As the child grows older, the authorship shifts gradually from the adult to the child in a spiral progression that includes the adult supplying new words the child needs to know; the child telling a story, and the adult writing the child's words; and the adult coaching the child as the child writes his/her own words and the adult suggests others. Ultimately, the child becomes a young adult who writes for him/herself to fulfill educational and personal communication goals. The LEB process may even prompt the young adult to keep a daily journal.

During the child's preschool and early elementary years, the LEB can go to the school in the child's bookbag to be shared with the teacher, thus informing him or her about the child's experiences and the words being used at home to describe them. As time passes, the medium can include digital formats in addition to the simple notebook or booklets. The accumulated LEBs also document the growth in the child's experiences and language abilities and further serve to impress on the child the importance of communicating with others in meaningful words. They also teach the child that books and writing come from people and that she or he can be part of this process. Please see Chapter 5, which also addresses making and using language experience books.

13.9 The Need for Higher-Level Thinking

Learning how to read and write must be thought of as continuous life-long processes for all literate people, including those with hearing loss. It is not enough to "crack the code," so as to identify words, or to amass a decent vocabulary, because the conceptual demands of reading and writing increase through the grades, higher education, and into a lifetime of activity. In the words of Smith, "Reading is thinking that is partly focused on the visual information of print; it's thinking that is stimulated and directed by written language."[27] Without access to ways of thinking that equip one for the evolving demands of language necessary to learn about and interpret an increasingly complex world, the child will not become an adult who consciously seeks new ideas, explanations, and questions. For this reason, those responsible for children becoming literate must take seriously the work of introducing them to and helping them navigate higher order thinking, also known as critical thinking.

Pearl

Parents and practitioners should guide children's critical thinking by asking questions that call for thinking beyond the concrete here and now.

13.9.1 Higher-Level Thinking: Critical Thinking for Children

Learning to apply higher order questions to experiences, whether those experiences take place in the natural or social world, or in text, enables children to pursue higher levels of educational achievement and to operate independently and creatively in their chosen endeavors.

Consider how the following questions[63] can be entertained by an elementary school child and by an adult engaged in solving a real-life problem. Being able to think critically in the presence of text makes for a critical reader and writer.

- How do I know?
- Why should I know it?
- How might my perspectives/assumptions be different from those of others? What are some other perspectives? How do others think about this?
- How would I solve the problem we're talking about?

Instruction, even before the formal teaching of reading begins, must go beyond asking questions whose answers appear literally in spoken language and written text. Auditory-Verbal therapy can give children many opportunities to think beyond the obvious and to make new connections using the materials and experiences at hand. As I watched Helen Beebe interact with my young child, I realized she was helping her think critically and abstractly in terms of ideas represented on paper in matrices and concept umbrellas. This pioneering A-V therapist was helping my daughter listen, categorize, remember, and make a novel response.

Critical thinking involves seeking evidence for making a claim, understanding where that claim fits into an argument, and then deciding how that argument compares to arguments made by others. Children can be challenged to think in these ways and to pull together many sources of information to solve a problem.

13.9.2 Higher-Level Thinking: Bloom's Taxonomy

The well-known hierarchy of thinking established by Bloom[64] is very helpful to practitioners and teachers in identifying how a child is thinking at a given time so as to make instructional decisions. Bloom's ascending categories begin with knowledge and extend up through comprehension, application, analysis, and synthesis to the pinnacle of evaluation. More recently, a slight reworking of the hierarchy has been proposed by Krathwohl[65]: remember, understand, apply, analyze, evaluate, and create. In either form, these categories aid in thinking about thinking, wherever that thinking is taking place. *Remembering* a concept and putting words to it is the basis for understanding it. *Understanding* it is necessary for *applying* it and then for *analyzing* and *evaluating* it. The culmination of these processes is *creating* something new, perhaps a new way of looking at something or a novel concept.[66] Knowledge of this hierarchy informs and reminds the practitioner that simply drilling children into remembering words and syntax is not sufficient; comprehension built on memory is the basis for listening, speaking reading, writing, and thinking.

13.9.3 Higher-Level Thinking: Metacognition—Thinking about Thinking

Even very young children can be challenged to monitor their comprehension, and they can be asked questions such as: "What makes you think that?"; "Why did you decide to do that?"; "How will you do it next time?" It is important that parents and practitioners engage them in increasingly complex conversations as they grow. Teaching metacognitive strategies equips children to progress in their reading comprehension.[67] Whether in response to an action, an experience, or a story in a book, children should be prompted to talk about what they understand and specify what they do not understand. They need help in sorting out their thinking and coming to a new understanding. Storyboards and storymaps can illustrate the sequence of steps and events in processes and experiences (steps in making a sandwich, taking the dog for a walk for example), as well as the events in a story book. Talking about how one circumstance leads to another establishes the principle of cause and effect. Older children are often presented at school and challenged to create graphic and semantic organizers and Venn diagrams that help them compare or contrast information from two or more sources.

13.9.4 Higher-Level Thinking: Fluency

Reading smoothly and without miscues is often thought of as the main goal in reading. More accurately, fluency is the successful end-product of many goals having been accomplished simultaneously during a given reading. Consider that a good voice synthesizer can deliver smooth oral readings that can almost sound human—but there is not a person behind that voice who is digesting and delivering language laced with meaning. The reader's schemas and their relevant vocabulary combine with word identification strategies and purposes for reading to produce fluency at any given moment, and it is possible for the same person to be able to read fluently on some occasions, but not others. Rasinski[68] holds that fluent readings are characterized by clear word identification, expression (rhythm and intonation), and phrasings based on the reader's construction of the text's meaning. When a listener is present, the expression and pace of the reading enable that person to construct meaning. Being able to identify words with good reliability (automaticity) is important, because being able to do so allows the reader more cognitive activity to deal with comprehension; therefore, working toward fluency can best be done by reading the same loved texts over and over again, because a well-known text is predictable in its vocabulary, structure, and overall meaning.

13.9.5 Auditory-Verbal Practice and Higher-Level Thinking

Auditory-Verbal practitioners can promote higher-level thinking from the first sessions in working with a child and his or her parents. Doing so involves learning about what the child already knows at whatever age and stage the child is and creating sessions that involve listening, speaking, reading, and writing done for authentic purposes. Authentic purposes can include identifying particular sounds and working one's way up a "ladder," identifying words that go with traffic signs while "driving" a toy car around a town on the table, taking "orders" for lunch and writing them down on a pad of paper, dictating or writing a letter to grandparents, answering who, where, when, why, and how questions, and talking about how to solve a problem at school or in the neighborhood. The prominent educational thinker John Dewey held that learning to reflect on one's experiences is the actual source of learning,[69] and practitioners and parents are urged to take the time to explore, question, problem-solve, discuss, and help a child apply new skills and concepts, thus enabling the child to come to new realizations.[2] Along the way, this kind of work helps the child build executive function marked by being attentive, holding information (both auditory and visual) in working memory, delaying gratification, and exerting self-control.[70] Auditory-Verbal practitioners have long worked in a tradition that nurtures these capabilities in children.

Pearl

Auditory-Verbal practitioners can intentionally build age-appropriate higher-level thinking into therapy sessions and help parents to stimulate such thinking in their children.

13.10 Conclusion

Literacy is complex and simple at the same time. Its complexity lies in the many processes and purposes laid out in theories. And then, such theory helps us step back and realize the simplicity of

making sure we help children with hearing loss learn to listen and speak, that we provide many meaningful experiences that build background knowledge and the language that goes with it, and that we read and write frequently with children using what they know. The Auditory-Verbal practitioner should focus on the present with a child and her/his family while keeping in mind the goals of higher-level thinking and literacy, all with the goal of a happy, productive life for the child. Helping a child with hearing loss become literate is an integral part of Auditory-Verbal practice. It can be a joyous experience.

Discussion Questions

1. Think about children with hearing loss with whom you have worked and are now working. What do you think is responsible for their academic success or lack of it? What could you use in the Auditory-Verbal approach to prevent learning problems?

2. Do you think it is important for children with hearing loss to attend schools designed mainly for children with typical hearing? Why? Why not?

3. Why is literacy achievement critical to academic and social success? What happens to children with hearing loss whose achievement lags behind? How would you talk with a parent about literacy?

References

[1] Hart B, Risely T. Meaningful Differences in the Everyday Experience of Young American Children. Baltimore: Brookes Publishing; 1995

[2] Beavers E, Orange A, Kirkwood D. Fostering critical and reflective thinking in an authentic learning situation. *J Early Child Teach Educ* 2017;*38*(1):3–18

[3] Suskind D. Thirty Million Words: Building a Child's Brain. New York: Penguin Random House; 2015

[4] Suskind D. (2020). Center for Early Learning and Public Health, University of Chicago. https://tmwcenter.uchicago.edu/ tmwcenter/who-we-are/history/

[5] Suskind DL, Leffel KR, Graf E, et al. A parent-directed language intervention for children of low socioeconomic status: a randomized controlled pilot study. *J Child Lang* 2016;*43*(2):366–406

[6] Pintner R, Paterson D. Learning tests with deaf children. *Psychol Monogr* 1916;20

[7] Farquhar G. A study of a reading test. *Am Ann Deaf* 1928;*73*:264–272

[8] Morrison W. The Ontario school ability examination. *Am Ann Deaf* 1940;*85*:184–189

[9] Walter J. A study of the written sentence construction of a group of profoundly deaf children. *Am Ann Deaf* 1955;*100*:235–252

[10] Wrightstone JW, Aronow MS, Moskowitz S. Developing reading test norms for deaf children. *Am Ann Deaf* 1963;*108*:311–316

[11] Qi S, Mitchell RE. Large-scale academic achievement testing of deaf and hard-of-hearing students: past, present, and future. *J Deaf Stud Deaf Educ* 2012;*17*(1):1–18

[12] Geers A, Moog JS. Factors predictive of the development of literacy in profoundly hearing-impaired adolescents. *Volta Review* 1989;*91*:69–86

[13] Goldberg DM, Flexer C. Outcome survey of auditory-verbal graduates: study of clinical efficacy. *J Am Acad Audiol* 1993;*4*(3):189–200

[14] Lane H, Baker D. Reading achievement of the deaf: Another look. *Volta Review* 1974;*76*:488–499

[15] Ling D. Auditory-verbal options for children with hearing impairment: Helping to pioneer an applied science. *Volta Review* 1993;*95*:187–196

[16] Moog JS. Changing expectations for children with cochlear implants. *Ann Otol Rhinol Laryngol Suppl* 2002;*189*:138–142

[17] Roberts S, Rickards F. A survey of graduates of an Australian integrated auditory/oral preschool, part II: Academic achievement, utilization of support services, and friendship patterns. *Volta Review* 1994;*96*:207–236

[18] Robertson L, Flexer C. Reading development: A survey of children with hearing loss who developed speech and language through the auditory-verbal method. *Volta Review* 1993;*95*:253–261

[19] Wray D, Flexer C, Vaccaro V. Classroom performance of children who are deaf or hard of hearing and who learned spoken communication through the auditory-verbal approach: An evaluation of treatment efficacy. *Volta Review* 1997;*99*(2):107–119

[20] Rattigan K, Reed V, Lee K. An investigation into the phonological processing and literacy skills of children using a cochlear implant in an oral educational setting. Paper presented at the meeting of the Alexander Graham Bell Association for the Deaf and Hard of Hearing, St. Louis, MO; 2002

[21] Geers AE, Hayes H. Reading, writing, and phonological processing skills of adolescents with 10 or more years of cochlear implant experience. *Ear Hear* 2011; 32(1, Suppl)49S–59S

[22] Madell J, Taylor Brodsky I. (2018) *The Listening Project*, a film interviewing 15 young adults who had hearing loss identified as children who are now in their 30's. *2018www.TheListeningProjectfilm.org*

[23] Robertson L. Literacy and deafness: Listening and spoken language. 2nd ed. San Diego: Plural; 2014

[24] National Council of Teachers of English. (2020). 2020 Children's Day, Book Day. https://ncte.org/get-involved/2020-cd-bd/. Retrieved April 24, 2020

[25] National Council of Teachers of English. (2019b). NCTE Statement on the Act of Reading: instructional foundations and policy guidelines. https://ncte.org/statement/the-act-of-reading/. Retrieved April 24, 2020

[26] Pearson P, Stephens D. Learning about literacy: A 30-year journey. In: Ruddell R, Ruddell M, Singer H, eds. Theoretical Models and Processes of Reading. Newark, DE: International Reading Association; 1994:22–42

[27] Smith F. Understanding Reading. 6th ed. Mahwah, NJ: Lawrence Erlbaum Associates; 2004

[28] Anderson R. Role of the reader's schema in comprehension, learning, and memory. In: Ruddell R, Unrau N, eds. Theoretical models and processes of reading. 5th ed. Newark, Delaware: International Reading Association; 2004:594–606

[29] Bransford J, Johnson M. Contextual prerequisites for understanding: Some investigations of comprehension and recall. *J Verbal Learn Verbal Behav* 1972;*11*(6):717–726

[30] Heath S. Ways with Words: Language, Life, and Work in Communities and Classrooms. New York: Cambridge University Press; 1983

[31] Rosenblatt L. The Reader, the Text, the Poem: The Transactional Theory of the Literary Work. Carbondale, IL: Southern Illinois University Press; 1978

[32] Freire P. Pedagogy of the Oppressed. New York, NY: Continuum; 1981

[33] Thorndike EL. Reading as reasoning: A study of mistakes in paragraph reading. *J Educ Psychol* 1917;*8*:323–332

[34] Scarborough H. Connecting early language and literacy to later reading (dis)abilities: Evidence, theory, and practice. In: Neuman S, Dickinson D, eds. Handbook of Early Literacy Research. New York, NY: Guilford Press; 2002:97–110

[35] Adams M. Alphabetic anxiety and explicit, systematic phonics instruction: a cognitive science perspective. In: Neuman S, Dickinson D, eds. Handbook of Early Literacy Research. New York: Guilford Press; 2002:66–80

[36] DeCasper A, Spence M. Prenatal maternal speech influences newborns' perception of speech sounds. *Infant Behav Dev* 1986;*9*(2):133–150

[37] Mintz TH. Language Development. In: Squire LR, ed. Encyclopedia of Neuroscience. Oxford, UK: Academic Press; 2009: Vol. 5, pp. 313–319

[38] Fry D. The development of the phonological system in the normal and the deaf child. In: Smith F, Miller G, eds. The Genesis of Language: A Psycholinguistic Approach. Cambridge, MA: The MIT Press; 1966:187–206

[39] Zipke M. Teaching metalinguistic awareness and reading comprehension with riddles. *Read Teach* 2008;*62*(2):128–137

[40] Cairns HS, Waltzman D, Schlisselberg G. Detecting the ambiguity of sentences: Relationship to early reading skill. *Comm Disord Q* 2004;*25*(2):68–78

[41] Wood A. *Quick as a cricket*. Boston: Houghton Mifflin Harcourt; 1982

[42] Clay MM. Concepts about Print: What Have Children Learned about Printed Language? Heinemann: N.Z.; 2000

[43] Goswami U. Early phonological development and the acquisition of literacy. In: Neuman S, Dickinson D, eds. Handbook of Early Literacy Research. New York: Guilford Press; 2002:111–125

[44] Snow C, Burns M, Griffin P, Eds. Preventing Reading Difficulties in Young Children. Washington, DC: National Academy Press; 1998

[45] Adams M. Beginning to Read. Cambridge, MA: MIT Press; 1990

[46] Hansen D, Bernstorf E. Linking music learning to reading instruction. *Music Educators J* 2002;*88*(5):17–21, 52

[47] Kamii C, Manning M, Manning G. Early Literacy: A Constructivist Foundation for Whole Language. Washington, DC: National Education Association; 1991

[48] Piaget J. Origins of Intelligence in the Child. London: Routledge & Kegan Paul; 1936

[49] Durkin D. Children who Read Early. New York, NY: Teachers College Press; 1996

[50] Peterson CC, Wellman HM. Longitudinal theory of mind (ToM) development from preschool to adolescence with and without ToM delay. *Child Dev* 2019;*90*(6):1917–1934

[51] Wellman HM, Peterson CC. Deafness, thought bubbles, and theory-of-mind development. *Dev Psychol* 2013;*49*(12):2357–2367

[52] Peterson C. Theory of mind development in oral deaf children with cochlear implants or conventional hearing aids. *Journal of Child Psychology and Psychiatry* 2004;*45*:1096–1106

[53] Remmel E, Peters K. Theory of mind and language in children with cochlear implants. *Journal of Deaf Studies and Deaf Education* 2009;*14*(2):218–236

[54] Dore RA, Amendum SJ, Golinkoff RM, Hirsh-Pasek K. Theory of mind: A hidden factor in reading comprehension? *Educ Psychol Rev* 2018;*30*(3):1067–1089

[55] Martin B, Carle E. Brown Bear, Brown Bear, What Do You See? New York: Henry Holt and Company; 1967, 2007

[56] Henkes K. A Weekend with Wendell. New York, NY: Harper Collins; 1986

[57] National Institute of Child Health and Human Development (NICHD). Report of the National Reading Panel. Teaching Children to Read: An Evidence-based Assessment of the Scientific Research Literature on Reading and Its Implications for Reading Instruction: Reports of the subgroups (NIH Publication No. 00–4754). Washington, DC: U.S. Government Printing Office; 2000

[58] Smith M. Reading Magic: Why Reading Aloud to Our Children Will Change Their Lives Forever. Orlando: Houghton Mifflin Harcourt.; 2008

[59] Smith F. Reading without nonsense. 4th ed. New York, NY: Teachers College Press; 2006

[60] Piasta SB, Justice LM, McGinty AS, Kaderavek JN. Increasing young children's contact with print during shared reading: longitudinal effects on literacy achievement. *Child Dev* 2012;*83*(3):810–820

[61] Dickinson D. Book reading in preschool classrooms. In: Dickinson D, Tabors P, eds. Beginning literacy with language. Baltimore: Paul H. Brookes; 2001

[62] Ozma A. The Reading Promise: My Father and the Books We Shared. New York, NY: Hatchette Book Group; 2011

[63] Halton M. Critical thinking is a 21st-century essential—here's how to help kids learn it. https://ideas.ted.com/ critical-thinking-is-a-21st-century-essential-heres-how-to-help-kids-learn-it/ (note: this website contains a useful TED Talk). Retrieved April 24, 2020

[64] Bloom B, Englehart M, Furst E, Hill W, Krathwohl D. Taxonomy of educational objectives: The Classification of Educational Goals. Handbook I: Cognitive Domain. New York: Longman; 1956

[65] Krathwohl DA. Revision of Bloom's taxonomy: An overview. *Theory into Practice*, 2002, *41*(4), College of Education, The Ohio State University

[66] Shabatura J. Using Bloom's Taxonomy to write effective learning objectives. https://tips.uark.edu/using-blooms-taxonomy/. Retrieved February 14, 2020

[67] Adler C. Seven strategies to teach students text comprehension. https://www.readingrockets.org/article/seven-strategies-teach-students-text-comprehension. Accessed March 1, 2020

[68] Rasinski TV. Why reading fluency should be hot! *Read Teach* 2012;*65*(8):516–522

[69] Dewey J. Experience and education (Kappa Delta Pi lecture). New York: Touchstone; 1938

[70] Stix G. (2015). How to build a better learner. *Scientific American*. https://www.scientificamerican.com/article/how-to-build-abetter-learner1/ Retrieved May 20, 2020

Recommended Reading

Fox M. Reading Magic: Why Reading Aloud to Our Children Will Change Their Lives Forever. Orlando, FL: Houghton Mifflin Harcourt; 2008

Ozma A. The Reading Promise: My Father and the Books We Shared. New York, NY: Hatchette Book Group; 2011

Trelease J. The Read-Aloud Handbook. 8th ed. New York, NY: Penguin; 2019

Yopp R, Yopp H. Literature-Based Reading Activities: Engaging Students with Literary and Informational Text. 6th ed. Boston, MA: Pearson; 2014

Recommended Website

Reading Rockets. https://www.readingrockets.org. Reading Rockets is a national public media literacy initiative offering information and resources on how young kids learn to read, why so many struggle, and how caring adults can help.

Recommended Sources for Children's Books

Children's Book Awards. https://www.infosoup.info/kids/awards-home. This site lists awards given by the American Library Association (ALA) and other organizations

Children's Books and Authors *https://www.readingrockets.org/books*

14 Dual Language Assessment and Intervention for Children with Hearing Loss

Michael Douglas

Summary

This chapter discusses dual language assessment and intervention for children with hearing loss. Dual language learning (two spoken languages or spoken and sign language) is possible for children with hearing loss with appropriate hearing technology allowing children to have good brain development. Assessment protocols need to be clear and appropriate for each language. Intervention requires good planning in both languages. Family centered protocols should be developed which include families, schools and other clinicians in working together to achieve the goals.

Keywords

dual language, bilingual, majority language, second language learning, monolingual, simultaneous bilingual, sequential bilingual, hearing age, intervention age, basic interpersonal communication skills, cognitive academic language proficiency, compensatory approaches, tag team, heritage language

Key Points

- Dual language learning (both spoken or one spoken and one manual) for children with hearing loss is possible if hearing is enhanced to an appropriate level and the environment is conducive to maintaining both languages.
- Proficient bilingual acquisition for children with hearing loss requires fair and accurate assessment as well as well-planned intervention in both languages.
- Partnerships between specialists, caregivers, and families who take particular roles in developing each language facilitate the most effective intervention.
- Auditory-verbal therapy principles as well as certain spoken language and literacy strategies have demonstrated enough compelling and promising evidence to be recommended for practice.

14.1 Introduction

The idea of young children with hearing loss learning two languages has been met with considerable skepticism among monolingual experts in hearing and speech sciences as well as deaf education.[1] Plagued by unfounded myths that learning a second language might

- interfere with the mastery of a majority language;
- confuse babies with hearing loss;

- cause further delay in the acquisition of a primary language; and
- precipitate language impairment

Clinicians and educators have, as a result, discouraged second language learning among this population for decades; negatively impacting the efficacy of families as well as the social-emotional and spoken language outcomes of these children with hearing loss.[2,3,4]

The truth is that a mounting number of studies have continued to emerge over the last 20 years reporting no inherent problems with supporting dual language learning for children with hearing loss provided that the environment is conducive to maintaining both languages. [2,4,5,6,7,8,9,10,11]

Most recent literature on outcomes in favor of dual language learning not only highlight that bilingualism is very possible for these children, preliminary evidence indicates that it even has the potential to accelerate expressive and total language skills as well as certain pre-literacy skills.[4,8] Literature on interventions for multilingual children with hearing loss indicate that learning environments where specific strategies (mentioned later in this chapter) are consistently implemented seem to be a promising ingredient towards achievement.[8,11,12,13,14,15,16,17] This chapter addresses the specific needs of children with hearing loss who are learning two spoken languages or are learning English while being exposed to a language other than English for a significant amount of their waking hours. Considerations that need to be made when conducting assessment and providing intervention with this population will be discussed. Methods of intervention that have demonstrated the potential to cultivate dual language learning will also be described.

14.2 Assessment Considerations

When conducting assessment on children with HL who are bilingual, standard protocols will likely have to be modified or extended to reflect the added considerations when HL is present.[18] Integrating these considerations starts with a comprehensive examination process that includes appropriate and fair speech and language assessment.

Pearl

Because recommendations will be based on a clinicians knowledge of therapy methods and their outcomes, it might be good for clinicians to contact centers who provide these services to develop a relationship to either observe or receive some kind of mentoring.

The American Speech-Language Hearing Association has identified three ways in which a child who is bilingual may be evaluated. This has been summarized as follows in previous publications:

Ideally, a bilingual speech-language pathologist (SLP) trained in dual language learning considerations and fluent in the individual's native language and English completes the assessment. If this option is not feasible, ASHA recommends the consideration of two other options. The first allows a trained monolingual SLP to conduct the assessment with assistance from a trained bilingual ancillary examiner. The ancillary examiner is one who has received in-depth training in the measures to be used and who administers testing in the native language in the presence of the SLP. The SLP is responsible for scoring and analyzing all testing data. The other method allows a trained monolingual SLP to conduct the assessment assisted by a trained interpreter.[3,18,19]

When hearing loss is present, a full audiological evaluation should preface all speech and language assessment so the clinician can consider audiological results during analysis of the child's spoken language capabilities. Knowledge about what the child can or cannot distinguish auditorily will help the clinician understand the child's responses and learning potential during assessment.

In preparing for assessment, best practice and the law has indicated it necessary to consider all the languages in which the child is exposed.[20] This is because bilingual children are not two monolinguals built into one mind. They are rather, children with two internalized languages that interact and influence each other.[21] Acknowledging this will allow the clinician to consider the impact of each language on the other, differentiate difference from disorder and avoid misdiagnosis. Furthermore, standard scores for some bilinguals may indicate below average performance because certain formal assessments have been designed for monolingual children.[18] There are several other considerations that need to be made before administering a fair examination.

Pearl

Be aware of bilingual phenomenon. Know what to look for so you understand when something is a mistake related to bilingualism, hearing loss, or language impairment.

Firstly, a thorough case history will be needed to capture supporting factors and expose areas of concern.[18] If another language is indicated on the child's case history, that language should be assessed to the extent that is feasible and appropriate.[20] Secondly, the distinction between simultaneous and sequential bilingual acquisition should be differentiated. The distinction between the two is important as each type of bilingualism may present with small differences in developmental patterns.[18]

This can be done based on the age the child began exposure to each language. Simultaneous language learners will be, have been exposed to, or have learned more than one language before the age of three. Sequential language learners have learned one language before the age of three and will begin, or have begun, exposure and learning of the second language after the age of three This information will also guide the selection of assessments for the examination. To make the most appropriate recommendations, the clinician will also need to discern whether the child being evaluated comes from a monolingual, other-language family, or a bilingual, English-speaking family. These distinctions are important, because each home environment may facilitate differing developmental patterns and guide the selection of tests as well. This information can be gathered through a home language survey.[18]

Thirdly, indices such as hearing age (HA) and intervention age (IA) will be important to calculate because they can provide clinicians better measurements to determine appropriate test selection rather than using chronological age alone.[18] For example, a complex sentence test would not be appropriate for a 5-year-old who has only had their cochlear implant or hearing aids for two years.

Standardized testing may be conducted in the native language, if appropriate measures and examiners are available. However, before executing a formal, standardized test in the native language, information needs to be gathered regarding language exposure, use, and proficiency in each language.[3,18] Furthermore, prior to assessment, clinicians must consider certain language proficiency levels in each language such as basic interpersonal communication skills (BICS) and cognitive academic language proficiency (CALP). This will help determine the appropriate measurement according to the child's level of development (i.e., preverbal, pre-sentence, simple, or complex sentence). BICS refers to the ability to understand and use basic words and phrases with context-embedded language in everyday conversational speech. This can take up to 1 to 2 years of exposure to develop. CALP refers to the capability to understand and use language in academic settings for the development of reading and writing. This can take from 5 to 7 years to develop when there is support for the language and up to 10 years without such support.[3] Obtaining preliminary information about an individual's BICS and CALP levels in both languages will assist in determining the extent to which skills in each language will need to be measured at either the pre-verbal, pre-sentence, simple sentence, or complex sentence level.

When formal, standardized assessment has been selected and administered, it's important to note the limitations of formal assessment and that it may not always be appropriate to use the test's norms.[2,18] This is especially the case when the match between the child and the standardization sample is questionable. Alternatively, the test can still be administered with the intention of listing strengths and weaknesses the child demonstrates on test tasks. It will be the examining professional's responsibility to select the most appropriate assessment and method for fair analysis, which may need to include a non-standardized, non-norm-referenced examination.

Such informal measures, done in a context where the child interacts most frequently, can be considered more accurate indicators of a child's linguistic function than standardized scores alone. There are several ways a clinician can utilize objective measurements to analyze informal linguistic skills. This data can be utilized to establish baseline abilities and compare post-intervention achievement. In this chapter, four, common methods are covered.

1. Review of existing data. This type of assessment considers evaluations and information provided by the parents of the child such as previous audiological, speech, language, and educational assessments and observations. Based on the input received from

the review, clinicians can identify what additional data, if any, are needed.

2. Authentic language sampling: Here the child's utterances are recorded while participating in a variety of familiar situations and linguistic tasks (narratives, conversations, etc.) and then documented. This data can be analyzed utilizing mean length of utterance and number of different words measurements.

3. Structured observation: Here the clinician observes and documents certain behaviors in a contrived setting, allowing the examiner to make observations of certain developmental milestones like early communicative intent or play skills.

4. Dynamic assessment. This method embeds treatment into testing, allowing the examiner to determine the child's response to an intervention and document what causes learning to occur. It consists of an informal pretest, intervention, and then a posttest. The more effort required to teach, the less likely the child will learn the skill on his own.

Pearl

If a child is limited English proficient but fluent in another language, this does not indicate a delay in the other language. Perhaps enlisting the services of an ESL teacher would be more appropriate than an SLP or Certified AVT. It's against the law to label someone as impaired or delayed when there is limited proficiency (which essentially means there hasn't been an opportunity to learn the other language).

After informal data is collected in both languages, results of the objective analysis can then be compared to general development and speech and language milestones as these are consistent across numerous languages.[22] In the case of formal or informal articulation or phonological assessment, interpretation of results compares each system to developmental milestones and considers the influence of each phonological system on the other(s).[18,19]

Overall, it's a combination of assessment tools (formal and informal, audiological, language, and articulation) that will accurately reflect the child's communicative capabilities and yield the most useful results. To avoid misdiagnosis, appropriate analysis requires the capability to not only consider the impact of each language on the communicative capabilities of the child, but the capability to differentiate patterns of progress for children with hearing loss and synthesize them into general milestone development and typical bilingual acquisition.[18,19] Either therapy, a trial period of therapy, a referral to a more appropriate professional, or a combination of all three will be recommended. Recommendations are often based on a clinician's knowledge of potential outcomes and intervention environments that generate such outcomes. They are based on fact and not opinion. For the remainder of this chapter, we consider evidenced-based environments and interventions that facilitate dual language learning.

14.3 Intervention Considerations

As with any intervention program for children with hearing loss, it's the partnership between specialists, caregivers, and families that facilitates the most effective intervention and allows

children with hearing loss who come from a home that speaks two languages or does not speak English to develop spoken languages.

Through partnership,

- audiological management provides access to the most up-to-date hearing technology, speech processing strategies, and careful monitoring of the hearing technology
- educational environments provide a consistent emphasis on developing speech, auditory, and spoken language skills in increasingly meaningful contexts
- roles and responsibilities are assigned for each language
- intervention environments are set up to make improvements in all the languages the child needs to communicate effectively

In setting up an individualized learning environment conducive to bilingual learning, decisions need to be made about whether the child will be a simultaneous or sequential bilingual language learner. While each approach has yet to be proven superior over the other, each situation requires a slightly different teaching approach and resources.[1,3] Simultaneous learners need to make improvements in both languages from the beginning. Sequential learners have already learned a language and need to learn a new one while maintaining the development of the first. Maintaining the first language is important to prevent loss of the first language and negatively impacting future learning; referred to as subtractive bilingual learning.[23] When making decisions regarding language(s) of intervention at certain time points (simultaneously or sequentially) clinicians need to consider:

- the child's and family's language proficiency,
- family language use, and
- the child's language environments.[1]

For infants, services should initially be provided in the home language or, if the child is older, the language in which the child demonstrates the most proficiency.[19] For families, providing services in their most proficient language makes it clear about what is needed for their children to achieve spoken language skills (e.g., device use, facilitative strategies, and consistence with the habilitation program). For children who demonstrate proficiency in one language, the use of the more proficient language can facilitate efficient learning of the second language.[24] In cases where no clear proficiency can be determined (which is often the case for bilingual children), individual instruction can be provided in two separate sessions. One in the home language to promote the development of first language skills (which can facilitate family involvement) while a second session in the second language can be held to help transfer skills learned in the first language to the second language.[19,24] Supporting the use of the family language will empower parents to provide the rich linguistic experiences required for a strong language foundation, ease generalization of skills across settings and preserve the overwhelmingly important social-emotional bond of the family.[3,25] Language environments are important to consider when determining the language of intervention because this information drives what children will need to learn to be successful communicators in their school, home, and neighborhood.[7] Considering language environments also facilitates the development of a thorough plan for adequate exposure and practice in each language. Afterall, dual language learning will only occur, if regular opportunities are provided for not only exposure to each language, but quality and intentional practice of both. [4,15]

If you don't consider both languages you could misdiagnose. Perhaps the child is learning Spanish quite well, but if you only consider English, and the English is below average, then you could misdiagnose delay from lack of proficiency.

14.4 Dual Language Intervention Methods

Currently, there is a profound lack of documentation on intervention efficacy for this population. However, auditory-verbal therapy as well as certain spoken language and literacy strategies have demonstrated enough compelling and promising strength to be recommended for practice.[14] According to Guiberson and Crowe,[14] strategies with compelling strength to recommend for use with bilingual children with hearing loss include, teaching key words, teaching frequently used words, teaching novel words, focusing on conceptual knowledge, narrative and story grammar, as well as teaching inferential strategies. Promising strategies include enhanced vocabulary instruction, enhanced/shared storybook reading, cross-linguistic referencing (mentioned later in this section), activating background knowledge, repetitive learning experiences, modeling and prompting, parental involvement, use of visual aids (gestures, pictures, objects, schedules, charts and graphs, etc.), and conversational or discourse skills. For literacy, strategies that have been documented to demonstrate compelling strength include phonics and spelling with visuals, phonological awareness, contextualized grammar instruction, reading and thinking activities, decoding instruction and explicit teaching of orthographic rules. Literacy strategies demonstrated to be promising for this population include book and print concept knowledge and collaborative writing approaches.

The remainder of this section will focus on implementing such intervention strategies via

- professional support;
- compensatory approaches; and
- coordinated support.

14.5 Professional Support

Professional support refers to intervention provided by skilled professionals trained in the spoken language needs of children with hearing loss. For children who are learning two languages simultaneously, a bilingual model, based on models for bilingual

children with typical hearing can be implemented.[1,4,25,26] In a bilingual model, the typical scope and sequence that is followed for monolingual learners is followed (pre-verbal, pre-sentence, simple sentence, complex sentence) in the home language (with either a bilingual therapist and a parent or an interpreter) while a deaf educator or speech-language pathologist takes the responsibility of teaching English. Each professional works in collaboration to parallel lesson plans, focusing on similarities between the languages. For example, in Spanish and English, there are cognates (e.g., *elephant* and *elefante*) and each language has noun + verb structure, a Subject-Verb-Object (SVO) structure and Subject-Verb Prepositional Phrase structure. Focusing on structures that are similar, increases opportunity for quick transfer of skills between languages because the child is essentially only having to focus on one thing at a time.[25] As the children advance in their skills (around the time they can talk about the use of language), bilingual intervention begins to focus on the teaching and facilitating practice in the differences between the languages. This is referred to as the cross-linguistic model.[25] In the cross-linguistic model, the differences between syntax elements in SVO sentences are explicitly taught. For example, in Spanish, the adjective comes after the noun. When a child says in English, *"I have a car blue!"*, the teacher might say, "Oh yes, that's how you say it in Spanish. In English we say, 'I have a blue car,' (and depending on their age) the adjective comes before the noun in English and the adjective comes after the noun in Spanish. Let's try it again with something else." When to use each model will depend on the teacher or clinician's knowledge of the child's capabilities as determined by regular assessment. Refer to Douglas[19] for a more explicit explanation of this model. For treatment of articulation errors, working in both languages is necessitated, because transfer of skills from one language to another does not occur spontaneously.[26]

An example of how the bilingual and cross-linguistic models might be utilized over time for developing simultaneous bilinguals with HL might go as follows (adapted from ref. 19):

1. Initially, during the pre-verbal stage of development, a bilingual speech-language pathologist (SLP) or a monolingual SLP uses a bilingual SLP assistant or interpreter to assist in providing service in the minority language. The main goal is for the parent to learn what they need to do for their child using the home language.

2. As the child demonstrates linguistic performance in the pre-sentence level and is old enough for preschool immersion, a monolingual deaf educator or speech-language pathologist works with the child at school in English and a bilingual SLP or bilingual SLP assistant works with the child and family on parallel lesson plans for individual therapy using the home language.

3. Later, as the child develops into more consistent use of simple sentences and demonstrates the ability to understand and talk about language, the cross-linguistic model can be initiated. During this phase, the child needs support in transferring skills between languages. The bilingual SLP or bilingual SLP assistant provides parallel services in both languages, using the stronger language to build on the weaker language as determined by regular language sampling in both languages.

4. As the language needs of the child become more complex, the monolingual SLP may provide individual instruction in English, the deaf educator may provide small group in English and the

bilingual therapist or assistant may provide services in the home language. All three professionals may work with the support of the bilingual SLP who can provide input during the design of the treatment plans.

This continuum of care could be followed until the child is determined by the entire team to be proficient enough to graduate from intervention.

14.6 Compensatory Approaches

Because there will never be enough professionals to fully support the hundreds of languages spoken in the United States, compensatory strategies are needed to serve families from low-incidence languages such as Farsi or Vietnamese or in a program where there is not a bilingual therapist. There are four types of compensatory support mentioned in the literature. These include services provided through interpreters, the "Tag-Team Approach, parent-centered integrated model, and heritage language programs.[1,19,26,27,28]

14.6.1 Support through Interpreters

For families who need services in low-incidence languages, every effort is made to find interpreters, train them regarding policies for sequential translation (interpreting what was said right after the speaker is finished versus simultaneous translation, where the interpreter speaks at the same time as the speaker), then brief them on the lesson prior to the interaction. During the interaction, the managing professional takes care to make eye contact with the client while respecting the limits of the translator's memory for sentences. After the therapy session, the managing professional and interpreter identify any issues about the session that need to be discussed and to arrange the next.[29]

14.6.2 Tag-Team Approach

If an interpreter is not available, the Tag-Team Approach, as defined by McConkey-Robbins,[30] can be utilized. Using lessons available in a variety of languages and English from resources like the John Tracy Clinic (JTC) Correspondence Course.[31] The Hanen Centre, www.languagelizard.com, or even free, downloadable resources from the rehabilitation page www.medel.com, the therapist selects the resource in both English and in a language spoken by the family to use as the interpreter. This, of course, requires that the family be literate in their first language. The therapist demonstrates the activity in English, then invites the family member to "tag team" or repeat the same activity in their language. Without knowing the language, the professional observes the parents' interaction style and provides nonverbal feedback (e.g., smiles, head nods, gestures, etc.). Linguistic boundaries are mutually agreed on between the parent and the professional, deciding on who takes responsibility for each language. These boundaries are built into the treatment plan in the Tag-Team Approach and applied as the child with hearing loss learns to interact with the professional in one language and with the parent in another. Implemented appropriately, the creation of linguistic boundaries can send the message to children that both languages are valued

and valuable while setting the stage for learning differences between languages.[25] The tag-team approach can be implemented with bilingual families and monolingual other-language families.

14.6.3 Parent-Centered Integrated Model

Another way to support parents who are proficient bilinguals (e.g., speaking English and another language fluently) and have chosen to develop both languages simultaneously with their young child with hearing loss, a parent-centered integrated bilingual model can be implemented. In this model, individual parent-centered therapy is provided with the help of a monolingual SLP.[3] The parent is enlisted to practice the strategies learned in the therapy session with their child at home in either the minority language or both languages. Immersion of the majority language through an auditory-oral or regular preschool with small student-teacher ratios is also recommended. As the child progresses in the parent-centered integrated bilingual model, professional support and coordinated models may be implemented to address the child's needs at each stage of bilingual development.[7] Some families who are fluent in two languages, or who have one parent fluent in one language with the other parent fluent in another language, may choose to have one parent speak to the child in one language and the other parent speak to the child in the other language, providing the child with bilingual language exposure.

14.6.4 Heritage Language Programs

Heritage language programs facilitate learning of a home or ancestral language. They may be found in in-school bilingual education program models, in-school foreign-language classes targeting heritage language speakers of the language (e.g., Hawaiian), and community-based programs outside of school hours.[28] Half-day preschool or weekend-based community heritage language programs may be a viable option for some children who have hearing loss and their parents who want to provide an opportunity for learning a second language. This support can be helpful for simultaneous learners as well as sequential learners. Families can find heritage language programs in all 50 states and review program profiles via the following website: http://www.cal.org/heritage/about/index.html.

14.7 Coordinated Support

Meeting the needs of children who are developing two languages sequentially can be achieved through coordination with professionals in the community (e.g., working with teachers in a heritage language program or individual tutors). After the child demonstrates proficiency in the first language, around the age of three or four, the second language can be introduced using a cross-linguistic model. Professionals work in tandem with teachers who specialize in English as a second language or the targeted language to effectively accommodate the needs of these children.[3] To prevent subtractive language learning of the first language, care should be taken to ensure that the skills of the first language are not sacrificed at the expense of learning the second language.[32,33]

14.8 Conclusion

Supporting the development of proficient bilingual acquisition for children with hearing loss requires fair and accurate assessment as well as well-planned intervention in both languages. This is accomplished through a variety of methods, implemented by a team of professionals, including the family, who take particular roles in developing each language. Doing so has the potential to set the foundation for future success both linguistically and socially-emotionally with these children and their families. While there is much work to be done on documenting the effectiveness of dual language interventions and outcomes, there is plenty of evidence to support these methods so children from bilingual and other language homes can be more effective as communicators and participate meaningfully across linguistic environments.[1,8,14,26]

Discussion Questions

1. 1. When you read or hear the idea of "dual language learning for children with hearing loss," what feelings come up for you? Are they tenuous feelings, feelings that indicate curiosity, or something else? How have your historic influencers contributed to these feelings?

2. What are the benefits of facilitating dual language intervention? What are some roadblocks? What are some potential solutions?

3. What kinds of adaptations, modifications, and additions might be required for a program to effectively deliver services to children and their families who are bilingual or are from other language homes?

4. Discuss potential testing materials you would consider for this population. How might you modify the interpretation of these tests based on the learner?

5. What additional training or readings might one need to better understand appropriate hearing, speech, and language diagnoses and treatment of children with hearing loss who are bilingual or come from a home where English is not spoken?

6. If you are bilingual, reflect and describe your proficiency in each language and how you became bilingual. How might your personal experiences impact your counseling?

7. If you are not bilingual, reflect and describe why you are not bilingual. Describe how your experiences may impact your counseling.

14.9 Case Studies

Case 1

Janette is 16 months old and has a profound sensorineural hearing loss in her left ear and a severe hearing loss in her right ear which was identified when she was 13 months of age. The cause of her hearing loss is unknown. She wears a hearing aid in her right ear and a recently activated cochlear implant in her left ear. Her parents speak only Spanish in the home. Both parents have a high school education. Dad is a farmer and reportedly knows "some" English. Mom stays at home and understands and speaks only Spanish. They have lived in a Spanish-speaking neighborhood for three years and have no plans to return to their home country, Mexico. Janette has normal health, normal cognition, and a gregarious personality.

They have access to a public-school system who contracts with a listening and spoken language infant, toddler, and preschool program that has Spanish-English service providers. She has been in early intervention, receiving services in Spanish since she was 14 months of age. The language of the public, mainstream school system is English. Her pure tone average with her cochlear implant is 20 dB HL and 30 dB HL with her hearing aid. Her language age in Spanish, based on criterion-referenced assessment, is 13 months.

Discussion Questions

1. Does this child come from a bilingual or monolingual other-language family?

2. Is the child limited English/other proficient or linguistically delayed? In which language? How do you know? Do you need further assessment? If so, what type and what would that entail?

3. Does she need to develop two languages? If so, why?

4. How could she do it? Simultaneously or sequentially? Explain your rationale.

5. By which process? Professional? Compensatory? Who's doing what?

6. What language of Individual Intervention would you recommend? What would be the language of Early Childhood School?

7. How would you help a family develop a plan and realistic expectations for Janette?

8. How would you structure a therapy program to make improvements in two languages?

9. After review of your recommended therapy program, do they have potential to facilitate improvements in both languages? How do you know?

Case 2

Noura is a 12-year-old girl with bilateral severe-profound hearing loss who recently immigrated to the United States with her family. The cause of her hearing loss was unknown, and her aided pure tone average bilaterally was 55 dB HL. Her parents and older siblings speak English and Arabic, but on the recommendations of past educators, audiologists, and speech-language pathologists, Noura speaks only Arabic. She is reportedly a graduate from an auditory-verbal therapy program and relies heavily on lip reading. She has normal health and cognition. She is polite and gregarious. Her most recent speech, language, and school reports indicate that she is an A and B student, is well liked by her friends and can converse in complete sentences on a variety of topics with intelligible deaf speech and has good spontaneous use of communication strategies when she misses the message. Her Dad works in the oil business and her mom stays at home. Her three older siblings have normal hearing and attend college. While establishing audiological care, her parents ask if she can learn English or if she should continue private tutoring in Arabic only. They plan to return to Saudi Arabia, where English is widely spoken and valued in universities and the workforce.

Discussion Questions

1. Does this child come from a bilingual or monolingual other-language family?
2. Is the child limited English/other proficient or linguistically delayed? In which language? How do you know? Do you need further assessment? If so, what type and what would that entail?
3. Does she need to learn another language? If so, why?
4. How could she learn another language? Simultaneously or sequentially? Explain your rationale.
5. By which process? Professional? Compensatory? Who's doing what?
6. What language of Individual Intervention would you recommend? What would be the language of Early Childhood School?
7. How would you help the family develop a plan and realistic expectations for Noura?
8. What would you recommend to the family to make improvements in a second language while maintaining the first? What other disciplines would you enlist?
9. After review of your recommendations, do they have the potential to facilitate learning of a new language? How do you know? What did you recommend for the family to do maintain the first language?

Case 3

48-year-old woman Daniela approached the author of this chapter after participating in a workshop on dual language learning for children with hearing loss. She explained that she was born to Italian immigrant parents and has two older siblings. When her parents immigrated to Canada, they moved into a neighborhood where most of the people spoke Italian. They spoke Italian to their children and English at a basic interpersonal communication level. Daniela was diagnosed with severe-profound deafness at 18 months of age because her mother recognized she was not developing speech like her older siblings did when they were young. The early intervention program professionals recommended that the family speak only English to her and that she needed to learn sign language. Her parents learned English and sign with Daniela and Daniela continued to learn spoken English and sign language in school through a total communication program. Daniela reminisced "I remember that at the dinner table my parents and siblings would speak Italian to each other and then they would switch to English with me. I remember not being able to understand them when they spoke Italian and feeling that it wasn't fair." She further explained that "no one in my family learned sign language very well. I learned sign language very well, I am fluent and am a teacher of the deaf. I can speak and sign, learning a language is not a problem for me." Sadly, Daniela's mother passed away two years before the conference from Alzheimer's disease. Daniela ended her story telling the author that she was glad to know about the dual language learning possibilities for children with hearing loss. As her mom's mind dwindled away, she reverted to using Italian only and Daniela was no longer able to "connect with her" mother in her final years. "I lost her more than two years ago," confessed Daniela.

Discussion Questions

1. At the time of her diagnosis, did Daniela come from a bilingual or monolingual other-language family?
2. How did the professionals' biases interfere with the treatment plan?
3. Did she need to develop two languages? If so, why? Which ones?
4. How could she have learned two spoken languages? Simultaneously or sequentially? Explain your rationale.
5. By which process? Professional? Compensatory? Who could have taken responsibility for which languages?
6. What language of individual intervention would you have recommended? What would the language of Early Childhood School be?
7. How would you have helped the family develop a plan and realistic expectations for Daniela?
8. How would you have structured a therapy program to make improvements in the languages Daniela needed to be a part of her family and school?

References

[1] Douglas M. Habilitation considerations for families who are linguistically diverse. In: Eisenberg LS, ed. Clinical Management of Children with Cochlear Implants. 2nd ed. San Diego, CA: Plural Publishing; 2017:651–663

[2] Werfel KL, Douglas M. Are we slipping them through the cracks? The insufficiency of norm-referenced assessments for identifying language weaknesses in children with hearing loss. *Perspect ASHA Spec Interest Groups* 2017;2(9):43–53. doi:10.1044/persp2.SIG9.43

[3] Douglas M. Teaching children with hearing impairment to listen and speak when the home language is not English. *Perspect Hear Hear Disord Childhood* 2011a;21:20–30

[4] Bunta F, Douglas M, Dickson H, Cantu A, Wickesberg J, Gifford RH. Dual language versus English-only support for bilingual children with hearing loss who use cochlear implants and hearing aids. *Int J Lang Commun Disord* 2016;51(4):460–472

[5] Phillips AH. (1999). Retrospective study of 48 hearing impaired children who participated in Montreal Oral School for the Deaf parent infant and/or nursery program (birthdates 1987–1993). Research Reports. Gouvernement du Quebec

[6] McConkey Robbins A, Green JE, Waltzman SB. Bilingual oral language proficiency in children with cochlear implants. *Arch Otolaryngol Head Neck Surg* 2004;130(5):644–647

[7] Thomas E, El-Kashlan H, Zwolan TA. Children with cochlear implants who live in monolingual and bilingual homes. *Otol Neurotol* 2008;29(2):230–234

[8] Bunta F, Douglas M. The effects of dual language support on the English language skills of bilingual children with cochlear implants and hearing aids as compared to monolingual peers. *Lang Speech Hear Serv Sch* 2013;44:281–290 10.1044/0161-1461(2013/12-0073)

[9] Deriaz M, Pelizzone M, Pérez Fornos A. Simultaneous development of 2 oral languages by child cochlear implant recipients. *Otol Neurotol* 2014;35(9):1541–1544 10.1097/MAO.0000000000000497

[10] Guiberson M. Bilingual skills of deaf/hard of hearing children from Spain. *Cochlear Implants Int* 2014;15(2):87–92

[11] Teschendorf M, Janeschik S, Bagus H, Lang S, Arweiler-Harbeck D. Speech development after cochlear implantation in children from bilingual homes. *Otol Neurotol* 2011;32(2):229–235

[12] Lund E, Werfel KL, Schuele CM. Phonological awareness and vocabulary performance of monolingual and bilingual preschool children with hearing loss. *Child Lang Teach Ther* 2015;31(1):85–100

[13] Alfano A, Douglas M. Facilitating preliteracy development in children with hearing loss when the home language is not English. *Top Lang Disord* 2018;*38*(3):194–201

[14] Guiberson M, Crowe K. Interventions for multilingual children with hearing loss: a scoping review. *Top Lang Disord* 2018;*38*(3):225–241

[15] Lund E, Douglas M. Teaching vocabulary to preschool children with hearing loss. *Except Child* 2016;*83*(1):26–41 10.1177/0014402916651848

[16] McDaniel J, Benítez-Barrera CR, Soares AC, Vargas A, Camarata S. Bilingual versus monolingual vocabulary instruction for bilingual children with hearing loss. *J Deaf*

[17] Werfel K, Douglas M, Ackal L. Small-group phonological awareness training for pre-kindergarten children with hearing loss who wear cochlear implants and/or hearing aids. *Deafness Educ Int* 2016;*18*(3):134–140 10.1080/14643154.2016.1190117

[18] Douglas M. Assessment considerations for children with hearing loss who are culturally and linguistically diverse. In: Bradham T, Houston T, eds. Assessing Listening and Spoken Language in Children with Hearing Loss. San Diego, CA: Plural Publishing; 2015:307–329

[19] Douglas M. Dual Language Learning for Children with Hearing Loss: Assessment, Intervention and Program Development. Innsbruck, Austria: MED-EL; 2014

[20] Individuals with Disabilities Education Act (IDEA; 2004), Federal Register, Volume 71, No. 156 Part V, Department of Education, 34 CFR part 300

[21] Pearson BZ. Raising a Bilingual Child. New York, NY: Random House; 2008

[22] Prath S. Red flags for speech-language impairment in bilingual children. Differentiate disability from disorder by understanding common developmental milestones. *ASHA Lead* 2016; 10.1044/leader.SCM.21112016.32

[23] Wright SC, Taylor DM, MacArthur J. Subtractive bilingualism and the survival of the Inuit language: Heritage versus second-language education. *J Educ Psychol* 2000;*92*(1):63–84

[24] Mattes LJ, Garcia-Easterly I. Bilingual Speech and Language Intervention Resource: Lists, Forms, and Instructional Aids for Hispanic Students. Oceanside, CA: Academic Communication Associates, Inc.; 2007

[25] Kohnert K, Derr A. Language intervention with bilingual children. In: Goldstein B, ed. Bilingual Language Development and Disorders in Spanish-English Speakers. 2nd ed. Baltimore, MD: Paul H. Brookes; 2012:311–338

[26] Douglas M. Teaching Children with CIs to Speak More than One Language. *hearSay.* 2011:7. Raleigh, NC: MED-EL. http://s3.medel.com/downloadmanager/downloads/bridge_us/Hearsay_Newsletters/en-US/HearSay_Issue_7.pdf

[27] Douglas M. The Center for Hearing and Speech: Bilingual support services through video-conferencing technology. *Volta Review* 2012;*112*(3):345–356

[28] Wright WE. Heritage language programs in the era of English-only and No Child Left Behind. *Heritage Language Journal* 2007;*5*(1):1–26

[29] Langdon HW, Quintanar-Sarellana R, Helm-Estabrooks N, Rainer NB, Whitmire K. Roles and responsibilities of the interpreter in interactions with speech-language pathologists, parents, and students. *Semin Speech Lang* 2003;*24*(3):235–244

[30] McConkey Robbins A. Clinical management of bilingual families and children with cochlear implants. *Loud and Clear!* 2007,1. https://amymcconkeyrobbins.com/PDF/Clinical_Management_of_Bilingual_Families.pdf

[31] The John Tracy Clinic Worldwide Parent Education. 2016. http://www.jtc.org/worldwide-parent-education/

[32] Anderson RT. First language loss and implications for clinical practice. In: Goldstein B, ed. Bilingual Language Development and Disorders in Spanish-English Speakers. 2nd ed. Baltimore, MD: Paul H. Brookes; 2012:187–212

[33] Waltzman SB, Robbins AM, Green JE, Cohen NL. Second oral language capabilities in children with cochlear implants. *Otol Neurotol* 2003;*24*(5):757–763

15 Children with Special Needs and Additional Disabilities

Elizabeth Tyszkiewicz and Sarah Hogan

Summary

Hearing loss can occur in isolation, or in the presence of a wide range of other challenges to development and learning. Where there is a demanding care situation, the management of audition may be low on the list of priorities for the family and team around the child. This chapter seeks to explore the ways in which hearing, and hearing technology, can take a valid, useful place in the life of a child who has a range of needs. Readers are encouraged to view each child and family individually, to examine their own attitudes, and to be creative in the way they tackle the problems to be solved to ensure that child, family and support team can incorporate the benefits of auditory learning into a comprehensive programme.

Keywords

additional difficulties, complex challenges, disability, family support, support team, collaboration, liaison, multi-disciplinary working, observation framework, communication, cognitive potential

Key Points

- Establish hearing baseline.
- Modify standard techniques, be "rigorous but flexible"; find ways to obtain accurate measures.
- Be creative about adapting equipment and fitting hearing technology.
- Support child's right to hear and be heard.
- Consider sensory deprivation and its interaction with other impairments—implications for assessment and for learning.
- Parents know their child best, so listen to them.
- View audition as "value added," not another problem to be manage.
- Assess and managed listening environment (e.g., in the UK, many "special school" settings routinely have music playing in the background)
- Embed therapy in real-life communication.

15.1 Introduction

Children who are hard of hearing or deaf frequently have other challenges that need attention. Demographic data over the last decades suggest that the prevalence of one or more additional disabilities is 30-40%.[1] It is understood that although we talk about "additional difficulties," the impact of these difficulties is not additive but multiplicative[2] and in some instances, the term "complex needs" better reflects the inter-relationship of the child's various challenges. The age at which deafness is identified in multiply challenged children is later, on average than for children with deafness alone for a variety of reasons including the necessity for medical interventions.[3] Medical intervention is sometimes needed because the complex difficulties can arise from chromosomal or genetic origins, prematurity, low birth weight, or from environmental teratogens.[4] The hearing loss may be diagnosed at the end of a list of other diagnoses or, by virtue of Newborn Hearing Screening Programs, the hearing impairment may be the first indicator of other yet undiagnosed difficulties. These additional needs can include medical, cognitive, physical, behavioral and emotional problems, as well as dual sensory impairment or specific speech and language disorders. Each additional difficulty can have a specific presentation from mild to severe which can interact in different ways in different children, giving rise to an extremely heterogeneous population. The wide variance in the children's needs highlights 1) an inadequacy in our vocabulary in applying appropriate descriptors that are understood across disciplines, and 2) the inability to make generalizations for children with similar etiologies.

In this chapter we have tried to make observations that apply universally to our interactions with the parents of children with multiple needs and suggest how we might best support them.

The expectations for children with complex needs are often guided by their developmental profile. For example, we know that speech recognition capabilities for children with complex developmental issues are highly related to their developmental profile.[5] By working effectively with professionals across many disciplines, we can offer strong supportive networks that will enable the child and will support the family to nourish their child's development.

15.1.1 Case Example

A therapist receives a referral from a pediatrician requesting support for a 6-month-old child who has profound hearing impairment. The letter begins with the following list:

Chronological age—6 months; corrected age—2 months

Second twin born at 25 weeks gestation

Birthweight 1 lb. 11 oz.

Duration on NICU/SCBU: 6 months

Patent ductus arteriosus (PDA)

Intraventricular haemorrhages (IVH)

Bronchopulmonary dysplasia (chronic lung disease)

Retinopathy of prematurity

Necrotising enterocolitis

Cerebral palsy

Hearing loss—profound

Cause of hearing loss—unconfirmed, likely extreme prematurity

This accumulation of clinical descriptions has the potential to create an image of a very sick and needy child. This in turn affects the therapist's expectation and attitude even before meeting the family. The profile of medical conditions describes one aspect of the child's experiences to date but is not the totality of the child's experience.

The parents of the child whose medical conditions just summarized have a conversation with their therapy practitioner just after the initial tuning of his bilateral cochlear implants. His father comments that he could envisage to a certain extent how his listening and spoken language would develop but it is harder to imagine how cerebral palsy would affect his son. Ten years later, his son is a proficient listener, talker, and lover of medieval history, a competent user of his electric wheelchair and a well-known personality at his mainstream school.

15.2 Flexibility in the Assessment of Hearing Potential

For most families, "multiple visits [to the Audiology clinic] are needed to define the exact configuration, degree, and nature of the hearing loss; monitor for possible changes; and alter management strategies as the child's auditory skills develop."[6] An investigation into the impact of the diagnosis of deafness for parents of children already known to have complex needs found that the most reported challenge was the assessment itself.[7] A child who is referred after the newborn period may have had other more urgent concerns overriding audiological assessment or, as a relatively older infant, may have been identified as "difficult to test." However, this is now the opportunity to support the child and family in optimizing hearing potential. By collaborating closely, and being both rigorous and creative, audiologists can seek to make sure that every child fulfils her or his hearing potential. Perhaps at the point when we meet the child, other issues have been at least partially resolved, and now the family is able to engage with audiology and auditory therapy services.

Sound offers connectedness to others and to the world. We need to ensure that the whole team of practitioners supporting the child sees this child's ability to hear, potentially leading to listening, understanding, and verbal communication, as a faculty that needs to be optimized. We also need to ensure that from the earliest days, parents' experience of the team supporting their child is positive and collaborative.

Pearl

Ask the parents about their observations. Listen to the answer.

What can the parents tell you about how to make their child feel at ease?

Will it be possible to conduct the assessment in a position that the parents advise?

How do parents interpret their child's responses?

What reactions to voice have parents noticed?

What responses does the child show to environmental sounds?

Audiology services around the world aim to meet guidelines to diagnose hearing loss by 1 month, to fit hearing technology by 3 months, and to enlist the family in early intervention programs by 6 months.[8] For children who have been born prematurely and who have had extremely stormy neonatal periods, the diagnosis of hearing loss may come at the end of a long list of other life-critical interventions. For other infants, for whom congenital hearing loss makes up one of many different attributes of a known syndrome, concerns for other aspects of their development may distract attention from the baby's ability to respond to sound. For yet other multiply challenged children, the onset of hearing loss is delayed (as can happen in congenital cytomegalovirus [cCMV], as a result of severe neonatal respiratory failure or bacterial meningitis) and because of the child's challenges with moving, verbalizing or maintaining attention, the lack of response to sound or speech in later infancy is not noticed. For these reasons and others, it may be that the child does not fit within the typical timeframe of testing.

With careful attention to the developmental stage of the child, an appropriate audiological assessment can be conducted.

Audiological assessment of children with additional challenges needs rigor but also flexibility. The rigor is maintained by following standardized protocols for audiological assessment as closely as possible,[9] while making thoughtful, appropriate adaptations. Additional information from informal assessments made either by the parents at home or by the wider multi-disciplinary team, perhaps using an early checklist for hearing behaviors (such as: https://www.aussiedeafkids.org.au/signs-of-hearing-in-babies. html, or from one of the many "Hearing Behaviours" checklists), will contribute to the emerging picture of the child's hearing status. It is likely that the full audiological picture will build up over time, with careful record keeping and information sharing contributing to its quality.

Pearl

Parents know their children best. If the parent has a concern, listen to them! (See https://www.babyhearing.org/resources/principles-family-centered-practice) Observing an infant's or child's responses to a specified sound will give insight into the minimum sound level required to stimulate a particular behavior. This is not the same as an auditory threshold but is useful information as a minimum response level.

Observation of auditory responses is greatly enhanced by ensuring parents and other close adults have the skills and awareness to collaborate with the audiologist. For example, we can share information about how a response can sometimes be provoked by another sensory input, such as smell or touch, but can be mistaken for a hearing response.

Colleagues from physical and occupational therapy services and specialist educators frequently have specific knowledge about the physical handling of a child with multiple challenges. An extremely helpful reference in this regard is a 1975 book by Nancie Finnie, referred to by Marie-Celeste Condon in her 1991 article "Unique Challenges: Children with multiple handicaps" and by Susan Wiley and Mary-Pat Moeller.[2] As described in Chapter 2. "Audiology: Building the Foundation," we need to ensure that the child's physical sense of himself or herself is one of being grounded and safe.

15.3 Practical Tips for Keeping Hearing Technology On

The tips given in Chapter 2, "Audiology: Building the Foundation," also apply to families for children with additional challenges but are set within a different context: For the family with a child with additional challenges, the hearing technologies are only one of the numerous interventions that the parents need to manage, as well as taking care of their family and meeting their own needs. One of the most important skills in which we can coach parents is how to look for behaviors that indicate their child is benefiting from hearing technology. If we can help parents to see that their child is accessing sound, that there are definite changes in behavior even though these changes may be very small, we can offer encouragement for them to persevere with the child's technology.

It is not uncommon for hearing technology to present challenges when used by children. Children after all are small, mobile, and not always open to rational argument when it comes to wearing assistive devices of any kind. Audiologists and parents need to be constantly seeking creative and effective means of ensuring comfort and audibility for this population. Where there are more complex involvements, this is truer than ever. It may not be possible for devices to be worn in the conventional way, and other solutions must be found. How can a cochlear implant coil be worn by a child who needs a helmet to protect his head from frequent falls? What type of fitting best suits a child with extreme sensitivity to touch around the ears and face? Can a wheelchair bound individual have part of the equipment fixed to the chair rather than the body, for greater ease and comfort?

This chapter cannot provide examples and solutions for every possible case. Rather, we would encourage, as always, collaborative observation, supporting the family and child in finding what works, and ensuring that there is close co-working within the multidisciplinary team. One size very definitely does not fit all, and sometimes a compromise (e.g., an unconventional approach rather than following strict standard guidelines) can yield significant benefit. A representative concrete example is the decision to provide a unilateral cochlear implant to a child who persistently rests his head to one side, to avoid pressure on the skin and subsequent difficulties in managing the equipment, even though the clinic policy may be to fit binaurally.

15.3.1 How Can We Improve?

Despite the widespread implementation of newborn hearing screening and early amplification provision, many children continue to have undetected, unconfirmed, or unassessed hearing loss through the early years of childhood. While this is true for all children, particularly those who are arriving from less developed countries, it is particularly true for children with complex needs: A study by Gregory and Harrigan in 2013, found that parents report that audiological assessment, which is vital to the process of assessment for cochlear implantation, can be difficult with this group of children and often takes a long time

and that because of the diversity of the group "it is often difficult to get assessments and support that recognizes the interaction of the deafness with the other disabilities."[10]

Non-verbal children in special schools whose various complex needs have masked significant hearing loss are at particular risk of being overlooked. By raising expectations for all deaf children,[1] it is more realistic to hope that identification of hearing loss in a multiply challenged child is seen as a right and positive step forward for the child's overall development.

15.4 Meeting the Child and Family

In his textbook on coaching, John Whitmore has this warning for all of us who have hard-earned knowledge: "It is (…) very hard for experts to withhold their expertise sufficiently to coach well."[11] We have painstakingly acquired expertise in our chosen clinical field. It guides our thoughts and actions in our encounter with our clients. There are benefits to being self-aware, because we can be making assumptions that get in the way of our capability to truly hear and see, especially when we receive a lot of information before we meet the people concerned. In the UK, children with multiple challenges often come to us preceded by reports that present a collection of health conditions, difficulties, and so-called "co-morbidities." It can seem that the parents are bringing not a child, but a cluster of problems, each one of which will make it harder for us to do the job we are competent to perform. We need to be alert to the assumptions that are unconsciously triggered in us by terms such as "epilepsy," "vision impairment," and "CHARGE syndrome." Do these terms begin to limit our view of the individual we are about to meet, based on our knowledge, our previous experience, our "expertise"?

We are reminded by Rush and Shelden[12] that:

Individuals who have previous experience as teachers or instructors tend to rely on or fall back into a directive mode when they are challenged by a particular situation (p. 9).

A parent comments:

I think because we'd taken Anna to so many appointments … audiology appointments and therapy appointments…and there's that real feeling that I used to get when I came out that she'd failed, we'd failed… you know there's always a lot of talking over the top of you like you're not there and just oh no, she can't do that, she can't do that, and just a horrible sense that we're getting it so wrong and that there's so much wrong with her.

For his or her family, the child is an individual, with a personality, a will, feelings, preferences, aversions, and desires. If we are open to their narrative, we are more likely to be able to work with them to optimize their child's auditory and communicative potential. We need to school ourselves in the following skills:

- Asking open questions
- Taking time to listen
- Asking for details and clarification so that we truly understand what we are hearing (for example, a parent might say "she doesn't like music and singing;" a clinician can avoid taking this at face value and simply writing it down in the notes, but

instead follow up with "How does she let you know that?" "Can you describe an example to me?" "What have you tried so far?")

All the information that emerges from the conversation is likely to improve the quality and specificity of the service the clinician can provide.

The family needs us to recognize their experience, and to try to see through their eyes. For this group of children, heterogeneous though it is, routines-based learning is even more than usually relevant. Children and their parents spend the day carrying out their activities while also navigating the challenges presented by his or her particular situation. As clinicians, we need to know the successes they experience, the aspirations they have, and the questions that are at the forefront of their minds.

15.4.1 Conversational Prompts

- *Describe ... for me*
- *What are your best times with ...?*
- *Can you talk about interventions you have had that you found helpful?*
- *What does ... like to do?*
- *Are there things that ... really does not like? How will we know?*
- *Who are the adults/children in ...'s life?*
- *How does ... let you know what she wants?*
- *How do you let ... know what's happening, or about to happen?*
- *What are your best times for communicating with ... ?*

If we can gain a realistic understanding of the family's situation, we have the best chance of devising a truly personalized and collaborative program for the child.

Rush and Shelden express this very clearly in their model that positions the parent as the "coachee": "an individual with knowledge and skills in a particular area applies a coaching interaction style to support the coachee in recognizing what he or she already knows and then builds on the previous knowledge or skills by sharing new information and developing new skills that are based on the coach's knowledge and experience."[12]

As a distinct and individual picture emerges, we learn from the family how they see listening and spoken language fitting into their lives. Our job is to work with them to establish baseline capabilities, latent skills, and available support. Then, together, we can create a tailored program to enable the child to fulfil his or her potential.

Children with hearing impairment routinely have many professionals on their team; family members, audiologists, otolaryngologists, speech and language therapists. Children with multiple challenges are often within a sizable network of professional practitioners who may or may not interact, or even know of one another's existence. This means that parents become a "walking archive" of their child's treatments and interventions. When they attend a session, they frequently have to summarize and report on all the assessments and inputs the child has received elsewhere. If we can find ways to make this less burdensome, we free up time for productive action.

The first people to consult about how to achieve this, of course, are those most closely involved.

Open questions, as always, are our friends.

Pearl

OPEN QUESTIONS

What is it important for me to know?

How would you like to share information about your child's team?

Can you tell me about your priorities for your child right now?

Turnbull et al.,[13] who write from a perspective as both parents and professionals, constantly remind their professional readers to question the influence of their own attitudes and behaviors on the dialogue they have with their clients, as in the extract below:

Responsiveness: You recognize that each individual has something unique and important to contribute; connection, rather than separation, is always the focus. You can begin to use some of the tools skilled dialogue offers by asking yourself:

What assumptions am I making about my power, ability, or knowledge as compared with the person with whom I am interacting?[13]

To what extent have I demonstrated a genuine interest in learning how the other person understands and feels about the current situation?

What am I doing or saying that promotes or sustains the current situation?[14]

For gathering more specific information, it may be possible to ask the family to bring to the appointment the names and contact details of their child's team. If writing is not efficient for them, can they photograph the contact details with their phones or make a short voice recording? We can then seek their permission to share and receive information, keeping them in the loop, without demanding that they take sole responsibility. We can mistake the useful idea of parents being "the experts on their own child" for one more like "you are responsible for explaining to me everything that other professionals have said and done in relation to your child."

Pearl

Respect and actively listen to the child's caregivers as your first source of information. Reduce the parental responsibility burden for information transmission by establishing working relationships with the wider team.

15.5 Encounter with the Child and Planning the Therapy Session

We need to try and put deficit-based observation (e.g., What problems can we identify? How are we going to solve them?) on hold, in favor of really meeting and listening to the child and family, being receptive to what their demeanor, words, and gestures convey.

In an example from practice, a six-year-old girl with severe hearing impairment and other involvements, responds to the question "What would you like to do today?" with "Do you know where the moon goes in the daytime?"

How can we interpret this irrelevant and conversationally inappropriate response? Who can help us understand it? What circumstances prompted it? What is a helpful next conversational turn from us? In this case, spending time with the child, and discussion with her parents suggested that her non-contingent conversational turns, and this phrase in particular, were a means of deflecting questions which made her feel under pressure. This in turn, indicated that it would be beneficial to support her in developing strategies for opting out or asking for clarification, rather than adopting the unusual and socially inappropriate means she had evolved for herself. Many behaviors that seem odd or unconventional may be the child's highly idiosyncratic way of solving a problem, and are worth spending time on for that reason. We can draw no conclusions until we have properly acquainted ourselves with the family and the individuals within it.

While we remain open to the individuality of the child and family we have in front of us, it is helpful also to have a structure on which to hang our observations. We need to establish a baseline of capabilities from which to start our therapy plan. Where a child has a "patchy" profile of communication capabilities because of hearing impairment and other involvements, it is helpful to have a detailed and specific framework in which to situate him or her, which allows us to agree with the family on a starting point for our intervention. We describe a structure later in this chapter that enables the therapist and parents to make fruitful observations within each of the spheres of influence, and to pool them to establish the listening and communication skills the child has already acquired, then to give direction for what to aim for next (see **Table 15.1**).

As supporters of auditory learning, what interests us most is the place of audition in this child's life. Do we have an accurate audiological evaluation? Do we have evidence that this child has optimal hearing technology? Has the technology been creatively adapted to the child's needs and behaviors?

If we can say "Yes" to all the previous questions, the next thing to consider is: Does audition have an important role at whichever level of auditory learning the child is currently working? Are the child's caregivers aware of what he or she hears, and how to provide auditory enrichment within their day-to-day interactions?

Auditory work for some children may start at the level of simply managing hearing technology; for others, the challenge may be the wide discrepancy between their capability to understand through listening, and to respond using speech. We may encounter yet other individuals whose potential for both receptive and

Table 15.1 Observation framework

Auditory access and auditory responses

Physical environment

Communication

Activities

Parental expectation—carry over at home

School setting—carry over at school

expressive spoken language has been underestimated, and who are held back by their communicative environment.[15]

There are also, of course, children with hearing impairment who listen and speak fluently, but whose challenges lie in the areas of pragmatics and social communication. Each one is a specific individual within a family structure, with preferences, dislikes, interests, emotions, and personality. Each one is so much more than the dispiriting list of "co-morbidities" that we find at the head of the referral.

Pearl

Ensure the physical environment does not interfere with the goal of the session by being inappropriate for the child. Liaise with others to gain information about what is needed. Prepare thoroughly.

15.5.1 Auditory Responses

Many physical and attentional factors can affect a child's auditory responses, and in the case of children with multiple involvements, hearing behaviors may be completely different from the ones we expect from uninvolved children who offer behaviors such as turning, eye widening, smiles, or showing understanding of speech. Sometimes, the challenges of keeping hearing technology on and working may be the principal goal for a time: e.g., a child with autism spectrum disorder (ASD) was fitted with cochlear implants at 2 years of age having had no previous auditory experience. This child removed the coils and/or processors 28 times within a 1-hour session. The child was closely observed and the removal of the technology was not associated with new sounds in the environment, with novel sounds, sounds of a certain pitch, or with loud sounds. The family and practitioners noted when the processors were removed and if there were any possible external triggers prior to their removal. They were aware of documenting not just the auditory environment but other aspects of the child's environment in case removal was a reflection of the totality of the child's sensory system. The parent felt supported by the practitioner's acknowledgement that it was hard to keep the hearing technology in place.

Where there have been slow, mis-timed, or unconventional responses, the people who care for the child have sometimes missed these responses and built up over time the conviction that there is no auditory perception to work with. For example, a child with severe visual impairment, even if provided with early amplification, may not display the developmentally expected alerting and localization behaviors, because turning to a sound provides no visual reward. This makes listening a less obvious behavior for the observers, who may go on to assume that the child is not perceiving sound. With a sensitive, collaborative approach, the therapist can support the family in setting up opportunities for the child to demonstrate that she is hearing and understanding, even if this is manifested in an unexpected way.

Whatever the baseline auditory ability is, that is our starting point, so it is crucial both to incorporate the information from audiological evaluations, and to recruit the child's parents and caregivers to collaborate in carrying out observations together with the therapist in controlled situations. Sometimes, the first therapy session that focuses on effective use of hearing technology to demonstrate detection, discrimination, or understanding can be a very joyful occasion for parents who have been toiling with hearing technology to what they may see as no avail. Success, however small, is a tremendous motivator.

Pearl

Be aware that response behaviors may be unusual or very slow.

Recruit parents as active observers.

Set up a successful listening experience as soon as possible.

15.5.2 Communication

The next information set that will help determine our therapy planning relates, of course, to the child's baseline communicative capability. In line with recent research findings[16] our therapy needs to be firmly anchored within serve-and-return interaction, with parents and caregivers at the center. The observations that we make, and the information that we seek, come under the following headings.

Pre-Verbal Communication

Is the child able to engage, and for how long? Does he or she attend to another person singly, or display joint attention, and the capability to track interaction in a group of people? Can the parent gain and hold the child's attention, and does the child initiate an exchange? All of these are strengths, and worth remarking on and supporting, particularly when the child has very low verbal capability. Parents and caregivers may not be aware of the many ways they support and facilitate communication learning as they engage in their day-to-day routines. For example, a father who held out his arms to his child in her car seat, looked directly at her, and asked "You coming up?" with an expectant expression, was not conscious of the many strengths his behavior demonstrated, and how much he was instinctively doing to help his child. Having this observed, described, and affirmed sets the scene for a coaching model of therapy, in which the therapist supports the development of existing skills and initiatives within the family.[17] As therapists, we need to take a keen interest in the content and level of complexity of the messages passing between the child and the parents, because this is the foundation we will work from as we aim to develop auditory and verbal skills. Functional everyday matters are often the most revealing. For example, when a child needs to use the bathroom, how is this conveyed? Does the parent simply ensure that the child goes regularly, or is taken when his or her behaviors indicate a need? Does the child convey the need? If so, how is this done? It could be a point, a gesture, a sign, a spoken word, or a phrase. Any of these is a mine of information for determining the way in which this family communicates in everyday life.

15.5.3 Auditory Understanding and Spoken Communication May Be Mismatched in Terms of Attainment

We need to establish what audition is contributing to this child's communication, and experience of the world. Where there are complex involvements, it is not unusual for a family to say that they do not know what, if anything, the child recognizes or understands through audition. This can be because many communications take place within a firmly established routine, and are supported by circumstantial, signed, pictorial or object-based information. A therapy session is the ideal safe setting in which to undertake the process, that may feel risky for them, of beginning to attach meaning to auditory information. Can the child detect his or her name being called? Does he or she recognize a familiar song or rhyme? Can he or she carry out simple spoken instructions? Is he or she able to follow more than one instruction, or enjoy a story? If there has always been visual or other support for communication, but the therapist sees unused auditory potential, these observations will be crucial to determining the starting level for intervention. People around the child may have assumed that he or she cannot carry out a Ling-sounds[18] based task (see Chapters 3, "Speech Acoustics: Strengthening the Foundation" and 8, "Toddler-type Language: Putting Words Together and Moving Up to Simple Sentences"). but creative adaptations may make it possible. This means the parents and therapist can work together to establish a more and more accurate hearing baseline and liaise with the audiologist to optimize technology.

15.5.4 How Does This Child Receive and Convey Messages, and What Are the Restrictions on This? What Is the Context and the Language Level?

We are also very interested in whether the child conveys messages to those close to him or her, and if so, how this is done (see previous bathroom example). Does the child use non-verbal means, vocalizations, a formal sign system, spoken words? What is the evidence for a range of communicative intents (initiating communication, drawing attention to something, asking for help, making a request, greeting, accepting or refusing, questioning, etc.)? Are caregivers giving verbal responses, expanding and developing the child's message? What are the caregivers' expectations of the quality of the child's communications, and are they clearly modelling the desired behaviors? Where care or behavior need is high, fulfilling it can become all-absorbing for the adults, and we need to be vigilant so that we make accurate observations, and set achievable, realistic goals based on what we have found out. The adults who care for the child are likely to be the most useful source of information about targets for communication intervention. Does this child need to be able to convey basic needs and requests? Take turns and listen to the contributions of others? Organize and convey a message? Name and talk about feelings and emotional responses? What is the level of intelligibility of the child's speech?

Close observation and discussion with the child's caregivers provide a detailed picture of the child's current communicative competence. Possibly, the developmental profile that emerges will be patchy. For example, a child with an extensive repertoire of receptive spoken language might have very limited spoken communication capabilities. This means that the therapy program needs to be designed to take this mismatch into account, and might have to incorporate forms of expression other than speech. These could include signs, picture systems, or Augmentative and Alternative Communication (AAC).[24] This, in turn, will create the need to establish co-working relationships with the relevant members of the child's team.

The goal is always to bring communicative competence into line with cognitive potential. A personalized program is built by all the people around the child, to ensure that the individual can participate as fully as is possible in the life of the family, community, and educational setting. If we don't work to provide optimal communication and language, this child may never be able to show what he or she is capable of.

15.5.5 Choice of Activities

What activities will give the child agency and independence as a communicator?

It is helpful to think of communication goals in terms of the level of agency and independence the target skills will give to the child. At the most basic level, being able to accept and refuse, to protest, and to request what one needs can make a remarkable difference to a child whose mobility and autonomy are limited. Being able to understand what is going to happen, and having a warning when it is imminent, is crucial to a sense of safety and peace of mind. For example, a severely visually impaired child whose verbal understanding enables her to monitor her environment, and understand speech, will live in a more secure and predictable world as a result. At higher levels of language, knowing how to question, discuss, negotiate, and narrate are crucial to social participation and educational attainment.

Pearl

First, establish an accurate hearing and communication baseline, with attention to the non-verbal precursors to meaningful interaction. Be open-minded as to what will be optimal for this particular individual, and co-work with other specialists. Aim to match communicative attainment with cognitive potential.

15.5.6 What Will be the Carryover at Home?

If the scenarios in therapy sessions are based on activities that have direct relevance to the family's everyday living, we can target functional vocabulary and skills that will be most effective for the child and allow the family to learn through successful interactions. Listening to the family, and exploring with them what they are experiencing at home, often gives clear pointers

for the selection of therapy goals. Sometimes, behaviors are indicators of a communicative need that can be instantly incorporated into the program. For example, does a child who climbs on the kitchen counters to raid the store cupboards know how to ask for a snack, or how to respond when offered a choice of things to eat?

15.5.7 What Will Be the Carryover to Daycare and School Settings?

Relationships with the child's key workers at day-care or school can be approached using the same broad principles as those outlined previously in work with parents. Understanding the hearing potential a child has, and learning to use a communicative framework for understanding behavior can be a tremendous motivator for staff in care or education settings. They know the child well. The child will benefit if support team members are included in the planning of goals, and given support to help the child develop appropriate skills.

15.5.8 Case Example

Nadia is 3.10 years old. Her therapist watches as her mother, Hanna, lifts her out of the car and she stabilizes herself on her walking frame. She has become gradually stronger and more proficient in using her frame, which has given her a new-found sense of independence. Nadia's vision, hearing, and balance are affected by CHARGE syndrome.[19] Nadia's therapist greets her at the door and asks Nadia and her mother to find the big balls, which is a way of directing Nadia to a space where she can stretch on the floor with sensory items within her reach. Hanna always builds in time for floor play before her AV therapy so that Nadia can have a break from sitting in her supported car seat before starting her session. The therapist accepts Nadia heading in the direction of the balls as her non-verbal turn in the conversation. This implies that Nadia has understood the spoken information. The therapist asks Hanna for her view: Hanna says she's not sure as she wonders if Nadia is remembering the situation in her previous session. The therapist asks about Nadia's energy levels at the moment and whether they should choose a floor-based session, a table-top session or a combination. Hanna thinks that it would be best to start at a table, as she finds it easier to gauge Nadia's listening attention when she is in a seated position.

The therapist tells Nadia that "It's time to find Mouse, ee-ee-ee." The toy "Angelina Ballerina" is a mouse and is Nadia's favorite toy from the toy cupboard. It waits on the table in the room where many of the activities will happen. The therapist has been careful not to give visual clues to this verbal communication as Nadia has recently had the initial tuning of her unilateral cochlear implant. It is a re-implantation as there was a device failure for her first implant: Nadia has no functional anatomical organs of hearing or balance in her other ear. Nadia alerts to the therapist's voice and looks toward the room where she expects Angelina to be. Hanna and the therapist both note that, although they had previously been conversing, Nadia appeared to alert to the auditory hook of "ee-ee-ee," made fleeting eye contact with the therapist and then looked toward her walking frame.

Nadia's parents have been advised to use a "say-sign-say" sandwich approach to communication with her. Just prior to device failure, Nadia started to put two signs together. However, as her device failed so her signing reduced and ultimately stopped. Nadia has had a period of one year during which she has not been using signs but, coincident with the initial tuning of her replacement implant, she is just starting to use signs again and currently has an expressive vocabulary of about ten signs.

On entering the therapy room, the therapist points to Nadia's chair and says with a finger point "Here's **your chair**!" but Nadia turns her whole body away from the chair. The therapist checks in with Hanna that this is a negation, meaning "I don't want to sit there," even though on other occasions Nadia has been happy to sit there. They agree that it would be an appropriate communication/pragmatic target for Nadia to be able to negate with a shake of the head and a modeled"uh-uh!" They also plan to build on Nadia's capability to make an affirmative choice from two items by using a finger point and vocalization. The close collaboration between the practitioner and the caregiver in pooling their observations and their thoughts, enables effective micro-adjustments to be made within the session that are appropriate in the moment for that activity, on that particular day. The act of collaboration maximizes the chance of effective learning within the session for all the participants.

As expressed by the following quotation, research confirms what families and early language practitioners have long known: Conversational exchange with a caring and attentive partner is the most powerful vehicle for a child's language learning. The "serve and return" model[20] needs to be the foundation of our therapy. In addition, recent research has shown conversational turns to be one of the most predictive metrics of child outcomes. Most importantly, a string of recent studies have indicated that conversations have more brain-building power than adult words alone.[21]

We know that these "serve and return" interactions need to be facilitated with the most important and constantly present people in the child's life, not with professionals, however skilled they may be: research has also shown that parent participation in intervention is key and that supporting parents in competently and confidently interacting responsively with young children during their daily routines is more critical to intervention effectiveness than the time children spend with professionals.[22,23]

For the children with multiple challenges under discussion here, just as for their peers in other situations, therapy needs to be relevant to the daily activities they undertake with their families: eating, traveling, care routines, interactions with relatives and friends, play, exercise, festivals and rituals, and anything else that is part of life, and does not come in a box from a supplier of educational toys!

Pearl

Embed goals in activities of daily life, and in serve-and-return communication.

15.5.9 Case Example

Anthony arrives with his mother and nanny, securely strapped into an adapted buggy. He uses bilateral cochlear implants as well as eyeglasses, and has a friendly, though slightly uncertain reaction to the new people he meets at the therapy clinic. He smiles and appears to enjoy going into the rooms that are recognizable as playrooms, but looks nervous when he sees any medical-looking equipment or devices such as audiometers. He is 18 months old, and it is eight weeks since his cochlear implants were activated. He has congenital profound hearing impairment, and severely restricted mobility resulting from intra-uterine stroke. Anthony is enrolled in an intensive program of physical and occupational therapy, as well as feeding advice and management from a specialist speech language pathologist (SLP).

Anthony's mother is very keen to begin work with his cochlear implant system, and relieved to feel he will now be able to access auditory information. She is able accurately to describe his range of movement, his weak and largely involuntary vocalizations, and the ways in which he expresses pleasure, dismay, or discomfort. In the course of the conversation, it emerges that a recent session with an AV (Auditory Verbal) therapist near her home has been a very significant experience for her and for Anthony: Anthony was able to learn to recognize his mother's utterance of "*Blow!*" and consistently turned his gaze to the bubble wand in anticipation. Both mother and nanny had observed this. The mother is able to share her goals, which are: to build on this early evidence of auditory understanding, and to explore Anthony's potential for vocal communication. Anthony's caregivers arrive with knowledge and experience that, if the therapist listens carefully, point to the direction the support program needs to go. This allows collaborative planning to begin, rather than the therapist viewing the situation only as a "blank slate" to be filled in by the professional's questioning and assessment.

Anthony goes on to make steady progress in his auditory understanding, and to work slowly on physical skills. As soon as he is old enough for this to be appropriate, he is assessed by a specialist team for Augmentative and Alternative Communication (AAC)[24] to identify the best option for his expressive communication.

15.5.10 Dealing with Sadness, Disappointment, Confusion—Your Own and Others'

In the handout material for her course "Assessment and Treatment of Sensorimotor, Attentional, and Emotional Problems in Infants and Young Children," held at Guy's and St Thomas' Hospital, London, UK in May 1998, Georgia Degangi, a pediatric occupational therapist and psychologist/child psychotherapist, makes this comment:

No developmental, behavioural or learning problem affects only the child—there is always a response or an adaptation that occurs in the family and parents. As professionals, we are part of the process.

We always have high aspirations, but we also accept that we cannot determine the outcome of our intervention. Our sadness, confusion and disappointment may be mirrored by that of the family, who came to us hoping that, as auditory verbal therapists routinely do, we were going to help their child develop verbal understanding and speech. For some, this is not an accessible goal. The way we handle our communication with the family and wider team throughout our involvement with them will determine the way in which painful realizations, or difficult decisions are experienced. On the other hand, the family may have a personal view of what would constitute success for them and for their child, and this might not be in line with our different, or higher aspirations. As ever, our view of the child within his or her family and support structures, and our attention to good communication are the resources we need to help us manage the encounter.

Pearl

Practitioners need honesty, resilience, and recognition of their own and others' emotions in offering services to complex populations.

15.5.11 Liaison with Other Professionals—Seeing the Bigger Picture

Children with additional needs usually have numerous practitioners and professionals who make up the team supporting both the child and the family. For some team members, the primary focus is the child, for others it is the parent-child interaction, for yet others the focus may be the family system, or the social situation. The societal intention is to ensure that the child and the family are supported in the very best way possible,[25] but the medical appointments and appointments for practitioners offering family support are also potential disruptors to every day family living. All practitioners aspire to add value to family interaction and to the quality of everyday living. To be a valued resource to the family, practitioners and professionals need to provide strong supportive networks.[26] What do we need to do to ensure that this is the case? Ideally, we practice the seven principles of family-professional partnerships identified by Turnbull et al.[13]: (1) effective communication; (2) professional competence; (3) respect; (4) trust; (5) commitment; (6) equality; and (7) advocacy. As part of the bigger picture, we can also signpost families to other support networks that are both local to the families and remote from them (on-line services), to family support groups, and to other resources that are likely to be of benefit by adding information or services.[13]

15.5.12 Case Example

Five-year-old Nabeela arrives at the therapy clinic looking uncertain, standing very close to her mother, holding a "blanky" (comfort blanket) and not meeting the gaze of anyone who approaches her. She is using bilateral hearing aids, which give her auditory access to speech across the frequency range. Her mother is using the transmitter for her remote microphone (RM). She is the youngest of three children. Her siblings, aged nine and seven, are typically developing. Nabeela has a diagnosis of Autism Spectrum Disorder and attends a specialist program within a mainstream primary school. During the session, she is quiet and compliant, in that she sits at the table, but does not engage with any communication or activity offered. She does not touch any of the items presented, but keeps both hands on her "blanky." After about 20 minutes, she suddenly removes her hearing aids, and becomes distressed when her mother attempts to reinsert the ear molds. Her mother is disappointed by this behavior, as she was hoping to gain benefit from the therapy session and go home with new strategies for supporting Nabeela's communication. She reports that Nabeela understands a range of verbal communication and can express herself though phrases and two- or three-word sentences. She has a strong memory and likes to recite passages from her favorite videos. She loves books with complex pictures and illustrations, and enjoys being out of doors.

The therapist listens carefully to the information Nabeela's mother conveys about her child. She asks about Nabeela's mother's thoughts on the withdrawn behavior they are observing. Information from this conversation points to the fact that Nabeela finds it hard to tolerate new situations and environments, and that she is at her best when she is well-prepared. The family always ensures that they use a range of strategies to provide her with support, including a calendar, photographs of people she will encounter, preliminary visits, an illustrated schedule for what will happen and in what order, opportunities to touch and handle any new materials, and modelling from her siblings. The therapy clinic is yet another new setting. Nabeela is showing signs that she is overwhelmed by the demands it places on her, and cannot co-operate.

In discussion, the therapist and Nabeela's mother arrive at a "lateral" solution for providing therapy services to Nabeela: rather than asking her to habituate to the therapy setting, they will arrange for the therapist to visit home and school as the "hearing advisor" within her known routines. Nabeela's mother takes a photo and a few seconds of video of the therapist, to use in preparing Nabeela for a visit to her home. The therapist gives Nabeela's mother some items from the clinic room (coloring sheets, stickers) to use as transitional objects to remind her of the visit. Nabeela's mother will mention to the school team that the therapist will be in touch about visiting the classroom. The therapy program is "exported" to home and school, so that the auditory work is founded on what has already been established for Nabeela, and energy can be directed to new learning, rather than expended in habituating her to yet another new environment.

15.6 Who Are You? Where Do You Fit In?

If we are clear in our own role and can define for the family what we propose to contribute, they will be in a position to decide whether this is what they need and desire. An auditory verbal practitioner, for example, supports and coaches them in prioritizing listening behaviors in their child. How this aspect is positioned within the child's program is dependent on the "bigger picture," which needs to include all its other components. Constant dialogue and feedback are the means to ensure that the inputs from each team member stay relevant for the family and support the child's overall goals. If we work in isolation, we are unlikely to be relevant. For example, auditory discrimination tasks, while certainly a valid input, may be irrelevant and difficult to implement, if the family's priority is behavior, sleep, feeding, or physical skills. If we can stay well informed about their daily tasks, and in touch with their wider support team, we are far more likely to come up with a realistic contribution. Some surprising connections can occur. For example, if a child needs daily physical therapy, many auditory and communicative goals may be incorporated into this process, perhaps covering turn-taking, following directions, auditory closure, songs, and vocalization. These things cannot happen unless there is good communication, and flexibility to accommodate the child and family's specific needs.

The information received from other professionals will help the auditory practitioner support parents by thinking of ways in which they can develop activities that target not only the language of the play activity but also a motoric goal identified by the physiotherapist or occupational therapist.

What are the auditory hooks, protowords, and language scripts that can be layered on to an exercise prior to and during the activity? For example, a 2-year-old child with bilateral cochlear implants is just learning to roll. Being able to roll his body is a target from the physiotherapist. The collaborating auditory therapist may suggest to the parents that they can set up a "serve and return" situation[20] in which the parent encourages the child to roll by putting a rewarding toy out of reach but within eyesight of the child. The parent can use an elongated vowel with an exaggerated pitch contour to ask the child to "ro-oll," (their serve—a request); the child will physically rotate himself (his return—nonverbal response); "Yeh!" (parent's return offering celebration—comment); child reaches for toy (return).

15.6.1 Introducing Yourself to Other Practitioners and Professionals and Seeking Information from Them

Written communication and clear records are of great value, always with a view to lifting the burden from the family of having to convey their child's entire history every time they encounter a professional. If we seek information from the family about who is on their team, and permission to liaise with them, all we then need to do is ensure that all correspondence is copied to the family in an accessible form. Providing a brief account of our qualifications, our professional role, and the services we have to offer, and giving our contact details is an efficient way to present ourselves to the network around the child.

The parents and the child are best supported when sessional records are clear and complete; when a copy is shared with the family; when each team member contributes observations to support clinical judgment (evidence-based advice) to team meetings; and when all team members share records collaboratively. If the child's support team is communicating well, the parents do not need to be the conduit of information. If the child's support team

is communicating well, the team is a resource to the parents and not a drain on their energies.

If all those involved have a complete picture of the child's developmental stage, it is possible to set appropriate and time-sensitive goals for listening and spoken language development but also to envisage how language can be used in play activities for the child and in the every-day experiences of the family.

Pearl

Our best work is done when we are part of a team.

15.6.2 Professional Boundaries

The LSLS Auditory Verbal certification process allows LSLS professionals the opportunity to both develop and consolidate their knowledge of child development with particular emphasis on communication, children's thinking and their learning. When sharing observations and describing behaviors, terminology and vocabulary may vary across disciplines: If we can avoid jargon but instead use specific non-judgmental language (accurately describing behaviors and their triggers), then we are using inclusive forms of communication that parents, specialists, and non-specialists can understand. Listening carefully to our colleagues, seeking information to help us to understand their goals and processes, providing them with unambiguous and evidence-based information about our observations, and respecting one another's professional status enables harmonious and productive working relationships. The better-informed each practitioner is about the expertise and referral criteria in other services, the more effectively the family can be oriented to additional supports. For example, many auditory practitioners benefit from working with pediatric occupational therapists, from whom they learn to spot the behaviors that warrant referral for assessment of possible sensory or regulatory disorder.

Pearl

In consultation with parents, make referrals to other specialists as needed.

15.7 From the Parents' Perspective

Parents are service users on behalf of their child. Any arrangement that lightens this responsibility frees up energy for the many tasks of family life. They may wish to have a key person within their team of professionals who liaises with them and then acts as a central point for disseminating information to the team. This person is frequently a pediatrician but can be any other member of the team who is likely to be alongside the family for a number of years including the LSLS Cert AVT practitioner, SLP, or specialist educator.

Parents are entitled to be involved in, or at least informed of, all conversations about their child taking place between professionals, other than where there are serious concerns of neglect or harm. Information relayed to the parent will be of most use if it is in accurate and accessible, non-specialist language. We can set up opportunities for families to challenge, to ask for clarification, and to question targets and strategies. As a professional team, we should welcome these opportunities to learn more about the child from the people who know this child best, and we should also be open to questioning or challenge.

As LSLS AV practitioners, SLPs or specialist educators, we aim to support parents in being the best service users and best advocates for their child and their child's needs. There are many books available that have been written by parents about the experiences of raising a child with special educational needs, nearly all of which are humbling and excruciating: humbling because of the dedication and determination of so many parents who know what is needed for their child and who wade through hell and high water to get it; excruciating because so often well-intentioned professionals portray themselves as experts and ultimately place unjustified confidence in their own expertise, or fail to listen to what parents are telling them. *Surviving the Special Educational Needs System—How to Be a Velvet Bulldozer* by Sandy Row (2009)[27] recounts one family's experience of long battles in obtaining correct diagnoses and then appropriate support for their four children, all of whom have special educational needs. The second part of the book's title, "How to Be a Velvet Bulldozer," refers to the parental advocacy described and is an apt aspiration! Are we supporting parents with the tools they need to become excellent advocates for their child, to become velvet bulldozers?

15.8 Concluding Remarks

In a hard-hitting 1987 article, the sociologist Simon Dyson asks us to examine the possible unspoken purposes of assessment, and to pay close attention to the language used in connection with so-called "special needs."[28] While many aspects have improved in over 30 years since the text was written, it still provides a useful prompt to practitioners to examine the unconscious limitations in our own thinking. Much has been written about the way in which an *impairment*, or loss of function, becomes a *disability* when it prevents a person from accomplishing an activity. The *handicap*, however, occurs as a result of the social context of the previous two. What are the structural, environmental, and social barriers to the achievement of the person's full potential? Even in the limited context of our therapy rooms and clinics, it can be enlightening and stimulating to consider these questions.

The family or social group we are encountering may also have very different conceptions of what their child's situation means, and how they wish to tackle it. One of the hardest things we have to attempt is to be truly open to points of view which may perplex us or, at worst, conflict with our own beliefs.

With thoughtful reflection, testing of ideas in discussion with colleagues and service users, and most of all, through active listening, we can attempt to tailor what we have to offer to each of the complex individual who seek our services.

Discussion Questions

1. Bearing in mind what you have read, imagine yourself as the parent of a multiply challenged child. Write five statements that express the characteristics you would like the professionals in your team to demonstrate, or how you would like them to act.

   I want my professionals to. . .

2. What information would you seek from the caregivers of a child who has severe hearing impairment and cerebral palsy, to prepare as effectively as possible for a therapy session? List five items.

3. A three-year-old child with severe developmental delay persistently removes her hearing aids, and her caregivers express that they are ready to abandon the use of amplification. How would you approach this difficulty?

References

[1] Hitchins ARC, Hogan SC. Outcomes of early intervention for deaf children with additional needs following an Auditory Verbal approach to communication. *Int J Pediatr Otorhinolaryngol* 2018;*115*:125–132

[2] Wiley S, Moeller MP. Red flags for disabilities in children who are deaf/hard of hearing. *ASHA Lead* 2007;*12*(1):8–29 https://leader.pubs.asha.org/doi/10.1044/leader.FTR3.12012007.8

[3] McCracken W, Pettitt B. Complex Needs, Complex Challenges: a report on research into the experience of deaf children with additional complex needs. Manchester, UK: University of Manchester; 2011

[4] Diefendorf AO, Corbin KR, Trepcos-Klingler R, Weinzierl AS. Audiologic considerations for children with complex developmental conditions. In: Tharpe A-M, Seewald R, eds. Comprehensive Handbook of Pediatric Audiology. 2nd ed. Plural Publishing; 2017:609–628

[5] Wakil N, Fitzpatrick EM, Olds J, Schramm D, Whittingham J. Long-term outcome after cochlear implantation in children with additional developmental disabilities. *Int J Audiol* 2014;*53*(9):587–594

[6] Sabo DL. Assessment of the young pediatric patient. In: The NCHAM eBook: A Resource Guide for Early Hearing Detection & Intervention. Utah: Utah State University; 2015:1–20

[7] Archbold S, Athalye S, Mulla I, et al. Cochlear implantation in children with complex needs: the perceptions of professionals at cochlear implant centres. *Cochlear Implants Int* 2015;*16*(6):303–311

[8] Joint Committee on Infant Hearing Year 2007 Position Statement. *Principles and guidelines for early hearing detection and intervention programs pediatrics* 2007;*120*(4):898–921 10.1542/peds.2007-2333

[9] Madell JR, Hewitt JG. Audiology: Building the Foundation. In: Madell JR, Hewitt JG, eds. From Listening to Language, Comprehensive Intervention to Maximize Learning for Children and Adults with Hearing Loss. New York, NY: Thieme; 2023:11–29

[10] Mulla I, Harrigan S, Gregory S, Archbold S. Children with complex needs and cochlear implants: The parent's perspective. *Cochlear Implants Int* 2013;*14*:S38–S41

[11] Whitmore J. Coaching for Perfomance: The Principles and Practice of Coaching and Leadership. 5th ed. London, Boston: Nicholas Brealey Publishing; 2017

[12] Rush DD, Shelden ML. The Early Childhood Coaching Handbook. 2nd ed. Baltimore, Maryland: Paul H Brookes Publishing; 2020

[13] Turnbull A, Turnbull HR, Erwin EJ, Soodak LC, Shogren KA. Families Professionals and Exceptionality, Positive Outcomes through Partnership and Trust. 7th ed. (subscription), USA: Pearson; 2015

[14] Barrera I, Kramer L. Using Skilled Dialogue to Transform Challenging Interactions: Honoring Identity, Voice, and Connection. Baltimore: Paul H Brookes Publishing; 2009

[15] Ritter K, Heyward DV, Estabrooks W, Kenely N, Hogan S. Children with additional challenges and auditory verbal therapy. In: Estabrooks, McCafffrey Morrison and MacIver-Lux, eds. Auditory Verbal Therapy Science, Research, and Practice. San Diego, California: Plural Publishing; 2020

[16] Romeo RR, Leonard JA, Robinson ST, et al. Beyond the 30-million-word gap: Children's conversational exposure is associated with language-related brain function. *Psychol Sci* 2018;*29*(5):700–710

[17] Bromwich R. Working with Families and their Infants At risk. USA: Pro-ed; 1997

[18] https://www.audiologyonline.com/articles/using-ling-6-sound-test-1087 accessed 29 June 2020

[19] Trider C-L, Arra-Robar A, van Ravenswaaij-Arts C, Blake K. Developing a CHARGE syndrome checklist: Health supervision across the lifespan (from head to toe). *Am J Med Genet A* 2017;*173*(3):684–691

[20] https://developingchild.harvard.edu/resources/5-steps-for-brain-building-serve-and- return/ Accessed 29 June 2020

[21] Proving the Power of Talk: 10 Years of Research on the Impact of Language on Young Children 2017; https://www.lena. org/conversational-turns/. Accessed June 29, 2020

[22] Mahoney G, Perales F. Relationship-focused early intervention with children with pervasive developmental disorders and other disabilities: a comparative study. *J Dev Behav Pediatr* 2005;*26*(2):77–85

[23] Mahoney G. Relationship focused intervention (RFI): enhancing the role of parents in children's developmental intervention. *Int J Early Child Spec Educ*, 2009;*1* (1): 79–94

[24] https://www.asha.org/public/speech/disorders/AAC/ Accessed May 2020

[25] Dunst CJ, Trivette CM, Starnes AL, Hamby DW, Gordon NJ. (1993). Building and evaluating family support initiatives: A national study of programs for persons with developmental disabilities. Paul H Brookes Publishing In: Wang M., Singer G.H.S Supporting Families of Children with Developmental Disabilities: Evidence Based and Emerging Practices New York: Oxford University Press; 2016:22

[26] McGinnis M. One practitioner learns to become family-centred. In: Rhoades EA, Duncan J, eds. Auditory Verbal Practice Family-Centred Early Intervention. Springfield, Illinois, USA: Charles C Thomas; 2017:289–302

[27] Row S. Surviving the Special Educational Needs System—How to Be a Velvet Bulldozer. London UK: Jessica Kingsley Publishers, 2009

[28] Dyson S. Reasons for assessment: rhetoric and reality in the assessment of children with disabilities. In: Booth T, Swann W, eds. Including pupils with disabilities. UK: Open University Press; 1988

16 Supporting Learners Who Are Deaf or Hard of Hearing (DHH) in the Educational Setting

Jenna M. Voss, Ellie White, Susan Lenihan, Paula E. Gross, and Dan Salvucci

Summary

This chapter focuses on learners who are deaf or hard of hearing (DHH), and the support needed for optimal development in communication, academics, and social and emotional skills through appropriate educational settings and professional services. How do parents and educators determine an appropriate placement for the learner who is DHH? This chapter describes the educational pathway for development and learning, identifies strategies, approaches and challenges, and emphasizes the importance of collaboration between professionals and caregivers in achieving successful educational experiences.

Keywords

deaf, hard of hearing, children, learners, preschool, early childhood, elementary, school-aged, educational settings, interprofessional practice, collaboration accommodations, modifications, communication, academic, social skills, emotional needs, inclusion, teacher of the deaf, itinerant teacher of the deaf, IEP, 504, advocacy

Key Points

- Children who are DHH can succeed academically in general education settings with appropriate support services.
- Utilizing a developmental approach, educators support learners who are DHH in varied educational settings by teaching the skills learners need to ultimately access their grade level curriculum independently.
- Supporting learners who are DHH and empowering them to reach their fullest potential is best achieved through intentional collaboration and information sharing between professionals and caregivers to ensure that education is accessible, appropriate, and addresses the needs of the whole child.
- In addition to attention to students' communication, academic abilities, and accommodations/modifications, professionals must also attend to learners' social and emotional needs.

In the last fifty years, technologic and legislative developments have dramatically changed the educational experiences of children who are deaf or hard of hearing. Early identification through newborn hearing screening, early intervention services and the development of more sophisticated listening technology including digital hearing aids, cochlear implants, and personal and classroom listening systems have increased the opportunity for the development of listening and spoken language in early

childhood.[1,2,3,4] Studies of children who are DHH receiving early intervention services have demonstrated that children are attaining language levels close to peers with typical hearing.[1,5,6] In the U.S., federal laws require that children with disabilities receive educational services in the least restrictive environment with the goal of access to the same curriculum as their peers with typical hearing with appropriate support from qualified professionals. But what is the least restrictive environment with regard to learners who are DHH? How do parents and educators determine an appropriate placement for the learner who is DHH? What supports are necessary in the educational setting to ensure the learner achieves successful outcomes across listening, language, communication, academic content, and social engagement?

Pearl

The proverb, "it takes a village to raise a child," is aptly evidenced when working with students who are DHH. The village comprises the students, their families, educators, medical professionals, and community stakeholders. Their collective voices ensure appropriate access in an environment that promotes success.

When children who are DHH have access to early identification, appropriate early intervention programs and appropriate hearing technology, they can achieve positive outcomes in communication and language development and are often able to succeed academically in general education settings with appropriate support services.[7,8] Conversely, children can experience delays in development in auditory, language, speech, pragmatic language, social, and literacy skills as a result of delays in identification, access to intervention, and access to sound through appropriately fitted hearing technologies.[6]

16.1 Listening and Spoken Language Practice Prior to School Entry

As described in earlier chapters of this text, auditory-verbal (AV) practitioners are responsible for promoting a learner's use of audition to facilitate the development of effective spoken language which allows one to communicate thoughts, questions, ideas, and emotions. Learners live, play, interact, and grow in a variety of environments including their homes, schools, playgrounds, and neighborhoods, to name a few. In these varied environments, learners communicate for a wide range of purposes. When the auditory verbal practitioner can keep the authentic, functional environments and varied purposes of communication in mind from the beginning, then the selection of strategies and activities to best support the learner's linguistic competence can be designed with the greatest efficiency. Though this chapter focuses primarily on the educational environments of learners, learning begins at or before birth, much before a child enters any formal educational system. The model of intervention that is most robust for learners aged birth through three, is that of family-centered early intervention (FCEI). Early intervention programs, typically serving children ages birth-three years and their families as dictated by Part C of the federal IDEA legislation, have a primary goal of supporting families of children who have, or are at risk for having, developmental delays by supporting caregiver capacity.[9]

Pearl

While a primary outcome for those engaged in AV practice is effective communication for a learner who is DHH, this does not come without consistent, specialized instruction which scaffolds a learner to develop finite skills in relatively structured settings and transfer these skills to the authentic communicative environments.

A transition from early intervention to early childhood education occurs in time for a child's third birthday, commonly known as transition from Part C to Part B, and may bring much change to a family's experience interacting with professionals. The early childhood programming may mark the beginning of a family's engagement with their child's public school district and brings their first experience with Individual Education Programs (IEPs), as opposed to Individualized Family Service Plans (IFSPs) which guided their experience in Part C. Note, some children continue to receive listening and spoken language intervention from auditory verbal practitioners outside of the school system, through services in clinics, university programs, audiology centers, hospitals, or private practices. Children whose support services are provided independently from their school system may not engage the educational models described in detail to follow, yet their intervention is still focused on supporting their full participation in school, community, and family life.

Children's development and achievement are significantly impacted by their school experiences. For students who are DHH, their experiences in educational settings can make the difference between outstanding achievement and academic underachievement. Effective support in inclusive settings is often high intensity and technical in nature, as professionals must provide support and information to general education teachers and parents.[10] This support also includes frequent, ongoing assessment of language development to ensure that high-intensity services are promoting positive outcomes and children are meeting developmental milestones.[11]

Pearl

For students who are DHH, their experiences in educational settings can make the difference between outstanding achievement and academic underachievement.

A student who requires support for delays as a result of hearing loss usually has an Individualized Education Program (IEP) to ensure equal access to the general education curriculum. The IEP can provide a range of services and supports to bridge access to the curriculum. Several factors influence the type, degree, and amount of services provided by the IEP. The student's audiologic profile (including functional listening skills), language and vocabulary level, academic performance, independence in classroom learning, personal attributes, and ability to advocate for one's self, with respect to the student's age and grade level should all be considered.[12] **Table 16.1** depicts a range of intervention models from most-to-least supportive. Descriptions of these models follow.

Additionally, see **Table 16.2** for terminology related to placements for students who are DHH.

16.2 Role of the Teacher of the Deaf

To fully understand effective placement settings for learners who are DHH, we must first acknowledge the contributions of the teacher of the deaf as the quality of a given placement is integrally tied to the teacher of the deaf who serves within it. Effective teachers of the deaf possess a multitude of skills related

Table 16.1 Models of Intervention for listening and spoken language deaf education*

	Early Childhood Programming AGE 3-5	School-Age Programming AGE 5+
Most Support ↑	Full time placement in self-contained preschool classroom	Full participation in self-contained school-age classroom
	Part-time self-contained preschool classroom and part-time general education preschool classroom	Part-time self-contained school-age classroom and part-time general education grade level classroom
	Full-time placement in general education preschool classroom with support from an itinerant teacher of the deaf or speech-language pathologist (push-in or pull-out services)	Full-time placement in general education grade level classroom with support from an itinerant teacher of the deaf or speech-language pathologist (push-in or pull-out services) or Full-time placement in general education grade level classroom with support from a teacher of the deaf in a resource room
Least Support ↓	Full time placement in classroom co-taught by a general education preschool teacher and a preschool teacher of the deaf	Full time placement in classroom co-taught by a general education grade level teacher and a teacher of the deaf
	Full time placement in general education preschool setting with private services outside of school from an AV practitioner	Full time placement in general education grade level setting with private services outside of school from an AV practitioner

Table 16.2 Placement terminology for students who are DHH

Placement	Definition	Characteristics
General Education Classroom	Typical preschool or grade level classroom	DHH student is taught beside typical same-age peers; DHH student can receive direct or indirect services (typically from teacher of the deaf and/or SLP) according to the IEP
Inclusion	Placement in general education setting regardless of disability or its impact	Accommodations and modifications are put in place to enable access to the curriculum according to the IEP
Mainstreaming	Placement in general education setting regardless of disability	No accommodations or modifications to the curriculum; DHH student can receive additional direct or indirect services (typically from a teacher of the deaf or SLP) according to the IEP
Resource Room	Separate classroom within general education building dedicated to supporting students with disabilities; Can be only for DHH students who are taught by a teacher of the deaf or can be for any students with disabilities and taught by a special educator	Students rotate in and out of this classroom individually or in small groups during certain classes or times to receive support dictated by their IEPs
Self-Contained Classroom	Separate special education classroom within a general education building serving a small group of students with similar educational needs	A small group of DHH students spends the day in this separate class taught by a teacher of the deaf
Co-Teaching Classroom	General education classroom teacher and a teacher of the deaf provide simultaneous and coordinated instruction to a group of students including typically developing and DHH	DHH students have full access to the general education setting (curriculum, teacher and typical peers) with communication facilitation from the teacher of the deaf; daily opportunities for specialized small group DHH instruction from the teacher of the deaf
Direct Service—Push-in	Support provided inside general education classroom (typically by the teacher of the deaf or SLP)	Specialized, individualized instruction and support specific to student need and content as dictated by IEP
Direct Service—Pull-out	Support provided out of the general education classroom away from peers (typically by the teacher of the deaf or speech-language pathologist [SLP])	Specialized, individualized instruction and support specific to student need and content as dictated by IEP
Indirect Service/ Consultation	Teacher of the deaf, SLP or educational audiologist provide support for school personnel regarding the DHH student's needs, or spend time with the student	Can include in-services for any staff working with the DHH child, in-services for peers, meetings with staff or parents, and time with the DHH student in the classroom to ensure needs are met or identify concerns; dictated by the IEP or 504 plan

to improving outcomes for learners who are DHH centered around the concept of *closing the gap* between students' delayed skills compared to typical skills for their age by making more than one year of progress in one year of time. The most notable gaps expected for learners who are DHH are in listening, language, and speech, though other areas including academic, pre-literacy/literacy, cognitive, motor, social, and emotional development are of equal importance for overall growth. To do this, teachers of the deaf support students while they access the curriculum, with the intent that the student will eventually fully close the gap and access the grade level curriculum independently.

The professional preparation of teachers of the deaf involves a developmental approach to teaching with respect to the impact of hearing loss on the learner. This preparation ensures learners in a variety of educational settings are taught the skills they need following the typical development trajectory. The knowledge of teachers of the deaf includes, but is not limited to, the following:

- various pedagogies and educational curricula
- auditory and neurological systems
- typical speech and language development
- impact of hearing loss on communication (auditory, receptive language, expressive language, pragmatic language, speech) and literacy
- academic and communication progress monitoring

- assessment and assessment interpretation for learners who are DHH
- benefits and limitations of hearing assistive technologies
- educational plans (IEP and 504)
- research and trends in deaf education
- audiology and speech pathology
- social and emotional development of learners who are DHH
- family engagement
- emotional impact of hearing loss on the family
- effective practice for instruction of listening and spoken language

This unique knowledge and skill set prepares teachers of the deaf to guide placement decisions, provide direct and indirect services, consult with professionals and parents, and provide other support necessary for learners who are DHH to succeed.

16.3 Models of Intervention and Placement Options in Early Childhood Education

Listening and spoken language (LSL) early childhood programming focuses on providing services that enable preschoolers to close the gap between their communication skills and the communication skills that are typical for their chronological age. Many placement options are available for children who are DHH during their preschool years including a wide range of supports, depending on the needs of the individual child. The IEP team develops a plan that includes goals written to address areas of need and minutes associated with services for meeting those goals. The IEP team decides on placement by determining the least restrictive environment that will allow for the provision of services and related minutes for goals outlined in the IEP. Some LSL preschool placement options are discussed in the following sections.

16.3.1 Full-Time Self-Contained LSL Classroom for Preschoolers Who Are DHH

Many options exist for LSL self-contained preschool classrooms in both public and private programs. These include a number of private schools belonging to an organization called OPTION Schools, described as "...an international, non-profit organization comprised of listening and spoken language programs and schools for children who are deaf or hard of hearing in Canada, South America, and the U.S."[13] In addition, LSL placements include a number of public school programs across the United States. Full-time placement in a classroom specifically designed for children who are DHH is determined by the IEP team. Placement in this setting, and any setting, is dependent on the individual needs of the student. Self-contained LSL classrooms for the deaf are most well-known for their wide-ranging focus on listening, spoken language, and speech development. In successful, self-contained LSL classrooms, teachers and staff provide constant listening, spoken language and speech instruction through the use of age-appropriate, play-based, engaging activities throughout the day. Every period in the schedule is intentionally planned to allow for two equally important aspects of instruction—*modeling* of the language related to the activity or routine and *prompting* of the language related to the activity or routine. To learn to listen and talk, children who are DHH must have a plethora of opportunities in every environment to practice listening and talking. They listen to the language modeled by those around them. Appropriate models allow children to hear the language of the activity including the vocabulary and grammatical elements necessary to provide meaningful and complete messages. Yet, learning to listen and talk is not only dependent on listening; it is also dependent on talking. Experienced teachers of the deaf are able to prompt children to use language meaningfully to verbally exchange ideas when they interact during planned activities and spontaneous opportunities. Prompting is the act of providing a cue or indication of what a child should say. The capability to appropriately prompt language is an art in itself—dependent on the situational context, ability of the child, and goals—and acquired by skilled teachers through a tremendous amount of practice and reflection.

A typical full-day LSL preschool program has a number of periods in the daily schedule to maximize listening, spoken language and speech development. This includes periods associated with a typical preschool day as well as periods for focused, deliberate, and intensive instruction of listening, spoken language, and speech. Typical preschool periods include circle time, centers, read-alouds and early literacy, playground or other gross motor periods, music, art, snacks, lunch, and rest time. In an LSL preschool program, these periods are built into the schedule as an opportunity to provide typical preschool experiences with the addition of a teacher of the deaf facilitating the listening, spoken language, speech, and social skills that are appropriate for preschoolers. In addition to those typical preschool periods, LSL preschool programming includes daily periods for explicit instruction in listening, spoken language, and speech. Explicit instruction refers to contrived, deliberate, intensive, repetitive, and sometimes drill-like instruction. It is intended for groups of 1–3 students who are alike in their capability and learning style. Explicit listening (or auditory skill development), language, and speech periods are essential in the daily schedule of an LSL self-contained preschool program. Frequently, explicit speech and auditory skill work are scheduled together and provided by the same professional. Explicit language lessons are one of the three components of the *Continuum of Language Instructional Settings.*

Pearl

A targeted, yet varied, set of learning language opportunities allows for efficient, effective, comprehensive language acquisition for DHH preschoolers.

16.4 Continuum of Language Instructional Settings

LSL preschool programs are heavily focused on spoken language acquisition through listening. Because language instruction is vital in these settings, teachers must dedicate the majority of the daily schedule to promoting language development using methods that work for a diverse group of preschoolers. The use of multiple and varied periods of language instruction allows for a systematic process of providing a great deal of support at one point in the day, a little less support later in the day, and then even less support after that to allow for children to experience a typical preschool setting (albeit with the educator's continued support including language facilitation). Though the amount of explicit teaching varies in these settings, no one setting is more important than another. The three settings work together to create an instructional system that promotes the support necessary to develop new language skills, practice previously learned language, and eventually generalize those skills to become independent users of that language.

- Explicit Language Lessons: contrived, deliberate, intensive, repetitive, and sometimes drill-like spoken language instruction. It is intended for groups of 1–3 students who are alike in their capability and learning style. Ideal for introducing and practicing new vocabulary and syntactic elements in authentic communication.

- Conversational Language Lessons: designed as a stepping-stone for practicing language learned in more structured lessons before using it proficiently in natural settings.[14] These are ideal for practicing vocabulary and syntax introduced in explicit language settings, but with the addition of typical preschool conversational skills, group skills and some play skills. These lessons are still teacher-directed, yet they require more students to allow for conversational skill development within a small group of about 4.

- Natural Language Lessons: Centers, which can also be referred to as learning centers or rotating centers, are the least structured and the most natural and versatile language period. It is a typical preschool period designed for exploration and engagement in various stations throughout the classroom, each focused on at least one age-appropriate learning goal in early childhood domains (communication, literacy, science, math, motor development, social development, and emotional development). It is imperative that preschoolers who are DHH have the same inclusive opportunities to engage in these activities as their same-aged peers do. Centers allow for practice using age-appropriate listening, spoken language, speech, and social skills that are typical for all preschoolers. In particular, it is an opportunity to use the spoken language skills they have acquired in more contrived settings. Yet, to be successful in centers, preschoolers who are DHH often require support from the teacher both beforehand (in explicit and conversational language lessons) and also during centers. Centers also provide the teacher of the deaf with ample data regarding a child's success at using listening, spoken language, and speech skills in the natural preschool environment. Teachers then use these data to guide future instruction in explicit and conversational language settings, allowing for more repetitive practice of certain skills, as well as future centers periods.

Pearl

Sample schedule from a Full-Day LSL Preschool

8:30–8:45	Arrival
8:45–9:00	Circle Time
9:00–9:30	Structured Language
9:30–10:00	Recess
10:00–10:15	Snack + Read Aloud
10:15–10:45	Conversational Language
10:45–11:30	Centers
11:30–1:15	Lunch, Recess, Rest
1:15–1:45	Early Literacy
1:45–2:15	Speech
2:15–2:45	Auditory Skill Work
2:45–3:15	Centers (with Pre-Academic Stations)
3:15–3:30	Closing Circle Time & Dismissal

16.4.1 Part-Time Self-Contained LSL Classroom for Preschoolers Who Are DHH and Part-Time Early Childhood General Education Setting

Most preschoolers who are DHH can benefit educationally from time spent with peers who are typically developing. Often, preschoolers who are DHH need to spend a significant amount of time in a classroom with a teacher of the deaf; yet they can also access time in the general education preschool setting. This enables preschoolers to experience typical preschool and the general education curriculum to the extent they are able to do so successfully, as well as interact with peers as communication partners. The IEP team determines the number of minutes per week the child will need to spend in special education to meet the IEP goals. In addition, the team will determine the number of minutes per week the child will spend in the general education preschool setting. This placement is often referred to as part-time/part-time. The numbers can vary significantly from child to child depending on individual needs. For example, if a child's school week consists of 1800 minutes, she might spend 1650 minutes per week in the special education setting to meet her listening, spoken language, and speech goals with the teacher of the deaf and speech-language pathologist. That same child would spend the remaining 150 minutes per week in the general education preschool setting. Other children may need less time in the special education setting and those minutes are determined by the IEP team based on the child's needs.

Pearl

Preschoolers who are DHH benefit from social interaction and language stimulation with their typically developing peers.

16.4.2 Placement in General Education Preschool with Itinerant Teacher of the Deaf or Speech-Language Pathologist Services

Some preschoolers who are DHH benefit from placement in the general education preschool setting yet are eligible for services based on need and critical learning period. These children often receive services from an itinerant teacher of the deaf and/or speech services from a speech-language pathologist with expertise in listening and spoken language instruction. This placement is often considered for preschoolers who are DHH who demonstrate typical or near typical listening, spoken language, and speech skills and developed those skills without intensive full-time listening and spoken language instruction. They can be removed from the typical preschool setting at scheduled times to receive these services, or the service provider can push into the more natural classroom environment to provide support there. Because preschoolers have not yet reached the typical age of fully developed listening, language, and speech skills, a teacher of the deaf or SLP with training in developing listening and spoken language is able to target these skills so the child's language can improve in a developmentally synchronous fashion. The IEP team determines the number of minutes per week the child will spend with the itinerant teacher of the deaf or SLP to meet the IEP goals. In addition to services for children in preschool settings, some children who are preschool age and attend daycare instead of preschool can also receive services from an itinerant teacher of the deaf or speech-language pathologist.

Pearl

Itinerant teaching support can allow preschoolers to succeed for a large percentage of the school day in the general education setting, while still receiving additional services for skills impacted by hearing loss.

Pitfall

Professionals may unknowingly place a preschooler inappropriately in the general education setting for most of the day with minimal itinerant services. For some children, this is significantly less special education than is needed to close the gap.

16.4.3 Placement in Classroom Co-Taught by a General Education Preschool Teacher and a Teacher of the Deaf

Some preschoolers who are DHH can benefit from placement in a classroom utilizing a co-teaching model with a general education preschool teacher as well as an early childhood teacher of the deaf. This is often established to allow for inclusion so children who are DHH have significant access to the general education setting; yet it also allows them the opportunity for specialized instruction. Co-teachers determine the schedule together to include all periods of the general education curriculum in the preschool day, along with specific time each day for the teacher of the deaf to provide explicit listening, spoken language, and speech instruction to children who are DHH. The teacher of the deaf also provides support as needed to facilitate communication between students during general education lessons. This placement requires a strong working relationship between the teachers including a similar teaching style and philosophy. In addition, this placement requires space for the teacher of the deaf to provide explicit lessons in a relatively quiet setting, which preschool classrooms are not known to be. Therefore, this setting is most effective for students who are DHH and who have typical or close-to-typical listening and language skills and thus require less explicit teaching in these domains.

Pitfall

Co-teaching is a well-documented style of teaching that requires significant training to be done well. Not all teachers can successfully execute a co-teaching environment that highlights the benefits of this placement. In some cases, co-teaching is the term used to erroneously describe two teachers leading two different classes in the same room, usually as a result of an issue with limited space, yet this is not at all the premise of a co-teaching model.

16.4.4 Full-Time Placement in General Education Setting

Some preschoolers who are DHH and their families have received consistent quality early intervention services from an auditory-verbal therapist, auditory-verbal educator, developmental therapist in hearing, speech-language pathologist or other hearing professionals since the hearing loss was diagnosed. These children may have already developed age-appropriate listening, spoken language, and speech skills by the time they are preschool age, and can therefore access the general education curriculum with no additional services or supports during the school day. Yet, because children who are typically developing continue to acquire foundational listening, language, and speech skills during and beyond the preschool years, we expect children who are DHH to need to continue progressing as well. Continued auditory-verbal therapy is essential for these children so they can maintain age-appropriate communication skills as they get older, and so they have consistent monitoring from a professional well versed in providing support for these children and their families. Frequent communication between this professional and the child's classroom teacher is suggested.

For other preschoolers who are DHH who do not receive auditory-verbal therapy outside of the school day, the IEP team could still decide to forgo any services or supports and place the child in a general education preschool setting. In this case, the risk of the child falling behind is certainly a consideration, as well as the risk of a general education preschool teacher missing the signs of a lag in development or regression. Therefore, transitioning the child from intensive services and supports before preschool to no services and support in preschool is not advisable.

16.5 Models of Intervention and Placement Options for School-Age Learners Who Are DHH

In the U.S., when children turn 5, they transition from IDEA Part B early childhood programs to IDEA Part B school-aged programs. Programs for school-age (kindergarten through 12th grade) students focus on academic curricula, as well as provision of services that allow students to close the gap between their communication skills (listening, spoken language, and speech) and the communication skills that are typical for their age. Current statistics indicate that approximately 75–87% of all students who are deaf spend a portion of the school day in general education settings.[11,15]

Despite research consistently showing academic and literacy skills of students who are DHH lagging behind their typically hearing peers,[16] specialized programs with specific and focused instructional strategies provide the necessary supports for meeting student needs. In effective programs, educators minimize these educational gaps, while recognizing that students who are DHH have a variety of language histories, learning needs, and communication preferences.[17] Addressing these educational gaps often requires that instruction is modified or augmented to support individual learner needs and facilitate growth, particularly in content areas as texts become increasingly complex and varied. Certainly, the shift from learning-to-read to reading-to-learn in third or fourth grade suggests the need for proficiency in foundational skills such as reading and language use.

Far too often, teachers assume that all students bring prerequisite skills to the classroom, but many learners who are DHH, especially those who have not had strong preschool listening, speech, and language instruction, do not possess these necessary skills, particularly for content areas and corresponding types of literature.[18] Indeed, the transition to complex and discipline-specific texts can be overwhelming. Many learning activities and tasks require abstract reasoning and other higher-level critical thinking skills which often necessitate explicit and systematic instruction. Learning about text structure and print features (e.g., boldface type, use of italics, headings, graphs, tables, figure, photographs, and captions) characteristic of these texts can prepare learners to engage with reading materials in the content areas. Additionally, there are other strategies that can help learners who are DHH.

With language skill development as the consistent underlying focus, teachers of the deaf can also implement strategies that foster language development within the context of academic content. Literacy skills that fall under English Language Arts in the general education curriculum, are necessary prerequisites for accessing *all* content areas. Strategies to support literacy development include promoting discussions, repeating questions and comments to fill in gaps for students, rephrasing as needed, asking open-ended questions, providing opportunities for making personal connections, predictions and inferences, presenting materials in multiple modes, using visuals and multimedia or multisensory formats, explicitly teaching background knowledge, using graphic and semantic organizers, the pre-teaching of targeted vocabulary, cooperative learning activities, summarizing material, using leveled texts, using technology such as captioning and other assistive technology, and promoting independent reading. These skills are required for successful access to curriculum in all content areas (**Table 16.3**).[19,20,21,22]

16.5.1 Full Participation in Self-Contained School-Age Classroom

Some options exist for LSL self-contained elementary classrooms, with less availability in middle and high school. Full-time placement in a classroom specifically designed for children who are DHH is determined by the IEP team. Placement in this setting, and any setting, is dependent on the individual needs of the student. In self-contained or blended classrooms, the teacher of the deaf is fully responsible for the academic progress and spoken language development of the student who is DHH. Many teachers of the deaf work with DHH students who are at multiple grade levels in the same classroom. In a classroom with several students who have different IEP goals and objectives, these teachers design a school year program that includes the scope and practice of all content areas and develop daily lessons within units that meet their state or common core standards. They collaborate with a variety of professionals who might also be serving the children in their classroom (including speech-language pathologists, occupational therapists, physical therapists, etc). Students in this setting do not have requisite levels of language to access the academic content. Thus, the instruction must provide both academic content as well as language support required for understanding and talking about that content.

16.5.2 Part-Time Self-Contained School-Age Classroom and Part-Time General Education Grade Level Classroom

Some students who are DHH benefit educationally from part-time placements in both typical grade-level classrooms and in specialized classrooms for learners with hearing loss. This enables students to experience the general education curriculum to the extent they are able to do so successfully, as well as interact with peers as communication partners. The IEP team determines the number of minutes per week the student will need to spend in special education to meet the IEP goals. In addition, the team will determine the number of minutes per week the student will spend in the general education setting. Students in this setting vary in their capability to understand academic content as a result of their delayed language skills. Thus, the instruction can provide both academic content as well as language support required for understanding and talking about that content.

16.5.3 Full-Time Placement in General Education Grade-Level Classroom with Support

Some students who are DHH benefit from placement in the general education setting yet remain eligible for additional services. These students receive services from one or more of the following professionals with expertise in listening and spoken language instruction: itinerant teacher of the deaf, teacher of the deaf in a resource room, speech-language pathologist, educational audiologist. Placement in a general education setting necessitates the student who is DHH has a sufficient language foundation to access the curriculum with minimal levels of support alongside typically hearing peers. However, as communication demands and independence expectations increase, the demands increase relative to the student's level of communication. A primary role of teachers of the deaf working in general education settings is to work with the student who is DHH and other professionals

221

Table 16.3 Specific strategies for instruction in content areas

Academic Content Area	Strategies
Math • Requires an understanding of symbols that represent concepts, vocabulary that has differing meaning from everyday language, and text structure that makes use of succinct writing[19] • Word problems can be difficult	• Using manipulatives • Drawing pictures or diagrams • Modeling think-alouds • Incorporating writing, such as poetry, to describe mathematical concepts
Science • Very technical vocabulary • Necessary use of critical thinking skills	• Using hands-on activities such as lab experiments and experiential activities
Social Studies • Vocabulary for abstract concepts (democracy, freedom) and concepts of time can be difficult • Pronunciation of unfamiliar places and people	• Using graphic and visual organizers • Using maps and manipulatives • Incorporating dramatization into instruction • Engaging in community service learning
Art • Expression of creativity and imagination	• Recognizing competing attention for auditory information versus hands-on or visual tasks during art instruction
Music • Vocal, choral or instrumental • Reading music promotes literacy skills • Increases auditory working memory, sound perception and discrimination, recognition of pitch, prosody and rhythm patterns, phonological awareness[21]	• Understanding directions or speech with music in the background, given competing auditory signals and diminished signal to noise ratios • Developing complex language or grammatical structures that are unfamiliar[20]
Physical Education • Physical skill (e.g., gross and fine motor, balance, agility, coordination) • Health (e.g., fitness, endurance, strength, body composition, flexibility, healthy lifestyle)[22] • Ensure listening devices are secured and not harmed (e.g., the use of sweat bands, tethering equipment, protective gear)	• Explaining complex or detailed rules and instructions as the acoustic environment of these activities may interfere • Recognizing the challenges of reverberations and background noise common in gymnasiums, playing courts, or outdoor fields, and activity spaces.

by ensuring the student develops the necessary skills to be independent in learning and to self-advocate. Collaboration is bi-directional and interprofessional. The teacher of the deaf and other professionals working with the student share information on the student's communication, academic capabilities, social supports, and accommodations or modifications to allow for full participation in the general education setting. Teachers of the deaf can provide direct service including push-in to the general education classroom or pull-out to another space with the student for individualized instruction. They can also provide indirect service that includes consultation for the general education teacher serving the student. An itinerant teacher of the deaf travels from building to building within a district or regional program to provide services to students who are DHH attending their neighborhood general education program. A resource room teacher of the deaf is comparable to an itinerant, but remains in one building and serves multiple students at multiple levels across multiple subjects in any given day. Frequently, students with various needs are scheduled for their resource room minutes at the same time as other students with very different needs. The resources room teacher of the deaf essentially finds a way to provide direct instruction to some while others work independently, alternating to support varied learners at varied levels. Resource room teachers are found in programs with a critical number of students who are DHH and who can benefit from part-time placement in general education, so the employer finds it worthwhile to employ an on-site teacher of the deaf to fulfill the students' special education services.

16.5.4 Full-Time Placement in Classroom Co-Taught by a General Education Grade-Level Teacher and a Teacher of the Deaf

Though rare, some programs implement a co-teaching model in which a general education classroom teacher and a teacher of the deaf provide simultaneous and coordinated instruction to a group of students including those who are typically developing as well as those who are deaf or hard of hearing. This is especially rare because it requires a critical mass of students who are DHH, who are at the same grade level, and have similar language and communication skills. Because deafness is a low incidence disability, it is uncommon to find a sufficient number of learners to justify this model.

16.5.5 Full-Time Placement in General Education Grade-Level Setting with Private Services Outside of School from an Auditory-Verbal Practitioner

Some students who are DHH in the general education setting do not receive educational support from specialists in their general education setting. These students fully participate in the general education setting, yet their parents choose to access services from an AV practitioner outside of the school day. Although the services and supports the student receives are not provided during the typical school day, it is beneficial that the parents, school educators, and private practitioners coordinate and collaborate about academics, self-advocacy, social development, and peer interactions. The decision for full-time placement in a general education setting necessitates the student have developmentally appropriate and age-appropriate language, listening, speech, social, and academic skills. To ensure full access to instruction, it is important that all DHH students have either a 504 plan or and IEP in place.

16.5.6 504 Plans for Students Who Are DHH

Pitfall

Students who have age-appropriate and developmentally appropriate communication and academic skills might no longer qualify for special education services through an IEP. These students instead receive a 504 plan. It is important to note that this means a student no longer receives special education services and is no longer covered by protections afforded by IDEA through the educational agency.

A 504 plan, under the jurisdiction of the Office for Civil Rights, is developed to ensure a student with disabilities (including deafness or hearing impairment) receives accommodations to the learning environment that will support academic success. For students who are DHH, 504 accommodations could include preferential seating, remote microphone systems (including FM, DM, or sound field systems), and captioned media, for example. The 504 plan is not intended to address skill development, but instead to address equal access to the curriculum. 504 plans can also include teacher of the deaf services such as observation, consultation, or case management. As students who are DHH have continually changing and increasing expectations for communication, academic learning, and socializing, a 504 plan that includes only a minimal amount of consultation can be insufficient for monitoring and providing supports that students who are DHH will inevitably need. Because of the risks associated with the reasons just stated, the authors favor IEPs for students who are DHH rather than 504 plans.

Pearl

The 504 plan is not intended to address skill development, but instead to address equal access to the curriculum. 504 plans can also include teacher of the deaf services such as observation, consultation, or case management. A 504 plan that includes only a minimal amount of consultation can be insufficient for monitoring and providing supports that students who are DHH will inevitably need.

16.6 Important Considerations to Support Learners Who Are DHH through Listening and Spoken Language

• *Educational Assessment, Eligibility, and Services*

The educational and related services for early childhood and school age students who are DHH continue to be guided by the IDEA. This law, which was originally passed in 1975 and most recently reauthorized as the Individuals with Disabilities Education Improvement Act in 2004, provides for the free, appropriate, and public education for children with disabilities. The current version places an emphasis on academic results by ensuring that students access the general education curriculum to the greatest extent possible.[23] Court rulings have reinforced that Individualized Education Programs (IEPs) must provide students with disabilities more than the minimal educational benefit, indicating that IEP teams must assess and provide reasonable services for the child to access curriculum and make progress.

To receive services, a student must meet eligibility criteria. Following a referral, an initial evaluation takes place that includes individual assessments and observations. According to IDEA, evaluation is defined as the process of determining eligibility and assessment refers to the specific tools used to gather relevant information about a child.[24] Assessment results provide the IEP team the needed information to determine specific goals and objectives for the development of an IEP. Eligibility criteria for services require that the child have one of the 13 disabilities as defined by IDEA and the impact of the disability must create a need for services.[25] In the case of hearing loss, in most states, the determination of disability requires the identification of special needs in two areas: one related to the hearing loss and one demonstrating the adverse educational impact of the hearing loss on areas such as sound-field word recognition, receptive and expressive language, or significant discrepancy between verbal and nonverbal performance on a standardized test.

• *Individualized Education Program (IEP)*

An IEP is a written statement for a child with a disability that is developed, reviewed, and revised in a meeting by the IEP team in keeping with certain requirements of U.S. law and regulations. At the meeting, which occurs at a mutually convenient time and place, hearing health and education professionals share the results of the evaluation, discuss its findings and give parents or guardians the opportunity to ask questions.[26] The IEP team must discuss specific information about the child, including the child's strengths, the parents' or caregivers' ideas for enhancing the child's education, the results of recent evaluations or reevaluations; and how the child has done on state- and district-wide tests. The format of the IEP document will vary in different states and districts but the components are delineated by IDEA.

• *Accommodations or Modifications*

For child with an IEP, the team determines what accommodations or modifications are necessary for a child to be successful in the educational setting. Accommodations are for changing *how* a child learns rather than *what* a child learns. **Table 16.4** lists accommodations and examples.

Modifications are for changing what the child is taught or expected to learn. This largely includes changes made to the curriculum and, for older children, assignments. Examples of modifications include changes in expectations, changes in levels and changes to evaluation criteria. The *IEP/504 Checklist* developed by DeConde-Johnson and Seaton can be found at the Hands and Voices website (https://www.handsandvoices.org/pdf/IEP_Checklist.pdf) and is an excellent resource for determining effective accommodations and modifications.

• *Consultation under Supports for School Personnel*

The IEP team may discuss the need for consultation to support any staff who works with the student to do so more effectively. These supports are provided to school staff to allow the student to meet IEP goals, support participation in the general education setting to the extent possible, or provide the staff with what they need to meet the specific needs of the student. Consultation for students who are DHH is often provided by a teacher of the deaf, speech-language pathologist or audiologist. This is written in the IEP under the category called *Supports for School Personnel.* Consultation does not include direct service minutes. Instead, it is stipulated in the IEP according to location (e.g., all areas) frequency (e.g., daily, weekly) and duration (e.g., begin and end dates). See **Table 16.5.**

• *Collaboration: Parents and Professionals*

Students who are DHH likely receive services from a number of professionals to meet the goals on their IEPs, provide audiologic management, and support the daily schedule. For example, a student in a full-time deaf education classroom might have a teacher of the deaf who targets multiple domains including spoken language, a speech-language pathologist for speech and auditory skill work, an educational audiologist who supports hearing technology and listening environments, and paraprofessionals who provide support throughout the day. Because a number of professionals could realistically work with any one student, the need for an effective team approach is paramount. The complexity of today's educational service delivery underscores the need for collaboration among staff that is better and more frequent than ever before.

Pitfall

A multidisciplinary team approach, in which providers work independently alongside one another to determine and meet the needs of the student, is not necessarily sufficient to deliver the most effective practice and best outcomes.

Pearl

True interprofessional collaboration occurs when the team simultaneously addresses concerns about the student, considers the student's needs, and establishes the steps to take for producing optimal outcomes.[27]

Collaborating with parents, guardians, or other caregivers, is also imperative for student success and is a critical component of IEP development and ongoing communication of progress on IEP goals. Parent interaction can come in many forms with various degrees of involvement. It can not only create open lines of communication, but it can also allow for parents to facilitate the carryover of learned skills at home. The need for a strong partnership between parents and school staff has become so evident that schools are now investigating ways for parents to not only be involved but engaged. When parents are simply involved, the school dictates the parents' activity level. However, to engage parents, schools facilitate opportunities for parents to take part in school functions, join in educational opportunities, and actively voice the amount and kind of involvement they would believe will most benefit their children's academic growth.[28] Because teachers are typically already familiar with the needs of the child and family, as well as having specialist training, they are likely in a

Table 16.4 Accommodations with examples

Accommodation	Definition	Examples
Presentation	the way information or materials are presented	Directions given in a variety of ways, provision of teacher notes/outlines, peer note-taking, concrete examples, verbal and visual cues, frequent check-ins for comprehension, pre/post-teaching, repeating what other students have said, study guides, captioned media, review of directions, untimed tests, highlight key directions, remote microphones/classroom amplification, captioned films, etc.
Response	the expected and acceptable responses from the child	Adjustments for speech intelligibility/fluency, use of sentence/language frames, graphic organizers or allow extra time for auditory processing
Setting	the environment in which a child learns or format for instruction	Preferential seating close to the teacher and away from noise, reduce auditory distraction through the use of sound absorbing materials (carpet, acoustic tiles and panels)
Timing	the additional timing allowed for completing tasks	Extended time for oral responses, allow extra time for tests and assignments
Scheduling	changes to the child's learning schedule	Allow frequent breaks and vary activities, provide extended school year services
Other		Frequent monitoring of hearing technology daily

Table 16.5 Examples of consultation

- In-services for any general education teachers, staff or students interacting with the child to explain about the child's hearing loss and resultant needs in any given setting, implications for instruction in the general education setting, hearing device use, monitoring, and care including hearing aids, cochlear implants, bone anchored hearing devices, remote microphone systems (including FM, DM, or sound field) and any other hearing devices or equipment the student might use
- Periodic meetings with the general education classroom teachers to provide input about the student's needs and suggestions for meeting those needs within the general education setting, including assistance implementing accommodations and modifications
- Time spent with the student to ensure unique needs are met and to identify any concerns, including planning of strategies for use with general education teacher or other school staff to address those concerns

prime position to offer appropriate guidance to parents and to act as a liaison between the school and home.

Pearl

An effective relationship among schools, parents, teachers, and related service providers can result in shared information and additional support within both the home and school, providing for a more positive educational experience. By facilitating home/school links and providing opportunities for parents to be involved in meaningful ways in their child's education, schools can capitalize on the support provided within the home.

Throughout the preschool years, communication among caregivers and professionals occurs on a regular basis through daily interactions in person, home/school journals, email, blogs, etc. As students transition from preschool to elementary school, the structure of school-age programs and the amount of parent involvement naturally decreases. This shift creates greater challenges in ongoing collaboration among parents and professionals as parents have less day-to-day contact with their child's educational team. Teachers of the deaf can be valuable resources in this time of transition, as their expertise and efforts may contribute to the development of the home/school relationship beyond the preschool years. Collaboration with parents continues to be an integral part of a student's educational success. The need for relationships among parents and professionals is important to the carryover of skill development from home to school and back to home.

• Hearing Assistive Technology (HAT)

The IEP team, which should include an educational audiologist, determines the assistive technology a child needs to be successful following the placement determination. When an educational audiologist is not part of the team, the clinical audiologist who works with the child will need to function as an educational audiologist to make HAT recommendations. This might include use of hearing aids, bone-anchored hearing devices, or cochlear implants, use of personal remote microphones (e.g. FM/DM

systems) for some or all of the day, and use of a sound field system for some or all of the day. Some school districts want to recommend HAT systems that are currently available in the school, however it is critical that the system chosen meets the needs of each specific child. See Chapter 2, "Audiology: Building the Foundation," for more detail about HAT. It remains important for learners who are DHH to have the capability to connect personal hearing assistive technology and integrate with classroom technology to achieve educational equity and ensure full access to the curriculum.[29]

• Auditory Learning and Fatigue

While teaching with auditory expectation, educators must address the physical classroom environment to ensure that background noise is minimized and visual access is provided to scaffold instruction for students who are DHH. The provision of assistive technology including classroom amplification or remote microphones, modifications to physical space to improve the signal to noise ratio, captioning and transcripts of video and audio information, lighting that allows for optimal visual access, peer notetakers, opportunities for collaborative learning, use of frequent comprehension checks, and efforts to ensure the speaker is facing the learner who is DHH are important.

Karen Anderson[30] describes a cascading impact of hearing loss with regards to a learner's capability to access school communication. Culminating elements of this cascade of impact include fragmented access to auditory information, increased effort, challenges with listening comprehension, listening fatigue, and a face-paced learning environment. When learners who are DHH have incomplete access to the spoken communication that occurs in a classroom environment due to distance from signal and competing background noise, their personal efforts to attend to key auditory information while simultaneously ignoring competing signals creates an increased tax on their executive function and auditory processing, resulting in higher levels of listening-fatigue.[31,32] These challenges are experienced by children with varying types and degrees of hearing loss. Children who are successfully able to use their hearing technology in quiet settings may find they experience significant listening challenges when listening in a noisy classroom setting where fast-paced peer-to-peer and teacher-student conversations occur. Educators and parents can tend to this challenge by assessing and asking children who are DHH to notice and identify their listening effort and subsequent fatigue. Learners who are DHH can use compensatory strategies, such as speech reading, to reduce their listening effort, but individual differences in visual processing, and working memory capacity result in varied success with listening and watching the speaker to gain key information. It is a fair assumption then that learners who are DHH work harder to listen and use more cognitive resources to understand classroom conversations than do their typically hearing peers, especially when factors such as background noise, reverberation, multiple speakers, and face-paced instruction are considered.

As learners who are DHH begin to experience listening fatigue, they are more likely to have slower mental processing, impaired decision making, and experience an inability to maintain attention and concentration. With increased cognitive demands and fatigue-related challenges, children who are DHH may experience reduced academic performance compared to their age and language-matched typically hearing peers. Thus, educators must recognize the potentially negative impact the fragmented access to sound, challenges to listening comprehension, and listening fatigue can have on otherwise, high achieving learners who are DHH. Educators are cautioned not to assume a learner who is DHH is able to be successful in a typical learning environment without close monitoring of listening comprehension and fatigue. When these factors are recognized, accommodations to the environment and instruction can be warranted to ensure the learner who is DHH maintains academic and social success.

- *Least Restrictive Environment (LRE)*

IDEA requires that a student with a disability participate in education to the maximum extent appropriate, with nondisabled peers. There is much debate about how to interpret this provision. Guidance from the Department of Education on the needs of students who are DHH states that "any setting which does not meet the communication and related needs of a child who is deaf, and therefore does not allow for the provision of FAPE [free and appropriate public education], cannot be considered the LRE [least restrictive environment] for that child."[33] General education settings are appropriate and adaptable to meet the unique needs of many learners who are DHH, while for others, a center or specialized school may be the least restrictive environment in which the learner's unique needs can be met.

- *Advocacy*

The intentional embedding of self-determination skills in all areas of curriculum and learning for students who are DHH can enhance independence, advocacy, and post-secondary transition outcomes. Learning that incorporates one's beliefs, values, and decision-making fosters the development of these skills. When students are actively involved in asking questions, making choices, demonstrating organizational and problem-solving capabilities, setting goals, and self-regulating their behavior, they are working towards the achievement of these goals and improvements in these capabilities. It is important to note that learners who are DHH may need explicit instruction to acquire the requisite language and skills for developing these skills.[34] Likewise, family involvement and support can help students generalize behaviors and skills to home or work environments outside the school setting. Indeed, such carryover advances those skills needed in adulthood. Similarly, participation in extracurricular activities provides opportunities for socialization and forming friendships. These interactions can cultivate leadership skills and enhance communication skills.[35]

Supporting learners who are DHH and empowering them to reach their fullest potential is the joint responsibility of families, teachers and other stakeholders. Collaboration ensures that education is accessible, appropriate, and addresses the needs of the whole child. Accordingly, professionals must address social and emotional needs as well as educational outcomes. Unfortunately, the road to success may have some bumpy roadblocks along the way. Children who are DHH are 3–4 times more likely than typically developing peers to experience any kind of maltreatment, from neglect to abuse.[36,37] In addition to child maltreatment,

children who are DHH may experience other types of adversity, including substance abuse, mental illness, or incarceration of family members, parental separation or divorce, separation from parents, or domestic violence. These, along with other examples of adverse childhood experiences (ACEs) can have long-term negative impacts on individuals across developmental areas including academics, behavior, social interactions, and even health outcomes.[38,39] The negative impacts of early adversity that can present during a learner's time within the educational system include acting out behaviors, withdrawal, anxiety, difficulties in learning, feeling unsafe, and even diminished physical health that makes one vulnerable to further maltreatment or failure in academic settings.

These effects can be mitigated when children have strong attachments with positive and caring adults.[40,41] Indeed, strong parent-child bonds foster trust and healthy emotional development. Similarly, strong positive relationships with educators are important and can help children who are DHH navigate the school setting. In addition to these strong bonds, parents and educators should be knowledgeable about developmental milestones for typically developing children as well as children who are DHH alike[42] and have consistent high expectations, for cognitive, academic, social, and emotional capabilities. Teachers and other school-based professionals should discuss the importance of personal boundaries and safety rules across settings (including, school, transportation such as school bus, and home). When these safety rules and healthy boundaries are observed, they will foster optimal learning environments for all. Finally, as mandated reporters, teachers and other professionals should be alert to physical and behavioral indicators of abuse or maltreatment and report their suspicions accordingly.

Pearl

Resources from the Parent Safety Toolkit from the O.U.R. Children's Safety and Success Project may be useful to identify opportunities to embed these safety guidelines into IEPs and 504 plans as well.[43] See **Table 16.6.**

- *Bullying*

Bullying that may occur among children is perhaps one of the biggest areas of concern for parents of learners who are DHH. Peers may target or victimize the child who is DHH because he or she looks different due to the use of listening technology, or because he or she talks differently or may not understand the subtleties of language such as sarcasm or figurative language. In fact, a 2011 study indicated that children who are deaf may be a greater risk for victimization by bullying than children with typical hearing, and reported that perpetrators often believe that their victims will not report the abuse.[44] A child who is DHH may have language usage issues or delays and may misinterpret social cues, which can compound trouble. In many ways technology can level the playing field between learners who are DHH and their typically hearing peers. However, technology must be used responsibly and carefully to limit opportunities for cyberbullying. Parents and educators should explicitly teach appropriate online communication skills, discuss the advantages and

Table 16.6 Suggestions for promoting advocacy and independence

- Provide requisite vocabulary for navigating specific situations and circumstances
- Enhance pragmatic skills, possibly including role-playing
- Teach how to care for listening technology as independently as possible
- Suggest participation in extracurricular activities, church groups, or sports
- Involvement in community service groups or projects
- Nurture positive working relationships
- Strengthen self-advocacy skills, gradually fading parental support
- Encourage participation in IEP meetings
- Promote volunteer efforts and opportunities
- Develop plans for secondary education, vocational skills, or employment

disadvantages of the cyberworld, and monitor online activity, including the use of possible filters or parental controls that limit inappropriate content. See the Resources section of this text for websites focused on the protection of school-age learners from bullying and maltreatment.

- *Transition to Post-Secondary & Careers*

All the work done by children, families, and professionals throughout the early intervention, early childhood, and school age years, in fact, prepares learners who are DHH for their adult life. One's early experiences continue to impact postsecondary and occupational outcomes, thus planning and preparation for the transition from educational settings into adulthood begins well in advance of high school graduation. Yet, the transition out of school-based services also provides a good time to reflect on the independent living, self-advocacy, and social skills needed to live a fulfilled life.[45] Just as accommodations, modifications, and technology were used to support learners who are DHH in school settings, these tools apply to post-secondary education environments and the workplace as well. See Reister[45] for a description of common solutions to communication challenges, including accommodations, in postsecondary and workplace settings. In the U.S., publicly supported vocational rehabilitation agencies are available to support individuals who are DHH in obtaining employment or securing the services and supports needed to be successful in the workforce. The Americans with Disabilities Act (ADA) is the federal law that includes provisions for workplace and public accommodations. This legislation requires employers to make reasonable accommodations for qualified employees. While the learner who is DHH can still receive special education services prior to the transition to postsecondary and workforce, professionals supporting these learners can begin to encourage the skills that will be necessary beyond the educational environment. These skills include helping learners understand their legal rights under ADA, how to utilize real-time captioning, interpreters, telecommunication relay services, and video remote interpreting. The development of self-advocacy skills, such as educating others about one's hearing loss, advance preparation, making use of anticipatory strategies, and persistence in pursuit of accommodations will support an individual's success in post-secondary and work environments.[45] In sum, "Self-determination skills—including communication, assertiveness, confidence in

self, negotiation, and problem solving—are important and need to be promoted and fostered in individuals with hearing loss in the school setting and also at home within families."[45]

16.7 Conclusion

For children who are DHH, their experiences in educational settings can make all the difference between outstanding achievement and underachievement. Along with support from parents, practitioners must strive to deliver the necessary and appropriate support for children to learn, flourish, and meet their full potential. Now, more than ever, with technological and pedagogical advances that support listening and spoken language development, children who are DHH have the opportunity to do just that. Indeed, the collective responsibility of each individual in a child's village is great in scale; yet the outcome of such great responsibility, coupled with deliberate and focused collaboration, makes all the difference in the life of that child.

Discussion Questions

1. Describe the conditions when a school-age learner who scores within normal limits on standardized assessment can still benefit from the support of a teacher of the deaf or associated professional?

2. Some itinerant educators find pre-teaching, post-teaching or teaching vocabulary is the *only or primary* role of the itinerant teacher. How would you describe other critical aspects of an itinerant's position? Why might these responsibilities be overlooked or neglected? What is the potential impact on the learner who is DHH when an itinerant only focuses on vocabulary or tutoring?

3. In some settings, teachers of the deaf and speech-language pathologists work in silos. Some professionals would even suggest that instruction provided by a teacher of the deaf and speech-language pathologists should not intersect but should focus on separate goals and targets. However, in the educational setting in particular, current evidence supports the intentional coordination of instruction among the complementary scope of practice. What might be the shared IEP goals and targets addressed by both professionals?

4. How would you explain the concept of *closing the gap* in preschoolers' communication skills to general educators? What placement options and instructional conditions are best suited to support closing the gap? Why?

5. In what way can educators, AV practitioners, listening and spoken language specialists and related service providers best support the social and pragmatic development of learner's while attending to their academic and cognitive priorities? How might intentional interprofessional practice support these learners who are DHH across a variety of instructional settings?

6. Compare and contrast the supports afforded by IEPs and 504 plans while considering what accommodations and modifications are necessary for a given learner who is DHH to access the general education curriculum.

7. What is the role of the family versus the responsibility of the professionals regarding advocacy and social emotional development of an early-childhood aged learner who is DHH? How do these roles and responsibilities shift as a learner ages?

8. How can a learner who is DHH develop strong social emotional competence and self-advocacy skills from early childhood through school-age learning environments? What services and supports will need to be in place to ensure optimal development of these skills? What pitfalls can be predicted throughout one's educational experience and which supports can be provided to bolster student success?

Case Studies

Case A: Ana is a 4 year 6 month old who has been utilizing bilateral cochlear implants since she was 11 months old. Her parents received weekly, in home, early intervention visits from a Certified Listening and Spoken Language Specialist (LSLS) since she was just one month old. Because she turned three, Ana has been attending her public school district's regional DHH preschool where she has been participating in intensive listening and spoken language instruction from a team of professionals. At her upcoming IEP meeting, her family plans to advocate for Ana to transition to her neighborhood elementary school when she begins kindergarten. What services and supports will Ana's team want to identify to ensure her continued success? What are the potential benefits and risks of transition at this time? How might the team ensure Ana's needs continue to be met in an inclusive educational setting?

Case B: Benny is an 11-year-old who utilizes a bone-anchored hearing aid due to bilateral microtia. He has good access to sound when wearing his device, but still struggles to perceive speech in noisy environments such as the cafeteria, gymnasium, and in all-school assemblies and extracurricular events. Benny's parents speak Spanish and Benny has developed linguistic competence in both spoken English (school) and Spanish. His educational team is proud of his academic success but remains concerned about the upcoming transition to middle school, where the school personnel may not be as aware of the impact of his hearing status on his communication. Further, the team is particularly concerned about Benny's social relationships as he is well-regarded by the peers who have attended school with him since kindergarten, but he is not particularly outgoing and lacks confidence in novel situations. How will you support Benny in preparation for the transition to middle school? How will you help to prepare the middle school team of professionals who will serve Benny over the next three years?

Case C: Ms. Cash is an itinerant teacher of the deaf who serves a cooperative of three rural public school districts in the Midwest. Ms. Cash's caseload of 23 students ranges in age from three through 19. Her students utilize a range of communication modalities and varied hearing technology. She has a strong collaborative relationship with the educational audiologist who also works for the co-op, and together they are able to service the hearing assistive technology and classroom amplification systems to ensure those learners who utilize hearing technology have consistent access to sound during the school day. Ms. Cash primarily serves learners on her caseload in independent pull-out interactions, as required by the IEPs. However, more recently, Ms. Cash has been concerned that the authorized IEP minutes are insufficient to support the language and communication development of several preschoolers and early elementary students on her caseload. While some of these learners also have minutes with speech-language pathologists and special educators, the authorizations are inconsistent, their practitioners work in different buildings and have limited time for collaboration, and their schools operate on different academic calendars and schedules. How might you design an educational program that more efficiently meets the needs of learners on Ms. Cash's caseload? What assessment data would you need to make recommendations for program development and ongoing monitoring? If met with resistance from district administration, how might you justify the development of more coordinated regional programming to support learners who are DHH? What would be on your *must-have, wish-list,* and *could-do-without* request for resources?

References

[1] Geers A, Moog J, Rudge A. Effects of frequency of early intervention on spoken language and literacy levels of children who are deaf or hard of hearing in preschool and elementary school. *J Early Hear Detect Interv* 2019;4(1):15–27 10.26077/7pxh-mx41

[2] Geers AE, Nicholas JG. Enduring advantages of early cochlear implantation for spoken language development. *J Speech Lang Hear Res* 2013;56(2):643–655 10.1044/1092-4388(2012/11-0347)

[3] Lenihan S. Trends and challenges in teacher preparation in deaf education. *Volta Review* 2010;110(2):117–128

[4] Moog J, Rudge A. 21st century teenagers and young adults who are deaf or hard of hearing: outcomes and possibilities. *J Early Hear Detect Interv* 2019;4(1):1–14 10.26077/jzyj-kz24

[5] Nittrouer S. Beyond early intervention: supporting children with CIs through elementary school. *Otol Neurotol* 2016;37(2):e43–e49

[6] Yoshinaga-Itano C, Sedey AL, Wiggin M, Mason CA. Language outcomes improved through early hearing detection and earlier cochlear implantation. *Otol Neurotol* 2018;39(10):1256–1263 10.1097/MAO.0000000000001976

[7] Berndsen M, Luckner J. Supporting students who are deaf or hard of hearing in general education classrooms: a Washington State case study. *Comm Disord Q* 2012;33(2):111–118

[8] Estabrooks W. 101 FAQs About Auditory Verbal Practice. Alexander Graham Bell Association for the Deaf and Hard of Hearing; 2012

[9] Voss J, Stredler-Brown A. Getting off to a good start: practices in early intervention. In: Lenihan S, ed. Preparing to Teach, Committing to Learn: An Introduction to Educating Children Who Are Deaf/Hard of Hearing.; 2019:8.1–8.18

[10] Ferrell KA, Bruce S, Luckner JL. Evidence-based practices for students with sensory impairments (Document No. IC-4). *Retrieved Univ Fla Collab Eff Educ Dev Account Reform Cent Website Httpceedar Educ Ufl Edutoolsinnovation-Config.* Published online 2014

[11] Luckner JL, Ayantoye C. Itinerant teachers of students who are deaf or hard of hearing: practices and preparation. *J Deaf Stud Deaf Educ* 2013;18(3):409–423

[12] Anderson KL, Arnoldi KA. Building Skills for Success in the Fast-Paced Classroom: Optimizing Achievement for Students with Hearing Loss. Butte Publications; 2011

[13] Schools OPTION. Inc. Published 2020. Accessed April 20, 2020. https://optionlsl.org/

[14] White E. Listening & spoken language preschool programs. In: Lenihan S, ed. Preparing to Teach, Committing to Learn: An Introduction to Educating Children Who Are Deaf/Hard of Hearing. National Center for Hearing Assessment and Management; 2019:9.1–9.30

[15] Reed S, Antia SD, Kreimeyer KH. Academic status of deaf and hard-of-hearing students in public schools: student, home, and service facilitators and detractors. *J Deaf Stud Deaf Educ* 2008;13(4):485–502

[16] Lederberg AR, Schick B, Spencer PE. Language and literacy development of deaf and hard-of-hearing children: successes and challenges. *Dev Psychol* 2013;49(1):15–30

[17] Dostal H, Gabriel R, Weir J. Supporting the literacy development of students who are deaf/hard of hearing in inclusive classrooms. *Read Teach* 2017;71(3):327–334

[18] Evans MB, Clark SK. Finding a place for CCSS literacy skills in the middle school social studies curriculum. *Clear House J Educ Strateg Issues Ideas* 2015;88(1):1–8

[19] Ming K. 10 Content-area literacy strategies for art, mathematics, music, and physical education. *Clear House J Educ Strateg Issues Ideas* 2012;85(6):213–220

[20] Chute PM, Nevins ME. School Professionals Working with Children with Cochlear Implants. Plural Pub.; 2006

[21] Torppa R, Huotilainen M. Why and how music can be used to rehabilitate and develop speech and language skills in hearing-impaired children. *Hear Res* 2019;*380*:108–122

[22] Klein E, Hollingshead A. Collaboration between special and physical education: the benefits of a healthy lifestyle for all students. *Teach Except Child* 2015;*47*(3):163–171 10.1177/0040059914558945

[23] Williams CB. No Limits: A Practical Guide for Teaching Deaf and Hard of Hearing Students. 2nd ed. Butte Publications; 2019

[24] Eskridge H, Wilson K. Language assessment of children with hearing loss. In: Assessing Listening and Spoken Language in Children with Hearing Loss. Plural Publishing; 2015:133–156

[25] Seaver L. Hands & Voices : Automatic Eligibility. A Question of Automatic Eligibility: Does My Deaf/HH Child Need an IEP? Published 2000. Accessed April 19, 2020. http://www.handsandvoices.org/articles/education/law/auto_elig.html

[26] AG Bell Association for Deaf & Hard of Hearing. AG Bell. Published 2020. Accessed April 20, 2020. https://www.agbell.org/

[27] Johnson A, Ed. Interprofessional education and interprofessional practice in communication sciences and disorders: an introduction and case-based examples of implementation in education and health care settings. American Speech-Language Hearing Association; 2016. Accessed February 17, 2017. http://www.asha.org/Practice/Interprofessional-Education-Practice/

[28] Fenton P, Ocasio-Stoutenburg L, Harry B. The power of parent engagement: sociocultural considerations in the quest for equity. *Theory Pract* 2017;*56*(3):214–225

[29] Peters K. Considering the classroom: Educational access for children fitted with hearing assistive technology. *Audiol Today* 2017;*29*(1):20–30

[30] The cascading impact of hearing loss on access to school communication. Central Institute for the Deaf. Published July 12, 2017. Accessed June 23, 2020. https://cid.edu/2017/07/12/cascading-impact-hearing-loss-access-school-communication/

[31] Bess FH, Davis H, Camarata S, Hornsby BWY. Listening-related fatigue in children with unilateral hearing loss. *Lang Speech Hear Serv Sch* 2020;*51*(1):84–97 10.1044/2019_LSHSS-OCHL-19-0017

[32] Pichora-Fuller MK, Kramer SE, Eckert MA, et al. Hearing impairment and cognitive energy: the framework for understanding effortful listening (FUEL). *Ear Hear* 2016;*37*(Suppl 1):5S–27S 10.1097/AUD.0000000000000312

[33] US Department of Education. Deaf Students Education Services; Policy Guidance. Published January 10, 2020. Accessed April 20, 2020. https://www2.ed.gov/about/offices/list/ocr/docs/hq9806.html

[34] Luckner JL, Sebald AM. Promoting self-determination of students who are deaf or hard of hearing. *Am Ann Deaf* 2013;*158*(3):377–386

[35] Luckner JL, Muir S. Suggestions for helping students who are deaf succeed in general education settings. *Comm Disord* Q 2002;*24*(1):23–30

[36] Hands and Voices. Observe, Understand and Respond: the O.U.R. Children's Safety Project. Published 2019. Accessed April 20, 2020. https://www.handsandvoices.org/resources/OUR/index.htm

[37] Johnson H. Protecting the most vulnerable from abuse. *ASHA Lead*. Published online November 20, 2012. Accessed January 9, 2013. http://www.asha.org/Publications/leader/2012/121120/Protecting-the-Most-Vulnerable-From-Abuse.htm

[38] Child Welfare Information Gateway. Adverse Childhood Experiences (ACEs). Published 2020. Accessed April 20, 2020. https://www.childwelfare.gov/topics/preventing/preventionmonth/resources/ace/

[39] Center for Disease Control and Prevention. Preventing Adverse Childhood Experiences: Leveraging the Best Available Evidence. National Center for Injury Prevention and Control, Centers for Disease Control and Prevention; 2019:40

[40] Bethell C, Jones J, Gombojav N, Linkenbach J, Sege R. Positive childhood experiences and adult mental and relational health in a statewide sample: associations across adverse childhood experiences levels. *JAMA Pediatr* 2019;*173*(11):e193007–e193007 10.1001/jamapediatrics.2019.3007

[41] Voss J, Lenihan S. Fostering resilience in children living in poverty: effective practices and resources for EHDI professionals. In: Schmeltz L, ed. The NCHAM EBook: A Resource Guide for Early Hearing Detection & Intervention (EHDI). National Center for Hearing Assessment and Management; 2014. http://www.infanthearing.org/ehdi-ebook/

[42] National Center on Birth Defects and Developmental Disabilities, Centers for Disease Control and Prevention. Milestones: Learn the Signs. Act Early. Published December 5, 2019. Accessed January 11, 2017. https://www.cdc.gov/ncbddd/actearly/milestones/index.html

[43] Hands & Voices. Parent Safety Toolkit: O.U.R Children's Safety and Success Project. Published online January 2020. https://www.handsandvoices.org/pdf/OUR-Toolkit.pdf

[44] Bauman S, Pero H. Bullying and cyberbullying among deaf students and their hearing peers: an exploratory study. *J Deaf Stud Deaf Educ* 2011;*16*(2):236–253

[45] Reister M. Career development & adult life. In: Lenihan S, ed. Preparing to Teach, Committing to Learn: An Introduction to Educating Children Who Are Deaf/Hard of Hearing. Logan, UT: National Center for Hearing Assessment and Management; 2019:16.1–16.16. https://www.infanthearing.org/ebook-educating-children-dhh/chapters/16%20Chapter%2016%202017.pdf

V
Completing the Structure

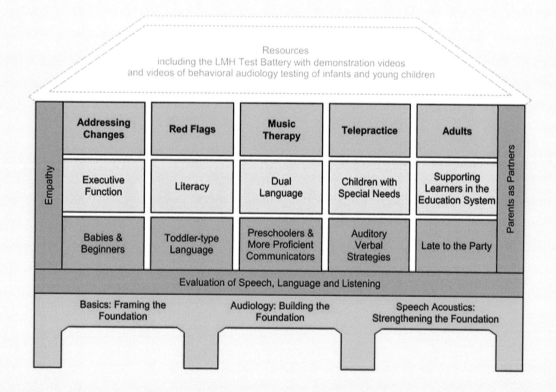

17 Addressing Changes in Auditory Access

Jane R. Madell and Joan G. Hewitt

Summary

The chapter discusses how to manage children who are experiencing changes in hearing and/or technology. The discussion includes children with borderline or unilateral hearing loss, children with progressive hearing loss moving to hearing aids and from hearing aids to cochlear implants, as well as children who did not rely on audition moving from hearing aids to cochlear implants after several years of hearing aid use. Children who move from hearing aids to cochlear implants will need auditory-based therapy to assist them in learning to listen to a different sound quality and to recognize and utilize frequency bands they have not heard before. Listening and spoken language therapy for children in the different categories will be discussed.

Keywords

auditory brain, borderline hearing loss, unilateral hearing loss, auditory memory, phonemic synthesis, language learning, auditory access, cochlear implants, sequential or simultaneous implantation, listening and spoken language therapy, children who are late identified,

Key Points

- Children who are identified late, or who, for some reason, have not used appropriate technology, will take longer to adjust to hearing aids and cochlear implants and, may not develop open set skills
- Children who receive technology late will need auditory based therapy to learn to use hearing technology successfully and develop auditory skills.
- Children who move from hearing aids to cochlear implants will need auditory based therapy to assist them in learning to listen to different sound quality and to recognize and utilize frequency bands they have not heard before.
- When children have been using hearing aids for several years, they may have difficulty adapting to hearing with the cochlear implant (CI). Removing the hearing aid (HA) and listening with the CI alone 2–3 hours a day will quickly build skills in the CI ear.

17.1 Introduction

Many children with hearing loss are identified within weeks and months of birth, are fitted with technology early, receive therapy and show progress with little difficulty. However, this ideal situation is not what happens with every child. Some children are not identified early, either because they were born in a place where screening for infant hearing loss is not taking place or

because their families did not participate. Other children have hearing losses that develop during infancy and childhood. Some families do not choose to use listening and spoken language for their children and do not provide hearing technology and/or auditory based therapies to their children when hearing loss is identified. Others do not have the financial ability to do so or live in a place where services are not available. Some families provide hearing aids initially but choose not to move on to cochlear implants when they are recommended. (See Chapter 11, "Late to the Party," for further discussion of reasons hearing loss may be late identified.) Finally, many children with hearing losses have changes in hearing that cause them to need changes in hearing technology. (See case reports at end of chapter.)

Pearl

Late-identified children will need technology and therapy to develop listening and spoken language skills.

17.2 Borderline and Unilateral Hearing Loss

Children with borderline or unilateral hearing loss may manage for some time, especially in the early years. But as language and learning become more critical, the effects of the hearing loss become more obvious. As children with borderline or unilateral hearing loss get older, some will start to struggle without hearing technology. For some, this happens when they are in preschool. For others, this does not happen until elementary school, and for a few, the difficulties may not become evident until high school. Families, clinicians, and educators recognize that the child is struggling and recommend having the child receive technology. As children start using technology, they will need assistance learning to use the technology and will require therapy to build auditory skills to permit them to use hearing to learn language and academics.

17.2.1 Listening and Spoken Language Therapy

While children with unilateral, borderline or mild hearing loss will have developed language skills, they will often be delayed. They may have difficulty with some specific language learning difficulties, such as problems with auditory memory, development of morphemes or phonemic synthesis, and can have speech production or perception errors due to problems with auditory access. Therapy will need to begin with assessments to identify the areas of weakness. It is important to use assessments that will show existing gaps in skills. Assessment will ensure that intervention begins from the appropriate starting point to build skills from the child's current level and must also fill in language "holes" the child may have. Many of these missing skills will develop readily with appropriately targeted intervention. These children may have speech production errors that are difficult to correct if they are habitual, automatic, and the result of many years of insufficient auditory access. If children have not heard high frequencies, they may be missing phonemes in their speech and morphemes in their language which are both dependent on high-frequency access. When technology is received, or when technology settings are improved, they may start hearing high-frequency sounds but still not be incorporating them into speech or language. Therapy for these children should not be long lived after technology is appropriately fitted and good auditory recognition develops.

17.3 Moving from Hearing Aids to Cochlear Implants

Many babies are now receiving cochlear implants early, but some children will continue to use hearing aids for several years and not receive cochlear implants until they are in elementary school, high school, or even later. It should not be assumed that receiving a cochlear implant alone will be sufficient and that no other services are needed after implantation for children to do well. Children who have developed good auditory skills with hearing aids should move relatively quickly to hearing with cochlear implants. Once they are implanted, all children (and adults), even those with well-developed language, will certainly benefit from auditory-based therapy. The better their auditory skills with hearing aids, the easier the transition to cochlear implants.

17.3.1 Realistic Expectations

Realistic expectations are critical. The audiologist will have counseled the family that, at first, a cochlear implant may sound like beeps and may be difficult to understand. In our experience, even though we tell families that children will not hear optimally when the implant is turned on, parents still often expect that children will hear very well. Older children who receive implants late will have the same reaction. We have had older children or families say *"I know you told me that it would sound like beeps but I thought I would understand speech right away."* We need to reassure families, that, in a relatively short period of time, children will begin to recognize voices and then some sounds and maybe some words. The more children listen with the implant the better they will hear and will develop skills not evidenced with hearing aids.

17.3.2 Sequential vs. Simultaneous Implantation

Most children who have been using hearing aids for several years will receive only one implant when moving from hearing aids to cochlear implants. If children have been using hearing aids, even if they have not heard optimally with the hearing aids, they will have become accustomed to hearing in a particular way. For a few weeks after surgery, prior to initial stimulation with the implant,

they will have to rely on hearing from only the hearing aid in the unimplanted ear. If we were to schedule simultaneous implantation, the children may have no hearing at all from surgery until the implants are turned on, and it might be several additional weeks to months before they hear well with the implants. For a child who is used to hearing, this would be very stressful, and sequential implantation may be preferable. For children who have not heard well enough with hearing aids to understand language, simultaneous implantation may be a better decision.

Pearl

For children who are used to hearing with hearing aids, and who have developed language with hearing aids, sequential implantation in one ear is recommended because losing hearing in both ears at the same time could be very stressful. For children who have not heard well enough with hearing aids to understand language, simultaneous implantation may be a better decision.

Adapting to the new implant.—We strongly recommend that new implant users try listening with the "new ear" alone 2–3 hours each day to build listening in that ear. The rest of the day they can and should listen with both ears. Children are likely to rely on the familiar sound from their other ear (hearing aid or CI) and "ignore" the hearing in the "new CI ear." Removing the familiar sound will help the child focus on listening with the new CI. In addition, long term hearing aid users may expect the implant to sound like a hearing aid and may be surprised when previously recognized low-frequency sounds are different and previously unrecognized high-frequency sounds are audible. They may also be surprised that the sound doesn't seem as loud as they were accustomed to with hearing aids. Again, listening with the implant alone for periods each day is essential to the child's adaptation to and recognition of the new sounds provided by the implant.

Pearl

When children have been using hearing aids, they may have difficulty adapting to hearing with the CI. Removing the HA and listening with the CI alone for 2–3 hours a day will quickly build skills in the CI ear.

17.3.3 Listening and Spoken Language Therapy

Therapy is critical. Even if a child has "graduated" from auditory-verbal therapy, it will be important to start therapy again now. The child's language and auditory skills determine the length of intervention. In general, as with all therapy, treatment has to be diagnostic. We need to start by assessing the child's areas of strength and weakness and use that information to develop an appropriate therapy-plan. The child who receives a cochlear implant will likely not have heard high-frequency sounds at all or only at a loud, probably distorted, level, or may have heard them at one time but, due to a drop in hearing, may no longer be hearing them. Initial therapy may be directed at helping the child discriminate and identify high-frequency sounds and use them in understanding speech. Nevertheless, it is important to recognize that, for children moving from hearing aids to cochlear implants, there is not one right developmental pattern. Some children may initially recognize high-frequency sounds and phonemes more easily; other may recognize low-frequency sounds and phonemes more easily. Moreover, development is not always linear so identifying and working with what a child can hear, rather than focusing on what the child cannot hear, is essential and encouraging to both the child and the family. For children who have not heard some part of the speech spectrum well prior to receiving an implant, we can expect that they can continue to have some speech production issues. While they may be hearing sounds well at this time, their capability to incorporate new auditory information into speech production may be limited. Some phonemes may develop spontaneously with the initial improvement of auditory access while some may require targeted intervention that matches perception and production. If the child has had poor perception and production for a long time, accurate production may not become automatic.

Typically, the longer the child has not heard well, the more difficult the problem will be to correct.

Pearl

In planning therapy, development is not always linear so identifying and working with what a child can hear, rather than focusing on what the child cannot hear, is essential and encouraging to both the child and the family.

17.4 Moving to Implants for Children Who Have Not Relied on Audition with Hearing Aids

Some families will decide to move children to cochlear implants, who either have not worn hearing aids before or have worn hearing aids but were enrolled in an educational program that relied on a sign system rather than listening and spoken language. Some families may make this decision because they feel that their child is not making good progress in a school for the deaf and they want to move them into a mainstream classroom. For others, a change in medical condition may suggest the need for a change in program, such as deteriorating vision with a diagnosis of retinitis pigmentosa or some physical condition that would make signing difficult. Finally, some parents may realize that they themselves are struggling to develop fluent signing skills and may wish to explore other avenues of communication with their child.

17.4.1 Realistic Expectations

For this population it is essential that both the child and the family have realistic expectations. If children have never used

audition for communication, it is not reasonable to expect that they will be able to rely on listening for communication. Children who have never had open set word recognition with hearing aids will not have open set word recognition within a short time after receiving an implant. Younger children, who have a more plastic auditory brain, will have a better chance of developing good auditory skills. Children who are implanted as teenagers or young adults and who have had little or no auditory access prior to receiving a cochlear implant will have less plastic auditory brains, so they will have a more difficult time developing auditory skills. Moreover, if the children have relied on visual communication and have no familiarity with the spoken language that is being introduced, even as auditory awareness develops, they will not be able to interpret spoken words and sentences because they are essentially listening to a foreign language.

17.4.2 Listening and Spoken Language Therapy

Auditory based therapy is critical for children who have used sign language for communication and are now working on developing auditory skills for the first time. While many of the therapy goals and techniques will be the same as those used for very young children, the activities will need to be more directed to the age and interests of the child. Goals should be practical, helping children to learn the skills they need to use to develop basic, but meaningful audition. Moreover, goals should focus on skills which will aid in the recognition and understanding of speech and language, rather than the recognition and identification of environmental sounds. How far a child progresses will vary depending on the age of the child and their brain plasticity at the time of implantation, the child's prior history of hearing aid use, and the child's history of participation in a therapy program which worked to develop auditory skills before implantation. Obviously, the younger the child, the greater the use of technology prior to receiving the implant, and the more the child has been in a therapy program that emphasizes audition, the more likely the child is to develop good auditory skills.

17.5 Children Who Are Late Identified

Some children are late identified because they are born in countries or communities without newborn hearing screening. Some are late identified because, for one reason or another, the family did not follow-up on a referral from newborn hearing screening, and some are late identified because the child has experienced a drop in hearing that was not recognized. In all cases, the child will need a lot of help to catch up. (See Chapter 11, "Late to the Party," for further discussion of reasons hearing loss may be late identified.)

17.5.1 Technology

Technology is the first step. For children to develop listening and spoken language skills, appropriate, quality amplification must be fitted as quickly as possible. Hearing aids are the typical first step. However, if a child is late identified with reliable audiological testing indicating a severe or profound hearing loss, we can know by looking at the audiogram that the child is not going to obtain good benefit from hearing aids. For this child, moving directly to cochlear implants is the appropriate next step. The original premise of cochlear implantation for profound hearing loss was based on a 95% confidence rate that a child with profound hearing loss would perform better with a cochlear implant than a hearing aid.[1,2,3] However, these researchers are suggesting that a child with a severe or even moderately severe hearing loss has a 75% probability of receiving more benefit from a cochlear implant than a hearing aid. Similarly, Dettman[4] and Boothroyd[5] report that for the development of oral communication, 70 dB is the basic "dividing" line. Children with hearing loss at 70 dB or more will perform better with a cochlear implant. Technology needs to be appropriately fitted as quickly as possible (see Chapter 2, "Audiology: Building the Foundation"). After technology is fitted, it is time to move on to therapy.

17.5.2 Listening and Spoken Language Therapy

Therapy for a late identified child has to start at the beginning. We need to start by assessing the current child's levels with the understanding that there can be inconsistencies in skill development. We must move through the process of identifying strengths and weaknesses, determining goals, and addressing them step by step through therapy as discussed in Chapters 1, "Basics: Framing the Foundation," and 11, "Late to the Party." When children come late to listening and spoken language, therapy activities will be different for an older child, but the goals are the same. We are not going to select an airplane to fly for a 10-year-old the way we would do for a 1-year-old, but we can do the same activity with paper and pencil.

Pearl

Children who are identified late or who have changes in hearing will need auditory-based therapy to develop good skills. The amount of therapy they will need will depend on what their auditory skills were prior to receiving new technology.

17.6 Summary

Even though a child has not received appropriate technology, every child deserves the right to receive good technology, appropriately set, and to receive therapy to build auditory skills, language, and literacy. The younger a child is, the more likely the child will develop good open set word recognition when appropriate technology is received. Children with unilateral, mild, and borderline hearing loss will receive benefit from appropriate technology and therapy. As with other children, the earlier the better. Children who are older, but have worn hearing aids and have auditory-based therapy would still be expected to receive good benefit from receiving a cochlear implant. Children who did not

use technology early will not have developed an auditory brain so, although they will receive some benefit from technology, they are not likely to develop open set word recognition and will continue to need a visual system (speech reading, cued speech, or a signed language) to communicate. (See Chapter 1, "Basics: Framing the Foundation" for discussion about communication systems.)

Discussion Questions

1. What can we expect in language and listening for a child with a unilateral hearing loss who is not using technology?
2. How do we determine what kind of habilitation (technology and therapy) a child who has hearing loss identified late requires?
3. How would you counsel a family of a 10 year old who has never used technology and has been enrolled in a signing program about expectations?

References

[1] de Kleijn JL, van Kalmthout LWM, van der Vossen MJB, Vonck BMD, Topsakal V, Bruijnzeel H. Identification of pure-tone audiologic thresholds for pediatric cochlear implant candidacy: a systematic review. *JAMA Otolaryngol Head Neck Surg* 2018;*144*(7):630–638 10.1001/jamaoto.2018

[2] Leigh JR, Dettman SJ, Dowell RC. Evidence-based guidelines for recommending cochlear implantation for young children: audiological criteria and optimizing age at implantation. *Int J Audiol* 2016; *55*(2, Suppl 2):S9–S18. doi:10.3109/14992027.2016.1157268

[3] Lovett RES, Vickers DA, Summerfield AQ. Bilateral cochlear implantation for hearing-impaired children: criterion of candidacy derived from an observational study. *Ear Hear* 2015;*36*(1):14–23 10.1097/aud.0000000000000087.0652

[4] Dettman SJ, Dowell RC, Choo D, et al. Long-term communication outcomes for children receiving cochlear implants younger than 12 months: a multicenter study. *Otol Neurotol* 2016;*37*(2):e82–e95

[5] Boothroyd A. Auditory capacity of hearing-impaired children using hearing aids and cochlear implants: issues of efficacy and assessment. *Scand Audiol Suppl* 1997;*46*:17–25

Case 1

Susan is 16 years old. She has a profound bilateral sensorineural hearing loss which was identified when she was 14 months of age. She has been enrolled in programs using American Sign Language (ASL) in schools for the deaf since her hearing loss was identified. She wore hearing aids for a few months as an infant but received very little benefit. The family made the decision to remove the hearing aids because she was not receiving benefit and because the family had made the decision to use signed communication. Both parents learned sign language and moved closer to the school for the deaf so Susan could live at home. Susan has good signing skills and is doing well in her school program.

Susan has recently been diagnosed with retinitis pigmentosa and is quickly losing vision. Because the vision loss is expected to progress, the family is anxious to try and build her auditory skills at this time. Susan and the family came to the center to see if Susan is a candidate for a cochlear implant. Susan wanted to know if she was going to be able to hear on the phone with a cochlear implant. Susan has not worn hearing technology since she was two years old. As a result, she has not developed an auditory brain and does not have good auditory skills. She does not alert to speech or to other sounds and does not use audition for understanding speech. She has not developed good auditory brain functioning so telephone use with a cochlear implant is not a realistic expectation.

Evaluation Results

Audiology—audiology testing confirms a profound bilateral sensorineural hearing loss. Susan was tested with hearing aids that were appropriately fitted using real ear measurements and testing performance in the test booth. Testing indicated aided thresholds at moderate hearing loss levels, indicating that Susan was not hearing soft speech and was hearing normal conversation at a very soft level. Speech perception was tested using pictures in a closed set format and was very poor, with scores below 20% monaurally and binaurally.

Speech-language-listening evaluation—Testing using signed language indicated that language skills were two years delayed at both expressive and receptive levels.

Recommendation to the Family

Test results were described and reviewed so both Susan and her parents understood the test results. We discussed that, because Susan had very poor speech perception, it was not likely that she would have good speech perception with the implant. We discussed that research indicates that children as old as Susan who have not had listening experience and who do not have open set speech perception prior to receiving an implant are not likely to have open set speech perception after receiving an implant. We discussed the kind of benefit that Susan could expect with an implant. We would expect her to have awareness of environmental sounds and, with therapy, she might develop some speech perception skills for closed set information but not likely open set speech discrimination.

Because of the need for Susan to know when people were talking to her, and to recognize environmental sounds, the family decided to proceed with cochlear implantation, understanding that expectations were limited.

Auditory-Based Therapy

The first therapy goal was to help Susan recognize when someone was speaking to her and to recognize environmental sounds, especially those which were critical for safety in real life situations. Therapy then would be designed around the results of diagnostic testing. Because Susan had never used audition, progress was slow.

Discussion Questions

1. How would you help a family develop realistic expectations for a child like Susan?
2. How would you structure a therapy program?
3. What would you recommend in addition to using the CI and therapy?

Case 2

Through the newborn hearing screening process, Robby was identified with a bilateral, symmetrical mild sensorineural hearing loss. His parents were counseled by the ENT that, because the hearing loss was mild, hearing aids were the only intervention needed. Robby was fitted with hearing aids at 2 months of age and referred by the audiologist for auditory-verbal services through the public early intervention program. For the first year of his life, Robby received auditory-verbal DHH services in his home 1 to 2 hours per month. At age 1, the services were increased to 1 hour per week.

Over the next 2 years, Robby's mother expressed concerns to the audiologist and early intervention DHH teacher that she was concerned about Robby's slow speech and language progress. At multiple appointments, his mother noted that he was not learning words quickly and that the words he did say were difficult to understand. While the audiologist was seeing the baby for testing every 6 months, she reported that he was "difficult to test" and told the parents that they needed to "input more language." The DHH teacher recognized Robby's mother's concerns, but said that "children develop at different rates."

Because no replicable behavioral hearing results had been obtained, when Robby was 2, the audiologist recommended sedated ABR testing. When Robby's mother discussed with the DHH teacher her concerns about sedation, the DHH teacher stated that the audiological clinic where Robby was being seen was not known to be good with pediatrics and admitted that she was extremely concerned about Robby's significant lack of progress with a mild hearing loss.

Robby's mother sought a second opinion at a pediatric audiological facility. Testing at age 2 years, 6 months revealed a moderate to moderately-severe hearing loss bilaterally, so the hearing aids were reprogrammed, and testing was recommended every 6 months. At this point, Robby finally began making progress in his speech and language development. Initially, progress was fairly rapid, but over the next year it slowed.

Audiological results obtained over the next year were inconsistent, but appeared to again indicate poorer thresholds than previously obtained. The audiologist recommended consultation with a pediatric ENT and a change to more powerful hearing aids with frequency shifting for better perception of high frequencies. The audiologist stated that, if the more powerful hearing aids with frequency shifting did not help, a cochlear implant might need to be considered. The pediatric ENT recommended a CT scan and MRI which were completed.

At this point, Robby's mother sought a third opinion from a different pediatric audiological clinic. On the way to the appointment, she received a call from the pediatric ENT who relayed that bilateral enlarged vestibular aqueduct syndrome (EVA) had been identified on the scans. Robby's testing at age 3 years, 6 months revealed even poorer results than those obtained at the second clinic (**Fig. 17.1** and **Table 17.1**).

Discussion Questions

1. Both the first and second centers recommended audiological testing every 6 months. Was this sufficient in this case? Why or why not?

2. Would you recommend a trial with more powerful hearing aids with frequency shifting prior to cochlear implantation? Why or why not? If yes, for how long?

3. If the family wants to consider cochlear implantation, would you recommend that Robby be simultaneously, bilaterally, or sequentially implanted? Why?

4. If Robby is implanted, what should the parents' expectations be for how he will hear at activation? How would you counsel them?

The Family's Decision

Based on the radiological findings, the audiological results, and the lack of consistent progress despite intensive appropriate intervention, cochlear implantation was recommended. Both the audiologist and cochlear implant surgeon counseled the parents that hearing aid technology would not be sufficient for Robby to develop age appropriate listening, speech, and language. While more powerful hearing aids with frequency shifting might make sounds more audible, they would introduce additional distortion and would not be expected to make speech and language more accessible or intelligible. Moreover, with the diagnosis of EVA, Robby's hearing loss would be expected to continue to progress. Finally, Robby was rapidly approaching the upper end of the critical 0 to 3 year period of language development. Ensuring that he had optimal access to develop speech and language prior to entering kindergarten was essential. Missing preschool because he was being implanted and then could not hear was much less consequential than missing academics after he entered the general education setting.

Although Robby would be without sound for 2 weeks after surgery and before activation, his parents made the difficult decision to have him simultaneously bilaterally implanted. Their reasoning included the facts that he was 3.6 years old and significantly delayed with a severe to profound hearing loss in both ears. Rather than extending a process that had already been significantly delayed, they chose to deal with the short-term challenges of his not hearing.

Robby was simultaneously bilaterally implanted at 3.9 years of age. Although the cochlear implant surgeon allowed Robby to try his hearing aids during the period between surgery and activation, he heard nothing with them and relied solely on speechreading and gestures to communicate.

At the initial activation, Robby's parents were concerned that, while he detected sounds, he did not recognize them. The first month of CI use was very difficult. Robby's parents had excellent AVT support through the preschool program in their school district, but still called the audiologist weekly with significant concerns that he was lipreading and not hearing. Their calls clearly indicated that they were struggling with the decision they had made to implant both ears simultaneously and completely change what he was hearing.

When Robby returned after 1 month for CI programming, his parents reported that, while he continued to ask for repetition of many things they said to him, they had recently noticed several times when he had responded to conversations near him that were not directed at him. By 2 months' post activation, Robby's parents and AVT reported that he, not only had open set listening,

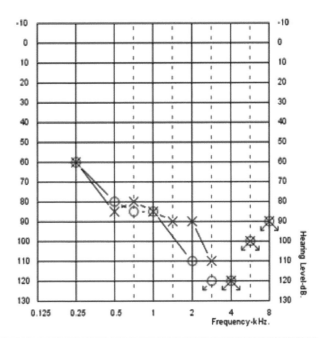

Fig. 17.1 Robby's behavioral thresholds at age 3 years, 6 months.

Table 17.1 Robby's behavioral thresholds at age 3 years, 6 months (CNT = could not test)

*NOTE: All testing was completed open set	Right Ear	Left Ear
Unaided SRT	105 dBHL	105 dBHL
Unaided NU-Chips at 105 dBHL	24%	48%
Aided SRT	CNT at 65 dBHL	50 dBHL
Aided NU-Chips at 50dBHL	CNT	0%

but was overhearing many conversations. Everyone, including Robby, reported that he was hearing better than he had heard with his hearing aids.

At the time of implantation, Robby's language was 18 months delayed. In the first year after implantation, he made more than 2 years' progress in his speech and language. With his current rate of progress (and a fall birthday, which allows him an extra year of preschool), Robby should enter kindergarten with language that is at or above the level of his hearing peers. Robby's parents strongly believe that making the very difficult decision to simultaneously bilaterally implant him was essential to remediating his delays and accelerating his progress to the level that would allow him to catch up with his peers.

Additional Discussion Questions

1. Does a mild hearing loss preclude the need for additional intervention other than hearing aids? If not, what other testing or interventions should be considered? Why?

2. What testing or interventions should be used to help prevent delays in diagnosis and delays in moving from hearing aids to cochlear implants?

3. If Robby's DHH teacher had concerns about his audiological clinic and his progress, should she have shared these with his mother? If so, how and when should she have shared these?

4. Would you consider Robby's hearing loss to be late diagnosed? Why or why not?

Case 3

Initial Audiological Information

Through the newborn hearing screening process, Sam was diagnosed with a bilateral moderate to severe sensorineural hearing loss. Connexin 26 testing was negative. Hearing aids were fitted by 3 months of age. Sam's hearing loss was stable until he hit his head at age 4 and reported that his hearing aids were quiet. Subsequent testing revealed a deterioration in hearing bilaterally. Two months later, Sam fell again and experienced further deterioration of hearing bilaterally, but worse in the right ear. See **Fig. 17.2** and **Table 17.2**.

A CT scan and MRI were then completed, which revealed enlarged vestibular aqueducts (EVA) bilaterally. Cochlear implantation of both ears was recommended, but the parents chose to implant the poorer (right) ear and continue with the hearing aid in the left ear so that Sam would not be without hearing after surgery.

Sam was implanted in his right ear at age 4.6. Although the recommendation was that aural habilitation focus on the development of listening with the right CI alone, Sam was somewhat uncooperative whenever the hearing aid was removed, so listening practice with the CI alone was discontinued at home and in therapy. Sam consistently reported that his implant was too quiet and did not sound like his hearing aid, but he also reported increased stimulation levels were painful. Moreover, programming measurements did not indicate that increased stimulation levels were necessary. Sam's parents were leery of a second implant because aided speech perception for the next 2 years was stable although it remained very poor in both ears. (See **Table 17.3.**)

Table 17.3 Comparison of Sam's speech perception results with his CI and HA 2 years after right ear implantation

	Right CI	Left HA
PBK at 50dBHL	36%	44%

Speech, Language, and Educational Development

Sam was enrolled in early intervention involving auditory-verbal therapy at 3 months of age. Until age 4, Sam's articulation was intelligible, but slightly immature sounding. His fricatives were distorted or stopped. His receptive and expressive language development progressed to within normal limits.

When Sam's hearing changed after the first 2 falls, his receptive language was significantly impacted and he began saying, "Huh?" or "What?" whenever he was spoken to. His articulation also deteriorated. His fricatives were more distorted or omitted. He also began speaking very quickly and quietly which impacted his intelligibility.

After a hearing aid change and implantation of the right ear, Sam again had access to receptive language although he said "huh?" and "what?" consistently. His expressive language was excellent and advanced for his age. His articulation improved, but the fricative issues continued. His rate of speech also remained fast.

In kindergarten, Sam was fully mainstreamed with DHH and SLP support, but each year his teachers reported that he struggled with attention and peer-to-peer communication.

Just before his seventh birthday, Sam slipped climbing out of the bathtub and hit his head. The next day, when he put on his hearing aid, he reported it was not working, even though his parents found it to be working properly. Sam also reported that his voice was "echoing in his head" and that he could not tell how loud he was talking without his CI. Although he noted no change with his CI, he refused to wear his hearing aid because it was "broken." Sam was seen for audiological testing 10 days after he hit his head. Testing revealed the results in **Fig. 17.3**.

Unaided left ear speech perception testing revealed an SAT at 105 dB, but no open set speech perception. Aided speech perception with the left hearing aid was 0% at 65 dB.

Table 17.2 Sam's speech perception results at age 4 after 2 falls

	Right Ear	Left Ear
Unaided PBK at 100dBHL	20%	48%
Aided PBK at 50dBHL	16%	44%

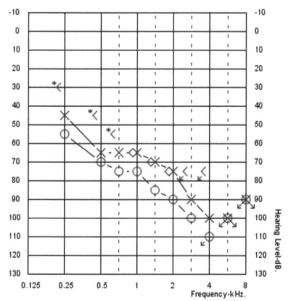

* Vibro-tactile response: Bone-conduction mastoid unmasked right @ 0.250 kHz;
Bone-conduction mastoid unmasked right @ 0.5 kHz; Bone-conduction mastoid unmasked r

Fig. 17.2 Sam's behavioral thresholds at age 4 after 2 falls.

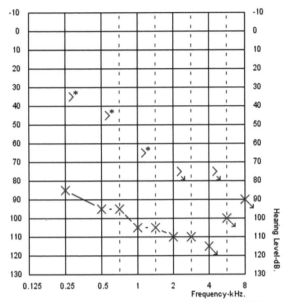

* Vibro-tactile response: Bone-conduction mastoid unmasked left @ 0.250 kHz;
Bone-conduction mastoid unmasked left @ 0.5 kHz; Bone-conduction mastoid unmasked le

Fig. 17.3 Left ear behavioral thresholds at age 7 after fall in bathtub.

However, the most interesting finding was Sam's speech perception with his right CI. Although the CI settings had not been changed, open set CNC testing was significantly improved. (See **Table 17.4**.)

Table 17.4 Sam's speech perception results at age 7 after falling in the bathtub (CNT = Could not test)

	Right CI	Left HA
CNC at 50dB HL	72%	CNT
CNC at 35dB HL	56%	CNT
PBK at 65dB HL		0%

Despite the loss of hearing in the left ear, Sam's parents and his DHH itinerant teacher reported that they had noticed a significant reduction in the number of "huhs?" and "whats?" in the previous week. In addition, his parents, DHH teacher, and audiologist all noted a marked improvement in articulation of fricatives.

Sam was subsequently implanted in his left ear. By the second day of activation, he was showing signs of some open set recognition. One month after activation, recorded CNC testing was completed with both CIs, and the results are presented in **Table 17.5**.

Table 17.5 Sam's speech perception results at age 7, one month after activation of left CI

	Right CI	Left CI
CNC at 50dBHL	80%	52%

Although Sam has always been conversational, he now has an ease of listening that is helping tremendously with classroom attention and peer interactions. Moreover, his articulation and rate of speech are improving with minimal intervention. Sam now reports that he hears "the best ever!"

Discussion Questions

1. As with Case 2, would other testing or interventions have been helpful when Sam's hearing loss was first diagnosed?
2. When Sam was tested 10 days after the fall in the bathtub, why do you think his speech perception with his right CI had improved so dramatically?
3. What do you think was impacting Sam's articulation and rate of speech before and why did they improve after the fall in the bathtub?
4. What do you think hindered his progress with his right CI for the first two years?
5. What techniques might be helpful for encouraging a child who is resistant to removing a hearing aid when learning to listen with a new CI?

Case 4

Jessica failed newborn hearing screening and was identified through ABR testing with a mild hearing loss; however, her parents did not feel a mild hearing loss would impact her, so they declined all intervention. Shortly after Jessica's second birthday, her parents contacted her pediatrician because they were concerned that she had less than 10 words. The pediatrician referred Jessica for an audiological evaluation. Through ABR and behavioral testing, a mild to moderate hearing loss was diagnosed. Again, Jessica's parents had difficulty accepting the diagnosis, so she was not fitted with hearing aids until age 3. The compilation of electrophysiological and behavioral thresholds is shown on **Fig. 17.4**.

By the age of 3 when the hearing aids were fitted, Jessica's language was significantly delayed. She used less than 50 one-word utterances, most of which were unintelligible to anyone except her mother. Because of her significant language delays, Jessica's IEP team provided placement in a regional auditory-oral DHH program outside her home district. Jessica was enrolled in self-contained auditory-oral DHH classrooms until first grade, when she returned to her home district and was mainstreamed fulltime in her home school. Although her receptive and expressive language remained 1 to 2 years delayed, the IEP team felt that, with significant support from the DHH itinerant teacher and the site-based SLP, Jessica could be successful in a mainstream first grade classroom.

After 2 months in the general education classroom, Jessica's teacher requested a meeting of the IEP team because she had significant concerns about Jessica's attention. She reported that Jessica always seemed to be watching her peers, rarely watched the person speaking, generally missed the instructions provided, and often completed assignments incorrectly. The teacher asked the parents to consider an evaluation for attention deficit disorder. While the IEP team was in support of this idea, the DHH itinerant requested that Jessica's hearing be evaluated by the contracted district audiologist prior to an assessment for attention issues. The IEP team agreed to refer Jessica for audiological evaluation.

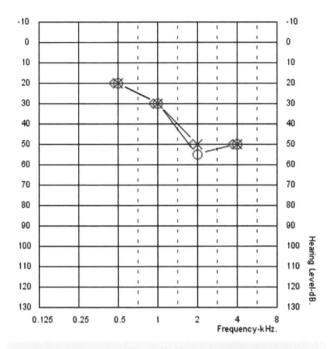

Fig. 17.4 Compilation of electrophysiological and behavior thresholds at age 2 years, 6 months.

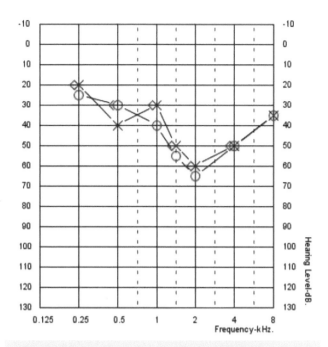

Fig. 17.5 Behavioral thresholds at age 6 years, 5 months.

The behavioral thresholds and speech perception results at age 6 years, 5 months are shown in **Fig. 17.5** and **Table 17.6**. In this testing, thresholds at more frequencies were obtained, which revealed a cookie bite configuration, rising in the high frequencies, rather than a sloping configuration indicated by the previous testing which only included four frequencies. In addition, the aided speech perception testing indicated that Jessica had very poor auditory access at both normal conversational and soft speech levels. When the audiologist reviewed the results and assessed the hearing aids, she noted that Jessica's hearing aids were a very low level of digital technology, with only four frequency band adjustments. With more information concerning the thresholds across the speech spectrum, the audiologist attempted to reprogram the hearing aids. However, with only four fixed frequency bands that could be adjusted, reprogramming of the hearing aids to fit the cookie bite configuration of Jessica's loss and optimize her auditory access was unsuccessful. By this time, Jessica's parents were extremely concerned about her delays and very frustrated that the hearing aids she had been wearing for more than 3 years did not provide her with optimal auditory access.

New digital hearing aids with a much higher level of technology and 16 frequency bands for programming to fit the cookie bite configuration were fitted. A comparison of Jessica's aided speech perception with her low-level (4 frequency bands) and high-level (16 frequency band) technology is presented in **Table 17.7**.

After the fitting of the new high-level hearing aid technology, many interesting events occurred. First, Jessica immediately exclaimed, "I can hear!" Because she had only experienced untreated hearing loss or poorly treated hearing loss, she did not know what it was like to hear easily with clarity. As a result of her improved hearing, Jessica's articulation improved very quickly. Although receptive and expressive language continued

Table 17.6 Speech perception results at age 6 years, 5 months

	Right HA	Left HA
Aided SRT	35dBHL	35dBHL
Aided PBK words at 50dBHL	48%	32%
Aided PBK words at 35dBHL	24%	20%
Aided HINT-C sentences at 50dBHL in quiet	52%	40%

Table 17.7 Comparison of speech perception results with Jessica's low-level (4 frequency band) hearing aid technology and new high-level (16 frequency band) hearing aid technology

	Low level HA—Right	High Level HA—Right	Low level HA—Left	High Level HA—Left
Aided SRT	35dBHL	20dBHL	35dBHL	20dBHL
Aided PBK words at 50dBHL	48%	56%	32%	72%
Aided PBK words at 35dBHL	24%	44%	20%	72%
Aided HINT-C sentences at 50dBHL in quiet	52%	67%	40%	58%

to be delayed, everyone working with Jessica reported that she was learning new words much more quickly and was beginning to use morphological markers that had previously been omitted. Jessica's parents were so astounded by the change in her rate of progress that they contacted the TODs and SLPs from her regional DHH program to ask if they had been aware that their daughter did not hear well with her hearing aids. All the professionals reported that they had been very aware that she did not hear well, but "thought that was what the parents wanted." This was exceptionally frustrating to the parents, who expressed that they had relied on the professionals and experts to guide them.

In addition to improvements in speech and language, Jessica's teacher noted improvements in her attention. She reported that Jessica was much more attentive during direct instruction and was completing more assignments correctly. However, she did note that Jessica continued to look to other students when she was unsure of instructions and rarely attended to other students when they were answering questions in class.

Finally, the district audiologist noted a significant improvement in speech perception with the new left hearing aid. However, while the right ear showed some improvement with the new hearing aid, speech perception remained much poorer than the left. Hearing aid programming changes and hearing aid technology changes did not improve the situation. Jessica has now been followed for more than 10 years. Although the cause of her hearing loss remains unknown, her hearing loss has slowly progressed over time. Throughout the progression, even though the unaided thresholds have remained fairly symmetrical, the right ear's speech perception has always been significantly poorer than the left. Recently, the thresholds in the right ear were noted to progress more than the left. The most recent behavioral threshold and speech perception results obtained at age 17 are presented in **Fig. 17.6** and **Table 17.8**.

Over the past 5 years as the performance of the right ear has declined, the audiologist has discussed possible right ear cochlear implantation with Jessica and her parents. Initially, Jessica was not open to the idea, but she has come to recognize that the speech in her right ear is not as clear as in the left and sometimes

Table 17.8 Speech perception results obtained at age 17

	Right HA	Left HA
SRT	30	25
CNC at 50dB HL	48%	68%
CNC at 35dB HL	4%	44%

interferes with her better hearing in her left ear, especially in noisy situations. Moreover, Jessica is keenly aware of how she has struggled and required support throughout her educational career. Even at age 17, she has vocabulary and comprehension deficits that impact her performance. Despite Jessica's interest in exploring implantation, her parents once again have declined to move forward with the evaluations or intervention.

Discussion Questions

1. How does identifying a hearing loss as "mild" interfere with families obtaining help for their children?

2. Does mild hearing loss require intervention? Why or why not? What are possible effects of untreated hearing loss in babies and toddlers?

3. How is sloping hearing loss (**Fig. 17.4**) different from a cookie bite hearing loss (**Fig. 17.5**)? How do they affect speech perception differently?

4. How would hearing aid programming be different with a cookie bite hearing loss as opposed to a sloping hearing loss? Why was the number of frequency band adjustments so important?

5. While Jessica's single word speech perception improved significantly after the fitting of the high level of technology, her ability to repeat HINT-C sentences improved only slightly (see **Table 17.7**). Why did her single word score improve significantly, but not her sentence score?

6. Why was Jessica's attention initially so poor? Why did she continue to observe other children when she was unsure of instructions and rarely look at other students when they were answering questions in class even after receiving the new hearing aids? Do you think she had attention deficit disorder? Why or why not?

7. Why did Jessica's articulation improve so rapidly after the fitting of the new hearing aids? Why did her rate of vocabulary development and language acquisition become more rapid?

8. What was the responsibility of the TODs and SLPs in the regional DHH program if they observed that Jessica did not hear well with her technology? How could they have broached this subject with the IEP team or the parents?

9. Why is cochlear implantation a consideration for the right ear? How would it benefit her? Would you support this? Why or why not? How would you discuss this with Jessica and her parents?

10. Jessica continues to struggle and require support at age 17. Review the decisions and intervention that she received. How did these early decisions and interventions impact and lead to her difficulties even in high school?

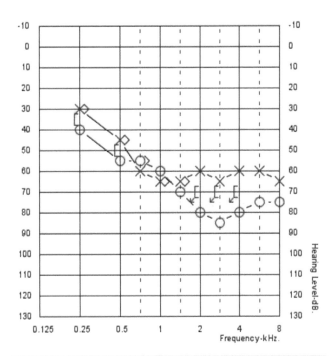

Fig. 17.6 Behavioral thresholds obtained at age 17.

18 Red Flags: Identifying and Managing Barriers to the Child's Optimal Auditory Development

Jane R. Madell and Joan G. Hewitt

This chapter is adapted from a chapter written by Madell, Hewitt, and Rothfleisch for *Pediatric Audiology: Diagnosis, Technology and Management*, 3rd edition, Thieme, 2019.

Summary

The responsibility of clinicians working with children with hearing loss is more than the diagnosis of hearing loss, evaluation of technology and planning therapy. All clinicians have the responsibility for studying the whole child, identifying concerns, and making appropriate recommendations for management. Some children fit with technology do very well. Others seem to struggle. When a child is struggling, it is incumbent on the clinicians to determine why. Speech perception testing—including language appropriate materials in different listening settings, assessing language and speech production—is critical for developing a treatment plan. This chapter will identify "red flags" that indicate when the problem is with technology settings, speech production, language development, or voice and discuss how to improve performance.

Keywords

red flags to auditory/neural development, hypersensitivity, behavioral control issues, vision as primary, insufficient progress, auditory support, intervention support, hearing aids, cochlear implants, BAHA, remote microphones, language development, speech and voice development

Key Points

- The audiologist's responsibility is greater than simply fitting and evaluating hearing aid technology; audiologists also have the responsibility of studying the whole child and making appropriate recommendations.
- The speech-language pathologist's responsibility is greater than teaching language. It includes developing the child's auditory brain and helping the family use audition to develop language and literacy skills
- Teachers of the deaf are responsible for more than monitoring academic performance. They must also monitor auditory, language, and social skills in and outside of the classroom
- All professionals are responsible for fully understanding the child's capabilities within their areas of specialization and for collaborating with other professionals to provide a comprehensive picture of the child and the child's capabilities.
- If an audiological evaluation does not include assessment of aided speech perception at normal and soft conversational levels in quiet and with competing noise using age-appropriate testing materials, professionals and parents will have an

incomplete picture of the child's auditory access to spoken language, which will limit their ability to plan appropriately for the child.

- A child's phoneme perception and production, voice quality, and language development can provide significant data concerning the child's auditory access and the appropriateness of technology settings.
- When a child has appropriate parental and interventional support, red flags point to the type of technology or the technology settings as the source of the child's lack of progress.
- Variability or delay in a child's progress in audition, speech or language should merit investigation into all aspects of the child's intervention.

Many children with hearing loss attain the listening and spoken language outcomes expected by family and professionals. Many children are fitted with technology and do well. They appear to hear sufficiently well to develop speech and language and learn. However, not every child with hearing loss is a superstar. Why is there a huge variation in performance among children who seem to be equal? We know that not all children achieve the same level of listening, spoken language, literacy, and academic proficiency, but why? Certain things are clearly a problem that will explain some differences in performance. For example, some children do not hear well with technology, some are not receiving appropriate therapy, some have parents and family who are not involved and not providing speech and language stimulation, and some have other developmental issues that interfere with progress. However, sometimes all variables seem to be managed in a positive fashion, yet the child still does not make the expected progress.

18.1 The Audiologist's Responsibility When a Child Is Not Attaining Expected Outcomes

The audiologist has a larger responsibility than simply evaluating hearing and fitting hearing aid (HA) and cochlear implant (CI) technology. As audiologists, we have the responsibility for monitoring performance with technology and working with other professionals to study the whole child. All professionals are responsible for fully understanding the child's capabilities within their areas of specialization. Each professional who works with a child with hearing loss needs to evaluate the child's use of auditory information. Audiologists need to obtain threshold information and assess speech perception with technology, while speech-language pathologists and listening and spoken language specialists (LSLS) need to monitor how well the child functions daily while wearing and using auditory technologies in all environments. Teachers of the deaf (TOD) need to monitor the child's use of hearing in the classroom, and parents are responsible for monitoring the child's performance at home and in social settings. The audiologist or other professionals may need to teach parents how to monitor the child's hearing and the child's use of technology so it can be checked on a daily basis.

We must accept and understand that a child's ability to hear is the fundamental basis for all speech and language development and that the success of intervention is reflected in the success of the child. "Success" should be defined as reaching the family's desired outcomes so that the child's spoken language, literacy, and academic skills are consistent with hearing peers. Each professional has the responsibility to understand, not only the data they collect, but the data collected by others as it pertains to the child's development in the critical areas of speech, language, functional listening, and social skills. If a child is not making one year's progress in one year's time, all team members are responsible and should be concerned. Clinicians must look at the overall progress of the child, beyond their own area of specialization. If clinicians look only to their own area of specialization and report that the problem is "not in their area," then the child's development is compartmentalized and the capability of one area of the child's development to positively or negatively affect others is ignored. All professionals must make the commitment to hold themselves accountable and take responsibility to recognize and examine issues in their own areas. To address red flags and improve the child's progress, we must each collaborate with other team members, understand the significance of the measures collected by colleagues in their areas of expertise, and evaluate how these data can contribute to analyzing test results in our own area of expertise. It is critical that the child's lack of progress be discussed with the entire team: all the professionals who work with the child and the family. Only by evaluating all aspects of the child's performance and being willing to accept that some of the responsibility might be ours can we determine what needs to be done to improve a child's outcomes.

Pearl

All clinicians must look at the overall progress of the child, beyond their own area of specialization.

18.2 Red Flags That Might Signal a Barrier to the Child's Optimal Auditory/Neural Development

18.2.1 Red Flag: Basic Behavioral Observations

Children Not Wanting to Wear Technology

If children hear well with their technology, they should want to wear their technology all day, every day. A child who does not

want to wear technology is demonstrating the most basic red flag. A child may not tolerate technology because it is too loud and uncomfortable or because it is too soft and he cannot hear with it.

Hypersensitivity

A red flag that should raise immediate concern is hypersensitivity to auditory stimuli. A child demonstrating eye blinks or facial sensation to auditory stimulation should provoke serious concern and prompt immediate professional action. Also, any reports of children who consistently remove their technology in the presence of loud noise should be investigated immediately.

Behavioral Control Issues

Occasionally, children refuse to wear technology because of their behavioral control issues; however, in the authors' experience, this is unusual. Other factors should be eliminated before reaching the conclusion that the child's own behavior is the source of the problem.

Poor Responses to Auditory Stimuli

Poor responses to auditory stimuli are a red flag. A child who has no responses or poor responses to sound (even as an infant) is a focus of serious concern.

Failure to Make One Year's Progress in One Year's Time

Children who are not making one year's progress toward desired outcomes in one year's time are demonstrating another significant red flag. Audiologists need to inquire about speech-language and academic progress. Speech-language pathologists, listening and spoken language specialists, and TODs need to ask about hearing soft speech with technology, and speech perception in quiet and in noise to be sure the child is performing as well as possible.

18.2.2 Red Flag: Ineffective Audiological Intervention

All professionals need to ensure that they are providing effective intervention, while parents need to ensure that their children are receiving effective intervention. Audiology services are ineffective if they fail to evaluate regularly how a child hears and understands speech with each piece of technology. Testing should include unaided thresholds and aided thresholds with the right and left ear technology individually and with the technology worn binaurally. Speech perception testing should be performed at normal and soft conversational levels in quiet and in competing noise.

Audiological red flags are indicated when aided thresholds are too soft (≤15 dB hearing level [HL]), aided thresholds are not soft enough (35 dB HL or poorer), poor speech perception scores (poorer than 80%) in any of the test conditions (normal and soft conversation in quiet, and normal conversation in competing noise), or speech perception results completed with inappropriate test materials (such as using a picture-pointing test for a main-streamed child in third grade).

Audiologists can support effective intervention by:

- understanding normal auditory skills development and the effect of hearing loss on auditory skills development,
- ensuring that technology is appropriately fitted through regular audiologic evaluations and programming visits,
- recognizing that only appropriately fitted technology can provide optimal auditory access to the brain,
- collecting data about auditory perception from other professionals who work with the child and from parents, and
- evaluating comprehensively any signs of difficulty noted by any of the professionals or parents.

18.2.3 Red Flag: Ineffective Speech, Language, and Listening Intervention

Red flags indicative of ineffective intervention would be noted in the delay of initial and basic auditory skill development. The clinician would primarily note a lack of clinical behaviors expected early in the auditory hierarchy. All interventionists should be concerned when children respond to fewer sounds with their hearing aids or cochlear implants on than with them off, responds to fewer sounds with their CI than previously with their HAs, or when skills acquired with their HAs do not transfer to their CI.

Red flags include, but are not limited to no response to a child's name; a lack of "listening attitude;" a poor voice quality; no evidence of improvement in speech production; an inability to discriminate or identify suprasegmentals, vowels, and consonant features; and limited comprehension of familiar phrases based only on suprasegmentals or key words.

18.2.4 Red Flag: Vision as Primary Modality

When a child's intervention does not primarily focus on audition and instead uses vision as the primary input modality for receiving spoken language, problems in the child's speech production often are observed. These speech errors are a consequence of the limited visual availability of acoustic speech features.

Indications of speech acquisition through vision and the resulting error patterns would include confusions of phonemes produced in the same place, voicing errors for cognate pairs, and poor control of suprasegmentals. Utilizing even minimal auditory cues would typically prevent most of these error patterns. To address or prevent visual speech errors, the intervention must focus on the child's use of audition and eliminate the child's reliance on vision for the reception of speech phonemes and spoken communication.

The child with hearing loss who is provided with optimal hearing technology that is appropriately set and receives appropriate intervention should develop auditory, speech, and language skills in the typical sequence and at an appropriate rate in a given time interval.[1,2,3,4]

Pearl

The child with hearing loss who is provided with optimal hearing technology that is appropriately set and receives appropriate intervention should develop auditory, speech, and language skills in the typical sequence and at an appropriate rate.

18.2.5 Red Flag: Child Making Insufficient Progress toward Attaining Desired Outcomes

When a child is not developing skills at the appropriate rate, weak areas of development and the rate of progress must be examined to detect the red flags revealing issues possibly affecting the child. Is the child hearing at a sufficiently soft level throughout the frequency range? Interventionists should be alert to any signs of deterioration of skills in the areas of comprehension, vocabulary, and language development (e.g., loss of capability in speech discrimination, identification, or production). These can be evidenced by the child's inability to demonstrate a previously emerging or mastered skill, regression, or plateau in a child's development. Regression or plateau in a child's auditory development is never acceptable and merits troubleshooting for cause.

18.2.6 Red Flag: Speech Production

Listening to the children's speech will indicate what they are hearing. Children speak what and how they hear. If a child is not producing a particular phoneme, it is as likely as not the child is not hearing that speech sound well enough or often enough to cement appropriate connections in the auditory centers of the brain. A red flag is indicated by children exhibiting poor voice quality, such as a gravelly quality or glottal fry, or by the inappropriate use of intensity demonstrated by the child who always whispers, is always too loud, or is unable to simulate a whisper in his productions. Additional red flags are noted in speech production with issues of oral or nasal balance (hyper- or hyponasality), lack of pitch control, and vocalizations that occur on inhalation rather than on exhalation of the breath stream.

Red flags are indicated when development of phonemes is atypical or does not follow the normal rate or sequence. When monitoring speech production, interventionists must be aware if the variety of manners or place of production is too limited. An inappropriate developmental sequence would be indicated when the child utilizes more advanced phonemes but demonstrates gaps in phoneme repertoire for earlier acquired phonemes. Another red flag would appear when a child is unable to produce phonemes with particular speech features, such as unvoiced consonants or bilabials.

18.2.7 Red Flag: Language Development

Interventionists must monitor the child for indications of appropriate emergence of language skills even prior to the initial expressive use of words. An overall lack of development of "conversational" babbling/jargoning is a concern. A child without intelligible vocabulary or language development who produces only canonical babbling and jargoning is not developing the next level of language abilities. Interventionists must be concerned when they observe receptive language development, but no parallel development of expressive language or speech production abilities by the child.

18.3 Recognizing Effective Auditory Intervention

If families have chosen listening and spoken language, the child's use of audition is fundamental. Intervention requires a defined auditory component such that the focus of therapy is auditory skill development in the appropriate sequence through the auditory modality.[5,6] In this auditory model, a sequence of auditory goals is determined through the knowledge of the normal progression of audition. The auditory verbal therapist or speech language pathologist must assess the child to determine baseline auditory capabilities and then progress through skills beginning at the appropriate level of difficulty. Intervention then moves through the sequence by incorporating auditory goals in every activity in every session. Effective intervention provides guidance and coaching to parents, enabling auditory goals to be incorporated throughout the child's daily life and in all settings.

18.4 Supporting Intervention through Auditory Demand

18.4.1 Auditory Support

All clinicians working with a child must determine whether the demand for the child to use audition extends across all environments—therapy, home, and school. Is the child wearing technology during all waking hours in every setting? Is there a consistent way to respond if the child removes her technology? Is the child expected to report age-appropriate issues with technology? Do adults interacting with the child have an expectation that the child will respond to sound, and have a clear understanding of what the child can and cannot hear in each specific environment?

18.4.2 Checking Technology

Effective intervention is impossible without appropriate and functioning technology. Technology must be aggressively monitored and checked correctly and thoroughly on a daily basis by the adults who have appropriate listening technology (HA stethoscope, CI earbuds, CI listening check) to determine when the child's technology is not functioning and to troubleshoot for issues such as a dead battery, a broken device, or intermittent use. Audiologists must make responding to equipment issues a priority by quickly facilitating repairs, replacement, or loaner equipment.

> **Pearl**
>
> All clinicians working with a child need to be able to monitor performance with technology daily and immediately refer to the audiologist if the child is not hearing well.

18.4.3 Parental Support for Effective Intervention

Parents must find knowledgeable, experienced professionals and actively participate in all intervention. Full participation in their child's intervention allows parents to reinforce all goals and objectives at home as well as ensure that all family members and caregivers are also able to do so. Parents must document observations about the child's auditory, speech, and language development so that they can provide feedback to all professionals. Parents do need to "trust their gut." If the intervention and progress do not seem optimal, then they probably are not. Professionals need to support parents in seeking a second opinion and not feel insulted when parents do so.

> **Pearl**
>
> Parents should be supported so that they can become strong advocates and competent medical consumers for their child. Professionals need to support parents in seeking a second opinion and not feel insulted when parents do so.

18.4.4 Interventionist Support for Effective Intervention

An auditory focus in intervention would ensure that input through sensory modalities other than audition is minimized; thus, professionals must model and coach strategies to maximize use of auditory input for parents. Expectations in therapy should be clear. The therapist's role is to teach carryover of these expectations into the child's daily life, allowing parents to have appropriate and consistent auditory expectations and knowledge of therapy targets and outcome goals.

18.5 Why Is Careful Monitoring of Red Flags Important?

Expectations for children with hearing loss should follow normal developmental patterns. If a child is fitted with appropriate technology early and receives appropriate therapy, we should expect one year's development in one year's time. However, if a child receives technology late, if technology is not providing sufficient auditory access, or if therapy intervention is not optimal, development will be impacted. Parents are novices and rely on professionals for guidance. Parents have reported that they do not feel professionals from different disciplines have the same expectations for their child's development. For example, audiologists may not always recognize a concern when auditory therapists report that a child cannot hear high-frequency phonemes from a distance. When members of different disciplines disagree, parents are put in a difficult position.

Pearl

If all clinicians applied information about use of audition and developmental milestones as a guideline, then they would all be using the same criteria for performance, leading to more cohesive expectations from all interventionists working with the child.

18.6 When Red Flags Point to Technology as the Source of the Problem

Speech-language perception issues result from one or more of four conditions experienced by the child with hearing loss: the sound was too quiet, too loud, not clear, or the child does not have sufficient language development.

Real-ear measures and CI programming are critical first steps, but they do not tell us what a child is hearing. Real-ear measures report the sound that is reaching the eardrum, not the sound that is processed by the auditory brain. Cochlear implant programming and neural response telemetry (NRT) values tell us how neural tissue responds to different levels of stimulation but, again, not what is being received by the auditory brain. Children provide us with accurate and reliable information about what they hear when we observe and understand their behavior, when we document their auditory skill development, when we listen carefully to their speech production and language, and when we verify their speech perception through audiological testing.

Table 18.1   When speech is too soft: signs of underamplification or understimulation

Hearing aids	Cochlear implants
Child consistently removes technology	Child consistently removes technology
Turns up volume	Turns up volume or sensitivity
Relies on visual input	Relies on visual input
Does not turn or respond to name	Does not turn or respond to name
Vocalizations do not change with technology	Vocalizations do not change with technology
Voice is loud	Voice is whispered
Listening/speech/language development is slow or nonexistent	Listening/speech/language development is slow or nonexistent
Speech perception at 70 dB HL is better (> 12%) than at 50 dB HL	Speech perception at 70 dB HL is better (> 12%) than at 50 dB H

Pearl

If a child does not clearly understand spoken language while wearing technology, something is wrong. The audiologist must act quickly to identify the source of the problem and modify the technology to enable the child to comprehend speech.

18.7 Evaluating Audiology Test Results

18.7.1 Red Flags That Indicate Speech Is Too Soft

When HAs are not providing sufficient amplification or CIs are not providing sufficient stimulation, children will exhibit a variety of behaviors that should indicate to the professionals and parents that speech is too soft. A lack of response to sound and a reliance on visual input are obvious indicators that speech may not be audible, but other behaviors are often present that provide further evidence that sound is too soft. **Table 18.1** provides a list of specific behaviors children may exhibit that indicate that speech is too soft. If the technology is too soft, a child will not have adequate access to speech and language. In our experience children who are receiving little benefit from their amplification will often remove the HAs or CIs because they serve little purpose. Speech perception testing can provide strong evidence that sound is too soft.

18.7.2 Red Flags That Indicate Speech Is Too Loud

From the authors' clinical experiences and from the reports of parents and educational professionals, overamplification and, especially, overstimulation are growing concerns with children. Moreover, the consequences of overstimulation and overamplification can be extremely detrimental to speech and language development.

Table 18.2 provides a list of specific behaviors children may exhibit when speech is too loud. Children should want to wear their technology if they hear well with it. Any time a child removes his technology or has a marked startle, involuntary eye blink, or facial stimulation in response to loud sounds, we should be very concerned. Children who are being overstimulated may appear to have a shortened attention span, agitated behavior, or both and exhibit poorly defined borders between their words and poor voice modulation with high-pitched sounds.[7]

If clinicians suspect that speech is too loud, they should ensure that all technology is functioning appropriately. Unilateral and bilateral assessment of aided speech perception of soft, conversational, and loud speech will provide information about the intensity levels at which speech is distorting or even becoming painful. For hearing aid patients, real-ear measurements performed at high intensity levels may provide information about frequencies that are being overamplified. While loudness scaling has long been a part of cochlear implant programming, its use with children should be carefully reviewed. Because hearing adults have been shown to be poor raters of loudness,[8] it is imprudent and even unrealistic to assume that children who are profoundly deaf are able to complete this highly subjective task accurately. On the other hand, the use of neural response telemetry (NRT), neural response imaging [NRI], and auditory response telemetry [ART]) can provide objective information for determining stimulation levels. Berger et al[7] found that for patients with the Cochlear device, reducing the comfort level stimulation to tNRT levels led to spontaneous resolution of the behavioral and interventional problems previously noted.

Pearl

Overamplification and overstimulation can have deleterious effects on wearing compliance, speech and language development, attention, and behavior.

18.7.3 Red Flags That Indicate Speech Is Not Clear

When speech is audible, but not clear, children will exhibit behaviors listed in **Table 18.3.** Children speak the way they hear, which means articulation errors may be "hearing" errors. Because a child's speech production should be the most accurate reflection of his speech perception, professionals and parents should make careful and accurate observations and note the child's consistent productions, omissions, and substitutions. After consideration is given for normal developmental patterns, the remaining errors provide us with significant information about the child's speech perception.

For children with hearing loss to acquire good speech production and morphemic functions in spoken English, they must be able to clearly perceive all the ~44 phonemes of the language. Although the Ling-Madell-Hewitt 10 Sound Quick Test[9] is helpful in determining whether a child has access across the speech spectrum, it provides us with a limited understanding of a child's phoneme perception. In a retrospective review of more than 230 cochlear implant mappings, Lochner, Hewitt, Owen, and Madell[10] found that the most common speech perception errors were not identified by the Ling detection test because of the extremely limited number of consonants that are assessed, and, when a child has widespread vowel errors, significant global programming issues can exist. Thus, to ensure that a child is able to perceive every phoneme in English clearly, identification, not detection, should be regularly assessed for all phonemes, with emphasis on consonant perception from distances of 3 feet and 10 feet.

Analysis of phoneme errors on informal and formal measures and review of a frequency allocation chart for speech phonemes can identify specific frequency bands to be adjusted. Making needed changes in specific frequency bands, rather than globally increasing or decreasing all bands, can improve speech perception for those sounds that are not clear to the patient without jeopardizing information that is already clear. Careful analysis of phoneme perception errors and specific programming changes targeted to improve perception can have an immediate impact on a child's speech perception and production.

Pearl

Careful analysis of phoneme perception errors and specific programming changes targeted to improve perception can have an immediate impact on a child's speech perception and production.

Table 18.2 When speech is too loud: signs of overamplification or overstimulation

Hearing aids	Cochlear implants
Consistently resists or removes technology	Consistently resists or removes technology
Turns down volume	Turns down volume or sensitivity
Startles, cries, or blinks to loud sounds	Startles, cries, or blinks to loud sounds
Has robust responses to very soft sounds	Has robust responses to very soft sounds
Is very quiet or withdrawn	Is very quiet or withdrawn
Voice is quiet	Voice is loud and/or gravelly; voices when whispering
Poor or deviant consonant development	Poor or deviant consonant development; produces only vowels and voiced consonants
Receptive language development without expressive language development	Receptive language development without expressive language development
Speech perception at 70 dB HL is poorer (> 12%) than at 50 dB HL	Speech perception at 70 dB HL is poorer (> 12%) than at 50 dB HL

Table 18.3 When speech is not clear: signs of poor clarity

Hearing aids	Cochlear implants
Relies on visual input	Relies on visual input
Poor or unusual voice quality	Poor or unusual voice quality
Inappropriate/unusual consonant development	Inappropriate/unusual vowel or consonant development
Consistent omission/substitution of specific consonants	Consistent omission/substitution of specific consonants
Speech production not improving	Speech production not improving
Hearing aid program is completely flat or heavily weighted to lows and highs	CI map is completely flat or heavily weighted to lows and highs
Very small or very large difference between gain for soft and normal conversation	Very small or large difference between T levels and C/M levels
Speech perception is poor at 35 dB HL, at 50 dB HL, or in noise	Speech perception is poor at 35 dB HL, at 50 dB HL, or in noise

18.7.4 Red Flags That Indicate Speech Is Not Balanced

The benefits of binaural hearing are well documented.[11,12,13] As a result of binaural summation, the auditory input from two ears will be louder and clearer than a monaural input. Furthermore, the auditory input to both ears should appear balanced to prevent binaural interference, in which the acoustic input from one device interferes with the capability to receive clear auditory input from the other device

While audiologists work to ensure that each ear individually is fitted with appropriately programmed technology, they must also determine whether the two devices together provide optimal binaural benefit. When a patient has been utilizing only one device, the programming or volume of that device will often be elevated to compensate for the lack of binaural summation. Often, HA programming algorithms automatically provide additional gain if a fitting is monaural only. However, when the patient receives a second device, the capability to fit the second device optimally will be compromised if the output of the first device is not readjusted and often reduced. When technology is not balanced or when binaural summation has created an overly loud input, children will often go to great lengths, such as removing the battery or turning off the loud or interfering device, to make the sound more tolerable. **Table 18.4** provides examples of behaviors noted in children when their technology is not binaurally balanced.

With the introduction of a new implant or HA, children should immediately begin receiving some of the benefits of binaural hearing, even if the listening capabilities in the ear with the new device are just developing. If the loudness is not balanced between the two devices, only the louder device may be audible, potentially causing auditory progress in the ear with the new device to be limited or rejection of the new device to occur.

One of the simplest ways to determine whether a child's technology is balanced is to ask, "Which ear is louder, this one or that one?" The correct answer is, "None" or "I don't know." Even preschoolers are often able to identify when one device is louder than the other. By asking the child, "Does this ear need to be louder or this ear need to be quieter?" the audiologist can obtain information to help guide programming changes. If parents or children report that one device appears to be bothersome, clear evidence of interference may be documented. If the technology is programmed and balanced appropriately, speech perception scores should improve in the binaurally aided condition when compared with the monaurally aided condition, especially in the presence of noise.

> **Pearl**
>
> With the introduction of a new implant or hearing aid, children should immediately begin receiving some of the benefits of binaural hearing, even if the listening capabilities in the ear with the new device are just developing. If both devices are reprogrammed and balanced, the sound quality of both, when worn together, should be good.

18.8 Summary and Conclusions

Different professionals can have conflicting viewpoints about a child's developmental expectations and outcomes. If certain professionals have lower expectations, they may discount the input of others and fail to assess objectively in their area of expertise, causing collaboration to be adversely affected. Resolution of legitimate concerns, and ultimately a child's progress, can be affected by professionals who have different viewpoints and are not willing to listen openly to colleagues. It is critical that all clinicians working with children listen with an open ear to colleagues and parents. Listening to the children also is essential; their speech production is a reflection of how well they are hearing.

It is essential that data be collected before making assumptions about performance. Returning to basic audiological principles, audiologists need to test to be certain children are hearing what we think they are hearing. Real-ear measures, NRT, and electrical stapedial reflex threshold (ESRT) are important tools, but they do not tell us what is reaching the brain. Only appropriate testing with technology including speech perception testing in multiple conditions will validate how a child is performing.

All professionals must have appropriate developmental expectations, collaborate fully with other interventionists, consistently assess a child's capability to clearly perceive speech and language, and actively pursue appropriate technology fittings and programming. If they do, they can and will positively impact the development of their young patients. Inappropriate technology or inappropriate technology settings are solvable problems. Audiologists can solve them, and the children we serve deserve to have them solved.

Table 18.4 When sound is not balanced: signs of unbalanced binaural technology

Consistently localizes to one direction
Consistently turns one ear to speaker/music/TV
Does not replace one device when it falls off
Startles, blinks, or asks for quiet when putting on 2nd device
Does not indicate when one battery dies
Original HA or CI is not reprogrammed when 2nd is added
Can tell that one device is louder than the other

> **Pearl**
>
> All professionals who have appropriate developmental expectations, collaborate fully with other interventionists, consistently assess a child's capability to clearly perceive speech and language, and actively pursue appropriate technology fittings and programming. If they do, they can and will positively impact the development of their young patients.

Discussion Questions

1. What red flags may be present for children who are not making optimal progress?
2. Why is carefully monitoring a child's speech perception and speech production essential in evaluating a child's benefit from hearing technology?
3. Why is the monitoring of red flags important for all professionals?
4. What information can be gleaned from collaboration with parents and other professionals about the child's overall progress?
5. What red flags indicate that the perception of speech through the child's technology is: (1) too soft? (2) too loud? (3) unclear? (4) unbalanced?
6. What speech production issues would merit cross-disciplinary assessment to determine the cause of the child's errors?

References

[1] Connor CM, Craig HK, Raudenbush SW, Heavner K, Zwolan TA. The age at which young deaf children receive cochlear implants and their vocabulary and speech-production growth: is there an added value for early implantation? *Ear Hear* 2006;*27*(6):628–644

[2] Geers AE, Nicholas JG, Sedey AL. Language skills of children with early cochlear implantation. *Ear Hear* 2003; *24*(1, Suppl):46S–58S

[3] May-Mederake B. Early intervention and assessment of speech and language development in young children with cochlear implants. *Int J Pediatr Otorhinolaryngol* 2012;*76*(7):939–946

[4] Tait M, De Raeve L, Nikolopoulos TP. Deaf children with cochlear implants before the age of 1 year: comparison of preverbal communication with normally hearing children. *Int J Pediatr Otorhinolaryngol* 2007;*71*(10):1605–1611

[5] Estabrooks W. Auditory-Verbal Therapy and Practiice. Washington, DC: Alexander Graham Bell Association for the Deaf and Hard of Hearing; 2006

[6] Madell JR, Hewitt JG, Rotfleisch S. Red Flags: Identifying and Managing Barriers to the Child's Optimal Auditory Development. In: Madell JR, Flexer C, Wolfe J, Schafer EC, eds. Pediatric Audiology: Diagnosis, Technology and Management. 3rd ed. Thieme; 2019

[7] Berger. Overstimulation in children with cochlear implants. 13th Symposium on Cochlear Implants in Children, Chicago, 2011

[8] Madell JR, Goldstein R. Relation between loudness and the amplitude of the early components of the averaged electroencephalic response. *J Speech Hear Res* 1972;*15*(1):134–141

[9] Madell JR, Hewitt JG. The LMH Test Protocol. https://hearinghealthmatters.org/hearingandkids/2021/3245/. HearingHealthMatters/Hearingandkids (blog), Published 2021

[10] Peters BR. Rationale for Bilateral Cochlear Implantation in Children and Adults. Sydney Australia; Cochlear Corporation: 2006

[11] Lochner L, Hewitt JG, Owen L, Madell JR. Analysis of Common Speech Perception Errors Prior to Cochlear Implant MAPping and Successful, Remedial Programming Changes. Washington DC: 2015

[12] Litovsky RY. Review of recent work on spatial hearing skills in children with bilateral cochlear implants. *Cochlear Implants Int* 2011;*12*(Suppl 1):S30–S34

[13] Litovsky RY, Goupell MJ, Godar S, et al. Studies on bilateral cochlear implants at the University of Wisconsin's Binaural Hearing and Speech Laboratory. *J Am Acad Audiol* 2012;*23*(6):476–494

19 Music, Listening, and All That Jazz

Christine Barton and Amy McConkey Robbins

Summary

Pioneers in the Listening and Spoken Language (LSL) approach identified the value of using music as part of the habilitation process in children with hearing loss, even before the advent of advanced hearing technologies. These authors have witnessed the changes brought about because of earlier implantation, intervention, and sophisticated technologies. Now, music perception is no longer the "final frontier" to be conquered but is central to the lives of many individuals with hearing loss. This chapter will support the reluctant practitioner in utilizing music to jumpstart listening, language, motor, social, and emotional development in children and adults with hearing loss. Music activities, case studies, and resources gleaned from years of these authors' practical experience and based on current research are provided in an easy-to-use and fun-to-try format.

Keywords

music, hearing loss, integrating music, listening, music and language milestones, Listening and Spoken Language (LSL), music intervention, music resources, activities, infant, toddler, school age child, teen, adult

19.1 Music Makes the World Go Round

When American poet, Henry Wadsworth Longfellow, wrote "Music is the universal language of mankind" he was on to something. While music scholars have debated this issue for years, there is now evidence that music is, in fact, universal. A study at the Harvard Music Lab[1] concluded that while music is diverse across cultures, there are several shared commonalities. First, all societies pair words and melody to create songs. Second, all societies dance to their music. Third, there is a tonality (albeit diverse) within all music. And fourth, music varies rhythmically and melodically from simple to complex. All societies also share musical forms such as lullabies, love songs, and dance music. This compelling research supports the claim of the universality and diversity of music. Thus, every known society has a body of music to call its own! Perhaps as Mithin proposes,[2] the instincts to speak and sing are inherently human. Through the millennia parents have relied on their sing-song voices to bond, play with, and calm their infants. That motherese or parentese voice, as it is known, is the place where music and language meet.[3] And some scholars argue that the capability to learn language and music is hardwired and is what sets us apart from other creatures on this planet.[4,5]

It's clear that music is prevalent in society. It accompanies us from the cradle to the grave. We use music to celebrate, mourn, support, teach, love, heal and in a myriad of other ways. In this current pandemic era, people around the world gathered daily to sing and play music from balconies, street corners, windows, and cars in an attempt to cheer on the first responders at the end of their shifts. National news featured stories of hospitals playing inspirational music selections as patients left after weeks of ICU care. Music has been and currently is a vital and integral part of our lives. But, what about for our children who are deaf or hard of hearing (DHH). Are they also wired to learn music and language? Can music be vital and integral to their lives? These authors believe it to be so and will try to make a compelling argument in support of integrating music into the Listening and Spoken Language (LSL) practice. This chapter will address and share:

- Current research on the connections between music, listening, and language development.
- Music and language developmental milestones.
- The importance of beat, rhythm, and melody to the music and listening experience.
- The social and emotional aspects of a music experience.
- Clinical case studies from years of practice pairing music with LSL in individual and group settings.
- Strategies for offering successful virtual music and LSL sessions.
- Culturally sensitive music experiences for all ages and stages of development.
- Resources to encourage and support inviting music into the LSL practice.
- Access to AudiTunes,[3] a music-supported approach designed to be implemented as part of the habilitation process for children with hearing loss currently enrolled in an LSL program. Video clips of both authors working clinically and MP3 song files are available gratis.
- Pearls and Pitfalls to guide the LSL practitioner.

Pearl

Music is a universal human trait that is culturally and geographically diverse. It is always wise to consider an individual's background and personal preferences when selecting music to use in sessions.

19.2 Time to Face the Music

One might assume that using music in an LSL practice is a relatively new idea. However, it has historical precedent in the work of LSL pioneers, Helen Beebe, Doreen Pollack, and Dr. Daniel Ling. In the halls of Saint Joseph Institute for the Deaf, Indianapolis, Indiana, there are photos of the nuns with groups of children gathered around the piano singing, playing bells, and even stringed instruments. This author remembers playing the piano for a dance group of deaf children in the 1960s. The piano was located on the stage and the children danced barefoot and felt the beat as the teacher directed them. This all before the advent of the sophisticated hearing technologies currently available. At the same time, music therapists Clive and Carol Robbins published their book *Music and the Hearing Impaired*.[6] Dr. Arthur Boothroyd, eminent audiologist, was a contributor to the textbook and wrote a chapter called *Audiological Considerations in Music with the Deaf*. These early pioneers in audiology, speech and language therapists, and music therapists understood the value of using music to support auditory, spoken language, and emotional development (**Table 19.1**).[7]

19.2.1 Importance of the Auditory Environment

Because music is primarily experienced as auditory, the same acoustic standards hold for music activities as for speech, language, and listening interventions. These authors describe musical activities with the underlying premise that children will be wearing state-of-the-art technology at home, in clinic and at school that provides optimum access to the features of music and singing. Likewise, the standards set for such things as frequent listening checks, a quiet classroom or therapy environment, and appropriate use of remote microphone technology are applicable whether the child is engaged in a speech/language session or a musical experience.

19.2.2 Similarities and Differences between Music and Spoken Language

Though music and language both convey information by modulating acoustic parameters, music is a more complex stimulus than language, demanding more complex processing mechanisms. This can be a detriment to those who access music via hearing technologies (hearing aids (HA) or cochlear implants (CI). Music may be thought of as containing more layers of sound, such as voice plus guitar, or several voices singing in harmony, that the listener's brain must process simultaneously. Music, compared to spoken language, requires resolution of a wider range of volume and pitch, a finding that presents challenges

to listeners wearing HA or CI, which provide a more limited dynamic range. Even though music and speech utilize different listening and processing strategies, improvements in one area often result in gains in the other.[9] Such specializations of music and speech processing strategies do not contradict the possibility of shared neural mechanisms,[10] thus making music and speech harmonious partners. Some have even proposed that music could function as a cross-modal training stimulus to enhance speech processing.[11] For these reasons, it is important for the reader to be mindful of the differences and similarities between spoken language and music (**Table 19.2**).[12]

Pearl

Music and speech processing have shared neural mechanisms, making them harmonious partners.

Research has also shown that children and adults who are involved in musical training of some kind, reap benefits in non-musical areas such as attention, memory, emotions, cognition, math, and hearing in noise.[13] They also maintain that listening to and making music is a way to achieve and maintain *auditory fitness*. Certainly, that is front and center to the LSL approach. It's important to note that one does not have to become a professional musician to gain these advantages, but music experiences are crucial.[14] For a complete literature review, see Robbins.[7]

If we acknowledge that music intervention can provide far reaching effects (better listeners, improved prosody, music and language synergy and social emotional connections with hearing peers), wouldn't we want to give our clients or students such an advantage? It's time to invite music into the practice.

Pearl

Current research has shown that music intervention can improve listening, prosody, memory, emotional connections, and cognition skills.

Table 19.1 The value of singing and music for children and parents in LS[8]

Listening to singing gives pleasure.
Singing to children helps develop their listening skills.
Good listening skills enhance speech perception.
Putting words to music helps children remember them (music is a memory magnet[2]).
Singing songs focuses on voice pitch and rhythm.
Perception of pitch and rhythm is essential to understanding spoken language.
Singing tunes enhances a child's control of intonation in speech.
Rhythm in song helps to develop rhythm in speech.
Singing helps to develop breath flow and breath control.
Singing can help to avoid speech disorders such as weak breath flow, hypernasality, pharyngeal tension, and the prolongation and neutralization of vowels.
Singing can be used in the remediation of many speech problems.
Music offers repetition, repeated practice, and rehearsal.*
Songs support executive functions, including planning, working memory and impulse control.*
Music enhances emotional discernment, including knowing the emotion of a speaker's voice.*
Singing or playing an instrument provides an outlet for feelings.*
Knowing the music of one's culture(s) allows for personal identity and group affiliation.*
Singing and musical experiences build children's confidence in listening.*

* Added by the chapter authors.

Table 19.2 Music and language similarities and differences[12]

Similarities	Differences
Both language and music are uniquely human and are found in every known culture.	Music encompasses a greater spectral range than speech.
Music and language follow a sequential developmental path whereby mastery is built on previously acquired skill sets.	Music can be instrumental, thus not requiring language.
Children are born with the capacity to learn both music and language.	Spoken language surrounds most children, where music may not.
Children must have access to spoken language and music to become fluent in each.	Music can transcend language in evoking an emotional response.
Music and speech share pitch, timbre, and timing.	
Music and speech have *prosody* or melodic contour.	

19.3 Jump on the Bandwagon

19.3.1 Your Voice Is the Most Important Instrument You Own[15]

Many speech-language and LSL practitioners have embraced music and are comfortable making it part of their therapeutic routine. Still, the authors hear regularly from reluctant clinicians who express hesitation at using music. Often, their reluctance is centered around three issues: They don't have a "good voice"; they don't have formal musical training; and they don't know where to start or what activities are developmentally appropriate for their students. Let's say a word about each one of these concerns. First, everyone has a singing voice. Everyone. Children don't know if a singer's voice is good or not. They judge the singing based on the pleasant feeling it evokes, the emotion of the person singing, the fun they are experiencing, and so on. Children only know a "bad" voice if it is labeled as such (e.g., "I have a terrible singing voice)." And because your voice is the most important musical instrument you own, let's agree that none of us will express that sentiment, about ourselves or anyone else. Second, formal training is certainly not a requirement for using music in your practice. We aren't trying to turn our children into opera stars. We are just using music as a mechanism to jumpstart the auditory system; to offer them a way to connect emotionally and socially with their peers and family; and, perhaps more importantly, to enhance their little lives.

Pearl

Singing to a baby is an enjoyable way to develop the emotional capacities that are required for later language development.

We have all grown up with music in our world, from our culture, our home, our interests. That experience with music is the primary source of your gift that you'll share with clients. In fact,

studies show that, along with music training, *informal musical experiences* confer impressive neurodevelopmental benefit and have the added advantage of encouraging emotional bonding between child and adult.[13] Finally, it is certainly true that you want to provide musical experiences that are age- and developmentally appropriate to your clients. With the resources we present in this chapter, and others that we recommend, readers will be able to identify appropriate musical activities based on such factors as the chronological age, listening experience, and language capability of children. One such tool we provide is the Music and Language Milestones Chart (**Table 19.3**)[16,17]. A clinician who knows the chronological and language age of the child will be able to find specific examples of appropriate activities to use.

19.3.2 Strategies for the Reluctant Practitioner to Incorporate Music

For those clinicians who would like a crash course in how to get going with music, we offer these four suggestions:

1. *Observe others in action.* Watch video clips from AudiTunes[3] to see the authors engaged in some of the activities described in this chapter. Or ask to observe a clinician in your area who has experience with integrating music into an LSL or SLP practice.
2. *Consult the Music and Language Milestones Table* (**Table 19.3**). Using this table, you can identify the age or stage of a child with whom you'll be using music. Locate some of the suggested activities there.
3. *Start with the familiar.* When starting out with musical activities, it helps to choose a song that you know well and that has a positive association for you. This way, you'll be more comfortable with the melody and words and can fully engage with the child.
4. *Learn to piggyback.* Piggyback songs are created by attaching new lyrics onto an existing, recognizable melody. One can create a novel song on the spot to meet a child's needs, fit a situation, or follow a classroom theme. For example, if you're having trouble keeping a child's focus during an auditory activity that involves a fishing game, you might piggyback new words onto the tune to "Row, row, row your boat" and start singing: "Fish, fish, fishing game/ Listen for the sounds/ Fish, fish, fishing game/ Listen for the sounds." Music often captures children's attention in a way that the speech stream does not. Note that your lyrics do not have to rhyme or even be clever. Simply sing what you would say. More examples of piggybacking can be found within the Let the Music Begin section of this chapter.

19.4 Strike Up the Band

Now that we have hopefully convinced you, the reader, that music should be part of your practice, let's try to figure out what music is.

- It is sound and silence.
- It can be simple or complex.
- It is humanly and culturally created.
- It has no physical form.
- It is a method of communication.
- It can be composed or improvisational.

Table 19.3 Music and language milestones in typical hearing children with associated music activities[12,16,17]

Age	Music Milestones	Language Milestones	Music Activities
Birth–3 months	Alerts and calms to music; prefers infant directed singing; coos/cries	Moves to the sound of a familiar voice; looks at speaker's mouth; coos/cries	Sing lullabies; gently rock and pat to music; narrate baby's day using "mama" interval
3–6 months	Musical babbling; repetitive movements in response to music; turns to the source of music; prefers higher pitched voices	Babbles; laughs; smiles; vocalizes pleasure and displeasure	Imitate baby's "musical" vocalizations; provide shakers, bells, and simple rhythm toys, bounce gently to music
6–9 months	Occasionally matches pitch; larger repetitive movements; recognizes familiar melodies; uses descending vocalizations	Smiles at speaker; uses voice and gestures to show displeasure; responds to own name	Imitate spontaneous songs; play pitch matching games using "la-la" or "loo-loo"; easy finger play songs; nursery rhymes with movement
9–12 months	"Sings "spontaneously; recognizes and attempts to sing along with familiar songs	Recognizes names of family members; waves bye-bye; says one–two words; responds to "no"; babbles with inflection	Provide songs for different activities like wake-up/bath time/bedtime; variety of recorded music; drums and xylophones
12–18 months	Dances to music; pays attention to lyrics; sings snippets of learned songs; more pitch matching; starting to match movements to music	Jargon-like utterances with some words included; follows one step directions; 20–100 words	Dance baby on your feet; sing simple songs/chants/nursery rhymes; songs with repetitive chorus like E-I-E-I-O and B-I-N-G-O
18–24 months	Looks for dance partners; spins, marches to music; spontaneous songs have steady rhythm; able to imitate songs; lyrics more accurate than pitch	Two-word phrases; uses question intonation; repeats overheard words; starts using pronouns; understands "where?" and "what's that?"; > 200 words	Experiment with different voices (big/little/high/low); make sounds with voice to encourage vocal range (sirens, birds, animal noises)
2–3 years	Learns singing vs. speaking voices; sings in different keys and meters; matches pitches consistently; some instrument discrimination	Three-word phrases; refers to self as "me"; starts to use verb endings; answers questions with yes or no; follows two step command; > 900 words	Play guessing games with familiar songs and instruments; repetitive rhythmic accompaniment to singing; sequential songs like "If You're Happy and You Know it"
3–4 years	Begins to discriminate between familiar instruments; uses rhythm instruments to accompany their songs; melodic contour is intact; makes up songs	Uses many more pronouns; names colors; sentences 5–6 words; tells stories; expresses feelings; enjoys poems; sense of humor starts to develop; > 1500 words	Marching band with rhythm instruments; high/low; up/down; play/stop; fast/slow; loud/soft; nonsense songs; read books based on familiar songs
4–5 years	Larger purposeful movements; imaginative songs and stories; beginning to recognize familiar melodies without lyrics; match beat to others	Asks what, who, where, why questions; answers why and how questions; uses future tense; tells name and address; uses longer sentences; > 2500 words	Rhythm stick games; movement songs using scarves, ribbons, etc.; story songs; group music experiences; xylophones, tone bars
5–6 years	Maintains steady beat while moving to music; sings melody with pitch accuracy; plays melodies on simple instruments; can remember songs in head; begins to read and write rhythmic notation	Uses past tense verbs, pronouns, prepositions correctly; sentences much longer; begins to read and write; knows time sequences; likes rhymes; > 2800 words	Sing rounds like "Row your boat"; practice singing; provide diverse genres and styles of music recordings/songs/games
6–7 years	Develops tonal center[1]; starts to sing harmony and rounds; vocal range focused around 5-6 notes; expands rhythmic and melodic written notation	Uses many more verb tenses; can tell right from left; makes comparisons; tells well crafted, imaginative stories; > 13,000 words	Build a repertoire of familiar songs; provide opportunities for music improvisation, reading and writing notation; music lessons
7–9 years	Vocal range expands; uses more complex meters and harmonies; demonstrates music preferences	Exaggerates; explains ideas in detail; likes vocabulary and word play; understands jokes, riddles and idioms; > 20,000 words	Offer individual and group music experiences; provide music games (computer, board) that focus on music terminology, notation and discrimination

[1]Tonal center is the "home key." When a child has a sense of tonal center, they can sing a song all the way through in the same key.

Music is made up of many different elements. It includes discriminating tones and rhythms, experiencing emotions and preferring the sound of a certain instrument or musical piece over another. Yet, not a single one of these features can describe the complex entity that forms music as a whole. Some indigenous cultures don't even have a word for music because it is synonymous with dance. In her book, *Music and the Child*,[18] Sarrazin defines music as an intentionally organized art form whose medium is sound and silence, with core elements of pitch (melody and harmony), rhythm (meter, tempo, and articulation), dynamics, and the qualities of timbre and texture. If this definition is a little too heavy for you, perhaps the thoughts of 107-year-old French pianist Colette Maze will ring true. She states, "In music there is everything—nature, emotion, love, revolt, dreams, it's like a spiritual food."[19] Of the elements listed in Sarrazin's definition we will consider rhythm/beat, pitch/melody, and timbre/tone color. We also explore the emotional qualities that music offers the listener and participant.

19.4.1 March to the Beat of Your Own Drum

Rhythm is the organization of music in time.[18] Beat is the steady underlying pulse of any kind of music, whether or not a drum or some kind of percussion is involved. When a mother sings a lullaby there is a pulse that is felt by the child and reinforced by the mother's rocking or patting. When we feel that beat, we begin to anticipate when the next beat will come. That "entrainment" allows us to move to music in a synchronized way alone and with others. When beats are organized into patterns, they make rhythms. Rhythm can exist without melody, but melody can't exist without rhythm, nor can speech.

> ## Pearl
>
> Rhythm can exist without melody, but melody can't exist without rhythm, nor can speech.

19.4.2 Change Your Tune

When individual pitches, tones or musical notes are strung together in a linear fashion it's called a melody. It is usually recognized as a separate entity. When only one singer or instrument is heard, it's called a melody. If two singers or instruments sing different melodies simultaneously, it's called harmony. For the purposes of this chapter, we will focus on melody, because children learn to sing melodies before they are able to harmonize. Not only do they have to sing it, they must also be able to "hear" the song in their head before they can add another part. Edwin Gordon, noted music educator, calls that skill audiation.[4] If you can sing a simple song like "Happy Birthday" in your head, then you have experienced audiation.

19.4.3 Toot Your Own Horn or Tickle the Ivories?

Timbre (rhymes with amber), also called tone color, refers to the unique characteristics of a particular instrument or voice and is how we are able to discriminate between them. It is how we know mother's voice from father's, a horn from a piano, and a bird from an airplane. It warns us of danger when a fire truck rushes by. Hearing children are able to identify timbre very early in life. As our children with hearing loss progress through the stages of LSL, timbre plays a large part in discrimination, the capability to tell one sound from another, and comprehension, what the sound is. It also plays a large role in how we form musical preferences.

19.4.4 Music Is the Shorthand and Connector of Emotion

Music embodies a wide range of emotions and has the capacity to evoke moods and feelings in the listener. Music can relate completely unrelated things and can convey emotions that can't be explained easily through words. What if we listen to a Jewish Cantor singing in Hebrew, or a rousing national anthem in a language unknown to us? Although the words may be a barrier, we can feel certain emotions through the way they sing and the tempo, or speed, of the piece and even its tonality. For this reason, Leo Tolstoy described music as "the shorthand of emotion."

Music is essentially a social activity, something people do in the company of others, either as co-creators or listeners. Among the reasons that the social functions of music are important is the emotional connection it provides.[20] When a child makes music with a parent and clinician, there is an emotional bond that forms. When children make music in a group, they are likewise bonding with each other within the emotional framework of the music, which might evoke happiness, sadness, anticipation, or other emotions. We make music with others just as we communicate with others. It is these authors' conviction that one never remove the emotional component of music that is used with children, even in a therapeutic setting.

19.4.5 Music Is a Jumpstarter across Developmental Domains

As clinicians working with children with hearing technologies, we see the potential that music has to jumpstart the mechanisms required to process and produce spoken language, as well as other important developmental skills.[21] The Oxford dictionary defines "jumpstart" as: "To give an added impetus to something that is proceeding slowly." Using this definition, we view music as valuable, not just at the initial stages of CI use, but across the lifespan of the listener. The fact that as humans we not only know music, but we also do music as a way of connecting with and engaging each other, speaks to the power of music in therapy and music as therapy. Even for listeners with less-than-optimal auditory resolution, the evidence confirms that music functions as a developmental jumpstarter, a language-learning tool, a cognitive enricher, a motivator, a perceptual booster, an attention enhancer, and a cultural connector.[7,21]

> ## Pearl
>
> The fact that as humans we not only *know* music, but we also *do* music as a way of connecting with and engaging each other, speaks to the power of music *in* therapy and music *as* therapy.

19.5 Let the Music Begin

Now it's time to provide you, the practitioner, with the tools necessary to include music as part of your practice. We will discuss musical skill sets from different ages and stages, as well as provide a plethora of music experiences to try with each population. There will be links to access recorded versions of many activities we share. Remember that these skill sets are based on typical hearing children and will need to be adjusted to a particular child's hearing age. But, they are benchmarks to guide you, so you may guide your child. So, let's start at the very beginning.

19.5.1 Infants/Babies/New Listener

From the beginning of human history, mothers and fathers have used music to soothe and cajole their unhappy babies. These lullabies, as they are known, are a universal song form. Singing to an infant in a slightly higher voice, using a slower rate of speech and sprinkled with emotional expressiveness is referred to as "motherese" or infant-directed singing.[22] It is this prosody of speech, or the sing-song nature of communication that conveys the emotional intent of the caregiver to the child and creates a bond, regulates affect, and sets the stage for both future language and music development.[16,17] These auditory patterns of phrases, rhythm, and grouping develop the baby's processing skills needed to decode speech.[23] Precisely why music should be part of daily life for a child with hearing loss.

Pitfall

Resist the temptation to play "background music" continually. It clutters the acoustic environment and teaches the baby to ignore it.

As soon as an infant has both auditory and environmental access to music they might:

- Alert and calm to the presence of music. Babies typically alert to playful songs and particularly when the caregiver is moving the child. Lullabies are universally used to calm infants.
- Move arms and legs repetitively to music (Baby Bop). As explained earlier, in the presence of music, the first response is motoric. While infants can't synchronize at this stage, they tend to move repetitively.
- Turn to the sound source.
- Babble musically (ascending and descending glides) in the presence of music. This is different from speech babble. It has greater range and sounds more like song and only occurs when music is presented to the baby.

As the baby nears the one-year mark they might:

- "Sing" spontaneously, especially when falling asleep. This acts as a self-regulator to help transition the baby from wakefulness into slumber.
- Move repetitively, but not synchronously to music. Babies are still trying to gain control over their movements. Synchronizing to the beat comes around 3–5 years of age.
- Recognize a familiar melody if sung correctly every time.

Baby Bop. One of the first responses hearing babies exhibit in the presence of music is a repetitive, bilateral, symmetrical movement; kicking legs, thrusting arms, and later swaying and rocking back and forth and nodding the head. The first author has dubbed this event the "Baby Bop."

Ma-Ma Interval. Also called the child's teasing song, these two pitches are the first interval a child will sing. Think *Rain, Rain Go Away*; *Ring around the Rosie*; *Na, Na, Na, Na, Boo, Boo*; *You Can't Catch Me*. Almost anything can be put to these tunes and be appealing to the young child.

Auditory Closure for Babies. Nursery songs are composed in a way that teaches the baby to anticipate the ending word of a phrase. They are often words that rhyme or are the same each time. Adults can model auditory closure by leaving off the final word of a phrase, pause and look expectantly at the baby, indicating that something is missing, then fill in the final word. For example, *Twinkle, twinkle, little...., How I wonder what you...*

19.5.2 Case Study: Piper

An otherwise healthy baby, Piper failed her newborn hearing screening and received a diagnosis of bilateral, severe sensorineural loss. She was fitted with hearing aids at three months and started LSL therapy shortly thereafter. Her parents noted that music was one category of sounds Piper responded to most readily. In LSL sessions with the second author, we focused often on music with Piper and gave the parents suggestions about using music at home.[7] Piper developed a "baby bop" response to the initiation of music, after we had modeled and reinforced this. As she grew, we used "Learning to Listen Musical Sounds"[3] to associate instruments with descriptive words (boom, boom, boom for a drum, shake, shake, shake for shakers, CRASH for a cymbal), through listening alone. At home, Piper's mother could always keep her attention if she narrated her actions using the "ma-ma" interval. Noting her strong attraction to music, her family also began to see the first author for weekly music therapy. There, auditory closure was addressed by the adult singing a song with the same word at the end of each of the four lines, stopping at that word (e.g., "Oh, my kitty, oh, my kitty oh, my kitty ....."). After the adult's expectant pause and eye gaze, Piper would eventually sing, "cat," completing each line. (See AudiTunes, Lesson 1 for a video clip of "baby bop" and Lesson 5 for "auditory closure.") With her strong auditory skills, she achieved music milestones at or slightly later than age expectations. She demonstrated a tonal center and capability to sing on tune at age five and a half. Piper sang with a choir and, at age seven, began violin lessons. As a teen and now a young adult, music continues to be an important part of her daily life (**Table 19.4**).

19.5.3 Toddlers

Gordon[4] maintains that at this age children learn through exploration and unstructured guidance from parents and caregivers. This method of learning helps to lay a foundation for formal instruction in the future. Singing and moving are the most basic requirements. Children also begin to recognize that music is different from speech in that we have a "singing voice" and a "speaking voice." Some words are now emerging and singing offers a fun way to practice their vocabulary. Do you ever wonder why some of the first songs children learn include animal sounds? They are easy one- or two-syllable utterances that encompass the entire vocal range, from the low growl of a lion, to the high-pitched meow of a cat. With repeated exposure to children's songs, they are beginning to pick up some of the rules that govern these songs. Things like a steady pulse and phrasing, which happens with predictability and often ends with a rhyming word. Soon, they will begin to anticipate when that

Table 19.4 Tuneful Toolbox infants/babies

Beat	Melody	Timbre	Emotion
Gently pat baby's back to the beat while chanting or singing nursery rhymes (seated, rocking, swaying or walking).	Sing baby's name using ma-ma interval.	Have various family members or caregivers sing, so baby can begin to discriminate between the individual voices. Some are high and some are lower.	Babies don't understand the words we sing, but they will understand the emotional intent. Singing baby's name is always welcome.
Hold baby on your lap facing away from you, with their head resting on your chest while singing (Hush Little Baby).	Sing finger play songs (Itsy Bitsy Spider, Twinkle, etc.).	Provide a few baby friendly rhythm instruments of different timbres (bells, shaker, drum).	Match songs with the baby's state of arousal. If sleepy, sing lullabies; if awake, sing play songs (Hush-a-Bye, Rickety, Rockety Riding Horse*).
Put baby on your knee and gently bounce to the beat of a nursery rhyme (This is the way the Ladies Ride) or listening to music.	Hum nursery songs/lullabies while rocking or patting baby's back.	Use the Learning to Listen Musical Sounds at AudiTunes to label the instrument sound (shake-shake and boom-boom, etc.).	Pair music with bath time (All the Fish Are Swimming in the Water), diaper changes (Slowly, Slowly), or putting on hearing devices (Put Your Ears On). Perhaps using the same song, or rhyme with each routine to help provide consistency and lessen distress.
Sit on the floor with baby resting on your knees. Gently move them up and down while chanting a rhyme.	Sing familiar songs on a single syllable, e.g., la or doo to highlight the melody.	Use different vocal ranges (high/low) when singing or reciting nursery rhymes.	Baby feels close to a caregiver or parent when singing, contributing to bonding and a sense of security.
Wiggle baby's fingers and toes while saying a rhyme (This Little Piggy went to Market).			Routines should be playful, never uncomfortable for the baby. They will associate these movements, chants, and physical contact with emotional trust (Up, up, up, into your chair).

* Songs in italics are available as MP3s at Tuneful Toolbox: https://www.sjiresources.org/.

word arrives and if the caregiver leaves it off, the child will fill it in as a sort of auditory closure.

Auditory Closure for Toddlers. After adults have modeled auditory closure by leaving off the final word of a phrase, pausing and then singing it, the child will be ready to fill in the final word. If not the actual word, then maybe a sound to take up that space. This simple example is what helps the child begins to learn the rules of the music of their own culture and environment.

Spontaneous Songs are also emerging when the toddler is at play. These are made up by the child and can be sung to a tune they already know, or may be entirely self-composed in the moment, often on the "ma-ma" interval. This is a developmental milestone for hearing children. So when parents witness it in their child with a hearing loss, it is something to celebrate.

At 18 months they might:

- Rock and "dance" to music. At this point the child is ambulatory and moving to music spontaneously. If seated on the floor or in a chair, the child will sway, maybe clap hands and rock head side to side.
- Ask for preferred songs or music. If the child has been provided a steady diet of songs, they will start to choose favorites and may ask for them by doing some finger motions (Itsy Bitsy Spider) or saying a word from the song (Old McDonald).
- Appear to be mesmerized by music. Language is emerging, but music is a more powerful stimulus and will hold the child's attention.
- Sing snippets of familiar songs. Caregivers should listen carefully for bits and pieces of songs the child has been exposed to and join them in singing.

At 24 months they might:

- Look for partners to dance with. Across cultures, people tend to dance with partners or in a group. Toddlers are also looking to share the experience.
- Pay closer attention to the words of songs. Language is a very strong motivator now and so children are listening intently to the words and connecting them to words they know.
- Provide the last word of a song phrase, anticipatory closure. Listen attentively to music.
- Attempt to sing along, even if it is unfamiliar.
- Experiment with pitch and expand vocal range. By now, the child has figured out that they have different ways to use their voice.
- Sing spontaneously while at play, either to narrate what they are doing or singing familiar songs.

If a child shows a particular attraction to music, consider enrolling in a family music class. See the Drum Up Support section of this chapter for more information.

19.5.4 Case Study: Len

Len was born with a rare genetic condition that involved bilateral profound deafness, craniofacial anomalies, and cognitive impairment. At age 18 months, an attempted CI surgery was aborted in Len's left ear due to anatomical anomalies. At 22 months, CI surgery was completed on the right ear. His left ear later underwent successful implantation. In spite of many developmental challenges, Len was a happy, affectionate toddler and his parents noticed immediately after initial CI activation that music captured his attention. After 6 months of device use, he clearly recognized music as a class of sounds different from speech. When he heard speech, he would pause and search, but when he heard music without visual cues, he would begin the baby bop by rocking and swaying to the beat. Before age three, he played musical auditory closure games with his mother, who sang familiar songs and paused at each line so that Len could supply the missing word. At age three, he was placed part-time in a community preschool where his favorite activity was music time. His mother bought the same children's CD that was used at preschool, and played it in the car. If other music played, Len would exclaim: "Play MY music, Mama!" Len's father is of Native American descent, and taught Len some musical chants he had learned as a child. These helped his father connect Len to his own cultural and linguistic heritage, an important function of music in multi-ethnic families. At every age, Len showed strong preferences for music, including the piece "The Four Seasons" by Vivaldi. His mother took Len to an open-air symphonic concert and told him that Vivaldi music was on the program. When another Vivaldi composition, "Concert for Two Trumpets" began, Len jumped up and protested, "That's not MY Vivaldi!" Now a young adult, Len has a service dog who is his constant companion. His mother wrote recently: "Len is standing in the middle of the kitchen, index fingers raised, eyes closed and humming Mozart as if conducting an entire symphony…tears of joy run from my eyes as I truly understand how much my deaf child loves music. With Len's multiple disabilities, his cochlear implants have been an amazing blessing." (See AudiTunes, Lesson 2 for a video clip of "baby bop" and "auditory closure.")

Pearl

Music can help multi-ethnic families connect their child to their own cultural and linguistic heritage (**Table 19.5**).

19.5.5 Preschoolers

Hopefully, by this age the children using hearing technology are now engaged in an LSL or integrated preschool setting. This milieu prepares the child for not only language, but social, emotional, fine, and gross motor skill acquisition. They may also be exposed to a group learning situation that has a daily schedule for the first time. An example of a school day routine might be: Arrive at School, Play, Attendance, Circle Time, Calendar, Recess, Lunch, Nap, and Home, which offer perfect opportunities to pair a song with each activity. It helps prepare the child for what's to come next in an efficient and fun manner.

At this age children might:

- Be able to move while playing an instrument. A child will enjoy marching, walking, spinning, dancing, and jumping through space with an instrument in hand.
- Match a common beat by patting knees. Not all children will be beat competent, but some will be able to pat bilaterally, symmetrical body parts to the steady beat of music. Clapping

to a beat is more difficult than patting knees because it involves crossing the midline.

- Play a rhythm instrument fast/slow; high/low; side to side; round in a circle, under/over, and quiet/loud.
- Sing along with the daily classroom songs and sing some at home.
- Develop preference for certain instruments and songs. As children are exposed to more instruments, genres of music, and performers, they begin to develop favorites. Songs related to certain movies or educational television shows may be chosen often.

In an LSL preschool, teachers and therapists use listening experiences to address auditory development in levels outlined by Erber[24]: detection, discrimination, identification, and comprehension.

- Most children who are DHH will progress through these stages in similar fashion as their typically hearing peers, although at a delayed pace. Individual learning differences create variability across children, as do age of technology fitting and constituency of device use. The children must acquire the skill sets associated with each level prior to moving to the next level. The "No Peeking" game, was developed by the first author to work on building these skill sets. To play, the teacher or therapist places six to eight markers (rings or dots) on the floor that show the child where to move when they hear the sound. The clinician stands out of view of the child, while the rest of the class reminds the child that there is no peeking. The clinician plays a single drumbeat and the child moves ahead to the next marker. When the child is able to hear and respond to a single instrument, a second instrument with a very different timbre such as a cymbal can be introduced. This time when the cymbal is heard the child moves back one marker. After the child successfully demonstrates the ability to discriminate between these two instruments, they are ready to move to the identification level by naming the instrument they heard. (See AudiTunes, Lesson 7 for a video clip of children playing the "No Peeking" game.)
- "Doggie, Doggie, Where's Your Bone?" is a game that can target voice identification. A doggie bone prop is required. Children sit in a circle with their hands behind their backs and eyes closed. One child walks around the circle and deposits the bone into a peer's hands as the children sing the song. When they sing the last phrase, "Who has the bone?" the child with the bone responds, "Me" or "I do." The children then guess whose voice they heard and the game begins again, with the child whose voice was heard moving around the circle and depositing the bone (**Table 19.6**).

19.5.6 School Age

By now, many students are in a supported classroom with typical peers. This affords them the opportunity to benefit from an abundant, language rich environment. Most likely, they are the only student with a hearing loss. Fortunately, by now they have learned to be advocates for themselves and are quite adept at

Table 19.5 Tuneful Toolbox toddlers

Beat	Melody	Timbre	Emotion
Put toddler on your feet facing you and hold their hands as you move to the steady beat of a nursery rhyme.	Sing finger play songs (The Wheels on the Bus, Itsy Bitsy Spider, *Whoops, Johnny**).	Expand instruments available to include drum, shaker, bell, and accompany a favorite song.	Sing lullabies substituting the child's name when possible or create one of your own.
Pat and name different body parts (knees, head, feet, etc.) while singing or listening to music. (Use instrumental music, so words don't interfere with your saying the body parts.)	Watch for toddler to start matching some pitches and singing snatches of learned songs, especially at play.	Sing songs or chants using different animal voices and vocal registers; a bear (low range), kitten (middle range), or a bird (high range).	Sing familiar songs and insert the child's name (Twinkle, twinkle, little [Child's name], or to the tune of BINGO, I knew a dad who has a girl and Grace is her name-o, G-R-A-C-E).
Put toddler on your knee and gently bounce to the beat of a nursery rhyme or slide them down your leg to the floor (*Riding to Boston*).	Sing songs that require the child to make animal sounds (Old MacDonald, Down on Grandpa's Farm, BINGO, *What Does the Kitty say?*).	Take a musical listening walk. Carry child or walk, activating "musical" sounds such as doorbell, rapping on wooden table, making a pinging sound on a glass. Describe what you hear: "That sounds tinny."	Pair music with the emotional state of the child. Name that emotion; you're happy, sad, mad, scared, etc.

* Songs in italics are available as MP3s at Tuneful Toolbox: https://www.sjiresources.org/.

Table 19.6 Tuneful Toolbox preschool

Beat	Melody	Timbre	Emotion
Provide drums, tambourines, shakers, rhythm sticks to emphasize the steady beat of a nursery rhyme or childhood song.	Provide a drum or shaker to accompany a favorite song.	Sing (*What's in the Bag?**) Then play a familiar rhythm instrument inside the bag and see if the child can name or point to the picture of that instrument.	Sing lullabies substituting the child's name when possible or create one of your own. Bedtime is an opportunity for bonding through closeness and music.
Model the body part to pat with your hands, rhythm sticks or small paper plates (bilaterally/symmetrically) and have the child copy. Can be with or without music (*Monkey See, Monkey Do*).	Sing movement songs (Hokey Pokey, Alouette, *Hoppity Hop**) Dance with scarves or streamers to familiar songs.	Expand to include several known instruments and play the same game. Label "singing" vs. "speaking" voices in a game and have the child identify.	Children often address fears through play, pretending to be a dinosaur, shark or monster (Baby Shark, We Are the Dinosaurs, and *Snap, Gulp*).
Switch roles and have the child be the leader. Different skills are required in the two roles.	Sing songs that have a freeze/stop component (*Two Feet*) Use a slide whistle or push-up puppet to work on up/down with both voice and body.	Pair a movement with designated instruments and have the child perform that movement when they hear the corresponding instrument (i.e. clap/shaker; jump/drum; turn/triangle, etc.).	Provide pictures of children expressing certain emotions (happy, sad, scared, mad, etc.) and piggyback a song to detail each emotion (If you're happy and you know it shout Hooray! If you're sad and you know it say boo-hoo, etc.).
Pat and say the syllables of the child's name on knees four times. Use other family members' names and call attention to same/different number of pats.	Model singing vs speaking voice.	Play the "No Peeking" and "Doggie, Where's Your Bone?" game as described in the text.	Pair music with daily routines, get dressed, clean up, brush teeth, wash hands, going to an appointment.

* Songs in italics are available as MP3s at Tuneful Toolbox: https://www.sjiresources.org/.

explaining and caring for their hearing technologies. Their peers will ask many questions and our children have the answers.

A child's expanding auditory and communicative capabilities enable a broad range of musical activities at this age and stage. Clinicians continue to use music to support LSL goals, to establish emotional connection with significant others and for the pleasure it brings. Activities are added that bolster academic learning, allow for expression of a child's individual personality and musical tastes, and address higher order thinking skills (HOTS) and social thinking.[25] School-aged children form opinions about their musical preferences and these are included as priorities for the music used in sessions. Here are some ways these authors use music in a classroom or individual setting.

Be My Echo. Clinicians use echo songs to focus on rhythm, pitch, and sung lyrics, using the format of imitation or echo. The leader sings a line, which is repeated by the follower(s). Traditional children's songs using echo include, "The Other Day I Met a Bear" and "Down by the Bay." This echo format also serves LSL goals in a "News of the Day" activity[26] using a clinician-created song. The adult does an auditory-only task while descending stairs or walking with the child just behind, allowing us to see how well he matches pitch and imitates lyrics (see Chapter 12, "Executive Function Therapy Integrated into Audioty-Verbal Practice"). Echo songs are also called Call-and-Response songs, a category that includes question and answer songs. Raffi's version of "Must be Santa" is an example of a call-and-response song, which is good practice for auditory routines and conversational turn-taking. As appropriate, the child is encouraged to be the leader who sings each question, "Who's got a beard that's long and white?" with the adult responding, "Santa's got a beard that's long and white!" This targets cumulative working memory because, after every other verse, the list of features is reiterated and the list grows longer. (See AudiTunes, Lesson 5 for a video clip of "echo song.")

Music in My Head. It is important to model and describe to children the phenomenon of "audiation,"[4] an important musical and listening landmark. As mentioned earlier, to audiate is to hear and comprehend music that is not physically present; the sound of the music is heard and experienced in one's head. Children with typical hearing can audiate around 5 to 6 years of age. Like other musical skills, exposure to adults who model this and use language to describe it is important for a child's learning. Clinicians should refer to "hearing songs in my head" or "hearing music in my mind" so children know this is something pleasant and expected with songs we know well. When celebrating a birthday in a session, for example, the clinician may close her eyes and say, "I hear the song, 'Happy Birthday' in my mind" (or use the term *audiate*, if appropriate). "Can you hear it in your mind, Mom? How about you, Gloria? Now that we hear it in our minds, let's sing it together." A six-year old with strong auditory skills shared, "My brain was singing that song" and described the process of audiation. Another shared that they kept hearing a song in their head for a couple of days. We used to call these "ear worms" or "ear candy." Audiation is only experienced by those with well-developed auditory cortical centers, so LSL practitioners should monitor how it develops over time. When a child demonstrates audiation, it's another moment to celebrate with parents.

Our Memory Magnet. [7] As an effective mnemonic device, music may be thought of as a "memory magnet" and recruited when recalling facts, academic rules or other rote information. It is appropriate to use piggyback tunes to teach children their address and phone number because these are important for a child's safety. A seven-year old boy with CIs wrote a song as a reminder of punctuation rules: "A sentence has an ending, an ending, an ending/It always has an ending: Period. Question mark? (sung with rising, questioning intonation), EX-CLA-MA-TION MARK!!!" (sung with enthusiasm and louder volume). The clinicians encouraged rehearsal when the child prepared to write, by asking, "What should you remember to do?" This song is now a memory magnet. The child sings it aloud or audiates it, which prompts him to use appropriate punctuation. Children who struggle to master math facts may be successful after they link them to music. Several programs offer chants and songs to retain academic facts (such as "Silly School Songs!" on YouTube). Identifying a child's interests will help the clinician know how to recruit the most appropriate resources. For example, if a child is interested in astronomy, he will be more motivated to learn facts about each planet by reciting a rap, "The Solar System Song" with a repeated chorus: "The sun, the moon and the stars [Pause]/Mercury, Venus, Earth and Mars."[27] Even a long passage such as the Preamble to the U.S. Constitution can be memorized if set to music, as the television series Schoolhouse Rock! did.

19.5.7 Music Promotes Literacy

Phonological Awareness. There are many songs that address phonological awareness, a broad skill that includes manipulating units of spoken language such as sounds, syllables, and onsets and rimes. The clinicians may sing the song, "Apples and Bananas" to work on sound substitution because each verse requires the singer to replace the vowels in the title phrase with another vowel such as "EE" or "OO" to become, "I like to eat, eat, eat, Ee-pples and Bee-nee-nees. I like to Oot, oot, oot, oo-ples and boo-noo-noos."

Spelling Words. Clinicians may encourage children to bring their spelling list to LSL sessions to review them together. Victor's adoption was an international placement. He did not speak English until five and was delayed in language and behind peers in school subjects, especially reading and spelling. This and other types of academic support require high parent involvement because the parents need to regularly promote literacy at home. His parents learned how to add rhythm and a musical beat to words that don't follow traditional phonics rules: "S-C-H (clap, clap)-O-O-L: **School**!" When breaking down a word into its individual letters, it should always be recombined afterwards, as is done in a spelling bee, so that the child knows what word he's spelling.

Parts of Speech and Grammatical Rules. Learning the names and functions of different parts of speech is a national academic standard and one that was difficult for Dorian, a nine-year-old boy with a CI and hearing aid. Music was used to make this information automatic and reduce working memory load. Using the popular word game, "Mad Libs," his mother asks him to name, "a verb ending in –ing." Dorian moves in a robust marching style and sings "The Verb Song." "I'm a verb, verb, verb, I'm an action word/So put me where the action is/'Cause I'm an action word."[27] Then he correctly offers the word, *kneeling*, and his mother jots the word in the Mad Libs blank. Chants from "Rap 'n Rock"[28] are catchy raps that help Dorian learn grammatical concepts such as the use of plural "s." Always check the fidelity of recorded songs to determine if the child can listen to them independently.

Musical Cousins. Poetry is a useful backdrop for many LSL activities and reminds children that "poetry and music are cousins."[26] Because they share features of rhythm, melodic intonation and often rhyming, I [Amy] have found that poetry can strengthen a child's musical skills and vice versa. Poetry also brings light-heartedness and whimsy to an LSL session. Aria, who is seven and wears bilateral hearing aids, listened as the clinician read the poem "Happy New."[29] We work on goals including: prediction (what word do you suppose is missing from the title?); phonological awareness (what word substitutes in the place of the key phrase?); auditory closure (how can we complete these silly greetings so they make sense?); rhyming (does my answer rhyme with the word it replaces?); and creativity (can we make up our own verses to extend the silliness?). As with music, parents are encouraged to contribute poems that are meaningful to them and to read them aloud with us, strengthening generational ties. Aria's mother brings her own childhood poetry book, given to her by her mother and suggests we read "The Swing" by R.L. Stevenson, which had been her favorite. Like a song, a poem may be associated with specific memories, eliciting emotion from its reader. Her mother told Aria how much it meant to her that they shared the experience. It was a moment to celebrate.

19.5.8 Executive Functions (EFs) and Music

EFs are a set of neurocognitive processes responsible for active management of cognitive resources, emotions, and behaviors to achieve a goal. Components include emotional regulation, controlled attention, planning, impulse control, and working memory. EFs are important in all the developmental areas needed for interpersonal, school, and life success. Children with CIs have been shown to have a two to five times greater risk of executive function (EF) deficits relative to hearing peers[30] meaning this is a priority focus for many children in LSL practice. Music is an effective way to improve EF deficits.[31] Six-year old Zamir is using *Social Thinking* materials[25] including T*he Social Explorers Curriculum*[32] which has an accompanying CD of music. Each Executive Function concept is reinforced by a book, teaching activities, and a song.[33] Zamir sings "The Plan" whose lyrics are a reminder that: "When it's you and only you/ you're alone, all on your own / But when it's you and me and we/There must be a plan." The clinician introduced Zamir to stories and songs about "Show Me what You're Feeling," "Your Brain's Where You Think a Thought," and "Size of the Problem." The automaticity afforded by these songs reduces working memory load and allows Zamir to have internalized rules for how to accomplish important interpersonal and academic tasks.

Boss Your Brain with Music. Meta-cognitive awareness allows us to think about how we think. With appropriate modeling, children learn that thinking is something they can get better at, but they have to practice it, to be the "boss of their brain" and to use specific strategies that help them think smarter, not harder. Robbins[34] described a set of strategies to help children boss their brain. The second author models the strategies with preschoolers but directly teaches them to children of school age. She also has created piggy-back songs for each strategy. These help Elvis, age seven, remember how to use them. Before we start an auditory memory game, Mom tells him, "You'd better boss your brain and re-auditorize what you hear. What does that mean? Elvis sings to the tune of *My Bonnie Lies over the Ocean*: I ne-ed to sa-y things out loud/That's how I re-auditorize/I say it out loud and repeat it/ My bra-ain can hear myself think! For the Finger Cues strategy he sings (to the tune *I've something in my pocket*): My fingers are like post-its /They remind me what to do / I remember when my fingers help / How about you? Singing each strategy to remember how he uses it helps Elvis increase his meta-cognitive awareness and be a more active thinker and learner.

Pearl

Music can be used to help develop many aspects of the school age child's life; from academic facts to literacy to executive functioning.

19.5.9 School Music Class

Many students will also have access to a general music class. This is where the support team can be invaluable. Set up a meeting with the music teacher to explain the child's equipment and hearing loss, if the teacher is required to wear a remote microphone, and the best place for the child to sit. It is recommended that a member of the support team attend music class with the child at first to trouble shoot any issues that can arise.

19.5.10 Case Study: Alejandro

Alejandro is an example of a child for whom an integrated LSL and music program resolved some significant oral motor planning deficits, resulting in dramatically improved speech intelligibility. He had received bilateral CIs by age 16 months and showed good progress in his auditory development. Alejandro was enrolled in an LSL preschool at age three, where the first author was on staff as music therapist. He was a spirited participant in music class, developing some music milestones close to age expectations. However, he had highly unintelligible speech, primarily due to motor programming deficits that resulted in very halting utterances. Alejandro had trouble sequencing speech sounds in words and feeding forward to combine words into phrases and sentences. This interrupted the natural rhythm of his utterances—the timing aspects of speech—which are so critical for intelligibility. These struggles had negative consequences for his communication and social interactions.

The second author began seeing Alejandro for LSL sessions, observing his oral motor issues and his use of "uhhhh" or "buhhh" between every word. These were verbal fillers he produced as he groped for the next sound. Goals were developed to improve his speech fluency and, in consult with the first author, combined work on speech rhythm and musical rhythm. Steady beat activities were used to establish an underlying beat and then, taking turns, chanted in rhythm to it, moving from rehearsed words to spontaneous ones. His mother was astounded at how this musical "entrainment" technique improved his speech. This technique was expanded to include more complex rhythms, such as those with syncopation, and concomitant improvements in his speech intelligibility were noted. These techniques worked because Alejandro enjoyed music and was motivated by it. Now age nine, Alejandro enjoys singing along with classic rock videos, including those of Elvis Presley, and has only one error in his speech: a "v" for "th" substitution.

19.5.11 Teenagers

Music is now a large part of everyday teen life. Perhaps CIs don't seem so foreign, as many of their peers have some kind of device hanging on their ears, while on the phone or listening to music. In fact, a hearing teen friend convinced his teacher that he had a hearing loss and was wearing hearing aids in class and the teacher believed him! Meanwhile, he listened to chess strategies for an upcoming match.

The music of teens is popular, trendy, visual, and rhythmic. In one day and out the next. Can be more about the artist and their costumes and sets than the actual music. Musically, it may be the rhythms our CI users latch on to, and certainly with captioning they catch the lyrics, too. In any event, music ties a lot of teens together and that can be a boon for our teens with hearing loss. Both authors have worked with teens who choreograph dance moves to pop songs with their hearing friends, and even play in bands. Listening to a piece of music with a teen during therapy is a way to establish a connection. What do they like about the piece? What instruments do they hear? What genre is it? What are the lyrics and what do they mean? How does the piece relate to their life right now? Many good conversation starters. Remember: we were all teens once upon a time, and the music we listened to back

Table 19.7 Tuneful Toolbox school age

Beat	Melody	Timbre	Emotion
By now, the child should be able to maintain a steady beat and demonstrate it by patting knees, playing rhythm sticks, or small paper plates to the music.	Sing familiar songs in different voices; high, low, middle.	Increase the number of instruments a child can identify through audition alone.	Use the song, *How Are You Feeling Today?* to ascertain the emotional state of the student.
Introduce rhythms by patting the syllables in the child's name. Provide pictures of different animals/bugs and pat the syllables of their name.	Use a slide whistle or push-up puppet to demonstrate the notion of up/down. Move the body up when the whistle or puppet goes up and vice versa (Grand Old Duke of York, *Noodles*). Have the child imitate the sound of the slide whistle with their voice.	Listen to a piece of music and ask the child to identify any instrument they hear.	Provide pictures of children expressing certain emotions (happy, sad, scared, mad, etc) and piggyback a song to detail each emotion. (If you're sad and you know it say boo-hoo, etc.).
Put two animals/bugs together and now you've made a rhythm. Ze-bra, El-e-phant. Chant it four times in a row and you've introduced the concept of a phrase.	Sing sequential songs (*My Aunt Came Back*, There was an Old Lady who Swallowed a Fly, Alouette).	Play the Instrument Lotto Game from *TuneUps*. Play Classroom Instrument Bingo by Harper and Instrument Lotto by Lavender.	Sing familiar songs in a voice associated with a certain emotion i.e., shy (sing softly), mad (sing loudly), scared (sing in a high voice).

*Songs in italics are available as MP3s at: http://www.sjiresources.org/

then had the same effect on parents as is does today. Mostly, they don't like it. You may not, either, but taking the time to dig a little deeper into their reasons for enjoying their music, can go a long way to building a caring, trusting relationship.

HOTS (Higher Order Thinking Skills) and Music. Aliyah, who is 14 and wears CIs, is well-integrated into her eighth grade class and has been invited to watch a movie, "Greatest Showman," with friends. She says she is nervous and wants help understanding what the songs mean. We listen to and analyze the lyrics of the song, "This is Me." Metaphor abounds. Helping Aliyah understand the cultural references, idioms, and use of slang within the song allows her to feel part of her peer group, as described in the "Hit Parade" activity.[35] Aliyah and her clinician discuss what it means in the lyrics when the singer responds to cruel criticism: "I'm gonna send a flood, gonna drown them out." Does it mean flooding them with water? What are "sharp words" and how do they "cut you?" The structure of this song also feels familiar to Aliyah because it tells a story and its chorus has a call-and-response element, a musical style she has practiced before. Like those in her peer group and beyond, she has been audiating, singing along to and inspired by this anthem to individuality and self-respect.

Fostering a Child's Musical Identity. As children develop their musical and spoken language competencies, it is rewarding to observe that they take on a musical identity[20] or self-description of their musical tastes. For all of us, musical identities develop and change across the life span. The second author shares with students that there are several songs she has taken as personal anthems and explained what that meant. She played for him the different songs that appeal to her in different moods. When she needs to strike a positive morning vibe, she plays Amy Grant's "Greet the Day." When she needs to put a struggle behind her, she sings Jimmy Cliff's "I Can See Clearly Now" and when she laments the fractious state of deaf education, she sings along with Nina Simone on "Please Don't Let Me Be Misunderstood." These three songs represent three different musical genres, yet each is a part of her musical identity. When children realize they may have multiple kinds of songs that appeal to them, their musical

horizons have permission to broaden. We nurture the growth of children's musical identities when we encourage them to talk about the music they like, to bring examples to sessions, to invite parents to do the same and to share our own reflections about the music that resides deep within us. In fact, some studies find that musical tastes are formed in the mid to late teens.[36] Others suggest there are subtle changes that take place with other life events, love, children, moves, etc.[37] In any case, the teenage years are all about the need to find identity and music is an effective vehicle.

19.5.12 Case Study: Noelle

Noelle was implanted at three and a half years, with a device failure in the first year. That device was quickly replaced. She functioned well for a number of years with a HA in the other ear. By 12 years of age, she no longer received benefit from her HA, so another CI was implanted. Noelle's largest complaint at the time was that music didn't have the same sound or appeal as it had in the past. So, her parents sought out the first author to see what might help her reclaim her enjoyment of music. This author took a music training approach and started Noelle on piano. She learned to read music, which added a visual component, she sang with solfege, a hand cue system that helps with singing, again another visual component. She used a pitch training software program that she could track visually to sustain individual pitches. After a couple of years, she was able to play a simple tune on the piano while singing along on pitch.

However, now she was a teenager and popular music was her passion. She and friends would choreograph and dance to favorite songs and put on shows for family members. Her enjoyment was back, but singing along to popular tunes was difficult because of the highly produced, fast-paced arrangements of popular music. At this point Noelle announced "Well, I may not be a singer, but I can be a composer!" And after a particularly difficult time with her (annoying) younger brother, she composed a song called Ants in My Pants.

I've got ants in my pants, and I'm going to France

With my family and my Lance, where my brother loves to run in his underpants

We're gonna dance, dance, dance, in France, France, France

And my brother in his underpants

Noelle is a college graduate working on the east coast for a large corporation. Music is still a love of her life!

Pitfall

Resist the urge to push a teen into a music activity that is not of their choosing.

19.5.13 Adults

Adults who participate in auditory-based sessions are commonly recipients of new hearing technology, either state-of-the-art hearing aids or cochlear implants. The authors have found that music is a valuable part of these client's auditory rehabilitation regimen for many reasons:

- Music is a welcome break from the more traditional speech-recognition activities.
- Music is a more gestalt listening task (perceiving the auditory experience and its meaning as one entity), whereas phoneme- or word-recognition activities are analytical listening tasks (perceiving small segments of sound as meaningful).
- Music may help adults access stored auditory memory of musical experiences.
- Music represents emotion, events, connection with people, rather than the blandness of word- or sentence-repetition tasks.

Given these features, motivation may be higher for listeners engaged in musical tasks.

At the initial session with an adult listener, it is important to inquire extensively about both past and present musical engagement. They are asked about preferred genres of music, if there were music lessons of any kind, instruments played, and the degree to

which music was a part of their childhood home and school environments. Then, they are queried about musical experiences that hold the deepest-seeded roots for them. In response to the latter, there is often a range of answers: the national anthem played at sporting events; hymns, a cantor's chanting, or organ music at worship; music associated with their children, especially when young, such as lullabies or music songs that the children enjoyed; a remembered song that was the special music of the listener and spouse. These expressed, deep musical experiences are almost always associated with an emotional connection to special people, to sacred events, to love of family or country (patriotic events). Because positive emotional events are highly memorable and retrievable, the astute clinicians will use these very experiences to build therapy activities.

19.5.14 Working with an Adult Shortly after Initial Stimulation of CIs

- Introduce a small set of four familiar songs, then sing the first lines, auditory-only, noting the percentage the adult correctly recognizes out of 10 presentations.
- Sing on the continuous vowel "ahhhh," sweeping in either a low-to-high pitch direction or a high-to-low pitch direction, using our singing voice. Provide feedback after each presentation ("Yes, that was high-to-low pitch, ahhhhhh") and note how often the correct response is given. Provide the visual cue of an upward-turning arc vs. a downward-turning arc to reinforce the direction of our pitch change.
- Practice music tracking. Provide the printed lyric to a highly familiar song. The clinician will sing the song while the client reads along. Then, stopping at random places in the song, have the client sing the next word or phrase.
- Play a short rhythm segment on a drum out of view from the client. Ask the client to match the pattern on their drum. Increase complexity as the client achieves success.

19.5.15 As the Adult Progresses in Listening Skills

- Assign the task of listening to an unfamiliar piece of vocal and instrumental music at home. We ask for written perceptions:

Table 19.8 Tuneful Toolbox teen-age

Beat	Melody	Timbre	Emotion
Steady beat is still important because to dance to music, which is what teens do, that beat must be felt. Use the teen's choice of music and tap the beat on a table, knees, or drum before moving to the music.	Identify who is singing the melody in a favorite popular song. Is it a male voice, female, does it change throughout the song?	Listening to a piece of music of the teen's choosing see how many instruments he or she can identify.	Teens are all about emotion. Check in with how the teen is feeling and have the teen choose and listen to a piece of music that matches his or her current emotional state.
Explore different genres of music and explore how beat and rhythm are similar or different.	See if the teen can follow the melody throughout the song.	Watch a YouTube video of the piece to see if musicians are playing instruments that can be identified.	Suggest the teen write a story while listening to music.
Talk about tempo, how slow or fast a piece of music is.	Choose a song to piggyback and have the teen write lyrics and sing it.	Play a music bingo or lotto game.	Suggest the teen draw or paint while listening to music.

What words were recognized? What are the impressions of the gender, age, and vocal timbre of the singer? What instruments were heard? Then replay the piece and experience the music together.

- Make music tracking more challenging by singing a familiar song without the printed lyric, while the client provides the next word, each time the practitioner stops singing.
- Sing from a set of four familiar songs, removing lyric cues by using "la" for each syllable. The client then relies on other musical elements (rhythm, melody) to identify the song.
- Isolate timbre cues. We play short recordings of different instruments, initially contrasting those with very different timbres (flute vs. tuba vs. drum), progressing to those with similar timbres (violin vs. cello vs. piano). We provide feedback and record accuracy (**Table 19.9**).

MOOZIC: Virtual Zoom Sessions for Students with CIs

For well over a year before vaccines were available, both authors conducted virtual sessions with students, teachers, and families. Some were conducted in the child's home as a typical LSL therapy session with a caregiver in attendance, others were zoomed into the classroom with the teacher there to facilitate. We coined the name "MOOZIC" for these, as a combination of CI and Zoom, spelled backwards. After becoming familiar with the virtual platform, sessions went better than either author expected and we were surprised that, in spite of the children wearing masks and hearing sound coming through a computer, they were able to follow and take part in the session. However, we did learn a number of things along the way. First, to plan sessions, the authors queried the parents about their child's musical interests, preferences, instruments available in the home and the importance of music to the family. A survey was developed and sent to each family (**Table 19.10**). Then, we realized that the setting of the environment was critical and created a guide for parents to maximize the effectiveness of the sessions. (**Table 19.11**) The children and family members were always eager for music time, so in that regard it could be considered successful. But, behavioral issues and listening and processing music are easier to address in the moment in person.

19.6 Resources

Drum up Support (Resources for parents and clinicians)

AudiTunes: A Music-Supported Approach to Spoken Language Development in Children with Hearing Loss. (2018)

This is designed to be a resource for parents and professionals caring for children with hearing loss currently engaged in a spoken language program. Each short video targets a specific aspect of music development and provides novel ways (and encouragement) for novices to include music in a home or therapy

Table 19.9 Tuneful Toolbox adult

Beat	Melody	Timbre	Emotion
Play recorded music and have the adult match the beat by patting knees, the table, or a drum. Model a short rhythm segment on a drum and have the client match the rhythm on another drum.	Using a familiar song, sing the melody without accompaniment.	Using rhythm instruments of different timbres, play out of sight and have the adult name the instrument they heard.	What is the adult's first memory of music? Can the client describe the feelings/associations connected with that memory?
Explore different genres of music and explore how beat and rhythm are similar or different.	Listen to or sing an unfamiliar song and explore how many lyrics the adult can pick out.	Can the adult discriminate between a female, male and child's voice singing a song?	Discuss the emotional intent of a favorite piece of music. What do the lyrics mean, and how does the music support the meaning?
Talk about tempo, how slow or fast a piece of music is.	Sing songs familiar to the adult on a single syllable, la, and see if the client can name the tune.	Listen to a piece of recorded music and have the adult name all the instruments/voices heard.	Explore the emotional connection to a familiar piece. What associations does the adult make with the music?

Table 19.10 Parent/caregiver music survey

In an attempt to optimize virtual music time (MOOZIC) with your child, I have a few questions I'd like to ask. Please reply to questions 6, 7, and 8 using the rating scale below.
1. Do you have any instruments at home? If yes, please list.
2. Does anyone in the family play an instrument? If yes, please list.
3. Does your child have a favorite song(s)?
4. Does your child have a favorite artist to listen to?
5. Does your child/family have a favorite genre/style to listen to?
6. How appealing would you say music is to your child?
7. How comfortable are you singing to and with your child?
8. How comfortable are you engaging in other music experiences with your child?

Not very				Very
1	2	3	4	5

Table 19.11 Suggestions for successful remote CI music sessions (MOOZIC)

Dear Parents or Caregivers,
I'm delighted to share music with your child this semester. We had many successful sessions last spring during the stay-at-home mandate. We also learned a number of things that will help maximize our time together. So please:
- Turn off the TV, radio, and any other audio or visual distractions during our sessions.
- Eat before or after the session so attention is focused on the ZOOM screen.
- Don't leave your child unattended during the sessions, as we are often moving to the music.
- Provide a shaker (can be as simple as beans, rice, or popcorn in an empty water bottle) and a drum (can be a coffee can, oatmeal container, or plastic food storage with a lid and a wooden spoon or pencil as a stick).
- Return the Parent/Caregiver Survey identifying what instruments are available to your child and I will include them in the sessions.
Siblings are welcome to join in the music making. I encourage your comments, as well.

setting. Printed materials for each lesson are available for download. The Learning to Listen Musical Sounds chart is also able to be printed. A core feature of AudiTunes is its use of multi-sensory music experiences within a diverse population and in a variety of settings. The series was developed by board certified music therapist, Christine Barton and speech pathologist, LSLS Cert. AVT, Amy McConkey Robbins. It is grounded on current research and evidence-based practice. AudiTunes is available at no cost to parents and professionals and is made possible through St. Joseph Institute for the Deaf, Indianapolis, Indiana, WFYI, and a private family foundation. Available at: https://www.sjiresources.org/.

Tuneups: A Music Program Designed to Foster Communication. (2008)

Winner of the Therapy Times 2009, Most Valuable Product Award. Developed by these authors, this music CD and habilitation program engages children in a listening, language, and learning experience. Available gratis from the Listening Room at Advanced Bionics.

19.6.1 Industry Resources

Advanced Bionics (AB) https://thelisteningroom.com/en/lessons/view/230. Sponsored by AB and Phonak. Registration is free, but required. Here you will find "TuneUps," "BabyBeats," and "A Journey through a Rainforest," all musical programs for children.

Cochlear www.cochlear.com. The Communication Corner site has rehab activities from birth through adult, plus a music program for Teens and Tweens. Cochlear App: "Bring Back the Beat"

MED-EL www.med-el.com. Hosts a blog called The Importance of Music in CI Rehabilitation for Adults.

19.6.2 Other Resources for Individuals and Families Dealing with Hearing Loss

www.agbell.org

www.HearingFirst.org

www.options.org

19.6.3 Music Resources

www.angelsound.emilyfufoundation.org/angelsound_music.html

www.musictogether.com

www.themusicplayhouse.com

www.kindermusic.com

www.little-folks-music.com

www.westmusic.com. Quality instruments and musical games like Classroom Instrument Bingo by Harper and Instrument Lotto by Lavender

19.7 It's Not Over Till the Fat Lady Sings

The authors trust we have made a reasonable case for including music, not only in the therapy setting, but in the lives of children with hearing loss. Our claim that music experiences enhance auditory and cognitive development in children with hearing technology is partly supported by research, but also a reasonable assumption based on what we have seen in practice, heard from parents, and know now.

In the years we have been LSL practitioners we have witnessed the amazing progress in new technology, earlier implantation and intervention. It gives us hope that music will no longer be the final frontier to be discovered through hearing technology, but rather a natural part of everyday life. As one little client said to his dad at bedtime, "Daddy, I can't hear your guitar when I take off my CIs, but I do hear music in my dreams!" We should all be so lucky.

References

[1] Mehr SA, Singh M, Knox D, et al. Universality and diversity in human song. *Science* 2019;22 November. 10.1126/science.aax0868

[2] Mithin S. The Singing Neanderthals: The Origins Of Music, Language, Mind, and Body. Cambridge, MA: Harvard University Press; 2006

[3] Barton C, Robbins AM. AudiTunes: A video resource of music activities to support listening and spoken language development. http://www.sjiresources.org. 2018

[4] Gordon E. A Music Learning Theory for Newborn and Young Children. Chicago, IL: GIA Publications; 2003

[5] Locke JL. The Child's Path to Spoken Language. Cambridge, MA: Harvard University Press; 1993

[6] Robbins C, Robbins C. Music for the Hearing Impaired: A Resource Manual and Curriculum Guide. New York, NY: MMB Music; 1980

[7] Robbins AM. Music and singing in auditory-verbal therapy. In: Estabrooks W, MacIver-Lux K, Morrison HM, eds. Auditory-Verbal therapy: Science, research, and practice. San Diego, CA: Plural Publishing; 2020

[8] Ling D. Introduction: speech and song. In: Estabrooks W, Birkenshaw-Fleming L, eds. Songs for Listening! Songs for Life! Washington, DC: Alexander Graham Bell Association; 2003

[9] Skoe E, Kraus N. A little goes a long way: how the adult brain is shaped by musical training in childhood. *J Neurosci* 2012;32(34):11507–11510 10.1523/JNEUROSCI.1949-12.2012

[10] Patel AD. Music, Language and the Brain. New York: Oxford University Press; 2008

[11] Patel AD. The OPERA hypothesis: assumptions and clarifications. *Ann N Y Acad Sci* 2012;*1252*:124–128

[12] Barton C. Children with hearing loss. In: Hintz M, ed. Guidelines for Music Therapy Practice in Developmental Health. Gilsum, NH: Barcelona Publishers; 2013:233–269

[13] Kraus N, Chandrasekaran B. Music training for the development of auditory skills. *Nat Rev Neurosci* 2010;*11*(8):599–605

[14] Williams KE, Barrett MS, Welch GF, Abad V, Broughton M. Associations between early shared music activities in the home and later child outcomes: findings from the longitudinal study of Australian children. *Early Child Res Q* 2015;*31*:113–124

[15] Barton C, Robbins AM. TuneUps™: A Music Program Designed to Foster Communication Development. Valencia, CA: Advanced Bionics, LLC; 2007

[16] Barton C. Music, Spoken Language, and Children with Hearing Loss: Definitions and Development, Part 1." SpeechPathology.com Published 2010. Accessed March 28, 2011

[17] Barton C. Music, Spoken Language, and Children with Hearing Loss: Using Music to Develop Spoken Language, Part 2. Speech Pathology.com 2010. Accessed March 28, 2011

[18] Sarrazin N. Music and the Child. New York, NY: Open SUNY Textbooks; June 15, 2016

[19] Beardsley E. This French Pianist Has Been Playing For 102 Years and Just Released A New Album. Morning Edition(NPR) 9-20-2021

[20] Hargreaves DJ, Miell D, MacDonald RAR. What are musical identities, and why are they important? In: McDonald RAR, Hargreaves DJ, Miell D, eds. Musical Identities. Oxford University Press; 2002:1–20

[21] Barton C, Robbins AM. Jumpstarting auditory learning in children with cochlear implants through music experiences. *Cochlear Implants Int* 2015; *16*(3, Suppl 3):S51–S62

[22] Trehub SE. 2013 Communication, music and language in infancy. In: Arbib, ed. Language, Music and the Brain. Strungmann Forum Reports. Vol. 10. Cambridge, MA: MIT Press; 2013

[23] Bergeson TR, Miller RJ, McCune K. Mothers' speech to hearing-impaired infants and children. *Infancy* 2006;*10*:221–240

[24] Erber N. Auditory Training. Washington, DC: AGBell; 1982

[25] Garcia-Winner M. Thinking of me thinking of you. Santa Clara: Think Social Publishing; 2007

[26] Robbins AM. Auditory-Verbal therapy: a conversational competence approach. In: Moeller MP, Ertmer DJ, Stoel-Gammon C, eds. Promoting language and literacy in children who are deaf or hard of hearing. Baltimore, MD: Paul H. Brookes Publishing; 2016

[27] Troxel K. Grammar songs. www.kathytroxel.com 1984

[28] Bryer J. Rap n Rock 2: More Musical Activities for Language and Literacy. Oceanside, CA: Academic Communication Associates; 1994

[29] Silverstein S. Everything on It. New York, NY: Harper Collins; 2011

[30] Kronenberger WG, Beer J, Castellanos I, Pisoni DB, Miyamoto RT. Neurocognitive risk in children with cochlear implants. *JAMA Otolaryngol Head Neck Surg* 2014;*140*(7):608–615

[31] Robbins AM, Kroenberger W. Principles of executive function intervention for children with cochlear implants. Paper presented at American Cochlear Implant Alliance meeting, July 11, Hollywood, FL, 2019

[32] Hendrix R, Palmer KZ, Tarshis N, Garcia Winner M. We Thinkers! Vol. 1 Social Explorers. Santa Clara: Think Social Publishing; 2013

[33] Chapin T, Galdston P. The Incredible Flexible You. The Last Music Co. and Kazzoom Music, Inc.; 2013

[34] Robbins AM. Bossing your brain: A history lesson with a middle school student who is hard of hearing. *Volta Voices* 2005; (July/August):38–40

[35] Robbins AM. Lesson plan for Lilly. In: Estabrooks W, ed. Cochlear Implants for Kids. Washington, DC: Alexander Graham Bell; 1998:153–174

[36] Stevens-Davidowitz, S. The Songs that Bind. https://www.nytimes.com/2018/02/10/opinion/sunday/favorite-songs.html 2018

[37] Bonneville-Roussy A, Rentfrow PJ, Xu MK, Potter J. Music through the ages: Trends in musical engagement and preferences from adolescence through middle adulthood. *J Pers Soc Psychol* 2013;*105*(4):703–717; Advance online publication 10.1037/a0033770

20 Telepractice for Children with Hearing Loss

Elizabeth A. Rosenzweig

Summary

This chapter on telepractice for children with hearing loss describes the use of teletherapy as a service delivery method to provide listening and spoken language therapy (LSL) or aural rehabilitation (AR) to children and adults with hearing loss. Telepractice terms, research, and professional issues (e.g., licensure) are explored to provide necessary background. Considerations for audiovisual technology, therapeutic techniques, child and caregiver engagement across distances, and assessment via videoconference technology are addressed. Special applications of telepractice, such as the use of videoconference technology for co-treating, professional mentoring and coaching, and supporting school-based teams, are explored, as are future directions for teletherapy.

Keywords

telepractice, teletherapy, listening and spoken language (LSL), aural rehabilitation (AR), children with hearing loss (CWHL)

Key Points

- There is strong evidence supporting the efficiency and efficacy of telepractice for a variety of populations, including children and adults with hearing loss.
- Practitioners must consider their capability to provide equivalent services via telepractice and work to build their competency in this modality.
- Patients and families need support in using both the hardware and software required for telepractice.
- Beyond direct patient care, telepractice has the potential to improve the state of the field by enabling more widespread professional education, more flexible parent or caregiver coaching, and connections between highly qualified professionals and families in underserved communities.
- The future of telepractice will involve emerging professional issues, such as HIPAA/FERPA compliance, remote audiology services, interstate licensing regulations, and reimbursement, as well as continued research on best practices and outcomes for this service delivery method.

There are roughly 1,000 Listening and Spoken Language Specialists (LSLS) certified worldwide, and other clinicians undoubtedly providing high-quality aural rehabilitation services to children with hearing loss (CWHL) and their families.[1] Still, many CWHL whose families have elected a listening and spoken language outcome do not have access to high-quality services. Provision of services to patients not physically present with the clinician via videoconference technology, or telepractice, is one solution that can help increase patients' access to specialist clinicians.

20.1 Background

20.1.1 Teletherapy Terms and Definitions

Telehealth, telemedicine, teletherapy, telespeech, teleaudiology, telerehabilitation—all of these terms have been used to describe the provision of health services via audiovisual technology. For the purposes of this chapter, the umbrella term "telepractice" will be used to describe the work of audiologists, speech-language pathologists, and teachers of the deaf who provide services in this modality. The American Speech-Language Hearing Association (ASHA) defines telepractice as "the application of telecommunications technology to the delivery of speech language pathology and audiology professional services at a distance by linking clinician to client or clinician to clinician for assessment, intervention, and/or consultation."[2]

Services provided via telepractice may be described as *synchronous* (practitioner and client(s) interacting in real time), *asynchronous* (practitioner and clients interacting with digital content and communicating at different times on their own schedules), or a combination of both synchronous and asynchronous content, known as a *hybrid* model. Practitioners may interact 1:1 with clients/families in *point-to-point* services, or may interact with groups of clients in *point-to-multipoint* visits (e.g., classes, group therapy sessions, or parent support groups where one professional is delivering content to clients in multiple locations at the same time). When videoconference technology is used to enable a client or professional to attend a meeting or appointment remotely (e.g., an educational audiologist employed by the school district conferences into a child study team meeting at a rural school), this can be called *telepresence*.

The technology used to deliver telepractice can be divided into two categories: *software* and *hardware*. The *software* is the telepractice platform used—the application or program that provides the videoconference technology. Telepractice *hardware* includes the physical technology, such as the desktop or laptop computer, webcam, speakers, and microphone. (Some professionals might utilize additional hardware, like document cameras or dual monitors, but this is not required for successful telepractice.) Recordings of telepractice sessions can be stored on the *local computer* (the practitioner's or client's device) or via *cloud* storage (managed by the telepractice platform or a third-party provider).

20.1.2 Evidence Base

While internet connectivity and videoconference technology have revolutionized the provision of medical and educational services via telepractice, the idea of providing speech, language, and hearing services via technology is not a new one. Gwenyth Vaughn, a speech-language pathologist at the Birmingham, Alabama Veterans Affairs (VA) Hospital, is credited with introducing speech-language services via telephone in the 1970s, providing treatment she called "tel-communicology."[3] In 1997, researchers at the Mayo Clinic compared the accuracy of speech and language evaluations conducted via telepractice versus those conducted in person and concluded, "[t]elemedicine evaluations can be reliable, beneficial, and acceptable to patients with a variety of acquired speech and language disorders, both in rural settings and within large multidisciplinary medical settings."[4] By 2005, improvements in audiovisual technology and internet access had made telepractice an emerging trend in the field of communication sciences and disorders, and ASHA issued a position statement endorsing telepractice as an appropriate service delivery model for speech-language pathologists and audiologists, stating that services rendered via this modality should be equivalent in quality to those provided in in-person treatment.[1]

In the broader field of communication sciences and disorders, telepractice has been used to deliver treatment for a variety of communication disorders. Grogan-Johnson et al. compared outcomes for children with speech sound disorders receiving treatment either via teletherapy or in a "side-by-side" (i.e., in-person) clinic setting and found no significant differences in post-treatment outcomes between the two groups, a finding substantiated in another study of children with speech sound disorders by Coufal et al.[5,6] For the Lidcombe Program, a parent-led early fluency intervention, researchers found fluency improvement among children randomly assigned to receive intervention via telepractice that was greater than or statistically equal to growth observed in the control (in-person intervention) group.[7,8,9] Metat-analyses and scoping reviews of telepractice for communication disorders in general and hearing loss in particular have demonstrated the feasibility and efficacy of this method of service delivery, while emphasizing the need for continued investigation.[10,11,12,13,14,15]

Studies of telepractice have illustrated unique difficulties and benefits specific to this service delivery model. Drawbacks of telepractice include a need for increased preparation time for each session, concerns about privacy and security of online platforms, and internet connectivity issues.[8,16] Despite these limitations, telepractice has many unique benefits for both professionals and clients as well. Telepractice is an effective tool to overcome challenges related to personnel shortages, particularly in rural areas.[17] Therapy delivered via telepractice can yield child outcomes equal to, or in some cases greater than, the gains made in in-person treatment, as well as improved caregiver participation and buy-in. In their randomized controlled study of telehealth versus community-based parent training in the Denver Early Start Model for autism, Vismara et al. found increased treatment fidelity and parent satisfaction among the telehealth group.[18] Telepractice may lead to fewer missed or cancelled sessions by eliminating concerns about transportation, illness, or childcare arrangements for children, families, and practitioners alike.[19] Most notably for listening and spoken language professionals who use a family-centered model of intervention, Poole et al. state that, "tele-intervention is naturally set up to support caregiver coaching, rather than a direct-service model".[20]

Similar to studies conducted on other pediatric populations, telepractice has been shown to be an effective method of service delivery for children with hearing loss and their families who have elected a listening and spoken language outcome. A multi-site study of telepractice outcomes for children with hearing loss also found comparable language outcomes for telepractice versus in-person intervention groups.[19] Children in the telepractice group had statistically similar scores on other language measures as well as family outcomes such as perceived support and knowledge for both treatment conditions.[19] Constantinescu et al. found comparable language outcomes for teletherapy versus in-person intervention groups.[21] Children who were two years post receipt of optimal amplification who received LSL therapy via teletherapy scored within normal limits when compared to typically hearing peers.[21] Practitioners' self-assessment of their use of coaching practices has not been found to differ between modalities.[22] Telepractice services for children with hearing loss have led to decreased treatment costs and increased parental engagement when compared to traditional home visit models.[23] Childhood hearing loss is a low-incidence disability, and there is a shortage of highly qualified professionals to provide listening and spoken language services to children and families who desire this outcome. Studies, such as those previously referenced, provide empirical support for the efficiency and efficacy of telepractice as a promising service delivery model to improve outcomes for this population.

Pearl

While research is ever-evolving, the current state of the literature suggests strong evidence for the efficiency and efficacy of telepractice services for people with hearing loss.

20.1.3 Professional Issues

Since 2005, the American Speech-Language Hearing Association (ASHA) has included telepractice within the scope of practice for both audiologist and speech-language pathologists.[2] The American Academy of Audiology (AAA), the professional organization for audiologists, does not include language on telepractice in its most recent scope of practice document.[24] No comparable nationwide professional credentialing associations exist for teachers in general or teachers of the deaf in particular. With the need for a rapid shift to remote service provision due to the Covid-19 pandemic, numerous professional organizations issued ad hoc guidance that will almost certainly be formalized in future scope of practice documents as telepractice becomes a more widely accepted aspect of practice for a variety of professions.

While providing therapy services, audiological treatment, or curricular instruction via telepractice may fall within the scope of practice for speech-language pathologists, audiologists, and teachers of the deaf, professionals must be cognizant of the difference between "scope of practice" and "scope of competence" to ensure they are providing high quality services to the children and families they serve. Scope of practice delineates all of the possible roles and responsibilities that fall under a particular occupational designation, credential, or licensure. An individual practitioner's scope of competence consists of the areas within their professional scope of practice in which they feel confident in their knowledge, skills, and capability to provide highly effective treatment. For example, while aural rehabilitation (AR) falls within the scope of practice for any certified speech-language pathologist, not all SLPs are highly competent in this area—one SLP might hold the LSLS Cert. AVT credential, while another might not have had coursework or clinical experience in AR since graduate school decades ago. Principle II of ASHA's Code of Ethics states, "Individuals shall honor their responsibility to achieve and maintain the highest level of professional competence and performance," further stating (in Principle II, Rule A) that professionals "shall engage in only those aspects of the professions that are within the scope of their professional practice and competence, considering their certification status, education, training, and experience."[25] As such, it is crucial that professionals who wish to engage in service provision via telepractice work to develop their skills in this modality and continually assess client benefit to ensure that they are practicing ethically and providing services that are both within their scope of practice *and* their scope of competence.

Pitfall

Just because telepractice falls within a professional's scope of practice doesn't mean it falls within their scope of competence. To practice ethically, professionals must evaluate their capability to provide treatment via telepractice equivalent to in-person treatment before beginning service delivery via this modality.

Licensure laws present another legal and ethical hurdle in the provision of telepractice services across jurisdictions. ASHA maintains an updated telepractice portal on the organization's website with guidance on professional licensure and state-by-state laws and regulations.[2] In general, professionals must be licensed in both their physical location and the patient's physical location. For example, a speech-language pathologist living in New York may provide services to a child with hearing loss and her family living in New Jersey only if the SLP is licensed in both states. Likewise, professionals wishing to provide service outside of the country in which they are located are obligated to research any applicable telepractice laws in the clients' country to stay in compliance with local regulations. In some countries with established licensing organizations for speech-language pathologists and audiologists (e.g., Canada), telepractice regulations regarding international service provision exist. In other countries where families with access to technology may seek auditory-verbal services from professionals abroad (e.g., Zambia), local regulations regarding telepractice do not exist and speech-language pathology and audiology may not yet be established as regulated professions. Jurisdictional regulations concerning teletherapy may include additional stipulations beyond licensure requirements, such as mandating in-person evaluations or a period of in-person treatment before commencing telepractice services, telepractice-specific documentation, or the need for teaching credentials for professionals providing services in the public school system.

Privacy and security must also be considered when providing services via telepractice. Telepractice is subject to the same regulations (e.g., HIPAA, FERPA) as in-person services. While some telepractice platforms may advertise their "HIPAA compliance," all technology is only as secure and private as the individuals operating it. Choosing a HIPAA-compliant telepractice platform is important, but it represents only the first step in delivering secure patient care. Professionals must also safeguard meeting notes, patient-family communication, session recordings, and other aspects of treatment to comply with regulations governing patient care and protected health information (PHI). Use of generally available videoconferencing features of mobile phones or tablets is not recommended. Additionally, just as professionals must obtain informed consent for general speech-language-hearing services, professionals and organizations should consider adding telepractice-specific information into their patient consent documents. Watzlaf et al. provide a HIPAA compliance checklist for telepractice technology, and Cohn and Watzlaf propose programmatic safeguards for privacy and security in telepractice.[26,27] As technology, internet privacy laws, and professional practice continue to evolve, so will professional issues regarding telepractice for speech-language pathologists, audiologists, and teachers of the deaf.

Pitfall

Professionals must be aware of relevant healthcare, education, and licensure laws that apply to telepractice. Consult your professional organizations and local/state/national legislative bodies.

20.2 Patient Considerations and Technical Considerations

20.2.1 Determining Patient Appropriateness for Teletherapy

Patients of a wide variety of ages, technological capabilities, and diagnoses have been found to benefit from intervention delivered via telepractice. Contrary to popular belief, no one is "too young," "too old," or "too technologically challenged" to benefit from this intervention modality. However, clinicians and service organizations must be cognizant of both the technology and user skills necessary to participate in telepractice and provide support for clients so that they can participate fully. Many decisions about patient appropriateness for teletherapy are made on a case-by-case basis by professionals relying only on their clinical judgment, while others are determined based on availability and location of service providers, not clients' preferences or needs.[28] In cases when telepractice is the only option for providing services to a child and the family, it might not be ethical to withhold treatment, even if it is determined that this is not the preferred or ideal modality for that particular client.

The American Speech-Language Hearing Association provides guidance on factors professionals must consider when determining whether or not a patient will benefit from telepractice, including physical, sensory, and cognitive abilities; access to technology; and availability of a parent, partner, or caregiver to assist the patient in navigating technology during treatment sessions.[2] Use of an "e-helper," or responsible party (e.g., teacher's aide, parent, caregiver) on the patient's end can help to facilitate telepractice sessions. Checklists establishing e-helper competencies, such as capability to assist with telepractice software, knowledge of patients' assistive technology, and behavior management, can help professionals determine families' or schools' capacity to assist children in benefitting fully from intervention delivered via telepractice.[29,30,31]

Culturally responsive practice, which encompasses student learning, cultural competency, and critical consciousness, should be at the forefront of any therapeutic or educational intervention, and telepractice is no exception.[32] While telepractice may advance equity by enabling clients and families to connect with service providers who share their culture or language, barriers due to lack of in-home technology and internet or lack of a safe, permanent home environment to receive services access can make telepractice sessions inaccessible for some children with hearing loss. Likewise, professionals should assess families' cultural beliefs and practices regarding engagement with technology and learn more about the family's home environment if telepractice sessions will be taking place there.[33] For example, some cultures place increased emphasis on face-to-face interactions and are less amenable to services delivered via telepractice.[34] Hilty et al. make the case that, in addition to competency with telepractice technology, and treatment techniques, professionals delivering telehealth services must also develop cultural competencies.[35]

20.2.2 Technical Considerations

While some general considerations (e.g., internet connectivity, privacy and security of the chosen platform, etc.) apply across patient populations, professionals working with children with hearing loss must pay special attention to the audiovisual environment when providing services via telepractice.

Low bandwidth and lagging internet speeds may cause a dyssynchrony between the audio and visual signals, making the use of visual cues that support receptive understanding of spoken language difficult. Poor microphone and speaker quality, on both the professionals' side and the clients', can make tasks such as auditory discrimination (for the client) or assessment of articulation quality (for the professional) more difficult. Children and families may need guidance to learn how to connect their hearing technology to the audio system of the computer, tablet, or phone (if applicable). This is especially relevant for children with single-sided deafness. These children, who have received a cochlear implant in one ear (and have hearing within normal limits on the contralateral side), can greatly benefit from teletherapy due to the capability to route computer audio directly to the implanted ear. This allows parents, caregivers, and professionals to provide targeted stimulation and (re)habilitation to the affected ear in isolation. In such telepractice sessions, the child can connect the device directly to the computer audio, the parent or caregiver present with the child can call in to the session on a phone or separate computer (so they also can hear the professional), and the professional can provide both auditory stimulation and coaching as usual from his or her end.

Professionals should consider the use of headphones with a built-in boom-style microphone, a setup that will eliminate background noise present in the professional's environment, ensure a consistent signal for the client regardless of therapist position, and provide maximum audibility of patient responses. On the child's end, use of a headset or microphone can limit child mobility and parent-child interaction. While having a child speak directly into a computer microphone can help professionals more accurately evaluate articulation, it is more important for the parent to be able to hear the professional's guidance and coaching and for the professional to see and hear the parent-child interaction than for the child to remain seated, focusing on the screen. Telepractice can be used very effectively to coach families in their natural environments, and one benefit of this technology is the capability for therapy to be "portable." Families can bring professionals along to the kitchen counter during cooking activities, put the professional on the shelf to observe parent-child playtime, or bring a phone or tablet along on a walk around the neighborhood.

Pearl

Telepractice is portable! When professionals provide family-centered coaching, children and their caregivers should not feel tethered to their devices.

20.3 Diagnostics and Intervention

20.3.1 Determining the Purpose of Teletherapy

While many different types of services fall under the broadly defined umbrella of "listening and spoken language," determining the purpose of services delivered may help professionals clarify the aims of telepractice sessions.

Traditional Auditory Verbal Therapy (AVT) takes place in a 1:1:1 situation, with one professional providing real-time guidance and coaching the parent(s) or caregiver(s) of a child with hearing loss. Children receiving this type of intervention are developing communication skills for the first time. AVT sessions focus on all domains of communication development, including audition, speech, language, cognition (play and academic skills), and social communication (pragmatics) using a developmental approach. In these telepractice sessions, point-to-point technology is used, and the primary objective is to deliver coaching to the parent(s)/caregiver(s) as they facilitate their child's listening, language, and speech development. Professionals delivering these services must be highly skilled in parent coaching strategies.

Educational programs can use telepractice to provide similar services to individual children and families or can utilize telepractice to deliver remote instruction ("teleschool") to groups of children. With groups, a point-to-multipoint configuration of technology is used that can necessitate additional troubleshooting time on the part of the professional. Professionals delivering intervention to groups via telepractice must provide differentiated instruction to meet the needs of children at various developmental levels. Goals for school-based services can include the achievement of curricular standards as well as listening, language, and speech development. In their discussion of school-based telepractice services, Walters et al. discuss the feasibility and efficiency of implementing telepractice services using extant technology in schools and school districts, while cautioning that additional professional preparation and collaboration between the remote professional and the school-based team is required for success.[36] Demographic trends for DHH students in many public school districts, such as increased demand for listening and spoken language services, dispersion of students into mainstream classes rather than grouped in self-contained settings, and lack of qualified service providers to meet their IEP mandates make telepractice an attractive and necessary innovation to be able to provide all students with appropriate access to education.[37]

While providers of AVT and listening and spoken language educational programs use a developmental, habilitative model to develop listening, language, and speech skills, telepractice can also be used to rehabilitate auditory capabilities in older children or adults who have already established a spoken language system. This type of therapy is commonly called aural rehabilitation (AR) and focuses on listening skills, not necessarily speech and language development. For example, consider the case of a child with a progressive hearing loss. This child may have worn hearing aids and received AVT services in early childhood. If the child's hearing loss progresses to the profound range during adolescence and he receives a cochlear implant, he may receive short-term AR services to relearn auditory skills with this new technology. Post-lingually deafened adults who receive hearing technology can also benefit from AR sessions. While family participation is recommended for optimal AR outcomes regardless of patient age, some AR clients can participate in telepractice sessions without an at-home "listening partner." In these cases, attention to the fidelity of the audio signal on both the provider's and client's end is especially important.

Determining the child's and family's needs can assist practitioners in making decisions about treatment frequency, duration, and goals.

20.3.2 Diagnostics

In general, most assessments that professionals administer in in-person treatment can be adapted to the virtual environment. Measurement developers have digitized their assessments for online administration (e.g., Pearson's *Q-global* digital assessment portfolio) and published white papers attesting to the reliability and validity of testing delivered in this form.[38,39] Werfel et al. calculated test-retest reliability for a variety of pediatric speech-language assessments for their study population of preschool and elementary school aged children with hearing loss and found that the reliability for most assessments was adequate (or higher), while noting that tests with time limits or timed items showed lower reliability.[40]

While many aspects of communication can be reliably assessed via videoconference technology, clinicians might want to obtain in-person information or recorded samples before making a definitive diagnosis of some aspects of speech and language production. For example, apraxia of speech is commonly characterized by inconsistent approximations and vowel errors (which can be assessed via telepractice), and groping mouth movements

(which might not be able to be assessed, depending on the quality of the video feed). Likewise, determinations regarding vocal quality made via telepractice (e.g., hypo/hypernasality) can be aided by corroborating evidence gathered from in-person observation or audio recordings conducted in the natural environment and sent to the clinician asynchronously. Pragmatic cues, such as eye contact, can be different with telepractice, as children may make "eye contact" with the screen image or the webcam, depending on hardware placement. Pragmatics are most accurately assessed by observing the child's interaction with others in their natural environment, not the child's interactions with the professional on the screen. In these cases, video recordings made of the child in the natural environment during daily routines or social interactions and sent to the clinician for analysis can be a more accurate indicator of the child's skills and needs than interaction during a telepractice session.

The Ling Six Sound Check and the Ling, Madell, Hewitt (LMH) test battery are daily measures of the functional access to the speech spectrum provided by a child's hearing technology.[41,42,43] Rather than a periodic means of assessing speech, language, and listening capability like the assessments previously discussed, this daily check should be conducted prior to any listening and spoken language intervention to provide a clinical verification of the child's hearing technology. Any errors or concerns should be reported to the child's audiologist as soon as possible. Spanning the range of sounds in spoken language, the Ling Six Sounds provide parents and professionals with a general approximation that the child has access to all of the sounds of speech. Developments in hearing technology and expanded auditory access have prompted professionals to add to the original Ling Six Sounds (/a, u, i, m, s, ʃ/). The LMH 10-Sound Quick Test (Ling-Madell-Hewitt/Low-Medium-High) adds phonemes /h, n, z, dʒ/ to the original six Ling. Sounds to probe the range of frequencies that should be expected of appropriately programmed hearing technology in the 21st century.[43] Because the human brain responds preferentially to live voice versus electronic audio, it is advised that a person (e.g., parent, teacher's aide, etc.) present with the child during the appointment conduct the sound check, with the professional observing and recording data.[44] Likewise, any auditory perception stimuli (e.g., minimal pair discrimination tasks) should be presented "live voice" by a person in the child's environment with coaching from the professional via telepractice if at all possible.

Pitfall

Even the best electronic signal is no match for live voice. Have a person present with the client conduct the listening check if at all possible.

Ongoing formal and informal evaluations are a key aspect of Auditory Verbal practice.[45] The data obtained from both formal testing and dynamic assessment within the context of intervention sessions allow professionals to monitor children's progress, provide families and caregivers with information about the child's development, and determine appropriate goals and treatment plans. Although assessment via telepractice may look slightly different from in-person diagnostic appointments, it is no less essential to the provision of high-quality listening and spoken language services in this modality. Thanks to the development of electronic test protocols and research establishing the validity thereof, clinicians can confidently administer and interpret a wide variety of assessments via videoconference technology.

20.3.3 Intervention

When planning a telepractice session, professionals should keep in mind the maxim that best practices in listening and spoken language intervention do not change based on the modality of service delivery. While materials can need to be adapted for telepractice, the foundational principles of auditory verbal therapy—the primacy of audition, the primacy of the family, and intervention that is developmental rather than remedial—remain unchanged.[46] This section will provide guidance on establishing rapport, providing parent and caregiver coaching, implementing auditory verbal strategies, and selecting therapy materials for telepractice interventions.

Pearl

Remember that telepractice is a service delivery modality, not a new type of therapy. If it wasn't best practice for an in-person session, it's not best practice for a teletherapy session!

Many professionals cite concerns about building rapport with children and families or caregivers as a reason they are concerned about the efficacy of telepractice.[47] Rapport can be conceptualized in many different ways, with Long and Long suggesting three key components: empathy, respect, and warmth.[48] Rapport is often established by nonverbal cues (nodding, mirroring of body posture, etc.) or physical reinforcement (e.g., giving a child a high five or shaking hands with a parent when introducing oneself at the beginning of an appointment) that may be less apparent, or altogether impossible, to convey across a screen. However, some aspects of rapport building are feasible via videoconference technology. In their qualitative investigation of children's experiences of their relationships with SLPs, Fourie et al. found common themes such as children seeing the SLP as playful and a source of fun and the importance of session routines and rituals as key to establishing and maintaining rapport.[49] While in-person sessions can be playful, telepractice sessions can be as well. Quantitatively, measures of therapeutic alliance have been found not to differ significantly between face-to-face and telepractice speech-language pathology sessions.[50] Incorporating activities children find enjoyable and building regular routines and rituals into telepractice sessions (e.g., beginning each session with a listening check, reading a book together each week, or ending with a goodbye song) can help facilitate the child's relationship with the professional. Regarding rapport with parents and caregivers, professionals providing services via telepractice stated increased communication (either during the videoconference sessions or by phone or email outside of session times) and sharing of session notes as practices that enhanced the relationship, while citing difficulty with collaboration on behavior management as one potential downside to developing rapport in this modality.[51]

Rush and Shelden describe parent or caregiver coaching as:

an adult learning strategy in which the coach promotes the learner's (coachee's) ability to reflect on his or her actions as a means to determine the effectiveness of an action or practice and develop a plan for refinement and use of the action in immediate and future situations.[52]

They include skills such as joint planning, observation, action, reflection, and feedback as parts of a successful coach's repertoire.[52] While Rush and Shelden's work focused on in-person intervention, subsequent research has been conducted on the adaptation of coaching practices to telepractice environments.[52] Snodgrass et al. discuss a hybrid approach to parent or caregiver coaching, pairing asynchronous video examples of language stimulation techniques and online learning modules with synchronous real-time observation of parents' implementation of strategies where professionals coached parents to mastery.[53] Parent coaching via telepractice has several benefits. It can enable parents who cannot attend in-person intervention (e.g., due to work schedules) to participate more fully in their children's education and for more equal sharing of home carryover tasks among caregivers.[54] Online intervention can allow for greater sharing of information between parents and professionals through the use of secure file sharing, shared documents that can be updated with observations and data from all team members, and sharing links to resources (e.g., articles of interest, video examples of strategies, websites for support services, connections to other parents of children with hearing loss, etc.

Fickenscher and Gaffney define auditory verbal strategies as,

a specific plan utilized to achieve a goal. It is a plan to move from Point A to Point B. In order to choose the correct listening and spoken language strategy, the therapist must be able to continuously analyze the child's strengths and needs, anticipate the child's response, and implement the correct strategy *at the correct time* while helping the parent to develop this skill as well. Knowledge of a variety of the listening and spoken language strategies is the first step in a learning trajectory. A professional must not only know which strategy to use to reach a determined goal, but must have the ability to model for parents and other professionals, and the ability to coach the appropriate use of the strategy.[55]

See chapter 10, "Auditory Verbal Strategies to Build Listening and Spoken Language Skills."

Most auditory verbal strategies, such as acoustic highlighting, whispering, repetition, extension/expansion, self and parallel talk, and the auditory sandwich can be implemented via telepractice. Others, like optimal position, may require some creative reimagining. "Optimal position" in a telepractice session can include both the professional coaching the adult on the child's end to sit closest to the child's best-hearing ear as well as determining the optimal position for the computer's speakers and microphone to provide the clearest auditory signal. While listening and spoken language practitioners usually encourage wait time, delivering an instruction auditorily just once and giving the child time to respond, poor internet connections can necessitate an in-person repetition of some instructions by the adult on the child's end, and this should be noted in session documentation. Auditory verbal strategies, and coaching thereof, can be among the easiest aspects of traditional listening and spoken language practice to adapt to a telepractice format.

In an in-person intervention session at a clinic or school, professionals are typically responsible for gathering the materials (e.g., books, toys, etc.) to be used in the session or lesson. Professionals used to home visiting services can also bring their own materials or use materials the family has on hand in the natural environment. Telepractice presents a new paradigm: how can professionals provide intervention when unable to physically interact with the same materials as the child and family? While some organizations with telepractice programs have established toy lending libraries or mail materials to families for use in telepractice sessions (see Constantinescu et al. for a sample protocol), this may encourage reliance on activities that would not be a part of the family's everyday interactions or otherwise accessible or culturally relevant for the family.[21] An initial assessment, such as a Routines-Based Interview, can assist professionals in familiarizing themselves with the family's normal pattern of interaction, daily routines, available resources, and activity preferences to serve as a springboard for session planning.[56] Then, professionals can coach families in how to use toys or other materials they have at their home (or wherever the services are provided, e.g., school, daycare).

Professionals can also use digital materials in telepractice sessions, but should do so with caution, keeping in mind best practices in early childhood development regarding screen media and the relevance and accessibility of digital materials to the children and families they serve. Literacy activities, such as shared reading, are a hallmark of auditory verbal practice.[46] In telepractice sessions, professionals can share ebooks on screen or coach families in reading materials already present in their homes. When compared to ebooks, a body of research suggests that parent-child communication is greater, and readers' comprehension is improved with traditional paper reading materials.[57,58,59] Professionals can elect to share digital reading materials for a variety of clinically valid reasons (e.g., to share with a family that does not have access to reading materials, to share a curricular text with a group of students during an educational session conducted via telepractice, or to share a book related to a specific theme or topic). When doing so, they should keep in mind research that indicates the deleterious effects of "enhanced" ebooks (i.e., those with additional animation, sounds, or interactive features beyond the static text and illustrations) on communication, attention, interaction, and comprehension.[60] For both typically hearing children and children with hearing loss adult interaction and incorporation of shared reading strategies is key to deriving maximum benefit from ebook activities.[61,62]

Professionals can make use of other digital activities or features of telepractice platforms to replicate activities traditionally used in in-person instruction. For example, digital whiteboards or platforms annotate functions that can be used to fill out digitized worksheets, complete graphic organizers, or play drawing games. While computerized games with animation or sound effects should be avoided due to concerns about screen time (see previous research in this chapter) and audibility, websites or downloadable materials that replicate physical manipulatives (e.g., games where children can decorate a digital cake, play with a digital dollhouse, or dress up digital paper dolls) represent a way to translate best

practices in play-based in-person intervention to telepractice. When professionals have materials on their end that they want to demonstrate or share with the child and family, they should be mindful of the size and reflectiveness of the materials, because both will affect their visibility on screen. Auxiliary technology to assist in materials sharing, like document cameras, dual-monitor computers, and ring lights, are helpful but not necessary for the provision of excellent telepractice services.

Pearl

The magic is in the talk, not the tech! Avoid introducing electronic stimuli that promote attention to a screen. Stick to simple activities that fit into the family's everyday routine and are likely to be practiced again and again between sessions.

20.3.4 Troubleshooting

Conducting a trial telepractice session, where intervention is delivered via videoconference technology but the professional and child and family are located in separate rooms in the same physical location, can help orient families to technology and allow for in-person troubleshooting assistance before moving to true telepractice sessions in the child's natural environment. Clinicians, or their employers (e.g., hospitals, clinics, schools, etc.), should establish telepractice-specific "attendance" policies, such as determining the amount of time that professionals will devote to assisting families with technological difficulties before requesting that the session be rescheduled for a later date. Use of email, texting, telepractice platforms' chat function, or platforms' online support centers can all be used to help professionals and patients with the technological demands of telepractice. The University of Maine's Speech Therapy Telepractice and Technology Program Manual provides a variety of checklists and handouts that can assist individual clinicians, organizations, and schools in anticipating, avoiding, or ameliorating common friction points in the development of telepractice programs.[63]

20.4 Special Applications

While the main focus of this chapter is the use of videoconference technology to provide direct therapeutic intervention or educational instruction to children with hearing loss (or their parents and caregivers), practitioners can also use telepractice to further listening and spoken language practice in other ways.

Previous sections of this chapter have addressed the importance of including telepractice skills as a key competency in personnel preparation programs for speech-language pathologists, audiologists, and teachers of the deaf. In addition to training future professionals in the use of telepractice, it can be used to prepare pre-service and in-service professionals for a variety of roles. When students in communication sciences and disorders programs have opportunities to participate in telepractice sessions with supervision from clinical mentors, they indicate greater comfort with this modality and a higher likelihood of incorporating it into their practice when licensed.[64] Neely et al. discuss how asynchronous online modules, self-evaluations, and feedback on taped intervention sessions delivered by an experienced clinician via videoconference can improve new clinicians' (and parents') incidental teaching skills.[65] When professionals providing family-centered intervention receive online guidance in their use of parent coaching techniques, they exhibit higher rates of parent coaching strategy utilization in their interventions in what Chung et al. call a "cascading coaching model."[66]

Professionals can use telepresence to attend staffings, case conferences, IFSP/IEP meetings or to provide inservices or professional development to colleagues located at a distance. This "telepresence" model enables highly qualified professionals with expertise in hearing loss and listening and spoken language to share their knowledge with colleagues at schools, day cares, camps, or other settings where listening, speaking children with hearing loss can be participating alongside their typically developing peers. Meetings of this type can be used to share information on communication strategies, necessary accommodations or modifications, hearing device troubleshooting, or other topics as applicable to the child and family in question.

Telepractice can also be used to provide parent education and coaching when parents are not a regular part of the child's intervention sessions (for example, providing parent education to caregivers of students who usually receive school-based services without family members present). Snodgrass et al. discuss how parent coaching practices common in early intervention can be expanded to benefit caregivers of children at other ages and stages using telepractice.[53] While parent coaching can be limited in traditional school-based intervention, telepractice ("teleschool") opens possibilities for incorporating families by "bringing school to them" and enabling parents and caregivers to videoconference into children's school-based intervention sessions from their places of employment. School-based professionals might struggle to plan parent education events during hours that are accessible to parents. Even evening or weekend events can be inaccessible to parents with nontraditional work schedules or those who have unmet childcare or transportation needs. While not all families will have access to the technology necessary to participate in virtual parent education events, use of telepractice platforms for synchronous or asynchronous parent education is one way to expand access to parents of children in schools.

Expansion of audiological services via telepractice is another exciting new direction for the field. Audiology telepractice can allow for real-time troubleshooting, use of remote computing technology for diagnostic testing, and remote programming of hearing aids or cochlear implant devices. This approach has great potential for delivering high-quality audiological care to under-resourced areas, though increased attention to the calibration and validation of testing and programming equipment will be needed to ensure parity of care between telepractice and in-person modalities.[67,68,69] Initial investigations of the quality of audiological testing delivered via videoconference technology have found suitable reliability.[70] For newborn hearing screening and early intervention programs, audiology telepractice has the potential to reduce loss to follow up rates for vulnerable children and families.[71] Videoconference technology has been used successfully for the remote fitting and verification of hearing aids with satisfactory patient outcomes in terms of audiological target matching, speech perception scores, and user wear time.[72] Likewise, cochlear

implant mapping conducted via remote technology has been found to be comparable to in-person services.[73,74,75,76,77] However, many training programs for future audiologists have yet to incorporate telepractice as a core competency for their graduates.[78] Inclusion of telepractice training for current and pre-service audiologists and continued development of technology to facilitate accurate and reliable testing and equipment maintenance can help improve and expand remote audiological services.

20.5 Future Directions

Professionals note lack of teletherapy-specific training as a barrier to successful provision of services via telepractice.[16,79] Inclusion of telepractice as a key competency in personnel preparation programs for new professionals, as well as providing ongoing professional development for those already in the field, can help improve providers' confidence in this service delivery modality. Blaiser and Behl outline resources available for current professionals who wish to build their telepractice competency, particularly for the provision of early intervention services for CWHL.[80]

Modernizing licensing and regulation laws will improve and expand telepractice availability, particularly to families living in states where there are no local Listening and Spoken Language Specialist certified professionals. Presently, clinicians must be licensed in both their location and the patient's. Other professions, such as nursing, medicine, and law, have successfully created interstate licensing compacts that professionals in communication sciences and disorders might want to replicate.[81] At the time of publication, some states have adopted the Audiology & Speech-Language Pathology Interstate Compact (ASLP-IC), legislation developed by ASHA that "facilitates the interstate practice of audiology and speech-language pathology while maintaining public protection."[82] The National Association of State Directors of Teacher Education and Certification (NASDTEC) maintains a similar registry for states that have established cooperative teacher licensing agreements.[83]

More stakeholder education will be needed to increase the adoption of telepractice as a service delivery modality. In an investigation of school-based telepractice services, Grogan-Johnson found misconceptions among both parents and school faculty regarding both the technical aspects of providing telepractice services as well as the reliability and efficacy of SLP services delivered in this way.[5] Stakeholders can be confused about how services will be delivered via videoconference technology or fear that telepractice services are a cost-saving measure of inferior quality. Professionals will need to explain both the mechanics of telepractice service provision (e.g., how technology will be set up, who will provide services, etc.) as well as the evidence basis that supports telepractice as being comparable to in-person treatment. Grogan-Johnson calls this public education regarding school-based telepractice services, "the five W's meet the three R's" (that is, the who-what-when-where-why of telepractice meet the traditional "reading, [w]riting, and [a]rithmetic" of primary education), and emphasizes that the rapid shift to remote instruction during the Covid-19 pandemic "is not the same as fully implementing a telepractice service delivery model."[84] Practitioners must continue producing and disseminating research on telepractice to build the evidence base and improve public understanding and acceptance of telepractice.

Insurance, funding, and reimbursement issues are another frontier for the future of telepractice. At present, more robust cost-benefit analyses are needed to demonstrate both the treatment efficacy and cost-saving potential of telepractice services to justify telepractice services.[28] ASHA maintains current information on state-by-state telepractice requirements, and reimbursement within the United States, with many states leaving reimbursement of SLP/audiology services delivered via telepractice up to the individual reimbursement source (e.g., private insurance companies, public assistance programs).[85]

In an increasingly digital and interconnected world where many children and families continue to struggle to receive high quality listening and spoken language service, telepractice represents the future of service provision in auditory verbal practice. More work is necessary, however, to make optimal use of this service delivery modality. Both pre-service and in-service professionals require training in telepractice implementation and additional research is needed to validate telepractice assessment and treatment. Limitations in access to technology, reimbursement, and cross-jurisdictional licensure represent significant barriers for both families and professionals who want to participate in telepractice. As stakeholders work to overcome these barriers and improve telepractice, they work to create a world in which any family who wants to pursue a listening and spoken language outcome for their child has access to highly qualified family-centered intervention.

References

[1] About the LSL Specialist Certification. AG Bell Academy for Listening and Spoken Language. n.d. https://agbellacademy.org/certification/ Accessed November 9, 2021

[2] Telepractice. American Speech-Language-Hearing Association. www.asha.org/Practice-Portal/Professional-Issues/Telepractice/ Accessed November 9, 2021

[3] Vaughn GR. Tel-communicology: health-care delivery system for persons with communicative disorders. ASHA 1976;18(1):13–17

[4] Duffy JR, Werven GW, Aronson AE. Telemedicine and the diagnosis of speech and language disorders. Mayo Clin Proc 1997;72(12):1116–1122 10.4065/72.12.1116

[5] Grogan-Johnson S. Getting started in school-based speech-language pathology telepractice. Perspect ASHA Spec Interest Groups 2018;3(18):21–31 10.1044/persp3.sig18.21

[6] Coufal K, Parham D, Jakubowitz M, Howell C, Reyes J. Comparing traditional service delivery and telepractice for speech sound production using a functional outcome measure. Am J Speech Lang Pathol 2018;27(1):82–90 10.1044/2017_ajslp-16-0070

[7] Bridgman K, Onslow M, O'Brian S, Jones M, Block S. Lidcombe Program webcam treatment for early stuttering: a randomized controlled trial. J Speech Lang Hear Res 2016;59(5):932–939 10.1044/2016_jslhr-s-15-0011

[8] Lewis C, Packman A, Onslow M, Simpson JM, Jones M. A phase II trial of telehealth delivery of the Lidcombe Program of Early Stuttering Intervention. Am J Speech Lang Pathol 2008;17(2):139–149 10.1044/1058-0360(2008/014)

[9] O'Brian S, Smith K, Onslow M. Webcam delivery of the Lidcombe program for early stuttering: a phase I clinical trial. J Speech Lang Hear Res 2014;57(3):825–830 10.1044/2014_jslhr-s-13-0094

[10] Cirrin FM, Schooling TL, Nelson NW, et al. Evidence-based systematic review: effects of different service delivery models on communication outcomes for elementary school-age children. Lang Speech Hear Serv Sch 2010;41(3):233–264 10.1044/0161-1461(2009/08-0128)

[11] Mashima PA, Doarn CR. Overview of telehealth activities in speech-language pathology. Telemed J E Health 2008;14(10):1101–1117 10.1089/tmj.2008.0080

[12] McCarthy M, Leigh G, Arthur-Kelly M. Telepractice delivery of family-centred early intervention for children who are deaf or hard of hearing: A scoping review. J Telemed Telecare 2019;25(4):249–260 10.1177/1357633x18755883

[13] McGill M, Noureal N, Siegel J. Telepractice treatment of stuttering: a systematic review. Telemed J E Health 2019;25(5):359–368 10.1089/tmj.2017.0319

[14] Wales D, Skinner L, Hayman M. The efficacy of telehealth-delivered speech and language intervention for primary school-age children: a systematic review. Int J Telerehabil 2017;9(1):55–70 10.5195/ijt.2017.6219

[15] Weidner K, Lowman J. Telepractice for adult speech-language pathology services: a systematic review. Perspect ASHA Spec Interest Groups 2020;5(1):326–338 10.1044/2019_persp-19-00146

[16] Behl DD, Kahn G. Provider Perspectives on telepractice for serving families of children who are deaf or hard of hearing. Int J Telerehabil 2015;7(1):1–12 10.5195/ijt.2015.6170

[17] Cason J, Behl D, Ringwalt S. Overview of states' use of telehealth for the delivery of early intervention (IDEA Part C) services. Int J Telerehabil 2012;4(2):39–46 10.5195/ijt.2012.6105

[18] Vismara L, McCormick C, Wagner A, Monlux K, Nadhan A, Young G. Telehealth Parent training in the Early Start Denver Model: results from a randomized controlled study. Focus Autism Other Dev Disabl 2016;33(2):67–79 10.1177/1088357616651064

[19] Behl D, Blaiser K, Cook G, et al. A multisite study evaluating the benefits of early intervention via telepractice. Infants Young Child 2017;30(2):147–161 10.1097/iyc.0000000000000090

[20] Poole ME, Fettig A, McKee RA, Gauvreau AN. Inside the virtual visit: using tele-intervention to support families in early intervention. Young Except Child 2020; (August): 10.1177/1096250620948061

[21] Constantinescu G, Waite M, Dornan D, et al. A pilot study of telepractice delivery for teaching listening and spoken language to children with hearing loss. J Telemed Telecare 2014;20(3):135–140 10.1177/1357633X14528443

[22] McCarthy M, Leigh G, Arthur-Kelly M. Practitioners' self-assessment of family-centered practice in telepractice versus in-person early intervention. J Deaf Stud Deaf Educ 2021;26(1):46–57 10.1093/deafed/enaa028

[23] Blaiser KM, Behl D, Callow-Heusser C, White KR. Measuring costs and outcomes of tele-intervention when serving families of children who are deaf/hard-of-hearing. Int J Telerehabil 2013;5(2):3–10. doi:10.5195/ijt.2013.6129

[24] Scope of Practice. American Academy of Audiology. https://www.audiology.org/practice-resources/practice-guidelines-and-standards/scope-of-practice/ January 2004. Accessed November 9, 2021

[25] Code of Ethics. American Speech-Language Hearing Association. www.asha.org/policy/ Published 2016. Accessed November 9, 2021

[26] Watzlaf VJ, Moeini S, Firouzan P. VOIP for Telerehabilitation: a risk analysis for privacy, security, and HIPAA compliance. Int J Telerehabil 2010;2(2):3–14. doi:10.5195/ijt.2010.6056

[27] Cohn ER, Watzlaf VJM. Privacy and Internet-based telepractice. Perspect Teleprac-tice 2011;1(1):26–37. doi:10.1044/tele1.1.26

[28] Theodoros D. Telepractice in speech-language pathology: the evidence, the challenges, and the future. Perspect Telepractice 2011;1(1):10–21. doi:101044/tele.1.1.10

[29] ASHA Facilitator Checklist for Telepractice Services in Audiology and Speech-Language Pathology. https://www.asha.org/siteassets/uploadedfiles/asha-facilitator-checklist-for-telepractice.pdf Accessed November 10, 2021

[30] Douglass H, Lowman JJ, Angadi V. Defining roles and responsibilities for school-based Tele-facilitators: Intraclass correlation coefficient (ICC) ratings of proposed competencies. Int J Telerehabil 2021;13(1):e6351 10.5195/ijt.2021.6351

[31] Grillo EU. Results of a survey offering clinical insights into speech-language pathology telepractice methods. Int J Telerehabil 2017;9(2):25–30 10.5195/ijt.2017.6230

[32] Ladson-Billings G. Toward a theory of culturally relevant pedagogy. Am Educ Res J 1995;32(3):465 10.2307/1163320

[33] Edwards-Gaither L. Cultural considerations for telepractice: an introduction for speech-language pathologists. Perspect ASHA Spec Interest Groups 2018;3(18):13–20 10.1044/persp3.SIG18.13

[34] Hiratsuka V, Delafield R, Starks H, Ambrose AJ, Mau MM. Patient and provider perspectives on using telemedicine for chronic disease management among Native Hawaiian and Alaska Native people. Int J Circumpolar Health 2013;72(1):21401 10.3402/ijch.v72i0.21401

[35] Hilty DM, Crawford A, Teshima J, et al. Mobile health and cultural competencies as a foundation for telehealth care: scoping review. J Technol Behav Sci 2021;6(2):197–230 10.1007/s41347-020-00180-5

[36] Walters SM, Bernis SA, Delvin-Brown MA, Hirsch SE. School-based speech-language services using telepractice. Interv Sch Clin 2021;57:103–110. Published online 2021:105345122110018

[37] Miller KJ. Trends impacting one public school program for students who are deaf or hard-of-hearing. *Comm Disord Q* 2014;36(1):35–43 10.1177/1525740114533380

[38] Pearsonassessments.com. https://www.pearsonassessments.com/content/dam/school/global/clinical/us/assets/telepractice/guidance-documents/telepractice-and-the-celf-5.pdf Accessed November 10, 2021

[39] Zhang O, Wang S. Equivalence of Q-interactive and paper administrations of a speech sound task, GFTATM–3 sounds-in-words. Pearsonassessments.com. https://www.pearsonassessments.com/content/dam/school/global/clinical/us/assets/q-interactive/GFTA-3-Equivalence-study.pdf Accessed November 10, 2021

[40] Werfel KL, Grey B, Johnson M, et al. Transitioning speech-language assessment to a virtual environment: Lessons learned from the ELLA study. *Lang Speech Hear Serv Sch* 2021;52(3):769–775 10.1044/2021_LSHSS-20-00149

[41] Ling D. Speech and the Hearing-Impaired Child: Theory and Practice. Washington, DC: Alexander Graham Bell Association for the Deaf; 1976

[42] Ling D. Foundations of Spoken Language for Hearing-Impaired Children. Washington, DC: Alexander Graham Bell Association For The Deaf; 1989

[43] Madell J. The LMH test for monitoring listening—Jane Madell and Joan Hewitt. Hearinghealthmatters.org. Published August 3, 2021. http://www.hearinghealthmatters.org/hearingandkids/2021/3245/ Accessed November 10, 2021

[44] Kuhl PK. Early language acquisition: cracking the speech code. *Nat Rev Neurosci* 2004;5(11):831–843 10.1038/nrn1533

[45] Principles of LSL specialists. Agbellacademy.org. https://agbellacademy.org/certification/principles-of-lsl-specialists/ Accessed November 10, 2021

[46] Rosenzweig EA. Auditory Verbal Therapy: A family-centered listening and spoken language intervention for children with hearing loss and their families. *Perspect ASHA Spec Interest Groups* 2017;2(9):54–65 10.1044/persp2.SIG9.54

[47] Tucker JK. Perspectives of speech-language pathologists on the use of telepractice in schools: quantitative survey results. *Int J Telerehabil* 2012;4(2):61–72

[48] Long L, Long T. TA and client-centered therapy. *Trans Anal Bull* 1975;5(2):139–140

[49] Fourie R, Crowley N, Oliviera A. A qualitative exploration of therapeutic relationships from the perspective of six children receiving speech–language therapy. *Top Lang Disord* 2011;31(4):310–324 10.1097/TLD.0b013e3182353f00

[50] Freckmann A, Hines M, Lincoln M. Clinicians' perspectives of therapeutic alliance in face-to-face and telepractice speech-language pathology sessions. *Int J Speech Lang Pathol* 2017;19(3):287–296 10.1080/17549507.2017.1292547

[51] Akamoglu Y, Meadan H, Pearson JN, Cummings K. Getting connected: Speech and language pathologists' perceptions of building rapport via teleplractice. *J Dev Phys Disabil* 2018;30(4):569–585 10.1007/s10882-018-9603-3

[52] Rush D, Shelden M. The Early Childhood Coaching Handbook the Early Childhood Coaching Handbook. 2nd ed. Brookes Publishing; 2019

[53] Snodgrass MR, Chung MY, Biller MF, Appel KE, Meadan H, Halle JW. Teleplractice in speech–language therapy: The use of online technologies for parent training and coaching. *Comm Disord Q* 2017;38(4):242–254 10.1177/1525740116680424

[54] Daczewitz M, Meadan-Kaplansky H, Borders C. PiCs: Teleplractice coaching for a parent of a child who is hard-of-hearing. *Deafness Educ Int* 2020;22(2):113–138 10.1080/14643154.2019.1587235

[55] Fickenscher SS, Gaffney E. Auditory verbal strategies to build listening and spoken language skills. In: CL Dickson. 2016

[56] McWilliam RA, Casey AM, Sims J. The routines-based interview: A method for gathering information and assessing needs. *Infants Young Child* 2009;22(3):224–233 10.1097/IYC.0b013e3181abe1dd

[57] Munzer TG, Miller AL, Weeks HM, Kaciroti N, Radesky J. Differences in parent-toddler interactions with electronic versus print books. *Pediatrics* 2019;143(4):e20182012 10.1542/peds.2018-2012

[58] Clinton-Lisell V. Reading from paper compared to screens: A systematic review and meta‐analysis: Screen and Paper Reading. *J Res Read* 2019;42(2):288–325 10.1111/1467-9817.12269

[59] Delgado P, Vargas C, Ackerman R, Salmerón L. Don't throw away your printed books: A meta-analysis on the effects of reading media on reading comprehension. *Educ Res Rev* 2018;25:23–38 10.1016/j.edurev.2018.09.003

[60] Reich SM, Yau JC, Warschauer M. Tablet-based eBooks for young children: What does the research say? *J Dev Behav Pediatr* 2016;37(7):585–591 10.1097/DBP.0000000000000335

[61] Lauricella AR, Barr R, Calvert SL. Parent–child interactions during traditional and computer storybook reading for children's comprehension: implications for electronic storybook design. *Int J Child Comput Interact* 2014;2(1):17–25 10.1016/j.ijcci.2014.07.001

[62] Wauters L, Dirks E. Interactive reading with young deaf and hard-of-hearing children in eBooks versus print books. *J Deaf Stud Deaf Educ* 2017;22(2):243–252 10.1093/deafed/enw097

[63] Walker JP. University of Maine, Speech Therapy Teleplractice and Technology Program Manual. University of Maine; 2015

[64] Watts KM, Willis LB. Teleplractice: A survey of AuD students pre- and post-teleplractice. *Perspect ASHA Spec Interest Groups* 2017;2(18):28–41 10.1044/persp2.SIG18.28

[65] Neely L, Rispoli M, Gerow S, Hong ER. Preparing interventionists via teleplractice in incidental teaching for children with autism. *J Behav Educ* 2016;25(4):393–416 10.1007/s10864-016-9250-7

[66] Chung MY, Lee JD, Meadan H, Sands MM, Haidar BS. Building professionals' capacity: The cascading coaching model. *J Posit Behav Interv* Published online 2021:109830072110392. doi:10.1177/10983007211039295

[67] Krumm M, Ribera J, Froelich T. Bridging the service gap through audiology teleplractice. *ASHA Lead* 2002;7(11):6–7 10.1044/leader.FTR2sb.07112002.4

[68] Swanepoel W, Hall JW III. A systematic review of telehealth applications in audiology. *Telemed J E Health* 2010;16(2):181–200 10.1089/tmj.2009.0111

[69] Swanepoel W, Clark JL, Koekemoer D, et al. Telehealth in audiology: the need and potential to reach underserved communities. *Int J Audiol* 2010;49(3):195–202 10.3109/14992020903470783

[70] Ribera JE. Interjudge reliability and validation of telehealth applications of the hearing in noise test. *Semin Hear* 2005;26(01):13–18 10.1055/s-2005-863790

[71] Hayes D, Boada K, Coe S. Early hearing detection and intervention by teleplractice. *Perspect Teleplractice* 2015;5(2):38–47. doi:10.1044/tele5.2.38

[72] Campos PD, Ferrari DV. Teleaudiology: evaluation of teleconsultation efficacy for hearing aid fitting. *J Soc Bras Fonoaudiol* 2012;24(4):301–308 10.1590/s2179-64912012000400003

[73] Eikelboom RH, Jayakody DM, Swanepoel DW, Chang S, Atlas MD. Validation of remote mapping of cochlear implants. *J Telemed Telecare* 2014;20(4):171–177 10.1177/1357633X14529234

[74] Hughes ML, Goehring JL, Baudhuin JL, et al. Use of telehealth for research and clinical measures in cochlear implant recipients: a validation study. *J Speech Lang Hear Res* 2012;55(4):1112–1127 10.1044/1092-4388(2011/11-0237)

[75] McElveen JT Jr, Blackburn EL, Green JD Jr, McLear PW, Thimsen DJ, Wilson BS. Remote programming of cochlear implants: a telecommunications model. *Otol Neurotol* 2010;31(7):1035–1040 10.1097/MAO.0b013e3181d35d87

[76] Ramos A, Rodriguez C, Martinez-Beneyto P, et al. Use of telemedicine in the remote programming of cochlear implants. *Acta Otolaryngol* 2009;129(5):533–540 10.1080/00016480802294369

[77] Wesarg T, Wasowski A, Skarzynski H, et al. Remote fitting in Nucleus cochlear implant recipients. *Acta Otolaryngol* 2010;130(12):1379–1388 10.3109/00016489.2010.492480

[78] Wilson NJ, Seal BC. Teleplractice in university Au.D. programs: Survey of program directors. *Perspect Teleplractice* 2015;5(2):27–37. doi:10.1044/tele5.2.27

[79] Tambyraja SR, Farquharson K, Coleman J. Speech-language teletherapy services for school-aged children in the United States during the COVID-19 pandemic. *J Educ Students Placed Risk* 2021;26(2):91–111 10.1080/10824669.2021.1906249

[80] Blaiser KM, Behl D. Teleplractice training for early intervention with children who are deaf/hard-of-hearing. *Perspect ASHA Spec Interest Groups* 2016;1(9):60–67 10.1044/persp1.SIG9.60

[81] Cohn ER, Cason J. Teleplractice, telehealth, and telemedicine: acquiring knowledge from other disciplines. *Perspect ASHA Spec Interest Groups* 2016;1(18):19–29 10.1044/persp1.SIG18.19

[82] ASLPCompact. Aslpcompact.com. https://aslpcompact.com/ Accessed November 10, 2021

[83] National Association of State Directors of Teacher Education and Certification. https://www.nasdtec.net/page/Interstate Accessed November 10, 2021.

[84] Grogan-Johnson S. The five W's meet the three R's: The who, what, when, where, and why of teleplractice service delivery for school-based speech-language therapy services. *Semin Speech Lang* 2021;42(2):162–176 10.1055/s-0041-1723842

[85] Teleplractice requirements and reimbursement. https://www.asha.org/siteassets/uploadedfiles/teleplractice-requirements-and-reimbursement.pdf Accessed November 10, 2021

21 Working with Adults

Lindsay Zombek

Summary

This chapter focuses on best practices for aural rehabilitation for adults who are deaf or hard of hearing who are receiving new amplification or are demonstrating challenges with current amplification. Hearing loss is associated with reduced quality of life for adults. Aural rehabilitation can help an adult improve functional listening and communication skills, lessening the impact of a hearing loss. This chapter will address assessment and treatment areas, special considerations, and goal setting for adults who are deaf and hard of hearing. Additionally, areas of assessment and treatment associated with cochlear implant use will be addressed. This chapter will identify areas in which similar skills are supported for adults and children who are deaf and hard of hearing, but will highlight specific differences for adults that promote maximal outcomes.

Keywords

adults, aural rehabilitation, deaf, hard of hearing, auditory skills, cochlear implant, auditory fatigue, environmental modification, assistive listening devices, counseling, music appreciation, goal setting, telephone use, listening in noise, suprasegmental

Key Points

- Adults need aural rehabilitation when they get new amplification or are reporting concerns despite appropriate amplification
- Assessment and therapy for adults with hearing loss can focus on areas including auditory skills development, communication skills and repair, improving the listening environment, and knowing one's rights

21.1 Introduction to Adult Aural Rehabilitation

Aural (re)habilitation is an immediate consideration when a child is diagnosed with a hearing loss and receives amplification. However, adults also face challenges related to hearing loss. This chapter explores the benefits of aural rehabilitation for adults with hearing loss.

21.1.1 Hearing Loss in Adults

According to the National Institute on Deafness and Other Communication Disorders (NIDCD), 50% of adults 75 years old and older have disabling hearing loss, defined as "hearing loss of 35 decibels or more in the better ear, the level at which adults could generally benefit from hearing aids."[1] Younger adults also can have hearing loss. The NIDCD found that around 2% of adults aged 45 to 54, 8.5% of adults aged 55 to 64, and almost 25% of adults aged 65 to 74 also have disabling hearing loss.

Adults can lose their hearing for many reasons. One of the most common etiologies, or causes, is age-related damage to the hearing system. Additional etiologies include noise exposure, trauma, autoimmune disorder, ototoxicity, and genetic differences.[2,3]

Adults can experience different types of hearing loss including conductive hearing loss (disorders of hearing occurring in the outer and middle ears) and sensorineural hearing loss (disorders of hearing occurring in the inner ear or nerve).[3] Forms of amplification include hearing aids, bone conduction hearing aids, and cochlear implants. Amplification options assist by providing improved access to sound but do not cure hearing loss.

The impact of hearing loss can be debilitating for adults. Hearing loss, particularly when not managed, is associated with reduced quality of life, including the decreased ability to communicate with family and friends, social isolation, challenges in the workplace and social community activities, increased rates of dementia and mental health issues such as depression, and increased risk of health problems.[4] Because of these negative impacts, it is important to identify and manage the hearing loss of adults of all ages.

Many adults may choose to pursue aural rehabilitation. For example, there may be a teen or an adult with a long term hearing loss that is transitioning from a hearing aid to a cochlear implant. Adults with sudden hearing loss may transition from no amplification to requiring a hearing aid or a cochlear implant. Receiving amplification, whether it is a hearing aid, cochlear implant, or bone conduction hearing aid, may indicate the necessity for aural rehabilitation.

21.2 Adult Aural Rehabilitation

When an adult gets appropriate amplification, additional education and skill training is needed to help the adult manage their listening and communication needs in their lives. Adults, regardless of age, rely heavily on hearing whether it is to communicate for jobs, with their families, or in their social networks. Aural rehabilitation is defined as the reduction of hearing-loss-induced deficits of function, activity, participation, and quality of life through sensory management, instruction, perceptual training, and counseling.[5] It can also be defined as "those professional interactive processes actively involving the client that are designed to help a person with hearing loss. These include services and procedures for limiting the negative effects of and compensating for the hearing impairment. They specifically involve facilitating adequate well-being and receptive and expressive communication (ASHA, 2001; WHO 2001)."[6] Aural rehabilitation services promote helping a participant achieve best quality of life by increasing the participant's knowledge and listening skills to equip them to best handle a given listening situation.

21.2.1 Common Concerns

When working with adults with hearing loss, it is clear that despite improvements with amplification, hearing challenges still remain. **Table 21.1** lists some common concerns stated by adults with hearing loss using amplification.

In this chapter, using aural rehabilitation to meet the communication and social needs of adults with hearing loss is explored. Common myths that prevent adults from receiving necessary aural rehabilitation are discussed. Furthermore, this chapter promotes best possible outcomes for adults with hearing loss through discussion of appropriate assessment and therapy. At the end of this chapter, the reader also learns how to work with the audiologist during adult aural rehabilitation and the role of communication partners in aural rehabilitation.

Pitfall

Myths about adult aural rehabilitation include the view that only struggling adults need or want aural rehabilitation, audiology programming can solve most issues, and there is limited coverage for aural rehabilitation.

21.3 Myths about Aural Rehabilitation

Despite reported concerns by adults with hearing loss, aural rehabilitation is not routinely recommended or provided for adults. There are many myths about aural rehabilitation that prevent access for adults to imperative services. Some of these myths will be discussed.

21.3.1 Adults Do Not Need Aural Rehabilitation

The danger in this myth is that the adult with hearing loss is led to believe that current outcomes with their technology are the best that can be achieved. Research has shown that adults can demonstrate benefit from aural rehabilitation.[7]

Table 21.1 Common concerns of adults with hearing loss

Adults arriving for aural rehabilitation often report:
I can hear talking but I do not understand what is being said
I cannot hear when it is noisy
I have trouble understanding on the telephone
I hear sounds but I do not know what they are
I get tired of saying "what," so I pretend to understand
If I cannot read lips, then I do not know what you are saying
Music does not sound the same with my cochlear implant
My amplification has buttons and options but I do not know how or when to use them

21.3.2 Advanced Audiology Programming Is All That Is Necessary

Programming does not address many of the other aspects of communication that can be targeted in aural rehabilitation. For example, advanced programming does not build auditory skills or promote communication repair strategies. Advanced programming is a critical part of aural rehabilitation but is not the only aspect that promotes better outcomes for adults with hearing loss.

21.3.3 Only Struggling Adults Need Aural Rehabilitation

Many professionals consider referring adults for aural rehabilitation only when the adult is struggling and audiological management efforts have been exhausted, leading to unnecessary frustration on the part of the adult with hearing loss. When aural rehabilitation is initiated immediately, the aural rehabilitation practitioner can identify and address challenges faced by the adult. The practitioner can assist the audiologist with referring back for device programming changes that are in the control of the audiologist. Additionally, the practitioner can begin targeting listening skills and communication techniques and strategies to help minimize challenges and maximize benefits and outcomes.

21.3.4 Adults Do Not Want Aural Rehabilitation

When adults understand what aural rehabilitation is, they are more likely to recognize value in the service. When the adult understands that a practitioner can help with development of listening skills and can address concerns such as listening in noise, listening in groups, or talking on the telephone, the adult is more likely to see a need and be interested in initiating services.

21.3.5 Lack of Insurance Coverage

Insurance coverage depends on the provider and type of the services. In the United States, a speech language pathologist can bill and receive reimbursement for providing education regarding device use where an audiologist could not bill and be reimbursed for the same service. In the United States, insurance coverage varies by plan by carrier by state; a service covered by a carrier in one state might not be covered by the same carrier in a different state. Additionally, an insurer's coverage can vary by individual employer plan. Many private insurance companies are covering aural rehabilitation. Often a letter of medical necessity and a report justifying the need for services is enough to secure approval for aural rehabilitation services. It should not be assumed that insurance does not cover or reimburse for aural rehabilitation; each person's coverage needs to be examined individually.

21.4 Adequate Case History Information

An important component of service provision and appropriate evaluation and therapy is to collect a thorough case history. Case histories must include the participant's audiology history including their current audiogram aided and unaided, speech perception testing completed by an audiologist, and information regarding etiology and duration of hearing loss. It is important to ascertain whether hearing loss was present at birth, sudden, or progressive. Current audiologic performance as well as knowledge regarding etiology and duration of hearing loss can help the practitioner shape recommendations, and guide the patient to successful motivation and expectations for aural rehabilitation.

Additionally, case history should include information about subjective functional hearing performance. **Table 21.2** lists some questions that may provide insightful information that would help with development of a plan of care.

Table 21.2 Sample functional listening questions for a thorough case history

How many hours a day do you wear your hearing aid or cochlear implant?

Do you have difficulty hearing sounds around you?

When you hear sounds around you, do you know what is making the sound?

Do you have trouble figuring out from what direction a sound came?

Do you frequently have trouble understanding what others are saying?

Do you need to be able to read lips in order to understand someone who is talking?

Is it hard to talk on the phone?

Do you have trouble hearing people talk when it is noisy?

Do you have difficulty hearing/enjoying music?

Do you have ringing in your ears?

Do you have difficulty with balance?

Do you have trouble or do not know how to use the buttons and accessories for your hearing aid or cochlear implant?

Describe how much talking is required in your daily routine.

What would you like to be the outcome of your aural rehabilitation therapy?

21.5 Considerations for Service Provision

When preparing to assess the auditory skills and communication skills of an adult, the practitioner must consider the physical layout and set up of the evaluation room to provide an environment conducive to demonstrating auditory skills.

21.5.1 Positioning of Patient

When preparing to assess auditory skills, it is imperative to consider the positioning of the patient before beginning the assessment. One consideration is distance from the examiner. It is important to remember that for doubling of distance away from a speaker, 6 dB of sound is lost.[8] Close proximity to the adult allows for the loudest, natural auditory signal. Space can be decreased by sitting next to the adult on their side with better amplification or across a small distance, particularly if the adult requires lip-reading cues to communicate.

21.5.2 Room Acoustics and Environmental Modification

To determine auditory skills, a participant will require an optimally quiet room, as background noise can be debilitating. The room should be free from others talking and should intentionally take place far from noise sources (whirring computers, buzzing lights, air conditioning/heating units, projectors, loud hallways, and more).

Some participants will have an assistive listening device in addition to their amplification. This can aid during assessment and therapy by helping the participant have better access to instructions. Use of the technology can help with hearing differences in sounds more clearly and in most situations should not be discouraged.

Most people use lipreading to aid in communication whether or not they have hearing loss and even if they do not realize they are doing so. Access to lipreading can help the participant better understand instructions in addition to making conversation easier and more natural. If the patient has an interpreter present, the interpreter should be located so that the participant has accessibility to the interpreter, therapist, and all testing protocols or therapy materials.

21.5.3 Computer Program vs. Trained Professional

As more professionals are recognizing the need for adult aural rehabilitation, the number of practitioners providing the service has not grown to sufficiently meet that demand. Furthermore, in person therapy is not always convenient for adults due to concerns about transportation, costs, time, distance, and other factors. As a result, computer programs targeting aural rehabilitation have emerged. While computer programs can serve as a convenient program for adults, they cannot identify the specific challenges held by a particular adult, provide counseling, and weave the adult's personal goals into the therapy goals. As stated by Plant and colleagues,[9] "Although self-directed training approaches are both time- and cost-effective, the reliance on this model of rehabilitation does not take advantage of the unique training and professional rehabilitation skills of audiologists and other communication specialists and might not always be the best method to improve communication difficulties for individuals with hearing loss." Computer systems can provide a way for adults to practice, but guidance and parameters for use should be determined by a treating practitioner.

Auditory Skill Assessment and Therapy in Adult Aural Rehabilitation

A comprehensive aural rehabilitation assessment requires evaluation of the auditory skills of an adult using their new amplification. The auditory assessment is imperative as it determines precisely how an adult is able to currently perform with their amplification and helps determine appropriate goals to increase auditory performance with the amplification. Goal setting can be a challenge, as one does not want to use a participant's time targeting skills that are already achieved (too easy) or skills that skip levels of development that the participant has not yet achieved (too difficult). Instead, thorough auditory skills assessment leads to development of a therapeutic plan that can systematically help someone progress with auditory skills.

After a comprehensive evaluation, therapy can be recommended for an adult with hearing loss. Therapy consists of training the brain to listen with a new amplification, counseling, practicing using technology including assistive listening devices, and many other areas. Through a comprehensive assessment, a practitioner can develop a plan of care that takes the participant's realistic personal goals into consideration and lay a foundation to help the participant make progress towards these goals.

Auditory skills for an adult are developmental. Developmental growth follows natural, predictable patterns of acquisition. Adults require the same foundational auditory skills as do children. These auditory skills develop through the building of neural connections. An adult who has lost hearing over time may develop these skills quickly as they have a neural network already programmed for auditory skills. Some adults may develop these skills very rapidly with hearing aids as hearing aids use the same hearing pathways and mechanisms for hearing as the person previously experienced. An adult listening through a cochlear implant is having the acoustic signal brought to the brain in a novel way and may require more assistance with developing auditory skills.

A common hierarchy for listening skill development created by Norman Erber consists of four stages: detection, discrimination, identification, and comprehension.[10] Detection indicates awareness of the presence or absence of sound. Discrimination is the capability to determine if two sounds are the same or different. Identification implies understanding and the ability to match a word or sound to an object or concept. Comprehension indicates understanding the meaning of a word in multiple contexts and in connected speech. These terms provide an easy to comprehend guideline to determine the level of independence one has with a particular auditory skill and the level of support needed and will be used when discussing auditory skills in this section.

21.5.4 Subjective Assessment of Self-Performance

Audiologists often define success with amplification as improved scores in thresholds and in speech perception testing.[11] However, one's capability to functionally hear in real world situations is not accurately represented by these measures. A person with a hearing loss could realistically be considered to be doing well with their amplification by professionals yet demonstrate a genuine difficulty in real listening situations.

Subjective measures have been created for adults to help quantify their level of impairment due to the hearing loss. The Hearing Handicap Inventory for Adults (HHIA) enables participants to indicate their areas of challenge and success in listening by answering "yes, sometimes, no" to a series of questions designed to determine whether a handicap exists.[12] Participants are asked

questions related to their psychological, social, and physical responses to situations due to hearing loss.

An additional self-report subjective measure is the TELEGRAM.[13] The TELEGRAM examines additional areas to determine the impact of hearing loss on a person including telephone communication, capability to participate in entertainment, knowledge of legislation related to rights for adults with disabilities, group communication, communication during recreation, and more. This test provides a rating in 8 areas on a scale of 1–5 to determine how a participant self-rates their experiences related to hearing loss.

A subjective test measure enables a professional to determine the participant's perception of their true functioning in real world situations. This information also enables for counseling to occur on areas most problematic and impactful to the adult with hearing loss, enabling appropriate goal selection and specifically tailored therapy. These subjective self-report measures help the practitioner become aware of issues important to the patient and areas, that when improved, will help the patient feel more satisfied with their amplification.

21.5.5 Suprasegmental Perception

One of the earliest auditory skills is the development of suprasegmental perception. Suprasegmental features are prosodic features that enable us ultimately to understand conversation, determine specific speech sounds, understand meaning of a speaker's tone and intent, and many other important purposes. These are features that assist an adult with truly understanding and participating in a spoken conversation. Collecting information on identification of duration gives the practitioner the opportunity to evaluate a base-level skill. A participant unable to determine duration needs to improve on this auditory skill to later achieve more advanced auditory skills.

Suprasegmental features traditionally are more likely to be more challenging for people who recently got a cochlear implant or have a long history of substantial hearing loss without appropriate amplification. This is less likely to be a target area for adults who have a recent hearing loss who are getting hearing aids or adults who have had hearing aids long term who are getting new hearing aids.

One key suprasegmental feature is duration. Duration is the length of a sound. The capability to distinguish between different durations includes being able to determine whether a sound is long or short (/a/ lasting 2 seconds versus /a/ as a quick burst), continuous versus broken (long /a/ versus /a a a/), and varying in number of syllables (one-syllable versus three-syllable word). Other suprasegmental features such as intensity (volume), pitch (frequency), and stress are important for conversational competence but are often excluded from testing. These areas, if challenging, may warrant informal assessment. Duration, however, is more commonly part of more formal auditory skills assessment.

Suprasegmental perception of duration is included as part of many tests and curriculums. Many of these tests were originally created and normed on children. Because adults follow a developmental sequence of acquisition of auditory skills, these tests can still be appropriate for the adult.

One test of suprasegmental perception focusing on duration is the Pre-Feature Identification Contrasts (PreFICs).[14] The PreFICS creates a numerical score on skills including detection of sound, long versus short, continuous versus broken, syllables of varying length, and same syllable identification. This numerical score can be used as a pre- and post-test to determine a change in skill ability.

Duration can also be assessed at phrase, sentence, and paragraph levels. Phrase and sentence length identification highlight a person's ability or inability to follow along with a phrase or sentence of varying lengths in a closed set. An example of phrase level identification would include carrier phrases such as "I want to buy a new" and then answer choices varying in number of syllables such as "car" (one syllable), "minivan" (three syllables), and "motorcycle" (four syllables). A sentence level task would similarly consist of full sentences varying in syllables such as "It is cold" (three syllables), "The cat played with yarn" (five syllables), and "Yesterday, he went to school" (seven syllables). The difference between length identification and true comprehension is that within the closed set, there are choices that contain different numbers of syllables. In theory, someone could not understand a word of the sentence but could identify the correct target by counting the number of syllables. Paragraph tracking is a closed set task that is a more complex suprasegmental assessment as the patient uses duration and rhythm to keep track of where a reader is reading. The task includes a reader reading a paragraph aloud and stopping at random words within the paragraph. When the reader stops reading, the participant identifies the last word said by the reader. Pre- and post-test scores can be calculated as a percentage consisting of the number of correct targets out of the number of trials.

The value of phrase, sentence, and paragraph length identification lies in whether the patient can maintain the capability to use durational cues beyond word level. This is a prerequisite skill for later conversation tracking that is needed for conversations in person, over the phone, while watching a movie, or other conversational situations. A person unable to complete these closed set tasks will likely not be able to complete more complex tasks such as comprehension of open set sentences without visual cues.

21.5.6 Therapy for Suprasegmental Perception

When a deficit in suprasegmental perception is noted in assessment, therapeutic intervention might be warranted. Many activities can work to target suprasegmental perception. The Erber model provides a natural scaffolding model to help make tasks incrementally more challenging to help a participant identify differences in suprasegmental features. **Table 21.3** provides examples of therapeutic activities (and the corresponding Erber hierarchy level) for common deficit areas for adults with needs in the area of duration perception.

21.5.7 Vowel and Consonant Feature Identification

An adult must able to perceive vowel and consonant cues such as vowel height, vowel place, consonant manner, consonant voicing, and consonant place to comprehend spoken words and sentences. The reader can review these cues as discussed in Chapter 3, "Speech Acoustics: Strengthening the Foundation."

An adult must be able to hear consonants and vowels correctly to hear words correctly. Adults use context clues to assist with comprehension of conversations. A word misheard could change the

Table 21.3 Recommended activities for suprasegmental features

Suprasegmental Area of Deficit	Recommended Activities
Presence Versus Absence of Sound	• Without visual cues, present a speech sound or no sound and the participant indicates whether a sound was presented (detection) • Set a timer to go off and the participant indicates when the sound is heard (detection) • Present a speech sound or environmental sound and have the participant indicate when the sound initiates and terminates
Long Versus Short Sounds	• Present two sounds and the participant indicates if they were the same length or different lengths (discrimination) • Present a long speech phoneme or short presentation of the same phoneme without visual cues; the participant indicates whether the sound was long or short (identification) • Have the participant repeat a pattern of long and short sounds (for example, using a vowel, see if the participant can imitate the pattern "short long long short" or "long short long long" (identification)
Continuous Versus Broken Sounds	• Present two sounds and the participant indicates if they were both continuous/broken or if two different sounds were presented (discrimination) • Present a continuous phoneme or a broken phoneme behind a hand cue or small screen; the participant indicates whether the sound was continuous or broken (identification) • Have the participant repeat a pattern of continuous and broken sounds; for example, using a fricative, see if the participant can imitate the pattern (identification)
Differing Number of Syllables	• Presenting two words, ask the participant to determine if the two words have the same or different number of syllables (discrimination task) • Present two targets to the patient differing in number of syllables; present one target and have the participant identify which target word was presented. A larger set of target words will make this more challenging. (identification task) • Have the participant identify two target words in a closed set of four or more words in which each potential word varies in number of syllables (identification) • All tasks should be attempted with words with greater variation in number of syllables (such as 1 vs 4 syllables) and work towards words more similar in length (1 vs 2 syllables).

meaning of a sentence. For example, an adult who mishears a consonant place cue could share a story about losing a "key" when really their conversational partner was wondering aloud about where they had misplaced their "tea." The adult who heard "key" would be perceived as off topic. Subjective reports suggest that adults with hearing loss often feel that they have misheard a word or sentence and say something that is inappropriate in the situation.

The Minimal Pairs Test is a test that captures a person's capability to identify vowel and consonant cues.[15] In this test, two pictures varying in one consonant or vowel feature are displayed and the adult identifies the target word.

21.5.8 Therapy for Vowel and Consonant Feature Identification

Therapy with vowels and consonant feature identification has been shown in research to benefit adults with hearing loss.[16] Vowels are often easier to hear for adults with hearing loss and are an appropriate starting place for therapeutic intervention. For consonants, generally manner of articulation is the easiest feature to identify, followed by voicing, and then place of articulation. Results from the assessment should guide where to start with a specific adult.

A direct way to target a person's capability to identify a particular feature is through the use of minimal pair contrasts. Minimal pairs are sets of phonemes that differ in a specific feature. For the purposes of adult aural rehabilitation, the most time should be spent with target minimal pairs differing in just one phoneme feature. For example, a word will vary in only one phoneme and that phoneme will vary in one feature such as manner. An example of a manner difference in a minimal pair contrast would be "mat" versus "bat" or "rice" versus "right." In both examples, manner differs in the initial or final consonant, but voicing and place of articulation are the same.

When targeting phoneme features, a specific feature should be targeted beyond isolation and word levels. **Fig. 21.1** shows a recommended progression from easiest to hardest to use when

practicing a specific feature. At the phrase level, note that sentences should be carrier phrases that do not convey context. If context is given, it will not be known if the participant arrived at the correct answer through context or through correct identification of the consonant feature. For example, if the sentence is "the man is wearing a ___", the answer is more likely to be a "hat" than a "cat." By providing no context, you ensure the participant was focused on identifying the consonant feature.

21.5.9 Closed Set and Open Set Comprehension

Of the targets discussed in this chapter, closed and open set comprehension is the area that best represents what adults face in typical real-life situations. Listening situations in the real world rarely depend on comprehension of a single sound, single word, or sentence with all possible answer choices known. Real conversations require the capability to use context clues and auditory skills to follow what, at times, are lengthy strings of communication. Closed set and open set comprehension practice can help move adults from analytic exercises to more functional synthetic practice. The analytic exercise such as minimal pair contrasts and duration identification help a person to comprehend parts of words and sentences. Synthetic practice with closed and open set comprehension tasks helps the participant to develop comprehension of the whole meaning of a message.

Open set sentence comprehension is an important part of a comprehensive aural rehabilitation assessment for adults. Adults with strong open set comprehension capabilities are more likely to be successful in face-to-face conversations as well as over the telephone when there are no visual cues (lip-reading, gestures, facial expressions, etc.).

The Common Phrases Test[17] can be adapted for adults. This test consists of lists of ten sentences that are not interrelated. A sentence is read by the practitioner without any visual cues and the patient repeats the sentence. Scoring is achieved by determining how many sentences were correctly repeated out of sentences presented.

21.5.10 Closed Set and Open Set Therapy

Closed set comprehension is an important step because it provides more context about a given message, helping to develop the bridge to open set communication. A closed set is when a patient has context and a limited number of possibilities for a correct target. Because of the limited possibilities, it is easier to predict the correct target answer. Closed set comprehension can occur at the word, phrase, sentence, or paragraph levels. **Table 21.4** lists some potential closed set comprehension activities at each of these levels.

Open set comprehension can take multiple forms when assessing an adult with hearing loss. A practitioner might want to determine whether a person is able to identify single words, phrases, sentences, or paragraphs. Open sets are targets that are not written for the patient and where a large to infinite number of possibilities exist. For example, a closed set might be a written set of four sentences where an open set can require a participant to understand a random sentence read aloud. Additionally, a closed

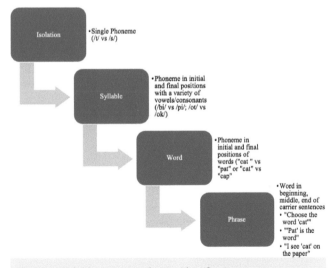

Fig. 21.1 Order for consonant feature identification.

Table 21.4 Closed and open set comprehension tasks

Communication Target Level	Closed Set Comprehension Tasks	Open Set Comprehension Tasks
Word	• Repeat a word within a known category with a small, finite group of answer choices, such as "taco fillings" • Select target from a list of 6 words	• Repeat a word within a category with many possible choices, such as "animals" • Repeat words from a random word list presented auditory only with no known category
Phrase	• Select a phrase from a set of 4 possible choices • Complete predictable phrases such as "Open the ____" or "Read the _____"	• Repeat common phrases without a known context • Repeat a chunk of three to four words from a written source read to the participant
Sentence	• Repeat target sentence from a list of 10 sentences • Repeat related sentences given a scenario such as "going to a restaurant"	• Repeat common sentences and questions without a known context • Repeat a sentence from a book or article read aloud
Paragraph	• Given three written paragraphs on either similar or different topics, indicate which paragraph was read • Answer a question about 2 or more sentences read with a picture demonstrating answer	• Repeat 2 or more sentences from an article without visual cues • Answer questions about a paragraph read aloud • Listen to an audiobook

set might consist of a category such as "pizza toppings" that has a limited number of choices versus an open-set task consisting of a larger category such as "animals," that has a vast number of possible answers. **Table 21.4** also lists examples of open-set comprehension activities for an adult.

21.5.11 Speech Assessment and Treatment in Adult Aural Rehabilitation

Speech assessment might not be necessary in all situations for adult aural rehabilitation. An evaluation should consider resonance, fluency, and voice in addition to production of speech sounds.

Resonance

Individuals with hearing loss can have differences in their resonance production. This could include either hyponasal or hypernasal speech. Adults might not hear themselves as clearly and inappropriately overuse or underuse velopharyngeal closure leading to a difference in resonance.[18] Resonance differences are most commonly found in adults with prelingual hearing loss. Assessment can be qualitatively measured with formal resonance software but can also be subjectively or informally tested.

Resonance therapy can include use of formal resonance software and tools that provides biofeedback to help a person develop appropriate production through vision and feel. Resonance differences can also be targeted through techniques addressing appropriate airflow. For an adult with hearing loss, resonance training must include an auditory component if there is no anatomical reason for the resonance difference. Nasality cues are available through audition at 500-100 Hz.[19] Hearing at these frequencies needs to be maximized to hear resonance cues.

Fluency

Common fluency disorders such as stuttering or cluttering are not known to be caused by hearing loss and should be considered an unrelated event. Prosody disorders can be noted in adults with

hearing loss, particularly adults with pre-lingual hearing loss who did not have appropriate technology and therapy as a child. Most prosody assessment measures are behavioral measures and are rarely, if ever, standardized.

Fluency therapy for a fluency disorder unrelated to hearing loss can be treated by a speech language pathologist certified in this therapy. For prosody, therapeutic intervention would include duration training and helping the participant to imitate appropriate duration.

Voice

Voice differences can be noted in adults with prelingual and postlingual hearing loss. These differences are thought to be related to adults not being able to hear and monitor their own voices. Voice changes can include strain, differences in vocal volume, as well as changes in fundamental frequency and pitch range. Many of these voice differences improve when people receive appropriate amplification.[20] However, some remain as habit and can be difficult to change. A speech language pathologist assessing voice should note whether the voice differences are consistent with the degree of hearing loss and refer for otolaryngology management when voice characteristics seem to not be related to hearing loss as a concurrent anatomical difference or true voice disorder could be present.

For voice quality differences due to hearing loss, a determination needs to be made on what aspect of voice quality or control is negatively impacted by the hearing loss. For an inappropriate pitch, a determination should be made whether the adult has appropriate access to frequencies between 250 and 500 Hz. This range gives access to appropriate fundamental frequencies and harmonics of voices.[19] The practitioner can coach the participant to match appropriate pitch if the person is able to hear pitch. If unable to hear pitch, exercises with a keyboard or other instrument and also the participant's voice can help the participant to learn to hear and match differences in narrowing ranges of pitch. Differences in vocal volume can also be taught through suprasegmental cue intensity and a participant can benefit from exercises teaching discrimination and identification of soft and loud volumes.

Speech Sounds

Many adults who have lost hearing over time or who have mild hearing losses may have no discernable differences in their speech intelligibility, their capability to have their speech sounds understood by others, and assessment might not be necessary. Adults with prelingual hearing loss can have predictable differences in speech production secondary to how the sound is perceived. For example, speech sounds not heard clearly might not be produced or might be produced with substitutions or distortions. Common errors for English speakers with hearing loss include specific phonemes such as fricatives, /r/ and /r/ colored vowels, affricates, and vowel differences and phonological processes including final consonant deletion.[21]

For adults who wish to target their speech intelligibility, formal testing can be completed. It is of note that most common formal articulation measures are standardized through the age of 21 only. These measures can be used for older speakers as speech sound development does not traditionally improve or decline after 21; that is to say that the standardized scores for an adult at 21 should hold true for an older adult as well. It should be noted in all reports when a formal test is used for someone outside of the known standardization age range.

Informal assessment can reveal which speech sounds are in error and which are stimulable (the capability to produce a specific sound). This creates a full picture of the sounds that the adult is not making in spontaneous conversation and if there are specific phonological patterns such as final consonant deletion or stopping of fricatives. Additionally, a patient stimulable for a specific sound is more likely to quickly be able to remediate the target sound.

Testing should include an auditory component. In this part of testing, the practitioner should ascertain whether the adult has access to hearing the sound with their amplification by comparing their amplified audiogram to speech frequency formants. The practitioner should determine whether the adult can discriminate and identify the speech sound from their error. For example, if the adult's error consists of the substitution of /t/ for /s/ the practitioner could use minimal pairs such as "sun" and "ton" to determine whether the adult can hear the acoustic property differences in /s/ and /t/.

Therapy for Speech Articulation

Speech sounds for adults with hearing loss should be taught through audition. It is likely that the adult is not producing the sound clearly due to how they are hearing the sound. The first step would be auditory skill development if the assessment indicated that the participant is not able to discriminate between the target speech sound and the erroneous production. The practitioner should target hearing the sound through the same vowel and consonant feature identification hierarchy previously described in this chapter. The reader is encouraged to follow the hierarchy with the target sound and the erroneous sound until the participant can easily identify the correct sounds in phrases. Practice even at the phrase level is important as the person will need to monitor their own productions automatically in spontaneous conversation.

When the person can accurately hear the features of a specific phoneme, remediation will continue in a traditional speech therapy format including cues to create correct placement of the speech sound and rehearsing the sound through a hierarchy consisting of producing the sounds in initial, medial, and final positions in isolation, syllables, words, phrases, sentences, and spontaneous conversation. Consideration should be paid to ensuring that the environment is quiet. Additionally, if the person uses an RM system, using the RM system during speech articulation training can optimize their capability to hear the target production and their own production of the sound.

Advanced Skills

Some adults will have no challenges with early developing auditory skills but can struggle in specific situations and environments. Testing of advanced listening skills can identify weaknesses and provide an opportunity to develop a particular skill that will increase communication success across environments or increase enjoyment of listening with new amplification.

21.5.12 Listening in Noise

Noise has long been known to be the enemy of listening comprehension.[22] One pitfall of modern amplification is that when someone is in a loud environment, the amplification picks up the noise in addition to the intended target. This makes hearing the intended target more challenging for someone with a hearing loss. Technology advances with hearing aids and cochlear implants have led to the development of programs and devices that allow some noise to be filtered out in noisy environments, but listening in noise remains a top complaint of most people with hearing loss.

There are speech-perception-in-noise tests that can be administered by audiologists in a sound booth. See Chapter 2, "Audiology: Building the Foundation," for additional details. Informal assessments can also be used. For example, the sentences from the Common Phrases Test used in open set testing can be used in noise to determine a person's difference in capability to comprehend sentences in quiet environments versus noisy environments. The comparison of similar sentences in quiet and in noise gives a strong picture of how the inclusion of noise impacts a particular person. Noise sources can be either environmental sounds or a competing speech signal. Competing speech noise has multiple speakers talking simultaneously and is a more challenging listening environment, but is more representative of problems in daily listening. The listener is asked to focus on the target voice despite the presence of other voices.

Therapy for Listening in Noise

Listening in noise can be improved with dedicated practice.[23] The practitioner provides therapeutic intervention using the same techniques, strategies, and hierarchies that are used for the development of open set comprehension. The activities listed in **Table 21.4** can be repeated in the same order with the addition of a noise source.

To provide more or less of a challenge, the volume of the sound can be altered; softer background noise will be easier for listening success than louder background noise. There is no research on the exact time to begin increasing volume, but it is recommended that if a participant is successfully comprehending 80% of the target at a given volume, the practitioner should consider increasing the volume of the background noise or making the speech signal softer.

An important technique when targeting listening in noise is to remember to not increase the volume of the practitioner's voice as the background noise increases. To make practice more efficient, the practitioner should maintain a consistent vocal volume in spite of increasing background noise, intentionally creating a more challenging signal to noise ratio.

Pearl

When doing practice listening in noise, practitioners need to remember not to increase their own voice as noise gets louder.

Therapy should include both environmental background noise and competing speech noise. Some adults might benefit from practice in the presence of music with lyrics playing, as this is a combination of environmental and competing speech sound, and is an experience frequently encountered in shopping centers, offices, and restaurants. When the practitioner's environment provides the opportunity to practice in functional, real world opportunities such as a cafeteria, lobby, or similar situation, practice outside of the therapy room may be highly beneficial. Feedback and suggestions can then be given to the participant in the privacy and quiet of the therapy room.

Pearl

Listening in noise is an excellent opportunity to practice using assistive listening devices such as microphones designed to improve the signal-to-noise ratio. These opportunities provide a safe environment to learn about and explore a new assistive listening while demonstrating the value of using the assistive listening device.

21.5.13 Telephone Use

The use of a telephone constitutes a challenging listening environment for many listeners with hearing loss. In addition to the challenges we all face with poor connections, conversational partners holding the receiver far from their mouths, and other trials, people with hearing loss experience additional hardships that make communication on the telephone more challenging. For adults relying on visual cues such as lip reading to comprehend conversation, a telephone call can be almost impossible because there may be no access to visual information. Additionally, phone signals are filtered which can alter how sound is heard through a cochlear implant.[24] An inability to use the phone can cause frustration for the person with hearing loss. While the world is increasingly moving towards texts and internet communication, many important functions such as making medical appointments, communicating with credit card or insurance companies, and interactions with businesses frequently relies on telephone communication. If a person must rely on another person to make telephone calls or listen to voicemails, it can be frustrating to the person and can lead to feelings of loss of autonomy.

Counseling is the starting point when working on telephone use and should include the myriad ways to participate in a telephone conversation through a person's particular amplification. The practitioner might need to research the individual participant's amplification to determine what telephone assistance options are available. These can include using speaker phone, telecoil, streaming directly to the amplification, streaming through a device, or other options. Conversations about text assisted conversations such as caption calling where the conversation is typed for a participant should also be counseled and explored. Counseling for telephone use should also include realistic expectations. Someone who struggles in face-to-face conversations is not likely to be successful on the telephone.

Testing skills on a telephone is not currently available in a formal test. Informal testing can reveal a person's skill level. A sample series of evaluation questions are listed in **Table 21.5** and can be used to assess a person's current experience with telephone use. A comprehensive evaluation of telephone skills should include technique, comprehension, and knowledge regarding communication options.

With technique, the practitioner should observe the participant holding the phone receiver or cell phone. Attention should be paid to whether the speaker of the phone is being held to the microphones of the patient's amplification. For example, recipients of cochlear implants may no longer have usable residual hearing through their ear, and the microphones for some companies can be on top of the ear instead of in the ear. If this is the case, a recipient

Table 21.5 Sample questions for telephone use assessment

Is speech over the phone too loud, a comfortable volume, or too quiet?

Which ear do you use for phone calls?

Do you use your amplification for phone calls?

How often do you need to talk on the phone in the course of your day?

Do you use your phone the same, more, or less than you did before your new amplification?

Do you use any assistive devices for phone calls (streamers, caption call, etc)?

Is speech over the phone sometimes, always, or never clear?

When the phone rings, do you answer the phone some, most, or none of the time?

Do you call family members?

Do you call doctor's offices to make appointments?

Do you recognize voices on the phone?

Can you understand a conversation without asking for repetitions or clarification most of the time, some of the time, or none of the time?

Can you understand a conversation with a friend or family member if you know the topic?

Can you understand a conversation with a stranger on the phone if you know the topic?

Can you understand a conversation with a friend or family member if you do not know the topic?

Can you understand a conversation with a stranger if you do not know the topic?

needs to hold the phone near the microphone to hear the speaker clearly. Furthermore, many hearing aids and cochlear implants have either Bluetooth streaming or telecoil options to use with telephones. Some adults might not be using these correctly, which could lead to decreased comprehension.

For comprehension, an informal assessment could include a conversation on the phone. The practitioner could assess whether the adult could identify a word in context (given a category, can the adult identify the target word), a sentence in context (such as things people say when making a doctor's appointment), and open set words and sentences. If the person can comprehend open set sentences, the capability to comprehend a read paragraph or a true conversation over the phone can be probed. Adults might not be familiar with technology such as captioned phone calls that aid in comprehension over the phone. Assessing an adult's knowledge and comfort with these additional technologies leads to recommendations that can help the adult communicate more successfully over the telephone.

21.5.14 Therapy for Telephone Use

Pearl

Therapy for telephone use consists of a blend of exercises and counseling.

A combination of exercises and counseling helps promote best outcomes with telephone conversations. Because telephones filter pitches and can distort the signal, the best practice is on the telephone.[24] Be prepared in a therapy session to have the participant call someone else and the practitioner can assist in helping the patient build skills. Before starting the call, make sure the practitioner clearly explains the instructions and provides any appropriate context.

Therapeutic exercises for the phone are developmental and follow the same developmental hierarchy as is used in developing open set communication. Telephone use operates as an adverse listening scenario rather than a completely unique skill set. Strategies for developing closed set and open set communication can be hierarchically practiced over a phone, starting with closed set word recognition and moving to open set paragraph comprehension. Many adults benefit from practicing and improving their skills with listening in noise before targeting listening on the telephone. Skills mastered in quiet and in noise can be targeted on the telephone.

Adults who cannot hear on the phone well enough to converse fluently could benefit from TTY services so they can speak and read responses from the person they are calling.

21.5.15 Music Appreciation for Cochlear Implant Recipients

Music appreciation is a challenge for some adults who get cochlear implants. Cochlear implants can change how a person perceives pitch or frequency (low or high sounds), timbre (the voice of instruments), duration/rhythm (the beat of the music), lyric comprehension (listening in noise), and other areas that might make music less enjoyable for some adults with cochlear implants. For some people, music does not hold big value and this might not be an area that bothers them. For others, music can play a large role in their life and they might be highly motivated to develop better music appreciation.

Music appreciation requires informal assessment as formal testing has not yet been developed. Resources such as the Munich Music Questionnaire[25] can provide guidance for determining a person's subjective experience with listening to music with a cochlear implant as well as to collect more information about how the person uses music (instruments played, participation in groups, etc.). Informal assessment should at minimum determine how a person subjectively experiences music. For example, a percentage of time that songs are enjoyable, a rating, or Likert scale indicating level of music appreciation can be used to gauge progress over time.

Therapy for Music Appreciation

Research shows the majority of participants in therapeutic exercises targeting music can increase their capability to understand and enjoy music.[26] For an adult struggling to hear music and motivated to hear music better, therapy offers a way of promoting better outcomes.

Music appreciation consists of counseling of how to best hear music as well as strategies and techniques to better develop music related auditory skills. The practitioner should remember that the instrumental music and lyrics of music are two separate tasks. If the concern of the participant is lyrics, strategies for listening in noise would be better suited to increase satisfaction. To target appreciation of the instrumental portion of music, recommendations are provided in **Table 21.6**.

21.6 Goal Setting and Frequency of Therapy

For goal setting with adults, an area of need should be determined and a measurable goal created to guide therapy and measure progress. With adults, there ia a primary need to determine what is important to each adult and tie goals into the adult's long term goal. For example, if an adult is not interested in music and has never listened to music, music appreciation therapy is not warranted. However, if the adult's goal is communication in groups, then all base skills should be appropriately targeted to help achieve that goal. The adult might need the practitioner to explain how each foundation skill brings the adult closer to their personal goal.

Table 21.7 will offer some potential goals in various target areas. This is not an exhaustive list, rather a suggestion of how to create measurable goals for multiple target areas.

Frequency of therapy varies depending on many factors. A specific person's current level of performance and personal goal can be close together and not warrant more than a session or two of aural rehabilitation therapy. Other people have a large gap between their current level of performance and their personal goal and want to participate in regular therapy sessions. Access to resources also influences therapy. For example, a person living hours from an aural rehabilitation practitioner might not have the capability of regular, weekly in person visits and can benefit from a tele-therapy program or a longer term home program with monthly or bimonthly sessions with the practitioner. The growing practice of teletherapy or telehealth can help overcome challenges with distance. Another consideration is if someone lives alone and does not have access to a communication partner for regular practice, this person can potentially benefit from additional aural rehabilitation sessions to meet personal goals. There are many computerized practice programs and resources available that can be used for practice, but many of these require a level of technology skill competence that cannot be assumed for all adults. A person with less access to practice materials can benefit from more frequent therapy; an adult who has access to a communication partner or individual practice materials can be appropriate for a longer home program and less frequent sessions with the practitioner.

21.6.1 Counseling Topics in Adult Aural Rehabilitation

Counseling plays a tremendous role in aural rehabilitation. Counseling paired with an opportunity to practice techniques and strategies gives adults the opportunity to gain knowledge and put the knowledge to immediate use. This section focuses on counseling opportunities for adults with hearing loss and includes the use of amplification and assistive listening devices, environmental modification, communication repair strategies, communication repair strategies, reducing auditory fatigue, and rights in public places.

21.6.2 Amplification and Assistive Listening Device Use

Amplification and assistive listening devices are technology and come with an inherent learning curve. Some participants will need basic information about how their amplification works and the basic settings such as volume control. As hearing aids and cochlear implants increasingly come with more advanced settings, participants benefit from learning about and truly understanding the purpose and function of these advanced

Table 21.6 Strategies and techniques for music appreciation for recipients of cochlear implants

Listen to Individual Instruments

- Find music featuring one instrument at a time (this can be found on the internet by searching a specific instrument name, or by borrowing CDs from the library)
- Try a variety of instruments: piano, keyboard, guitar, electric guitar, drums or any instrument commonly found in music you typically enjoy

Listen to familiar music

- Try music that you have enjoyed for a long time and know very well

Listen to new types of music

- Different types of music might be easier to understand with a cochlear implant and you can enjoy them more—try folk music, country, rock, orchestral music (with few instruments)

Listen for Rhythm

- Try to "tap out" rhythm of songs
- Look for visual cues, such as watching people playing an instrument or watching a computer media player that has a visual representation of the music

Pitch Training

- Practice with a partner. Have the partner play two keys on either a keyboard or keyboard app. Tell whether the sounds are the same or different. When that is easy, tell your partner whether the second pitch is lower or higher than the first pitch.

General Music Tips

- Listen with your implant directly connected to the music source or through the regular speakers to see if one way is better for you
- Talk to your audiologist about whether creating a music program is appropriate
- Listen to music at a normal volume; too loud or too soft will distort the sound
- For music with lyrics, read the lyrics while listening to the music
- Try listening to songs from your childhood, these songs are often more familiar and have a strong beat/rhythm
- Listen to music with all of your amplification (both implants, a hearing aid and a cochlear implant, whatever you have)

functions. By truly comprehending the purpose and knowing how to use a given function, the adult can better take advantage of resources available through their amplification. Additionally, many amplification types use remotes or apps on telephones to

Table 21.7 Sample goals for aural rehabilitation

Identify	Comprehend	Produce	Demonstrate
	"target below" WITH ___% ACCURACY IN ____ MONTHS		
words varying in number of syllables	word/sentence/paragraph in environmental noise	fricatives	capability to change volume on amplification
phrases/sentences of differing lengths	three paragraphs in competing speech noise	specific phoneme	understanding of when to use amplification programs
common phrases in a known/ unknown context	sentences over the phone with a predetermined topic	appropriate volume in a conversation	understanding of preferential seating across multiple environments
consonants varying in place of articulation	conversation with a family member on the phone	appropriate pitch in a sentence	knowledge of rights under the law
instruments in a closed set of four	lyrics with music	words with appropriate nasality	conversational repair techniques

control the settings of the amplification. Adults benefit from a review of how to use the remote or app. Learners appreciate a labeled picture of buttons that were newly learned for easy practice and review at home.

Adults might come to aural rehabilitation having already acquired assistive listening devices. A practitioner should not assume that having a device and wearing the device means that it is functionally or optimally being used. Practitioners should verify that devices are on and connecting or streaming appropriately and, if necessary, teach the participant how to use the device. Labeled pictures with clear, large font are also appropriate here to give a person a reminder of how to replicate the procedure at home.

Through counseling and conversation, the practitioner can become aware of an assistive listening device that will benefit the participant. Counseling about available resources helps the participant find an assistive aid that benefits a specific concern area. Participants may not be aware of available amplification options or their specific benefit. Independent assistive listening devices exist to help with areas such as communication on the telephone, listening in noise, listening in meetings and groups, and other areas. Patients should be encouraged to discuss with their audiologist which types of assistive devices might be helpful.

21.6.3 Environmental Modification

Most listening environments will have an element such as background noise, competing voice, distance, or reverberation of sound that could potentially make listening more challenging. Through counseling, adults can be taught to identify these difficult situations and use strategies and techniques to minimize the impact of the challenge. These strategies and techniques may not make the listening situation completely ideal but give the participant the best possibility to create the best possible listening environment by changing controllable factors.

Adults can be counseled to identify sources of noise around a given room. Noise sources in an office include but are not limited to music, coworkers, hallway noise, parking lot noise, heating and air conditioning units, whirring of computers or projectors, and printers. Restaurants also have noise such as kitchen noise, server stations, music speakers, and other guests. Home noise sources include dishwashers, washer and dryer, refrigerators, televisions, and people in the home.

When an adult can identify potential noise sources, techniques and strategies can be taught to reduce the impact of sound. One highly beneficial tool is strategic seating. Strategic seating involves analyzing the room in each situation and determining where to place oneself to optimize the listening condition.

Pearl

Each new situation presents its own ways to limit noise. Identifying the noise source can help determine how to reduce the effect of noise.

Office Meeting Room: the best seat might be near the meeting leader, away from the projectors.

Restaurant: the best seat might be in a corner booth with no people behind the participant, across the room from the kitchen, away from a server station, and away from the front door.

Conversation with a spouse: the best location might be out of the kitchen in a quiet room with the television turned off.

Party/gathering: the best location might be on the edge of the room with no one behind, away from music speakers.

Medical appointment: can be improved if the participant tells the doctor to face him or her while talking and to wait to turn on any machines until after instructions have been given.

Counseling about environmental modification can also include identifying and using assistive listening devices. Learning about assistive listening devices and how to incorporate them into given situations might help reduce the challenge of a given situation. For example, a restaurant might be less difficult if the participant uses an FM/DM system. A doctor's visit can be improved with a speech-to-text app on a phone, tablet, or computer. These devices probably will not remove all challenges associated with hearing loss in these environments but help empower the adult to create the best possible listening environment by manipulating the factors that can be controlled.

21.6.4 Reducing Auditory Fatigue

Auditory fatigue occurs when a person experiences fatigue from listening experiences and can appear as exhaustion, headaches, avoidance, and other presentations. Adults with hearing loss are more likely to report more effort and concentration on typical auditory experiences than adults without hearing loss.[27] Fatigue is known to negatively impact people with hearing loss at work, cause changes in social relationships, and decrease quality of life.[28] Adults can only process information in their working memory intently for 10 to 20 minutes before experiencing mental fatigue[29]; an adult with hearing loss additionally has a degraded auditory signal and has to work harder to decipher and process the information leading to increased mental fatigue. Adults can be counseled to know and recognize auditory fatigue and techniques to reduce the impact of auditory fatigue.

The best way to combat auditory fatigue is to identify ways to reduce the cognitive load and energy used in processing a message. One way is to maximize the quality of the listening environment through strategic seating, environmental modifications, appropriate amplification and use of appropriate assistive listening devices. By increasing the quality of the communication environment, the brain might not have to work as hard to process a message because the message arrives more clearly.

Another strategy would be to reduce the amount of time the brain has to process information. Breaks in listening, when practical, can give the brain time to rest and recharge before being ready to listen again. Taking a break after 20 minutes, or when feeling fatigued, reduces the cognitive load and helps reduce auditory fatigue. When a person is taking a break, it is important for the person to not be responsible for auditory information during that time period. These breaks can happen during a heavy auditory task, but can also be planned into an adult's day before and after heavy auditory tasks. For example, if an adult knows he or she needs to listen intently through an afternoon meeting, then he or she could consider a quiet break during lunch without being responsible for auditory information. Similarly, time could be saved after the meeting for a period of quiet rejuvenation.

21.6.5 Communication Repair Strategies

Communication repair strategies are those strategies that can attempt to fix a communication breakdown. Communication breakdowns occur when one party in the communication dyad either misses or misunderstands information shared. Failed communication can be frustrating to both communication partners and is often cited by adults as reasons why they feel isolated with hearing loss. Because people with hearing loss are more prone to missing or misunderstanding information, tools can be taught to the adult and to key communication partners to help fix communication breakdowns more quickly and with less frustration.

Sometimes information is missed by a person with hearing loss due to the delivery of the message by the communication partner. People do not naturally, innately know how to speak to increase the likelihood of communication success with someone with hearing loss. Direct, specific pointers can be helpful. These pointers include: speak slower or faster; speak louder or softer; look at me when you speak to me; do not cover your mouth when you speak to me; please turn down the radio so I can hear you more clearly; and speak normally—you do not need to exaggerate your speech.

Pearl

Communication partners need to be encouraged not to say "never mind" when the person with hearing loss misses some communication. This increases the feeling of isolation.

Information can be missed when a person with hearing loss does not hear a detail presented in the sentence. Repeating what you did hear or requesting a specific piece of information can be helpful. The communication partner knows an attempt to listen was made and knows exactly what detail to repeat. Participants can ask questions such as "Where did you say we should meet at 3 o'clock?" When important, key details are shared, it is beneficial for the person with hearing loss to repeat the key details to verify the correct message. Verification statements such as "I will be there Wednesday at 10 AM" allow early opportunities for errors to be corrected.

21.7 Rights in School, Workplace, and Other Places

Many people with acquired hearing loss are not aware of their rights as an adult with a diagnosed medical condition. Different countries have varying rights for citizens with hearing loss in the workplace, schools, and community. A practitioner should become familiar with the rights of people in their practicing country. Knowing rights and accommodations available is important for job security, capability to do one's job with reasonable accommodations, and access to curriculum and job training.

21.8 Communication Partners in Aural Rehabilitation

Because aural rehabilitation is about communication, there is an imperative role for a communication partner. This can be a spouse, partner, family member, friend, or other person with whom communication frequently occurs. Communication partners play an important role as practice partner, trusted provider of feedback, and motivator. People who spend more time wearing their cochlear implant are correlated with better listening outcomes[30] and communication partners can encourage increased wear time of amplification, and provide motivation and encouragement. Communication partners can help identify successes and weaknesses that might not be known to the participant.

Communication partners can help with carrying out a home program. A familiar voice is sometimes easier to understand. However, it is common that a person finds someone in their home challenging to hear, especially voices of women and children. Practicing together provides a low pressure situation to gain structured experience with listening to the other person's voice. Communication partners attending aural rehabilitation sessions can learn strategies and techniques for practice at home.

A major benefit of communication partners in aural rehabilitation occurs during the counseling piece of aural rehabilitation. While relationship issues are not within the scope of practice of aural rehabilitation practitioners, communication strategies and techniques do fall under the appropriate purview and the communication habits of both partners can be addressed.

Some people live alone, do not regularly see a specific person, have schedules that do not allow time to practice with other home members, or do not wish to involve a communication partner in practice. When someone does not have a communication partner, a home program can be created for independent practice. Focus should include giving the person access to conversational level speech and promoting appropriate wear times of the cochlear implant. Participants should be encouraged, as their situation allows, to interact with others in communication.

21.9 Communication with Audiology During Adult Aural Rehabilitation

Some audiologists are providing aural rehabilitation, but when the practitioner is not an audiologist or is not the audiologist managing all of the participant's amplification, it is imperative that the practitioner be in regular communication with the audiologist. Audiologists have the ability to address many areas of concern with technology and need to be aware of changes in performance and progress. A positive impact after the audiologist has made a change in technology settings indicates successful remediation of a problem. A negative change or lack of progress is a red flag for the audiologist that there is room for change in programming or early warning signs of device failures, or technology in need of repair. The practitioner can share specific auditory skill development areas of weakness such as specific phoneme confusions. Understanding how a participant is struggling helps the audiologist to recommend specific settings or programming, the addition of assistive listening devices, or re-evaluate current programming settings. Audiologists can benefit by sharing challenges with programming or equipment with the aural rehabilitation practitioner who can develop practice programs for technology use to help educate the participant.

21.10 Conclusion

Adult aural rehabilitation is necessary for adults receiving new amplification, or a change in technology, as in moving from hearing aids to cochlear implants, and should be considered as part of the process of getting new technology. Adults can benefit from many aspects of aural rehabilitation and can be anticipated to make progress in their overall communication. Adult aural rehabilitation is a valuable service and serves a large role in helping adults with hearing loss achieve optimal outcomes with their amplification.

21.11 Case Studies

21.11.1 Case Study 1

A 58-year-old man reported for aural rehabilitation. Case history revealed a moderate sensorineural hearing loss beginning 2 years ago, suspected to be related to noise exposure. He received new hearing aids 2 years ago and had lasting complaints of lack of comprehension when he cannot lip-read and severe challenges in noise. This reportedly negatively impacted him at work and in social situations. Testing results were as follows:

Initial Goals that were selected:

1. Comprehend open set sentences with 90% accuracy in 2 months
2. Comprehend open set sentences in environmental and competing speech noises with 90% accuracy in 4 months
3. Comprehend paragraph in noise with 80% accuracy in 6 months
4. Demonstrate comprehension of when to use hearing aid programs and capability to select program in 90% of opportunities in 1 month.

Counseling topics: education on hearing aid programs, assistive listening devices such as DM/FM system, strategic seating, environment modification, legal rights for the workplace in this country for people with a disability, ear protection for noise exposure

21.11.2 Case Study 2

A 72-year-old woman reported for aural rehabilitation. Case history revealed a severe sloping to profound sensorineural hearing loss progressive over 10 years. She wore hearing aids for 10 years and then received a cochlear implant 1 month ago. She reported hearing robotic speech sounds and not understanding people who are talking. Testing results were as follows:

Initial Goals that were selected:

1. Identify consonants varying in place of articulation in beginning, middle, and end of words in beginning, middle, and end of sentences with 90% accuracy in 3 months
2. Identify the target phrase in a closed set of 4 with phrases of varying number of syllables with 90% accuracy in 2 months
3. Identify the target sentence in a closed set of 4 sentences with sentences varying in number of syllables with 90% accuracy in 3 months
4. Independently change volume on cochlear implant with 90% accuracy in 1 month.

Counseling topics: education on cochlear implant volume buttons, education on assistive listening devices that came with her cochlear implant, and communication strategies

---

Discussion Questions

1. What information can be collected and assessed in a thorough case history and assessment to determine an appropriate aural rehabilitation plan of care that meets the needs of an adult with hearing loss?
2. What are advantages of including communication partners in aural rehabilitation?
3. Discuss the role counseling plays in aural rehabilitation.
4. Explain the order for the auditory skill consonant feature identification.
5. List two activities a practitioner could do with an adult with hearing loss that is exhibiting challenges with comprehension of sentences.

Resources

[1] NIDCD. Quick Statistics about Hearing. https://www.nidcd.nih.gov/health/statistics/quick-statistics-hearing Published 2016
[2] Zahnert T. The differential diagnosis of hearing loss. *Dtsch Arztebl Int* 2011;*108*(25):433–443, quiz 444
[3] Michels TC, Duffy MT, Rogers DJ. Hearing loss in adults: differential diagnosis and treatment. *Am Fam Physician* 2019;*100*(2):98–108
[4] Cunningham LL, Tucci DL. Hearing loss in adults. *N Engl J Med* 2017;*377*(25):2465–2473
[5] Boothroyd A. Adult aural rehabilitation: what is it and does it work? *Trends Amplif* 2007;*11*(2):63–71
[6] Schow RL, Nerbonne MA. Introduction to Audiologic Rehabilitation. 5th ed. Boston, MA: Pearson; 2007
[7] Harris MS, Capretta NR, Henning SC, Feeney L, Pitt MA, Moberly AC. Postoperative rehabilitation strategies used by adults with cochlear implants: a pilot study. *Laryngoscope Investig Otolaryngol* 2016;*1*(3):42–48
[8] Boothroyd A. Characteristics of listening environments: benefits of binaural hearing and implications for bilateral management. *Int J Audiol* 2006;*45*(Suppl 1):S12–S19
[9] Plant G, Bernstein CM, Levitt H. Optimizing performance in adult cochlear implant users through clinician directed auditory training. *Semin Hear* 2015;*36*(4):296–310
[10] Erber NP. Auditory Training. Alexander Graham Bell Association for the Deaf and Hard of Hearing; 1982
[11] McRackan TR, Bauschard M, Hatch JL, et al. Meta-analysis of cochlear implantation outcomes evaluated with general health-related patient-reported outcome measures. *Otol Neurotol* 2018;*39*(1):29–36

[12] Newman CW, Weinstein BE, Jacobson GP, Hug GA. The Hearing Handicap Inventory for Adults: psychometric adequacy and audiometric correlates. *Ear Hear* 1990;*11*(6):430–433

[13] Thibodeau LM. Plotting beyond the audiogram to the TELEGRAM, a new assessment tool. *Hear J* 2004;*57*(11):46–51

[14] 14. DeVault Otologic Research Laboratory of the Department of Otolaryngology-Head and Neck Surgery at the Indiana University School of Medicine. Pre-Feature Identification Contrasts. 1999

[15] Robbins AM, Renshaw JJ, Miyamoto RT, Osberger MJ, Pope ML. Minimal pairs test. Indianapolis, IN: Indiana University School of Medicine; 1988

[16] Zeh R, Baumann U. [Inpatient rehabilitation of adult CI users: Results in dependency of duration of deafness, CI experience and age]. *HNO* 2015;*63*(8):557–576

[17] Osberger MJ, Robbins AM, Miyamoto RT, et al. Speech perception abilities of children with cochlear implants, tactile aids, or hearing aids. *Am J Otol* 1991;*12*(Suppl):105–115

[18] Kim EY, Yoon MS, Kim HH, Nam CM, Park ES, Hong SH. Characteristics of nasal resonance and perceptual rating in prelingual hearing impaired adults. *Clin Exp Otorhinolaryngol* 2012;*5*(1):1–9

[19] Ling D. Foundations of spoken language for hearing-impaired children. Washington, DC: Alexander Graham Bell Association for the Deaf and Hard of Hearing; 1989

[20] Ubrig MT, Goffi-Gomez MV, Weber R, et al. Voice analysis of postlingually deaf adults pre- and postcochlear implantation. *J Voice* 2011;*25*(6):692–699

[21] Ellis L. Articulation characteristics of severely and profoundly deaf children and approaches to therapy: a review of the electropalatography literature. *Lang Linguist Compass* 2009;*3*:1201–1210

[22] Kochkin S. Why my hearing aids are in the drawer: The consumer's perspective. *Hear J* 2000;*53*(2):34–42

[23] Sullivan JR, Thibodeau LM, Assmann PF. Auditory training of speech recognition with interrupted and continuous noise maskers by children with hearing impairment. *J Acoust Soc Am* 2013;*133*(1):495–501

[24] Ihler F, Blum J, Steinmetz G, Weiss BG, Zirn S, Canis M. Development of a home-based auditory training to improve speech recognition on the telephone for patients with cochlear implants: A randomised trial. *Clin Otolaryngol* 2017;*42*(6):1303–1310

[25] Brockmeier SJ. Munich Music Questionnaire (MUMU). Innsbruck, Austria: MED-EL GmbH; 2000

[26] Gfeller K, Guthe E, Driscoll V, Brown CJ. A preliminary report of music-based training for adult cochlear implant users: Rationales and development. *Cochlear Implants Int* 2015; *16*(3, Suppl 3):S22–S31

[27] Dwyer RT, Gifford RH, Bess FH, Dorman M, Spahr A, Hornsby BWY. Diurnal cortisol levels and subjective ratings of effort and fatigue in adult cochlear implant users: a pilot study. *Am J Audiol* 2019;*28*(3):686–696

[28] Bess FH, Hornsby BW. Commentary: listening can be exhausting—fatigue in children and adults with hearing loss. *Ear Hear* 2014;*35*(6):592–599

[29] Sousa DA. How the Brain Learns. Thousand Oaks, CA: Corwin; 2017

[30] Schvartz-Leyzac KC, Conrad CA, Zwolan TA. Datalogging statistics and speech recognition during the first year of use in adult cochlear implant recipients. *Otol Neurotol* 2019;*40*(7):e686–e693

VI
Storing Treasures in the Attic

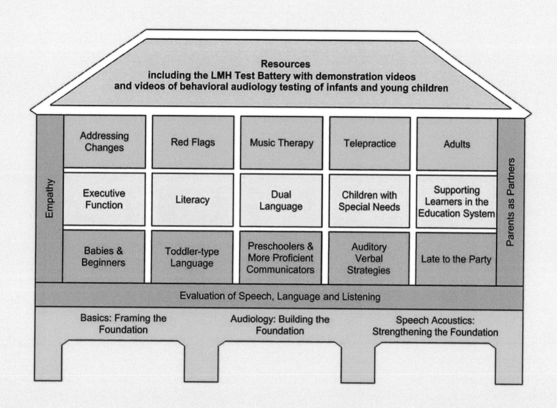

22 Resources

Section 1: Creating a Firm Foundation

Chapter 1: The Basics: Framing the Foundation

Resource 1.1: Resources for Individuals and Families Dealing with Hearing Loss

- www.agbell.org
- www.HearingFirst.org
- www.options.org

Resource 1.2: Information for Professionals Considering Listening and Spoken Language (LSL) Certification

Listening and Spoken Language Specialist (LSLS®) Certification Responses to Frequently Asked Questions AG Bell Academy for Listening and Spoken Language The AG Bell Academy for Listening and Spoken Language (the Academy) is the certification body that administers the LSLS® certification process. A subsidiary of the Alexander Graham Bell Association for the Deaf and Hard of Hearing, the Academy has offices in Washington, D.C. and Madrid, Spain. The Academy envisions a future where all individuals and families will have access to a certified Listening and Spoken Language (LSL) professional who provides listening and spoken language services. The Academy's mission is *to advance listening and talking through standards of excellence and international certification of professionals.*	**Certificación de Especialista en Escucha y Lenguaje Hablado (LSLS®) Respuestas a las preguntas más frecuentes AG Bell Academy para la Escucha y el Lenguaje Hablado** La AG Bell Academy para la Escucha y el Lenguaje Hablado (la Academia) es el organismo de certificación que administra el proceso de certificación LSLS®. La Academia, que es una filial de la Asociación Alexander Graham Bell para Personas con Sordera o Hipoacusia, tiene oficinas en Washington D.C. y en Madrid, España. La Academia imagina un futuro en el que todas las personas y familias tengan acceso a un profesional certificado en Escucha y Lenguaje Hablado (LSL) que proporcione servicios de escucha y lenguaje hablado. La misión de la Academia *es potenciar la escucha y el habla a través de estándares de excelencia y certificación internacional de profesionales.*
What is Listening and Spoken Language (LSL)? LSL is one of the options parents/caregivers choose to help their child who is deaf or hard of hearing learn and communicate. LSL is provided according to the Principles of Listening and Spoken Language. Strategies for developing listening and spoken language are called LSL strategies and these strategies are used to help the child learn to listen and talk. Families should consider what they desire to see as outcomes for their child as they evaluate which of several communications options are available for their child to use. Basic information about the primary communication options can be found on AG Bell's website (https://www.agbell.org/Families/Communication-Options), but families and professionals are encouraged to find other in-depth information in books and online and in-person courses.	**¿Qué es la Escucha y el Lenguaje Hablado (LSL)?** La LSL es una de las opciones que los padres/cuidadores eligen para ayudar a su hijo con sordera o hipoacusia a aprender y comunicarse. La LSL se proporciona de acuerdo con los Principios de la Escucha y el Lenguaje Hablado. Las estrategias para desarrollar la escucha y el lenguaje oral se denominan estrategias LSL y se utilizan para ayudar al niño a aprender a escuchar y hablar. Las familias deben tener en cuenta los resultados que desean para su hijo cuando evalúan las diversas opciones de comunicación disponibles para su hijo. La información básica sobre las principales opciones de comunicación se puede encontrar en la página web de AG Bell (https://www.agbell.org/Families/Communication-Options), pero se anima a las familias y a los profesionales a buscar otra información más detallada en libros y cursos *online* y presenciales.
What is LSLS Certification? LSLS certification is a credential that is pursued, earned and maintained by professionals who work with families who wish to pursue the option of LSL. Audiologists, speech-language pathologists and teachers of children who are deaf and hard of hearing can seek certification. Certified LSL professionals, when engaged in LSL practice, typically focus on teaching the child, and modeling, guiding and coaching his/her caregivers and educators (if in a school environment), on how to develop LSL. Intentional and timely pursuit of excellent pediatric audiology services, early fitting and use of hearing technology during the child's awake hours, and ongoing LSL services with sequenced goals, objectives and use of LSL strategies help the child develop and maximize his/her capability to listen and talk as part of natural, everyday life.	**¿Qué es la certificación LSLS?** La certificación LSLS es una credencial que buscan, obtienen y mantienen los profesionales que trabajan con familias que desean aplicar la opción de LSL. Audiólogos, logopedas y profesores de niños con sordera o hipoacusia pueden solicitar la certificación. Los profesionales certificados en LSL, cuando se dedican a la práctica del LSL, se centran en enseñar al niño y en modelar, guiar y entrenar a sus cuidadores y educadores (si están en un entorno escolar) en cómo desarrollar el LSL. La búsqueda intencionada y precoz de excelentes servicios de audiología pediátrica, la adaptación y el uso tempranos de tecnología auditiva durante las horas de vigilia del niño y los servicios continuados de LSL con metas y objetivos secuenciados y el uso de estrategias de LSL ayudan al niño a desarrollar y maximizar su capacidad de escuchar y hablar como parte de la vida natural y cotidiana.
Who can pursue LSLS certification? LSLS certification is a highly regarded qualification that can be earned by professionals who have a professional degree (either a bachelor or graduate-level degree that allow a professional to practice) in audiology, deaf education or speech-language pathology. Administered by the Academy since 2005, LSLS certification is considered the defining qualification of a professional who has specialized in and can competently guide the development of LSL in children who are deaf or hard of hearing and their families. Professionals pursue one of two LSLS designations; either the LSLS Cert. AVT® or the LSLS Cert. AVEd®. These credentials each have a set of Principles to which LSL professionals are expected and agree to adhere to as part of their practice. Professionals typically pursue the designation that is the best fit for the work environment they are employed while pursuing LSLS certification. Professionals who are employed in a clinical, medical, or public or private therapy/intervention setting might find pursuit of the LSLS Cert. AVT designation to be the better fit for them. Professionals who are employed in public or private educational/school settings might find pursuit of the LSLS Cert. AVEd designation to be the better fit for them. Regardless of the designation, both the LSLS Cert. AVT and LSLS Cert. AVEd designations indicate competence by the professional in helping children who are deaf or hard of hearing develop LSL.	**¿Quién puede obtener la certificación LSLS?** La certificación LSLS es una cualificación de gran prestigio que pueden obtener los profesionales que tengan un título profesional (ya sea una licenciatura, grado o un título de postgrado que permita el ejercicio profesional) en audiología, educación para sordos o logopedia. Administrada por la Academia desde 2005, la certificación LSLS se considera la cualificación que define a un profesional que se ha especializado y puede guiar de forma competente el desarrollo de la LSL en niños con sordera o hipoacusia y a sus familias. Los profesionales pueden obtener uno de los dos certificados LSLS: el LSLS Cert. AVT® o el LSLS Cert. AVEd®. Cada una de estas credenciales tiene un conjunto de Principios a los que se espera que los profesionales de LSL se adhieran como parte de su práctica laboral. Los profesionales suelen optar por la designación que mejor se adapte al contexto en el que trabajan mientras obtienen la certificación LSLS. Los profesionales que trabajan en un entorno clínico, médico o de terapia/intervención pública o privada pueden encontrar que la búsqueda de la designación LSLS Cert. AVT es la mejor opción para ellos. A los profesionales que trabajan en entornos educativos/escolares públicos o privados les puede resultar la designación LSLS Cert. AVEd como la mejor opción. Independientemente de la designación, tanto el LSLS Cert. AVT y LSLS Cert. AVEd indican la competencia del profesional para ayudar a los niños con sordera o hipoacusia a desarrollar la LSL.

Where do families and professionals find a certified LSL professional?
Currently, more than 1,000 individuals in 30 countries are certified LSL professionals. The Academy's *Locate a Listening and Spoken Language Specialist (LSLS) Directory* is one way to find a certified LSL professional who provides LSL services. This directory also indicates which professionals offer mentoring services to aspiring LSL professionals: https://www.agbell. org/Membership/Membership-Search. Families seeking a certified LSL professional are not limited to services within their own borders. Many LSL professionals provide services remotely, so children in many countries or in remote areas can receive support. Parents who have a computer or tablet can receive services from willing certified LSL professionals located anywhere in the world. Professionals who want to find a certified LSL professional who can act as their mentor during the LSLS certification process are fortunate that many mentors can provide mentoring from a distance.

What is unique about a certified LSL professional?
It is normal for someone to ask, "What is so special about a certified LSL professional?" Can we just say, "The knowledge and skills set is not just aspirational! It's achievable and enviable when you see it in a professional!" The Academy worked with Kryterion, Inc., to identify the following knowledge and skills set (https://agbellacademy.org/wp-content/ uploads/2018/12/LSLS-Certification-Exam-Blueprint_FINAL.pdf). The LSLS Certification Exam Blueprint is a wonderful resource and guide to what a LSLS Cert. AVT and LSLS Cert. AVEd knows and can put into practice! Professionals who pursue LSLS certification tend to be highly motivated people who believe in others and are capable of guiding, encouraging, supporting, and standing beside them as they reach towards their own goals. As life-long learners, LSL professionals join a community of other professionals who want to make the world a better place for families with children with hearing loss through their commitment to new knowledge, innovative practices, and impactful relationships!

Ten benefits to the professional who earns LSLS Certification and utilizes the credential

1. **Acknowledgment of competence** in the specialized knowledge and skills set of LSL and related areas (e.g., parent coaching) by parents and other professionals.

2. Listing of the LSLS Cert. AVT or LSLS Cert. AVEd credential following your name helps parents, professionals and society **identify you as a professional who knows how to teach LSL to children who are deaf or hard of hearing.**

3. **Promotion of you as a certified LSL professional** in the "Locate an LSLS Directory" on the Academy's website, which could lead to new opportunities.

4. **New opportunity** for employment or promotion to higher positions.

5. **Possibility of** pay increase (depending on employer), other compensation or **recognition for your exceptional knowledge and skills.**

6. **Personal thrill and pride** of knowing you have succeeded at what you may consider one of your life goals—to reach a high level of happiness and meaning in your work and to know that you and your work impact the lives of others in a positive and intangible way!

7. **Professional satisfaction** of having achieved one of your long-term professional goals. Congratulations, you did it! You are now a certified LSL professional/LSLS Cert. AVT/LSLS Cert. AVEd!

8. **Increased opportunity to participate** in your field through invited presentations and appointments to committees, task forces and boards.

9. **Giving back** by becoming a **mentor** to aspiring professionals in the future or contributing **financial support or other supports** to aspiring LSL professionals.

10. **Networking** in the larger professional world through **participation and connection to the worldwide community of certified LSL professionals.**

¿Dónde pueden encontrar las familias y los profesionales un profesional certificado en LSL?
Actualmente, más de 1.000 personas en 30 países son profesionales certificados en LSL. El directorio de la Academia "*Localice a un especialista en audición y lenguaje hablado*" (LSLS) es una forma de encontrar a un profesional LSL certificado que preste servicios de LSL. Este directorio también indica qué profesionales ofrecen servicios como mentores a los aspirantes a profesionales de LSL: https://www.agbell.org/Membership/ Membership-Search. Las familias que buscan un profesional LSL certificado no están limitadas a optar por servicios en su país. Muchos profesionales de LSL prestan servicios a distancia, para que los niños de muchos países o de zonas remotas puedan recibir apoyo. Los padres que disponen de un ordenador o una tableta pueden recibir servicios de profesionales de LSL certificados dispuestos a ello y situados en cualquier parte del mundo. Los profesionales que deseen encontrar un profesional de LSL certificado que pueda actuar como mentor durante su proceso de certificación de LSLS ahora tienen la suerte de que muchos mentores pueden ofrecer tutoría a distancia gracias a la tecnología.

¿Qué tiene de único un profesional de LSL certificado?
Es normal que alguien pregunte: "¿Qué tiene de especial un profesional certificado en LSL?". Podemos decir: "¡El conjunto de conocimientos y habilidades no es sólo un sueño! Es alcanzable y envidiable cuando lo ves en un profesional". La Academia trabajó con Kryterion, Inc., para identificar el siguiente conjunto de conocimientos y habilidades (https://agbellacademy. org/wp-content/uploads/2018/12/LSLS-Certification-Exam-Blueprint_ FINAL.pdf). El LSLS Certification Exam Blueprint es un recurso maravilloso y una guía de lo que un LSLS Cert. AVT y LSLS Cert. AVEd sabe y puede poner en práctica.
Los profesionales que obtienen la certificación LSLS suelen ser personas muy motivadas que creen en los demás y son capaces de guiarlos, animarlos, apoyarlos y estar a su lado mientras alcanzan sus objetivos. Aprendiendo de por vida, los profesionales de LSL se unen a una comunidad de otros profesionales que quieren hacer del mundo un lugar mejor para las familias con niños con pérdida auditiva a través de su compromiso con nuevos conocimientos, prácticas innovadoras y relaciones con mayor impacto.

Diez beneficios para el profesional que obtiene la certificación LSLS

1. **El reconocimiento,** por parte de los padres y de otros profesionales, **de la competencia profesional** en el conjunto de conocimientos y habilidades especializadas de LSL y áreas relacionadas (por ejemplo, el entrenamiento de los padres).

2. La inclusión en la lista del LSLS Cert. AVT o LSLS Cert. AVEd con su nombre, ayuda a los padres, a los profesionales y a la sociedad a identificarle como un **profesional que sabe cómo enseñar LSL a niños con sordera o hipoacusia.**

3. **Promoción** para usted como profesional certificado en LSL en el "Directorio de LSLS" de la página web de la Academia, lo que podría dar lugar a nuevas oportunidades laborales.

4. **Nuevas oportunidades** de empleo o promoción a puestos superiores.

5. Posibilidad de aumento de sueldo (dependiendo del empleador), otras compensaciones o **reconocimiento por sus conocimientos y habilidades excepcionales.**

6. La **emoción y el orgullo personal** de saber que ha tenido éxito en el que puede considerar uno de los objetivos de su vida: alcanzar una gran felicidad y dar sentido a su trabajo sabiendo que repercute en la vida de los demás de forma positiva e intangible.

7. La **satisfacción profesional** de haber alcanzado uno de sus objetivos profesionales a largo plazo. ¡Enhorabuena, lo ha conseguido! ¡Ahora es un profesional certificado en Terapia Auditivo-Verbal (LSLS Cert. AVT) o Educación Auditivo-Verbal (LSLS Cert. AVEd)!

8. **Más oportunidades de participar en su campo** a través de presentaciones, designaciones a comités, grupos de trabajo y reuniones.

9. **Cerrar el círculo, convirtiéndose en mentor** de los aspirantes a profesionales en el futuro o contribuyendo con **apoyo financiero u otros apoyos** a los aspirantes a profesionales de LSL.

10. **Establecer una red de contactos** en el mundo profesional a través de la participación y la conexión con la comunidad mundial de profesionales certificados de LSL.

What is required to successfully earn the LSLS certification?

Many professionals become a LSLS Cert. AVT or LSLS Cert. AVEd after they have gained some professional experience through their work settings. Most professionals do not learn or even hear about LSL during their formal education years. For this reason, most professionals who pursue LSLS certification will benefit immeasurably (as will the children and families they serve) by engaging in a mentor-mentee relationship with a professional who is currently a certified LSL professional.

General Information Regarding Initial LSLS Certification

Completed and accepted LSL Registry Enrollment application (requires essential personal and demographic information and provision of documentation related to that professional's education/degrees), one professional letter of reference and a letter of commitment from a certified LSL professional who has agreed to be the candidate's mentor: https://agbellacademy.org/certification/lsl-registry/.

Professional degree (or equivalent) that enables a professional to practice in one of the following fields: Audiology, Deaf Education, or Speech-Language Pathology.

Professional license or credential that enables a professional to practice with children and others (if required in that professional's location).

Selection of which designation will be pursued—either **LSLS Cert. AVT or LSLS Cert AVEd**—and a **signed commitment to the Principles** of the LSLS AVT or the LSLS AVEd practice (whichever one has been selected as the designation of pursuit) https://agbellacademy.org/certification/principles-of-lsl-specialists/.

Professional continuing education that totals, at least, 80 hours. Forty (40) of these hours can be obtained prior to the beginning of the certification process.

Observation of 10 sessions provided by one or more certified LSL professionals and completion of the Academy's related documentation.

Provision and documentation of direct LSL services with children who are learning to listen and talk and developing LSL as their primary mode of communication. Professionals must provide **900 hours of LSL services** during their certification period (for a minimum of 36 continuous months and up to 72 months). Most of these hours should be with children who are infants, toddlers or preschoolers and whose families are participating in parent coaching. Up to 10 percent of these hours can be with adult clients who are receiving services after obtaining a new cochlear implant or other hearing device. Some hours of indirect services (e.g., parent groups, audiology appointments or meetings related to a child) can be counted towards the total number of hours.

Ongoing mentoring during the certification process by one or more certified LSL professionals for a total of 20 LSL sessions led by the candidate. These sessions can be observed either live or via video by a mentor, and feedback must be provided on the Academy's approved form (F-1) for each of the mentored sessions.

A formal, self-written description of the candidate's LSL practice (completed near the end of the 36- to 72-month certification period).

Professional letters of recommendation provided by two (2) professionals familiar with the candidate's work related to direct or indirect LSL services.

Parent letters of recommendation from two (2) parents whose children have received direct LSL services from the candidate.

Passing score on the LSLS Certification Examination (provided in English and Spanish). The candidate can choose to take the exam at any point during the certification process, provided that the candidate has applied and been accepted into the LSL Registry.

Muchos profesionales se convierten en un LSLS Cert. AVT o LSLS Cert. AVEd una vez que han adquirido cierta experiencia profesional en su entorno laboral. La mayoría de los profesionales no aprenden o ni siquiera oyen hablar de LSL durante sus años de educación formal. Por esta razón, la mayoría de los profesionales que desean la certificación LSLS se beneficiarán enormemente (al igual que los niños y las familias con las que trabajan) al participar en una relación de mentor-alumno con un profesional certificado LSL.

Información general sobre el Inicio de la certificación LSLS

Solicitud de inscripción en el Registro LSL completada y aceptada (que requiere información personal y demográfica esencial y aportar documentación relacionada con la educación y títulos del profesional), una carta de referencia profesional y una carta de compromiso de un profesional LSL certificado que haya aceptado ser el mentor del candidato: https://agbellacademy.org/certification/lsl-registry/.

Título profesional (o equivalente) que permita ejercer en uno de los siguientes campos: Audiología, Educación para Sordos, Fonoaudiología, Logopedia o Patología del Lenguaje.

Licencia o credencial profesional que permite a un profesional ejercer con niños y otras personas (si se requiere en el lugar en el que se ejerza).

La **selección de la designación que se dese obtener**, ya sea LSLS Cert. AVT o LSLS Cert AVEd y un compromiso firmado con los Principios de la práctica LSLS AVT o LSLS AVEd (la que haya sido seleccionada como la designación deseada) Principios LSL Auditivo-Verbales - AG BELL International

Formación profesional continua que sume, como mínimo, 80 horas. Cuarenta (40) de las cuales pueden obtenerse antes del inicio del proceso de certificación.

Observación de 10 sesiones impartidas por uno o más profesionales certificados en LSL y cumplimentar la documentación relacionada con la Academia.

Prestación y documentación de servicios directos de LSL con niños que están aprendiendo a escuchar y a hablar y que están desarrollando el LSL como su principal modo de comunicación. Los profesionales deben **proporcionar 900 horas de servicios de LSL durante su período de certificación** (durante un mínimo de 36 meses continuos y hasta 72 meses). La mayoría de estas horas deben realizarse con niños que sean bebés, niños pequeños o preescolares y cuyas familias participen en la terapia. Hasta el 10% de estas horas pueden ser con clientes adultos que estén recibiendo servicios tras un nuevo implante coclear u otro(s) dispositivo(s) auditivo(s). También pueden contarse para el número total de horas algunas horas de servicios indirectos (por ejemplo, grupos de padres, citas de audiología o reuniones relacionadas con un niño).

Tutoría continua durante el proceso de certificación por parte de uno o más profesionales certificados para un total de 20 sesiones de LSL llevadas a cabo por el candidato. Estas sesiones pueden ser observadas en directo o por video por un mentor, y se debe proporcionar retroalimentación en el formulario aprobado por la Academia (F-1) para cada una de las sesiones tuteladas.

Una descripción formal, escrita por el propio candidato, de su práctica de LSL (realizada cerca del final del período de certificación de 36 a 72 meses).

Cartas de recomendación profesionales proporcionadas por dos (2) profesionales familiarizados con el trabajo del candidato relacionado directa o indirectamente con los servicios LSL.

Cartas de recomendación de dos (2) padres/madres cuyos hijos hayan recibido servicios de LSL directamente del candidato.

Puntuación de aprobado en el examen de certificación LSLS (en inglés y español). El candidato puede optar por realizar el examen, una vez preparado, en cualquier momento del proceso de certificación, siempre que haya solicitado y sido aceptado en el Registro LSL.

Is there a continuing professional education requirement that certified LSL professionals must meet?	¿Existe algún requisito de formación profesional continua que deban cumplir los profesionales certificados en LSL?
Certified LSL professionals are nearly always highly motivated professionals who engage in ongoing education as a way to provide excellent LSL and other services. When certified, a professional is required to participate in 15 hours of Academy-approved hours and provide evidence of completion of those continuing education units (CEUs) every two years. A course or activity that is Academy-approved for LSLS CEUs must have content that is related to one or more of the Nine LSLS Domains of Knowledge: https://agbellacademy.org/certification/lsls-domains-of-knowledge/. Professionals and organizations who are interested in becoming an LSLS CEU Provider so they can offer LSLS CEUs can find information on the Academy's website: https://agbellacademy.org/continuing-education/for-ceu-providers/.	Los profesionales certificados en LSL son casi siempre profesionales muy motivados que se implican en la formación continua como forma de proporcionar una excelente LSL y otros servicios. Una vez certificado, el profesional está obligado a participar en 15 horas aprobadas por la Academia y proporcionar evidencia de haber completado esas Unidades de Educación Continua (CEUs) cada dos años. Un curso o actividad aprobado por la Academia para obtener CEUs de LSLS debe tener un contenido relacionado con una o más de las Nueve Áreas de Conocimiento de LSLS: 9 Domains_Spanish.pdf (agbell.org) Los profesionales y organizaciones que estén interesados en ser proveedores de CEUs de LSLS para poder ofrecer CEUs de LSLS pueden encontrar información en la página web de la Academia: https://agbellacademy.org/continuing-education/for-ceu-providers/ Link with information in English
Is there someone I can talk with about LSLS certification, certification renewal or LSLS continuing education?	¿Puedo hablar con alguien sobre la certificación LSLS, la renovación de la certificación o la formación continua LSLS?
If a professional is unable to find the information they need on the Academy's website (www.agbellacademy.org), they should reach out to the Academy by email at Academy@agbell.org (English) or Academia@agbell.org (Spanish). The Academy has a small staff who works first through email to respond to questions, resolve issues and provide guidance. If email proves to be ineffective and a question or issue is unresolved, individuals are encouraged to request a WhatsApp call or Zoom meeting that can be conducted in English or Spanish.	Si un profesional no puede encontrar la información que necesita en la página web de la Academia (www.agbellacademy.org), debe ponerse en contacto con la Academia mediante correo electrónico escribiendo a academy@agbell.org (inglés) o academia@agbell.org (español). La Academia cuenta con equipo reducido que trabaja fundamentalmente a través del correo electrónico para responder a las preguntas, resolver los problemas y proporcionar orientación. Si el correo electrónico resulta ineficaz y una pregunta o problema no se resuelve, se anima a las personas a solicitar una llamada de WhatsApp o una reunión de Zoom que pueden realizarse en inglés o en español.

Chapter 2: Audiology: Building the Foundation

See **Video 2.1** Introduction to Testing Techniques.

See **Video 2.2** Introduction to Behavioral Observation Audiometry.

See **Video 2.3** Testing Using Behavioral Observation Evaluation.

See **Video 2.4** Introduction to Visual Reinforcement Audiometry.

See **Video 2.5** Testing Using Visual Reinforcement Audiometry.

See **Video 2.6** Introduction to Conditioned Play Audiometry.

See **Video 2.7** Testing Using Conditioned Play Audiometry.

See **Video 2.8** Introduction to Speech Perception Testing.

See **Video 2.9** Speech Awareness Threshold (SAT) Testing.

See **Video 2.10** Speech Reception Threshold (SRT) Testing.

See **Video 2.11** Closed-Set Speech Perception Testing.

See **Video 2.12** Open-Set Speech Perception Testing.

Resource 2.2: Suggestions for improving hearing aid and cochlear implant retention:

- *My Child Won't Keep His Hearing Aids/Cochlear Implants On/* posted July 10, 2019: https://soundspeechnj.com/blog/2019/7/3/my-child-wont-keep-his-hearing-aidscochlear-implants-on
- https://www.babyhearing.org/devices/help-baby-adjust-hearing-aids
- *Meeting the Challenge: Keeping Hearing Devices on Young Children* from OTICON Pediatrics: https://www.oticon.com/-/media/oticon-us/main/download-center/family-support-materials/professional-all/35537-keeping-hearing-aids-on-young-children.pdf

- Free downloadable *Keeping Hearing Aids On* brochures for families: https://successforkidswithhearingloss.com/strategies-for-keeping-hearing-aids-on-young-children/

Resources for individuals and families dealing with hearing loss: see Resource 1.1

Chapter 3: Speech Acoustics: Strengthening the Foundation

Resource 3.1: String Bean Audiogram. (See **Fig. 3.3**.)

Resource 3.2: The LMH (Ling, Madell, Hewitt or Low, Mid, High Frequency) Test Battery: The LMH Test Battery is a series of functional listening assessments that increase in difficulty as the child's speech perception and capability to respond grow. As with all functional listening assessments, all tests in the battery are presented through audition only with no visual input.

Goals of the LMH Test Battery are:

1. Progression from rudimentary screening (LMH 10 sound quick test) to all individual phonemes to more detailed testing (medial consonants) to formal speech perception testing (see **Fig. 22.1**);

2. Progression from clinician administration to caregiver administration (see **Fig. 22.1**);

3. Notation of consistent errors by parents and clinicians that are then shared with audiologists to ensure optimal programming and speech perception.

Part 1 of the LMH Test Battery: Detection, Identification, and Imitation of the LMH 10 Sound Quick Test: The first test, the LMH 10 sound quick test, is used to quickly assess a child's perception across the speech spectrum. Madell and Hewitt (2021) added four additional consonants (/z/, /h/, /n/, and /dʒ/) to the six Ling sounds to provide additional information about mid-frequency perception. (See **Fig. 22.2**.)

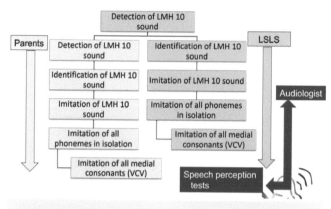

Fig. 22.1 Progression of LMH Test Battery from LMH 10 Sound Quick Test to medial consonants and from clinician administration to caregiver administration.

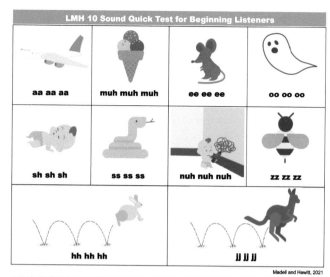

Madell and Hewitt, 2021

Fig. 22.2 LMH 10 Sound Quick Test pictures (English)

The test is administered by the parent or professional who presents the sounds in random order and with varying intervals of silence between sounds. Each sound is presented three times in quick succession (e.g. [a a a], [muh, muh, muh], [h h h], or [z z z]), and children indicate that they heard (or detected) the sound. It is important when presenting the sounds to produce each sound with the same duration so that no clues are given.

Testing begins with detection. Babies demonstrate detection by alerting, by starting or stopping sucking, or by localizing. Toddlers respond by dropping a block into a bucket or building a tower. As children develop their auditory skills, they should quickly move from detection to identification of the 10 sounds by either pointing to the appropriate picture or repeating the sound.

Part 2 of LMH Test Battery: Imitation of All Individual Phonemes
The LMH Test Battery does not end with the LMH 10 quick sound test. English has ~44 phonemes. To truly understand how well a child hears all the phonemes, it is essential to begin testing every phoneme, not just the LMH 10. Evaluating perception of all consonants will enable clinicians to know what children hear and what they do not hear. Children progressing from the LMH 10 sound quick test to all phonemes can be asked to imitate all phonemes using the same three quick presentations (e.g. [ba ba ba] or [t t t] or [f f f]). (Note that voiceless consonants are not presented with a vowel.)

Part 3 of LMH Test Battery: Imitation of Medial Consonants
When children's imitation skills have advanced to the point that they can imitate vowel-consonant-vowel (VCV) combinations, the LMH Test Battery moves to perception of all consonants in this manner (e.g. [aba], [ata], [afa]) Children with hearing loss as young as 2 years of age can begin to participate in this level of assessment that provides the most realistic perception information for running speech.

Resource 3.3: Videos of the LMH (Ling, Madell, Hewitt or Low, Mid, High Frequency) Test Battery

See **Video 3.1** 18-month-old with normal hearing—LMH 10 Sound Quick Test identification.

See **Video 3.2** 18-month-old with normal hearing—LMH 10 Sound Quick Test identification and beginning imitation.

See **Video 3.3** 2 1/2-year-old and parent demonstrating LMH 10 Sound Quick Test repetition.

See **Video 3.4** 4-year-old with profound bilateral hearing loss from cochlear nerve deficiency, received bilateral cochlear implants at 13 months—Individual phonemes with left CI (no cochlear nerve on imaging).

See **Video 3.5** 4-year-old with normal hearing—Medial Consonant Test.

See **Video 3.6** 4-year-old with profound hearing loss, received bilateral cochlear implants at 3 years—Medial Consonant Test.

See **Video 3.7** 8-year-old misdiagnosed as being on the autism spectrum at 1 year, diagnosed with profound hearing loss at 5 years, received bilateral cochlear implants at 6 years—Medial consonants with right CI before programming changes.

See **Video 3.8** 8-year-old misdiagnosed as being on the autism spectrum at 1 year, diagnosed with profound hearing loss at 5 years, received bilateral cochlear implants at 6 years—Medial consonants with right CI after slight increase on electrodes corresponding to 1500 Hz and 4500 Hz.

See **Video 3.9** 8-year-old misdiagnosed as being on the autism spectrum at 1 year, diagnosed with profound hearing loss at 5 years, received bilateral cochlear implants at 6 years—Medial consonants with right CI after slight increase on electrode corresponding to 4500 Hz and slight decrease on electrode corresponding to 6000 Hz.

Resource 3.4: Consonant Energy Bands (see **Fig. 3.3** in Chapter 3)

Section 2: Framing a Strong Structure

Chapter 4: Empathy: Changing the Culture of Communication

Resources for individuals and families dealing with hearing loss: see Resource 1.1

Resource 4.1: Unconscious Bias Exercise Tool (UBET), Individual Version

Intent: *Understanding Others, Gaining Insight, Experiencing Greater Empathy* by Johnnie Sexton (2020)

Background: Unconscious bias is a neutral term, the beliefs held outside of a person's consciousness.

Intent: The Unconscious Bias Exercise Tool (UBET) is designed to allow the individual completing it to look inward at how one defines oneself based on upbringing, background and life experiences. In addition, the exercise is designed to take the individual completing it to a different or more opposite perspective, enabling a closer look at how individuals view those who are not like them. The desired outcome is to gain a deeper and broader perspective of oneself and others.

Audience: Please complete the first section (YOU), listing things about YOU.

Then go to the next section (DIFFERENT THAN YOU) and describe someone who is or could be different than you in terms of background, upbringing, etc. using the same categories.

Please know that you are not required to answer any item with which you are uncomfortable. Thanks.

Section 1

- **YOU**
  - Race/ethnicity
  - Gender
  - Sexual identity
  - Age
  - Children
    - Yes
    - No
  - Hearing status
    - Deaf
    - Hearing
    - Hard of hearing
  - Communication mode
    - Spoken language
    - Visual language
    - Combined spoken and visual language
  - Parents
    - Living
    - Deceased
  - Siblings
    - Yes, if so, how many?
    - No
  - Educational level
    - High school
    - College
    - Graduate Degree
    - Doctoral Degree
  - Religion
  - Socioeconomic status
  - Geography
    - Where did you grow up?
    - Where dyou currently live?
  - Marital status
  - Occupation

Please share how completing this section made you feel about yourself.

_____

_____

_____

Section 2

- **DIFFERENT THAN YOU: Using the same categories as the previous section, describe a person whis the opposite of you, different from you, not you.**
  - Race/ethnicity
  - Gender
  - Sexual identity
  - Age
  - Children
    - Yes
    - No
  - Hearing status
    - Deaf
    - Hearing
    - Hard of hearing
  - Communication mode
    - Spoken language
    - Visual language
    - Combined spoken and visual language
  - Parents
    - Living
    - Deceased
  - Siblings
    - Yes, if so, how many?
    - No
  - Educational level
    - High school
    - College
    - Graduate Degree
    - Doctoral Degree

o Religion
o Socioeconomic status
o Geography
  ▪ Where did you grow up?
  ▪ Where dyou currently live?
o Marital status
o Occupation

Take time to consider how you felt about this person who is different than you. Was there any part of this that upset you? Did anything make you feel glad that you are not this person. If so, why? Be honest and write your feelings below.

_____

_____

_____

Please share any additional comments.

_____

_____

_____

Chapter 5: The Parent as a Critical Team Member: Creating a Partnership for Learning

Resource 5.1: Resources to aid parent coaching and creation of language-rich environment: Some parents are apprehensive when it comes to talking to their baby or toddler after the hearing loss has been identified. Exceptional resources for auditory and early language development that can assist in demonstrating listening and language concepts include the following:

• Handouts from www.asha.org
• Handouts from A.G. Bell (www.agbell.org)
• John Tracy Clinic (www.jtc.org)
• Supporting Success for Children with Hearing Loss (https://successforkidswithhearingloss.com)
• HELP for Home - Hawaii Early Learning Profile:(https://www.vort.com/home.php?cat=1)
• Hanen program (www.hanen.org)
• Rehabilitation information from Med El (www.medel.com/support/rehab),

Advanced Bionics (www.advancedbionics.com/us/en/portals/professional-portal.html) and Cochlear websites (www.cochlear.com/us/en/professionals/resources)

• Learn to Talk Around the Clock (www.learntotalkaroundtheclock.com)
• Hearing First (www.hearingfirst.org/learning-growing-lsl/lsl-strategies-techniques)

• Articles from Carol Flexer (www.continued.com/early-childhood-education/articles/to-grow-young-child-listening-22841)
• Articles from Jane Madell (www.audiologyonline.com/articles/counseling-support-for-children-with-13758, www.audiologyonline.com/articles/helping-families-accept-technology-829)
• www.audiologyonline.com
• www.thelisteningroom.com

Resource 5.2: Coaching parents to use cognitive questions: Providing parents with lists of sample cognitive questions to ask at home helps their child improve higher level thinking skills as well as aids carryover into inferential reading comprehension skills. Some excellent resources for additional cognitive work with an older student include:

• Cognitive Skills Chart for Parent / Therapy Intervention based on Leahea Grammatico's *Cognitive Curriculum and Bloom's Taxonomy* (see Resource 5.2).
• *Manual of Exercises for Expressive Reasoning* (MEER) by Zachman
• *Handbook of Exercises for Language Processing (HELP for Language)* by Lazzari
• No-Glamour Language and Reasoning Cards by Bowers
• No-Glamour Auditory Processing Cards by LoGiudice

Resources for individuals and families dealing with hearing loss: See Resource 1.1

Suggestions for improving hearing aid and cochlear implant retention: See Resource 2.2

LMH (Ling-Madell-Hewitt or Low, Mid, High) Test Battery: See Resource 3.2

Resources to aid parent coaching and creation of a language-rich environment: See Resource 5.1

Coaching parents to use cognitive questions: See Resource 5.2

Informal auditory checklist: See Resource 6.2

Assessments to identify possible gaps in language and cognitive skills for students with hearing loss (ages 6+): See Resource 6.5

Functional Listening Checklists and Assessments: See Resource 6.6

Auditory Learning Guide in English: See Resource 7.1

Auditory Learning Guide in Spanish: See Resource 7.2

Revised CAP (Categories of Auditory Perception) Scales and Integrated Scales of Development: See Resource 7.3

Early Listening Function (ELF): See Resource 7.4

Current Level of Functioning (CLF)—Verbal: See Resource 7.6

Expectations of Skill Development for HA & CI Users by Jane Madell, Joan Hewitt, and Sylvia Rotfleisch (2018): See Resource 7.7

Resources for additional learning on LSL Strategies: See Resource 10.1

Video examples of LSL strategies: See Resource 10.2

Recommended website for information on how children learn to read, why some struggle, and how adults can help: See Resource 13.2

Recommended sources for children's books: See Resource 13.3

Children Who Are Deaf or Hard of Hearing with Additional Learning Needs by Susan Wiley: See Resource 15.1

Suggested websites for children with hearing loss and additional needs: See Resource 15.2

Recommended websites for planning and education: See Resource 16.1

Suggested Roles of Educational Audiologists, Teachers of the Deaf and Hard of Hearing, and Speech-Language Pathologists (2018): See Resource 16.2

Resources for parents and clinicians to encourage integrating music in intervention: See Resource 19.1

Chapter 6: Evaluation of Speech, Language, and Listening in Children with Hearing Loss: Knowing the Level at Which Children Are Functioning

Resource 5.2: Cognitive skills chart for parent and therapy intervention
Based on Leahea Grammatico's Cognitive Curriculum and Bloom's Taxonomy

Taxonomy Level	Questions	Sample Activities
Observe/Inquire Parents ask questions to inquire what child is observing or what he knows; parents can add new info different perspective	"What do you see?" "What happened?" "Tell me about…" "What do you know about…?"	-Looking at a book, creations from shapes, looking out windows, on a walk—Play-Doh, sand play, rice table -Picture scenes, family photos -Real experiences, familiar items
Create, Organize, Association Parents present activities which help child learn to associate, organize, and sort	"What goes together?" "Where does this belong?" Do any of these belong together?" (categories presented) "Where could we find this?" "How can we organize ___?"	-Match animals: babies, homes -Sort items by color, shape, size -Sort vehicles that fly; go in water -Sort stories: characters, settings -Unload groceries into frig, freezer, pantry -Put toys away -Map items in a bedroom, bathroom, school, grocery store -Find items from grocery list -Create map for pretend zoo -Sort toys into containers and label -Plan a birthday party -Make home chore schedule
Evaluate, Compare and Contrast, Classification Parents ask questions to teach relationships - comparisons with similarities and differences; parents help determine categories, but understand children can have different categories, classifications	"How are these alike?" "How are these different?" "Can you find a way these belong together? and "Why?" *no categories presented (true classification) "What does not belong? Why not?" and "How are the others alike?" "What would we need for…?"	-Compare clothing of children (pockets, sleeves, zippers) -motorcycle and bicycle? -Compare 3 Little Pigs and 3 Bears -Classify animals: how they move, where they live, attributes -in toolbox? backpack? suitcase? -Estimate shopping cart or basket needed for shopping list
Analyzing/Problem Solving Parents ask questions to engage child in solving problems	"What should we do?" "What do we need?" "How could they help…?" "What could we use to …?" "What's wrong?"	-to find Mom when lost? -when the car won't start? -if the milk carton is empty? -if the tire on the bike is flat? -if holiday lights are too short? -when it is too cold in the house? - if no electricity at school? -if the shoes are too small ? -calm the baby down? -get the ball on the roof? -set table and leave off forks; put baseball in lunchbox
Applying/Inference Parents ask questions and help child use partial information to form generalizations or conclusions	"What would you find in a …" "What do we need to make a …" "How would ___ feel if…" "What do we need to …?" "What will we see when …?" "Where would I go to…?" "How will you…?" "Why did he say ___?"	- refrigerator? garage? purse? - pizza? cookies? birthday party? pretend flower shop? shoe store? - someone took his lunch? her brother broke her favorite doll? - act out this story?, fix our dinner? - we go on our walk in our neighborhood? go to the pond? - buy Mom a present? borrow a book, purchase some groceries? adopt a pet? - take care of new pet?, earn money for Dad's gift? -"Get out of the house!"?, "I'm tired"?, "I need help!"?
Understand/Prediction Parents ask questions and use everyday activities and books to help child understand future events	"What would happen if…" "What might happen?" "What might happen next?" (using events and books – ask before turning page) "How will the story end?"	-you got lost while shopping? - the car was locked with keys inside? - you left caps off the markers? - I forgot to water plants? - you get a cavity in your tooth? - you mail a letter without a stamp? - Predict items - sink or float?

| Knowing/Sequencing
Parents ask questions to help child put logical steps of an event together; prompt describing and naming | "Can you put these in order?"<br>"Which one happened first?" "Which one happened last?"<br>"What should I do next?"<br>"What's missing?"<br>"What do you see?" | -Sequence pictures: plant seeds, make sandwich, brush teeth
-Tell how to carve a pumpkin, wash the car, organize a party
- with baking, making bed, clearing table, helping with laundry
-House: door, chimney, window, doorknob, doorbell, porch
-Part to whole: show partial pictures (horn, paw, whiskers) |
| Evaluation
Parents prompt child to think and discuss a story or experience | "What did you think about…?"<br>"What did you like about…?"<br>"What important lesson can we learn from…?"<br>"What could we have done differently?" | -field trip? visit to Grandpa's farm?
-birthday party? park? story? new pet?
- story? hurt feelings? lost homework? |

Resource 6.3: Sample Speech-Language Evaluation/Functional Listening Assessment: Preschool Case (see Chapter 6)

Resource 6.4: Sample Speech-Language Evaluation/Functional Listening Assessment: School-Aged Case (see Chapter 6)

Resource 6.5: Assessments to identify possible gaps in language and cognitive skills for students with hearing loss (ages 6+):

Resource 6.1: Classification of Auditory Responses

Auditory Process	Underlying Skill	Auditory Demand
Detection	Presence or absence of sound	Auditory awareness Auditory attention Distance listening Localization
Discrimination	Distinguishes between two or more sounds	Change vs. No Change Same vs. Different
Identification	Recognition of what is heard and is able to repeat it back	Auditory association Auditory analysis Sound-blending Sequential memory
Comprehension	Demonstrates understanding and able to act on what is said	Auditory processing Auditory comprehension Auditory closure

Resource 6.2: Informal Auditory Checklist

Detection	Sampling task: While visually attentive to parent and/or while actively engaged, noisemakers and speech will be introduced to assess detection level responses	
Noisemakers	Loud	Soft
Clacker or Banging on drum (low)	__ of 3	__ of 3
Musical Toy (Mid)	__ of 3	__ of 3
Bell or Squeaky toy (High)	__ of 3	__ of 3
Discrimination		
Duration	Sampling task: Pushing a vehicle, spinning a toy, shaking a scarf or burp cloth in prolong vs. short durational patterns, while producing the low-frequency vowel "ah"	
Intensity	Sampling task: Can determine from response to above detection level noisemakers	
Syllable Number	Sampling task: Shaking burp cloth/scarf or bouncing the child or a stuffed animal in accordance with varying syllabic patterns, while producing the syllabic sequence "bah"	

Ling Vowels	ah, ee, oo Sampling Task: Observe any change in ongoing behavior indicative of detection of these vowel sounds when presented from both the right and left side. For older infants and toddlers, may elicit imitation of these vowels, suggesting identification level response.
Ling Consonants	sh, s, m Sampling Task: Observe any change in ongoing behavior indicative of detection of these consonant sounds when presented from both the right and left side. For older infants and toddlers, may elicit imitation of these vowels, suggesting identification level response.
Sustained Attention	Sampling Task: Observe and comment about visual attention to speakers and toy manipulation as well as to the environment in general
Localization	Sampling Task: Observe any searching behaviors for the sound source
Onset of voicing	Sampling Task: Pretend play with a stuffed animal and a blanket or burp cloth. Pretend to rock and put the stuffed animal to sleep. Cover the toy and wait a bit before moving your mouth with reduplicated pattern of "bah-bah-bah"(without voicing), then add voicing while simultaneously removing the blanket. Sample 3 times. Confirm the consistency of response to the onset of voicing with responsiveness observed during the assessment when baby is talked to.
Conditioned Response	Sampling Task: Observe and comment on whether the child has a "listen and drop" response; can hold a toy and wait for a speech stimuli before making a response (like putting cookies into the mouth of a Cookie Monster toy in response to Ling sounds or "yum-yum".

- The Listening Comprehension Test-2/The Listening Comprehension Test Adolescent, which assesses main ideas, details, reasoning, vocabulary and understanding messages
- The Test of Problem Solving 3, which assesses inference, problem solving, prediction, negative questions, and sequencing.
- Both assessments are normed on hearing peers and provide the clinician with a good amount of information regarding how the child with hearing loss is utilizing his/her auditory skills, language and cognitive skills.

Resource 6.6: Functional Listening Checklists and Assessments:

- LittlEARS Auditory Questionnaire can be completed at www.medel.com/en-us/about-hearing/hearing-test/little-ears-auditory-questionnaire
- Parent Evaluation of Aural/Oral Performance in Children (PEACH), retrievable from www.outcomes.nal.gov.au/_files/ugd/13b4ea_5e0d3bfed263472d9638dcfab76aa34d.pdf
- Parent Evaluation of Aural/Oral Performance in Children+ (PEACH+), retrievable from www.outcomes.nal.gov.au/_files/ugd/13b4ea_5b3eb01864cb4822960ab4fe6e9f8d37.pdf
- Teacher Evaluation of Aural/Oral Performance in Children (TEACH), retrievable from https://uw-ctu.org/wp-content/uploads/2020/05/teach.pdf
- Children's Auditory Performance Scale (CHAPS), retrievable from www.phonakpro.com/content/dam/phonakpro/gc_hq/en/resources/counseling_tools/documents/child_hearing_assessment_childrens_auditory_performance_scale_chaps_2017.pdf
- Functional Auditory Performance Indicators (FAPI), retrievable from www.phonakpro.com/content/dam/phonakpro/gc_hq/en/resources/counseling_tools/documents/child_hearing_assessment_functional_auditory_performance_indicators_fapi-V1.10.pdf
- Listening Inventory for Education—Revised (LIFE-R), retrievable from https://successforkidswithhearingloss.com/wp-content/uploads/2011/08/LIFE-R.pdf

LMH (Ling-Madell-Hewitt or Low, Mid, High) Test Battery: See Resource 3.2

Section 3: Building the First Floor

Chapter 7: Babies and Beginners: Starting with Nothing and Building up to Words

Resource 7.1: Auditory Learning Guide in English by Beth Walker Wooten (2008) (see **Fig. 22.3**)

Resource 7.2: Auditory Learning Guide in Spanish by Beth Walker Wooten (2009) (see **Fig. 22.4**)

Resource 7.3: Revised CAP (Categories of Auditory Perception) Scales and Integrated Scales of Development, retrievable from adipcochlearimplant.in/ADIP_PDF/CAP%20and%20ISD%20scales.pdf

Resource 7.4: Early Listening Function (ELF), retrievable from https://successforkidswithhearingloss.com/wp-content/uploads/2011/08/ELF-Oticon- version.pdf

Resource 7.5: Current Level of Functioning (CLF)—Pre-Verbal by Cheryl Dickson, adapted by Elizabeth Tippette (see **Fig. 22.5**)

Resource 7.6: Current Level of Functioning (CLF)—Verbal by Cheryl Dickson, adapted by Elizabeth Tippette (see **Fig. 22.6**)

Resource 7.7: Expectations of Skill Development for HA & CI Users by Jane Madell, Joan Hewitt, and Sylvia Rotfleisch (2018) (see **Fig. 22.7**)

Developed for FIRST YEARS (http://firstyears.org/) - Listening Spoken Language Development Intervention
© Beth Walker, 2009

Auditory Learning Guide

SOUND AWARENESS (Speech and Environmental Sounds)	PHONEME LEVEL** (Speech Babble)	DISCOURSE LEVEL (Auditory Processing of Connected Speech)	SENTENCE LEVEL	WORD LEVEL
Step 1 - Detect* the presence of any speech syllable.	**Step 1** - Imitate physical actions (before speech imitations).	**Step 1a** - Imitate motions of nursery rhymes/songs with accompanying vocalization.	**Step 1** - Identify familiar stereotypic phrases or sentences.	**Step 1a** - Identify and imitate approximations of "Learning To Listen" sounds varying in suprasegmentals and vowel content. e.g., (a-a-a)/*airplane*, (u)-(u)/*train*, (oi) (oi) *pig* in isolation, at the end, and then in the middle of a sentence.
Step 2 - Detect* vowel variety, [u] [a] [i] and raspberries [b-r-r]	**Step 2** - Imitate any phoneme that child produces spontaneously when given hand cue (or other cue).	**Step 1b** - Identify nursery rhymes or songs.	**Step 2** - Recall two critical elements in a message.	**Step 1b** - Identify one, two, and three syllable words in isolation, e.g., *cat* vs. *chicken* vs. *kangaroo*.
Step 3 - Detect* consonant variety, e.g., [m-m-m], [b^] [b^] [b^] and [wa] [wa]	**Step 3** - Imitate varying suprasegmental qualities in phonemes (vary intensity, duration, and pitch) aeeee (long) vs [ae ae] (pulsed); [ae-ae] loud/quiet/whispered; [ae] high/mid/low pitch.	**Step 2** - Answer common questions with abundant contextual support, e.g., "What's that?", "Where's mama?", "What is ________doing?"	**Step 3** - Recall three critical elements in a message.	**Step 2** - Identify words having the same number of syllables but different vowels/diphthongs and consonants, e.g., *horse* vs. *cow* vs. *sheep*.
Step 4 - Detect* the presence of environmental sounds at loud, medium, and soft levels at close range, at a distance of 6-12 ft. and at a distance of greater than 12 ft.	**Step 4** - Imitate vowel and diphthong variety, e.g., [u], [ae], [au], [i], etc.	**Step 3** - Identify a picture that corresponds to a story phrase in a three or four scene-story.	**Step 4** - Complete known linguistic messages from a closed set (ex: nursery rhymes, songs, familiar stories).	**Step 3a** - Identify words in which the ***initial*** consonants are the same but the vowels and final consonants are different, e.g., *ball* vs. *bike*.
Step 5 - Detect* whispered [hae] [hae] and [p] [p] [p]	**Step 5** - Imitate alternated vowels and diphthongs, e.g., [a-u] [e-i] [a-i]	**Step 4** - Identify an object from several related descriptors (closed set).	**Step 5** - Answer common questions about a disclosed and familiar topic: a) without pictorial cues b) over the telephone c) on audio/video-	**Step 3b** - Identify words in which the ***final*** consonants are the same but the vowels and initial consonants are different, e.g., *food* vs. *card*.
Step 6 - Detect* the sounds of the Six Sound Test.	**Step 6** - Imitate consonants varying in manner (fricatives, nasals, and plosives). Use phonemes previously produced, e.g., /h/ vs. /m-m-m/ vs. /p/	**Step 5** - Follow a conversation with the topic disclosed.	**Step 6** - Recall four or more critical elements in a message to follow multiple element directions.	**Step 4** - Identify words in which the initial and final consonants are identical but the vowels/diphthongs are different, e.g., *book* vs. *back*.
Step 7 – Detect* the sounds of the Six Sound Test at various distances.	**Step 7** - Imitate consonants differing in voiced vs. unvoiced cues, e.g., [b^] [b^] vs. [p] [p] and then with vowel variety, [bobo]	**Step 6a** - Answer questions about a story with the topic disclosed.	**Step 7** - Complete known linguistic messages (open set).	**Step 5a** - Identify words in which the vowels & final consonants are identical but the ***initial*** consonants differ by three features - manner, place of articulation, and voicing, e.g., *mouse* vs. *house*.
Step 8 – Locate the direction of sound if amplified binaurally.	**Step 8** - Alternate consonants varying in place cues, first with varying vowels, e.g., /ma-ma/ /no-no/; /go-go/ bi-bi/, etc.	**Step 6b** - Answer questions about a story with the topic disclosed; story is teacher-recorded.	**Step 8** - Follow open set directions and instructions (disclosed).	**Step 5b** - Identify words in which the vowels & initial consonants are identical but the ***final*** consonants differ by three features - manner, place of articulation, and voicing.
	Step 9 - Alternate syllables with varying consonants and same vowel, e.g., [bi], [di], [ho] [go]	**Step 7** - Recall details of a story (topic disclosed).	**Step 9** - Recall specific elements in a sentence by answering questions about an undisclosed but familiar topic.	**Step 6** - Identify words in which the vowels and the final/initial consonants are identical but the initial/final consonants differ by two features: (a) manner and place (voicing in common), *moat* vs. *goat*; (b) manner and voicing (place in common), *man* vs. *pan*; (c) place and voicing (manner in common), *boat* vs. *coat*.
		Step 8 - Sequence the events of a story (topic disclosed)	**Step 10** - Repeat each word in a sentence exactly. a.) predictable sentences "I'm going to the grocery store to buy cereal and milk." b.) less predictable sentences "A woman hit me so I told her to calm down."	**Step 7a** - Identify words in which the vowels and final consonants are identical but the ***initial*** consonants differ by only one feature - manner of articulation, e.g., *ball* vs. *mall*.
		Step 9 - Retell a story with the topic disclosed, recalling all the details in sequence.	**Step 11** - Recall specific elements in a sentence by answering questions on an undisclosed topic.	**Step 7b** - Identify words in which the vowels and initial consonants are identical but the *final* consonants differ by only one feature - manner of articulation, e.g., *cloud* vs.
		Step 10 - Make identification based on several related descriptors (open set).		**Step 8a** - Identify words in which the vowels and final consonants are identical but the ***initial*** consonants differ by only one feature - voicing, e.g., *coat* vs. *goat*.
		Step 11 - Follow a conversation of an undisclosed topic.		**Step 8b** - Identify words in which the vowels and initial consonants are identical but the ***final*** consonants differ by only one feature - voicing, e.g., *bag* vs. *back*.
		Step 12 - Retell a story about an undisclosed topic, recalling as many details as possible.		**Step 9a** - Identify words in which the vowels and final consonants are identical but the initial consonants differ by only one feature - place of articulation, e.g. *bun* vs. *gun*.
		Step 13 - Process information in noise and at various distances.		**Step 9b** - Identify words in which the vowels and initial consonants are identical but the ***final*** consonants differ by only one feature- place of articulation, e.g. *sheep* vs. *sheet*.
		Step 14 - Process group conversations		

The color codes in the chart designate auditory behaviors to be mastered by the end of the specified year, given optimally fitted hearing devices.

KEY
YEAR 1
YEAR 2
YEAR 3
YEAR 4

This guide is intended to aid professionals in the *beginning* stages of learning an auditory-based approach. As professionals acquire more experience in auditory teaching, children should progress more rapidly.

The information on this chart was adapted from Judy Simser's article in the *Volta Review* (1993) (** items), from the Auditory Skills Program, New South Wales Department of School Education, from the Foreworks Auditory Skills Curriculum (1976, North Hollywood, CA), and from teacher input.

Notes:
* A detection response could include turning head, pointing to ear, clapping, dropping a toy in a container, etc.

Reference:
Simser, J.I. (1993). Auditory-verbal intervention: Infants and toddlers. *Volta Review* 95(3): 217-229.

revised: 4/3/09

Fig. 22.3 Auditory Learning Guide in English by Beth Walker Wooten (2008).

Resources for individuals and families dealing with hearing loss: See Resource 1.1

Suggestions for improving hearing aid and cochlear implant retention: See Resource 2.2

LMH (Ling-Madell-Hewitt or Low, Mid, High) Test Battery: See Resource 3.2

Resources to aid parent coaching and creation of a language-rich environment: See Resource 5.1

Functional Listening Checklists and Assessments: See Resource 6.6

Resources for additional learning on LSL Strategies: See Resource 10.1

Video examples of LSL strategies: See Resource 10.2

Recommended sources for children's books: See Resource 13.3

Children Who Are Deaf or Hard of Hearing with Additional Learning Needs by Susan Wiley: See Resource 15.1

Suggested websites for children with hearing loss and additional needs: See Resource 15.2

Recommended websites for planning and education: See Resource 16.1

Suggested Roles of Educational Audiologists, Teachers of the Deaf and Hard of Hearing, and Speech-Language Pathologists (2018): See Resource 16.2

Resources for parents and clinicians to encourage integrating music in intervention: See Resource 19.1

Chapter 8: Toddler-Type Language: Putting Words Together and Moving up to Simple Sentences

Resources for individuals and families dealing with hearing loss: See Resource 1.1

Suggestions for improving hearing aid and cochlear implant retention: See Resource 2.2

LMH (Ling-Madell-Hewitt or Low, Mid, High) Test Battery: See Resource 3.2

Resources to aid parent coaching and creation of a language-rich environment: See Resource 5.1

Coaching parents to use cognitive questions: See Resource 5.2

Functional Listening Checklists and Assessments: See Resource 6.6

Auditory Learning Guide in English: See Resource 7.1

HEARING FIRST
Powering Potential

Guía del Aprendizaje Auditivo

CONCIENCIA DEL SONIDO (Sonidos del Habla y Ambiente)	NIVEL DEL FONEMA** (Balbuceo del Habla)	NIVEL DE DISCURSO (Procesamiento Auditivo del Habla Conectada)	NIVEL DE ORACIÓN	NIVEL DE PALABRA
Paso 1 - Detectar * la presencia de cualquier sílaba de habla.	**Paso 1** - Imitar acciones físicas (antes de imitaciones del habla).	**Paso 1a** - Imitar movimientos de rimas / canciones infantiles acompañadas de vocalización.	**Paso 1** - Identificar frases o oraciones estereotípicas familiares	**Paso 1a** - - Identificar e imitar las aproximaciones de los sonidos "Aprendiendo a Escuchar" variando en suprasegmentales y vocales, por ejemplo, (a-a-a) / *avión*, (u) - (u) / *tren*, (oi) (oi) / cerdo en aislamiento, al final, y luego en medio de una oración.
Paso 2 - Detectar * variedad de vocales, [u][a] [i] y las pedorretas	**Paso 2** - Imitar cualquier fonema que el niño produzca espontáneamente cuando se le da una señal manual (u otra señal).	**Paso 1b** - Identificar rimas infantiles o canciones	**Paso 2** - Recordar dos elementos críticos en un mensaje.	**Paso 1b** - Identificar palabras de una, dos y tres sílabas aisladas, por ejemplo, *pan vs. pollo vs. canguro.*
Paso 3 - Detectar la variedad de consonantes, por ejemplo, [m-m-m], [b ^] [b^] [b ^] y [wa] [wa].	**Paso 3** - Imitar diferentes cualidades suprasegmentales en fonemas (variar intensidad, duración y tono) aeeee (largo) vs [ae ae] (pulsado); [ae-ae] fuerte / silencioso / susurrado; [Ae] alto / medio / bajo paso.	**Paso 2** - Responder preguntas comunes con abundante apoyo contextual, por ejemplo, "¿Qué es eso?", "¿Dónde está mamá?", "¿Qué está haciendo?"	**Paso 3** - Recordar tres elementos críticos en un mensaje.	**Paso 2** - Identificar palabras que tengan el mismo número de sílabas pero diferentes vocales / diptongos y consonantes, por ejemplo, *caballo vs. sandia vs. oveja.*
Paso 4 - Detectar * la presencia de sonidos ambientales a niveles altos, medios y bajos a corta distancia, a una distancia de 6-12 pies y a una distancia mayor de 12 pies.	**Paso 4** - Imitar las vocales y la variedad de diptongos, por ejemplo, [u], [ae], [au], [i], etc.	**Paso 3** - Identificar una imagen que corresponda a una frase en una historia de tres o cuatro escenas.	**Paso 4** - Completar los mensajes lingüísticos conocidos de un conjunto cerrado (por ejemplo: canciones infantiles, canciones, historias familiares).	**Paso 3a** - Identificar palabras en las que las consonantes **iniciales** son las mismas, pero las vocales y las consonantes finales son diferentes, por ejemplo, *bola vs. bici.*
Paso 5 - Detectar * susurró [je] [je] y [p] [p] [p].	**Paso 5** - Imitar vocales y diptongos alternados, por ejemplo, [a-u] [e-i] [a-i].	**Paso 4** - Identificar un objeto de varios descriptores relacionados (conjunto cerrado).	**Paso 5** - Responder a preguntas comunes sobre un tema divulgado y familiar: a) sin señales pictóricas b) por teléfono c) en audio / video.	**Paso 3b** - Identificar palabras en las que las consonantes **finales** son las mismas pero las vocales y las consonantes iniciales son diferentes, por ejemplo, *miror vs. tomar.*
Paso 6 - Detectar * los sonidos de la Prueba de Seis Sonidos.	**Paso 6** - Imitar consonantes que varían en forma (fricativas, nasales y plosivas). Utilizar fonemas producidos previamente, por ejemplo, / h / vs / m- m-m / vs / p /.	**Paso 5** - Seguir una conversación con el tema revelado.	**Paso 6** - Recordar cuatro o más elementos críticos en un mensaje para seguir direcciones de múltiples elementos.	**Paso 4** - Identificar palabras en las que las consonantes iniciales y finales son idénticas, pero las vocales / diptongas son diferentes, por ejemplo, *pan vs. pon.*
Paso 7 - Detectar * los sonidos de la Prueba de Seis Sonidos a varias distancias.	**Paso 7** - Imitate consonants differing in voiced vs. unvoiced cues, e.g., [b^] [b^] vs. [p] [p] and then with vowel variety, [bobo] [pae-pae].	**Paso 6a** - Responder a preguntas sobre una historia con el tema revelado.	**Paso 7** - Completar los mensajes lingüísticos conocidos (abierto).	**Paso 5a** - Identificar palabras en las que las vocales y las consonantes finales son **idénticas**, pero las consonantes iniciales se diferencian por tres características: forma, lugar de articulación y expresión, por ejemplo, *ratón vs. botón.*
Paso 8 - Localice la dirección del sonido si se amplifica de manera binaural.	**Paso 8** - Las consonantes alternativas varían en lugar de las señales, primero con vocales variables, por ejemplo, / ma ma / / no no /: / go go / / bi bi /.	**Paso 6b** - Responder preguntas sobre una historia con el tema revelado; La historia está registrada por el maestro.	**Paso 8** - Seguir las instrucciones e instrucciones del juego abierto (divulgadas).	**Paso 5b** - Identificar palabras en las que las vocales y las consonantes iniciales son idénticas, pero las consonantes **finales** difieren por tres características: forma, lugar de articulación y expresión, por ejemplo, *conoces vs. conocen*
	Paso 9 - Sílabas alternativas con consonantes variables y la misma vocal, por ejemplo, [bi], [di], [ho], [go].	**Paso 7** - Recordar los detalles de una historia (tema revelado).	**Paso 9** - Recordar elementos específicos de una oración respondiendo preguntas sobre un tema no revelado pero familiar.	**Paso 6** - Identificar palabras en las que las vocales y las consonantes finales / iniciales son idénticas, pero las consonantes iniciales / finales difieren por dos rasgos: a) manera y lugar (expresión en común), *bote vs. elote*; b) la manera y la entonación (lugar en común), *von vs. pon*; c) lugar y entonación (manera en común), *correr vs. barrer*
		Paso 8 - Secuencia de los eventos de una historia (tema divulgado).	**Paso 10** - Repetir cada palabra en una oración exactamente. a) frases previsibles "Voy a la tienda de comestibles a comprar cereales y leche" b) frases menos previsibles "Una mujer me golpeó así que le dije que se tranquilizara."	**Paso 7a** - Identificar las palabras en las que las vocales y las consonantes finales son idénticas, pero las consonantes **iniciales** difieren por una sola característica: modo de articulación, por ejemplo, *mar vs. bar.*
		Paso 9 - Repetir una historia con el tema revelado, recordando todos los detalles en secuencia.	**Paso 11** - Recordar elementos específicos en una oración al responder preguntas sobre un tema no revelado.	**Paso 7b** - Identificar palabras en las que las vocales y las consonantes iniciales son idénticas, pero las consonantes **finales** difieren por una sola característica: modo de articulación, por ejemplo *paren vs. pored*
		Paso 10 - Hacer la identificación basada en varios descriptores relacionados (conjunto abierto).		**Paso 8a** - Identificar palabras en las que las vocales y las consonantes finales son idénticas, pero las consonantes **iniciales** difieren por sólo una característica - entonación, por ejemplo, *paso vs. baso*
		Paso 11 - Seguir una conversación de un tema no revelado.		**Paso 8b** - Identificar palabras en las que las vocales y las consonantes iniciales son idénticas, pero las consonantes **finales** difieren por sólo una característica - entonación, por ejemplo, "*vivas vs. vivaz*"
		Paso 12 - Revelar una historia sobre un tema no revelado, recordando tantos detalles como sea posible.		**Paso 9a** - Identificar palabras en las que las vocales y las consonantes finales son idénticas, pero las consonantes **iniciales** difieren sólo por una característica - lugar de articulación, por ejemplo, *paso vs. caso*
		Paso 13 - Procesar la información en ruido ya varias distancias.		**Paso 9b** - Identificar palabras en las que las vocales y las consonantes iniciales son idénticas, pero las consonantes **finales** difieren sólo por una característica - lugar de articulación, por ejemplo, *pop vs. pot (en Inglés)*
		Paso 14 - Procesar conversaciones de grupo.		

CLAVE

Año 1 / Año 2 / Año 3 / Año 4 — Los códigos de colores en el gráfico designan los comportamientos auditivos que se dominarán al final del año especificado, si se otorgan los aparatos auditivos apropiados.

Esta guía pretende ayudar a los profesionales en las etapas *iniciales* del aprendizaje de un enfoque basado en la audición. A medida que los profesionales adquieren más experiencia en la enseñanza auditiva, los niños deben progresar más rápidamente.

La información en esta gráfica fue adaptada del artículo de Judy Simser en *Volta Review* (1993) (** elementos), del Programa de Habilidades Auditivas del Departamento de Educación Escolar de Nueva Gales del Sur, del Currículo de Destrezas Auditivas de Foreworks (1976, North Hollywood, CA), y del aporte del maestro.

Notas:
* Una respuesta de detección podría incluir girar la cabeza, apuntando a la oreja, aplaudiendo, dejando caer un juguete en un contenedor, etc.

Referencia:
Simser, J.I. (1993). Auditory-verbal intervention: Infants and toddlers. Volta Review 95(3): 217-229.

Reconocimiento:
Desarrollado originalmente para First *YEARS*, un programa de capacitación para profesionales de la audición y el lenguaje hablado desarrollado en asociación y ofrecido por la Universidad de Carolina del Norte en Chapel Hill y la Alexander Graham Bell Asociación para Sordos y Personas con Dificultades Auditivas con fondos de la Fundación Oberkotter. © Beth Walker, 2009

Revisado el 15/09/16

Fig. 22.4 Auditory Learning Guide in Spanish by Beth Walker Wooten (2009).

Current Level of Functioning
Verbal

Name:	Date of Birth:	Chronological Age:	Today's Date:
Device:	Age at amplification:	Age at initial activation (if CI):	Duration in AVT:

Ling-Madell-Hewitt/Low-Mid-High (LMH) 10 Sound Test: **Hearing Loss:**

Detect:	Distance:	Degree/Configuration:
Identify:	Distance:	Etiology:
Imitate:	Distance:	Additional Condition(s):

Audition *[describe highest level of auditory memory, tracking of songs, questions understood, etc]:*

Audition Age:

Language:

Language Age:

Receptive Vocabulary:	
Expressive Vocabulary:	
MLU:	
Bloom & Lahey Phase or CASLLS Band:	

Speech Production: *[isolation, syllables, words (initial/medial/final), phrases; imitative, spontaneous]*

Speech Age:

Vowels & Diphthongs:		Level:
Consonants:		Level:
Intelligibility:		
Vocal Quality:		

General Development:

Fine Motor:		Gross Motor:	
Non-Verbal Cognition:		Language:	
Self Help:		Social Emotional:	

Concerns:

CLF Age (average of Audition, Language, and Speech ages above):	Therapist:

Cheryl L. Dickson, M.Ed., LSLS Cert. AVT, copyright pending ©
Adapted by Elizabeth Tippette, MSP, CCC-SLP, LSLS Cert. AVT; Used with permission.

Fig. 22.5 Current Level of Functioning (CLF)—Pre-Verbal by Cheryl Dickson, adapted by Elizabeth Tippette.

Current Level of Functioning
Verbal

Name:	Date of Birth:	Chronological Age:	Today's Date:
Device:	Age at amplification:	Age at initial activation (if CI):	Duration in AVT:

Ling-Madell-Hewitt/Low-Mid-High (LMH) 10 Sound Test: | **Hearing Loss:**

Detect:	Distance:	Degree/Configuration:
Identify:	Distance:	Etiology:
Imitate:	Distance:	Additional Condition(s):

Audition *[describe highest level of auditory memory, tracking of songs, questions understood, etc]:*

Audition Age:

Language:

Language Age:

Receptive Vocabulary:	
Expressive Vocabulary:	
MLU:	
Bloom & Lahey Phase or CASLLS Band:	

Speech Production: *[isolation, syllables, words (initial/medial/final), phrases; imitative, spontaneous]*

Speech Age:

Vowels & Diphthongs:		Level:
Consonants:		Level:
Intelligibility:		
Vocal Quality:		

General Development:

Fine Motor:		Gross Motor:	
Non-Verbal Cognition:		Language:	
Self Help:		Social Emotional:	

Concerns:

CLF Age (average of Audition, Language, and Speech ages above):	Therapist:

Cheryl L. Dickson, M.Ed., LSLS Cert. AVT, copyright pending ©
Adapted by Elizabeth Tippette, MSP, CCC-SLP, LSLS Cert. AVT; Used with permission.

Fig. 22.6 Current Level of Functioning (CLF)—Verbal by Cheryl Dickson, adapted by Elizabeth Tippette.

Children Who Are Deaf or Hard of Hearing with Additional Learning Needs by Susan Wiley: See Resource 15.1

Suggested websites for children with hearing loss and additional needs: See Resource 15.2

Recommended websites for planning and education: See Resource 16.1

Suggested Roles of Educational Audiologists, Teachers of the Deaf and Hard of Hearing, and Speech-Language Pathologists (2018): See Resource 16.2

Resources for parents and clinicians to encourage integrating music in intervention: See Resource 19.1

Chapter 9: Preschoolers and More Proficient Communicators: Using Complex Language to Communicate and Think

Resources for individuals and families dealing with hearing loss: See Resource 1.1

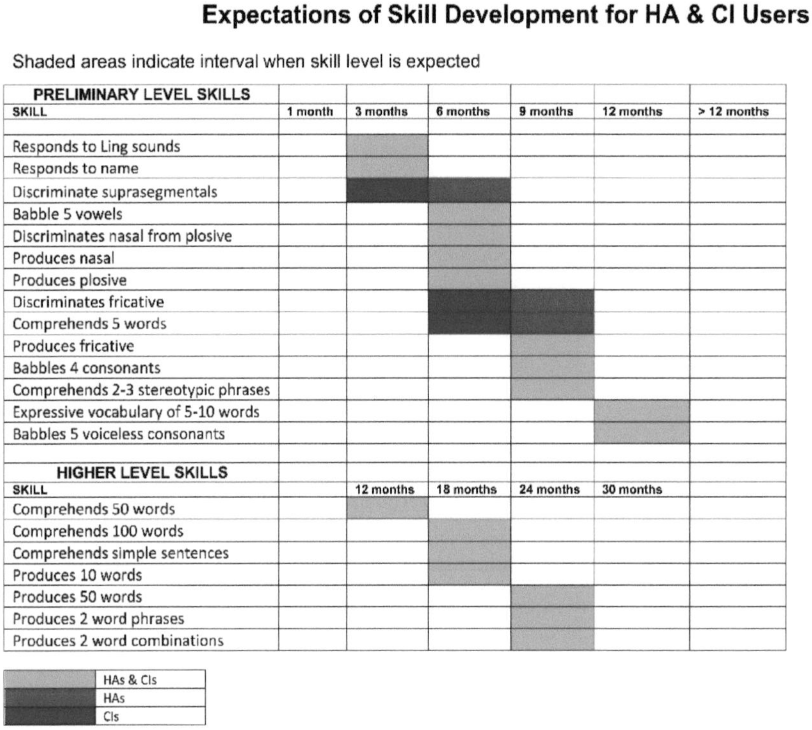

Expectations of Skill Development for HA & CI Users

Shaded areas indicate interval when skill level is expected

PRELIMINARY LEVEL SKILLS

SKILL	1 month	3 months	6 months	9 months	12 months	> 12 months
Responds to Ling sounds						
Responds to name						
Discriminate suprasegmentals						
Babble 5 vowels						
Discriminates nasal from plosive						
Produces nasal						
Produces plosive						
Discriminates fricative						
Comprehends 5 words						
Produces fricative						
Babbles 4 consonants						
Comprehends 2-3 stereotypic phrases						
Expressive vocabulary of 5-10 words						
Babbles 5 voiceless consonants						

HIGHER LEVEL SKILLS

SKILL	12 months	18 months	24 months	30 months
Comprehends 50 words				
Comprehends 100 words				
Comprehends simple sentences				
Produces 10 words				
Produces 50 words				
Produces 2 word phrases				
Produces 2 word combinations				

	HAs & CIs
	HAs
	CIs

Madell, J.R.; Hewitt, J. G, and Rotfleisch, S (2018) Chapter 25: Red Flags: Identifying and Managing Barriers to the Child's Optimal Auditory Development; in *Pediatric Audiology: Diagnosis, Technology and Management, 3rd Edition.* Thieme NY-Stuttgart

Fig. 22.7 Expectations of Skill Development for HA & CI Users by Jane Madell, Joan Hewitt, and Sylvia Rotfleisch (2018).

Suggestions for improving hearing aid and cochlear implant retention: See Resource 2.2

LMH (Ling-Madell-Hewitt or Low, Mid, High) Test Battery: See Resource 3.2

Resources to aid parent coaching and creation of a language-rich environment: See Resource 5.1

Coaching parents to use cognitive questions: See Resource 5.2

Assessments to identify possible gaps in language and cognitive skills for students with hearing loss (ages 6+): See Resource 6.5

Functional Listening Checklists and Assessments: See Resource 6.6

Auditory Learning Guide in English: See Resource 7.1

Auditory Learning Guide in Spanish: See Resource 7.2

Current Level of Functioning (CLF)—Verbal: See Resource 7.6

Resources for additional learning on LSL Strategies: See Resource 10.1

Video examples of LSL strategies: See Resource 10.2

Suggested Materials for Use in Integrated Executive Function, Speech-Language and Auditory-Verbal Intervention Activities: See Resources 12.1, 12.2, and 12.3

Recommended website for information on how children learn to read, why some struggle, and how adults can help: See Resource 13.2

Recommended sources for children's books: See Resource 13.3

Children Who Are Deaf or Hard of Hearing with Additional Learning Needs by Susan Wiley: See Resource 15.1

Suggested websites for children with hearing loss and additional needs: See Resource 15.2

Recommended websites for planning and education: See Resource 16.1

Suggested Roles of Educational Audiologists, Teachers of the Deaf and Hard of Hearing, and Speech-Language Pathologists (2018): See Resource 16.2

Resources for parents and clinicians to encourage integrating music in intervention: See Resource 19.1

Chapter 10: Auditory-Verbal Strategies to Build Listening and Spoken Language Skills

Resource 10.1: Resources for additional learning on LSL Strategies:

- AGBell Academy for Listening and Spoken Language Exam Blueprint
- AGBell Academy for Listening and Spoken Language Certification
- *Auditory Verbal Strategies to Build Listening and Spoken Language Skills* by Sherri Fickenscher and Elizabeth Gaffney. Retrievable from www.clarkeschools.org/AVstrategiesBook

- *Auditory-Verbal Therapy: Science, Research, and Practice* by Estabrooks, Morrison, & MacIver-Lux (2020). Chapter 15: Strategies for Developing Listening, Talking, and Thinking in Auditory-Verbal Therapy.
- Hearing First offers Learning Experiences specifically on LSL strategies; the catalog of Learning Experiences can be viewed at https://www.hearingfirst.org/learning-experiences
- Parent friendly handouts of LSL strategies: https://www.hearingfirst.org/what-to-do/strategies-techniques
- *Preparing to Teach, Committing to Learn: An Introduction to Educating Children Who Are Deaf/Hard of Hearing* by Lenihan (2020). Chapter 7: Listening and Spoken Language Strategies. Retrievable at: https://www.infanthearing.org/ebook-educating-children-dhh/chapters/7%20Chapter%207%202020.pdf

Resource 10.2: Video examples of LSL strategies can be viewed at the following websites:

- https://www.jtc.org/ideas-advice/video-tips/
- https://www.jtc.org/es/ideas-y-consejos/consejos-en-video/
- Welcome To Rehab At Home | The MED-EL Blog

Chapter 11: Late to the Party: When Children Come Late to Listening and Spoken Language Therapy

Resources for individuals and families dealing with hearing loss: See Resource 1.1

Suggestions for improving hearing aid and cochlear implant retention: See Resource 2.2

LMH (Ling-Madell-Hewitt or Low, Mid, High) Test Battery: See Resource 3.2

Resources to aid parent coaching and creation of a language-rich environment: See Resource 5.1

Coaching parents to use cognitive questions: See Resource 5.2

Assessments to identify possible gaps in language and cognitive skills for students with hearing loss (ages 6+): See Resource 6.5

Functional Listening Checklists and Assessments: See Resource 6.6

Auditory Learning Guide in English: See Resource 7.1

Auditory Learning Guide in Spanish: See Resource 7.2

Current Level of Functioning (CLF)—Pre-Verbal: See Resource 7.5

Current Level of Functioning (CLF)—Verbal: See Resource 7.6

Expectations of Skill Development for HA & CI Users by Jane Madell, Joan Hewitt, and Sylvia Rotfleisch (2018): See Resource 7.7

Resources for additional learning on LSL Strategies: See Resource 10.1

Video examples of LSL strategies: See Resource 10.2

Suggested Materials for Use in Integrated Executive Function, Speech-Language and Auditory-Verbal Intervention Activities: See Resources 12.1, 12.2, and 12.3

Recommended website for information on how children learn to read, why some struggle, and how adults can help: See Resource 13.2

Recommended sources for children's books: See Resource 13.3

Children Who Are Deaf or Hard of Hearing with Additional Learning Needs by Susan Wiley: See Resource 15.1

Suggested websites for children with hearing loss and additional needs: See Resource 15.2

Recommended websites for planning and education: See Resource 16.1

Suggested Roles of Educational Audiologists, Teachers of the Deaf and Hard of Hearing, and Speech-Language Pathologists (2018): See Resource 16.2

Resources for parents and clinicians to encourage integrating music in intervention: See Resource 19.1

Section 4: Adding the Second Floor

Chapter 12: Executive Function Therapy Integrated into Auditory-Verbal Practice

Resource 12.1 Suggested Materials for Use in Integrated Executive Function, Speech-Language and Auditory-Verbal Intervention Activities: Games and Toys

- *Blurt* (www.educationalinsights.com)
- *Bubble Talk—the Crazy Caption Boardgame* (www.technosourceusa.com)
- *Buzz Word and Buzz Word, Jr.* (www.patchproducts.com)
- *Chess* (www.wikihow.com/Play-Chess)
- *Concept* (Repos Production)
- *Dinkee Linkee for Kids* (bananagrams.com)
- *Fast 5* (www.educaborras.com)
- *Headbanz for Kids* (www.patchproducts.com)
- Learning Well board games: *Predicting Outcomes, Getting the Main Idea, Inference, Cause and Effect, Reading for Detail, Following Directions* (www.eaieducation.com)
- *Line Up—The memory game of quick looks and tricky crooks* (www.mindware.com)
- *Simon* electronic toys (www.hasbrogaming.hasbro.com)
- *Sloth in a Hurry—an Improv game* (www.eeboo.com)
- *Sort it Out!, Jr.* (www.universitygames.com)
- *Super Mind Pack: Negotiation Game, Word Planning Game* and others (de Bono, 1998, DK books)
- *Taboo* (www.hasbrogaming.hasbro.com)
- *Three for Me* (www.patchproducts.com)
- *Tribond* and *Tribond Kids* (www.patchproducts.com)
- *Watch This Face—An Emotional Literacy Activity* (www.eeboo.com)

Resource 12.2: Suggested Materials for Use in Integrated Executive Function, Speech-Language and Auditory-Verbal Intervention Activities: Books and suggested readings

- *Coaching Students with Executive Skills Deficits* (Dawson & Guare, 2012)
- *See Time Fly—Visualizing and Verbalizing History Stories* (Bell, 2001)
- *Smart but Scattered* (Dawson & Guare, 2009)

- *Smart but Scattered for Teens* (Guare, Dawson & Guare, 2013)
- *Social Explorers Curriculum* (Tarshis et al, 2016.)
- *Superflex—A Superhero Social Thinking Curriculum* (Madrigal & Garcia Winner, 2008)
- *Thinking about You Thinking about Me* (Garcia Winner, 2007)
- *Thinking for Action* games (de Bono, 1998; www.dk.com)
- *Visualizing and Verbalizing for Language Comprehension and Thinking* (Bell, 1991)

Resource 12.3: Suggested Materials for Use in Integrated Executive Function, Speech-Language and Auditory-Verbal Intervention Activities: Additional suggestions

- *642 Things to Write About—Young Writer's Edition* (www. chroniclebooks.com)
- Graphic Organizers (downloadable online or found in *Graphic Organizers* (www.teacgercreated.com)
- Joke books, including knock-knock jokes, puns, play on words, double meanings
- *Six-Way Paragraphs* (Pauk, 2000)
- *Specific Skill Series,* including *Main Idea, Drawing Conclusions, Using the Context* and others.
- *The Expressionary—The Ultimate Dictionary Companion for Idioms, Everyday Phrases and Proverbs* Schmidek, M. (2003) (www.acadcom.com)
- *Time Tracker* visual timer and clock (www.learningresources. com)

Chapter 13: The Auditory-Verbal Approach and Literacy

Resource 13.1: Recommended Readings

- Fox, M. (2008). *Reading Magic: Why Reading Aloud to Our Children Will Change Their Lives Forever.* Orlando, FL: Houghton Mifflin Harcourt.
- Trelease, J. (2019). *The Read-Aloud Handbook* (8th edition). New York: Penguin.
- Ozma, A. (2011). *The Reading Promise: My Father and the Books We Shared.* New York: Hatchette Book Group.
- Yopp, R. & Yopp, H. (2014). Literature-Based Reading Activities: Engaging Students with Literary and Informational Text (6th edition). Boston: Pearson.

Resource 13.2 Recommended website for information on how children learn to read, why some struggle, and how adults can help: Reading Rockets https://www.readingrockets.org

Reading Rockets is a national public media literacy initiative offering information and resources on how young kids learn to read, why so many struggle, and how caring adults can help.

Resource 13.3: Recommended Sources for Children's Books

- Children's Book Awards: https://www.infosoup.info/kids/ awards-home: This site lists awards given by the American Library Association (ALA) and other organizations

- Children's Books and Authors: https://www.readingrockets. org/books

Chapter 15: Children with Special Needs and Additional Disabilities

Resource 15.1: Children Who Are Deaf or Hard of Hearing with Additional Learning Needs, by Susan Wiley, Retrievable from https://www.aucd.org/docs/Reading%201%20(Wiley).pdf

Resource 15.2: Suggested websites for children with hearing loss and additional needs:

- Hearing Loss PLUS Additional Disability(ies): https:// successforkidswithhearingloss.com/hearing-loss-plus-additional-disabilityies/
- Deaf Students with Disabilities: https://clerccenter. gallaudet.edu/national-resources/info/info-to-go/deaf-students-with-disabilities.html
- Communication Considerations: Deaf Plus: https:// handsandvoices.org/comcon/articles/deafplus.htm

Resources for individuals and families dealing with hearing loss: See Resource 1.1

Suggestions for improving hearing aid and cochlear implant retention: See Resource 2.2

LMH (Ling-Madell-Hewitt or Low, Mid, High) Test Battery: See Resource 3.2

Resources to aid parent coaching and creation of a language-rich environment: See Resource 5.1

Coaching parents to use cognitive questions: See Resource 5.2

Assessments to identify possible gaps in language and cognitive skills for students with hearing loss (ages 6+): See Resource 6.5

Functional Listening Checklists and Assessments: See Resource 6.6

Auditory Learning Guide in English: See Resource 7.1

Auditory Learning Guide in Spanish: See Resource 7.2

Current Level of Functioning (CLF)—Verbal: See Resource 7.6

Resources for additional learning on LSL Strategies: See Resource 10.1

Video examples of LSL strategies: See Resource 10.2

Suggested Materials for Use in Integrated Executive Function, Speech-Language and Auditory-Verbal Intervention Activities: See Resources 12.1, 12.2, and 12.3

Recommended website for information on how children learn to read, why some struggle, and how adults can help: See Resource 13.2

Recommended sources for children's books: See Resource 13.3

Recommended websites for planning and education: See Resource 16.1

Suggested Roles of Educational Audiologists, Teachers of the Deaf and Hard of Hearing, and Speech-Language Pathologists (2018): See Resource 16.2

Resources for parents and clinicians to encourage integrating music in intervention: See Resource 19.1

Chapter 16: Supporting Learners Who Are Deaf or Hard of Hearing (DHH) in the Educational Setting

Resource 16.1: Recommended websites for planning and education

- IEP Checklist—Recommended Accommodations, Hands & Voices: https://www.handsandvoices.org/pdf/IEP_Checklist.pdf

- Our Children Safety Project—Parent ToolKit, Hands & Voices: https://www.handsandvoices.org/pdf/OUR-Toolkit.pdf
- Protecting learners who are DHH from bullying:
  - https://www.kidpower.org/bullying/
  - www.cartoonnetwork.com/promos/stopbullying/index.html
  - www.StopBullying.gov
  - www.pacer.org/bullying
  - http://www.abilitypath.org/areas-of-development/learning-schools/bullying/

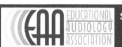

Supporting Students who are Deaf and Hard of Hearing: Shared and Suggested Roles of Educational Audiologists, Teachers of the Deaf and Hard of Hearing, and Speech-Language Pathologists

(Approved by the Board of Directors of the Educational Audiology Association February 2018)

Educational audiologists, teachers of the deaf and hard of hearing, and speech-language pathologists are critical partners on the school education team. Together, they address the needs of students who are deaf and hard of hearing and promote language and communication access that is essential for participation and learning in today's educational environments. The Individuals with Disabilities Education Act (IDEA), Section 504 of the Rehabilitation Act, and the Americans with Disabilities Act (ADA) all contain regulations pertinent to the services and accommodations contained in this guidance document.

Language and Communication Regulations (Title II and IDEA)

Title II of the ADA includes the following requirements for schools:

- Communication for students who are deaf and hard of hearing must be "as effective as communication for others" [ADA Title II 28 C.F.R. §35.160 (a)(1)].

- Provision of appropriate aids and services "affording an equal opportunity to obtain the same result, to gain the same benefit, or to reach the same level of achievement as that provided to others" [ADA Title II 28 C.F.R. §35.130 (b)(1)(iii)].

- Students who are deaf and hard of hearing should be able to participate in and enjoy the benefits of the district's services, programs, and activities" (DOJ-DOE p14)[1].

- These requirements apply to all school-related communications, and when a public school is deciding what types of auxiliary aids and services are necessary to ensure effective communication, it must give "primary consideration" to the particular auxiliary aid or service requested by the person with the disability. (DOJ-DOE p27).

IDEA (2004) "Special Factors" regulations specify that schools must provide the following supports for students who are deaf or hard of hearing [34 C.F.R. §300.324(a)(2)(iv)]:

- Opportunities for direct communication with peers in the student's language and communication mode.

- Opportunities for direct communication with professional personnel in the student's language and communication mode.

- Opportunities for direct instruction in student's language and communication mode.

IDEA (2004) also requires:

- Routine checking of hearing aids and external components of surgically implanted medical devices to ensure they are functioning properly [34 C.F.R. §300.113(a)(b)(1)]

- Audiology Services [34 C.F.R.§300.34(c)(1)]

- SLP Services [34 C.F.R.§300.34(c)(1)]

- Assistive Technology Devices and Services [34 C.F.R.§300.34(c)(15)]

- Highly Qualified Special Education Teachers [34 C.F.R.§300.18]

To assist schools in meeting the language and communication requirements above, the following checklist describes supports to be considered for each student who is deaf or hard of hearing and those with other auditory learning needs. This checklist was developed and field-tested with input from all three professional groups via focus group meetings and online surveys. Categories are described as "student assurances" with activities and expected outcomes that should be addressed by the student's team of educational professionals, including educational audiologists (Ed. Aud), speech-language pathologists (SLP), and teachers of the deaf and hard of hearing (TODHH). Because student needs change over time, this checklist should be completed at least annually.

[1]. U.S. Department of Justice & U.S. Department of Education (2014, Nov 12). *Frequently Asked Questions on Effective Communication for Students with Hearing, Vision, or Speech Disabilities in Public Elementary and Secondary Schools.* http://www2.ed.gov/about/offices/list/ocr/docs/dcl-faqs-effective-communication-201411.pdf

| Educational Audiology Association | www.edaud.org | 1-800-460-7EAA (7322) |

Fig. 22.8 Suggested Roles of Educational Audiologists, Teachers of the Deaf and Hard of Hearing, and Speech-Language Pathologists (2018).

Continued on page 312

- *Smart Kids Learning Disabilities:* general, testing and assessment, behavioral: www.smartkids withhold.org
- Success for Kids with Hearing Loss: https://successfor-kidswithhearingloss.com/for-professionals/accommodations-for-students-with-hearing-loss/
- Wright's Law: https://www.wrightslaw.com/

Resource 16.2: Suggested Roles of Educational Audiologists, Teachers of the Deaf and Hard of Hearing, and Speech-Language Pathologists (2018) (See **Fig. 22.8**.)

Resources for individuals and families dealing with hearing loss: See Resource 1.1

Suggestions for improving hearing aid and cochlear implant retention: See Resource 2.2

Information for Professionals considering Listening and Spoken Language (LSL) Certification: See Resource 1.2

LMH (Ling-Madell-Hewitt or Low, Mid, High) Test Battery: See Resource 3.2

When the student's team is designating primary responsibility for each activity listed, the professional scopes of practice and state licensure/certification requirements, as well as training and experience, should guide considerations for specifying responsible personnel. Areas with direct scope of practice implications are checked.

Student Assurances: Audiological and Equipment Needs	Ed Aud	TODHH	SLP	Other
1. Audiological evaluations that include recommendations to enhance communication access and learning.	✓			
2. Diagnosis of auditory processing disorders (APD) with recommendations to manage APD issues provided to school personnel for the classroom and to parents for out of school consideration.	✓			
3. Management of auditory access in all educational environments				
4. Assessment of classroom acoustics with recommendations made to improve classroom listening environments where necessary.				
5. Evaluation and fitting for personal hearing instruments, classroom, and other hearing assistive technology.	✓			
6. Management of hearing assistive devices including maintenance and troubleshooting.				
7. Provision of training for school personnel and students, when appropriate, to perform listening checks and basic troubleshooting to maintain proper functioning of personal hearing instruments and hearing assistance technology.				
8. Provision of hearing assistive technology services including educating students, teachers of the deaf/hard of hearing, and other school personnel regarding technology performance and expectations.				
9. Use of daily listening checks to monitor functioning of hearing technology used by students.				
10. Other:				
Student Assurances: Communication - Speech, Language, Auditory, Visual Needs	Ed Aud	TODHH	SLP	Other
11. Evaluation of current speech production skills including articulation, fluency, voice, and resonance, as appropriate for the student's preferred language and communication mode.			✓	
12. Evaluation of current language skills in the student's preferred language and communication mode, including: • Comprehension, expression, and language processing in oral written, graphic and manual modalities • Phonology, semantics, syntax, morphology and pragmatics/social aspects of communication • Pre-literacy and language-based literacy skills, including phonological awareness • Description and interpretation of specific language communication skills and needs identified through appropriate formal and informal, standardized and non-standardized assessments.				
13. Evaluation of communication-related visual and/or auditory skills and needs as appropriate in the student's preferred language and communication mode.				
Student Assurances: Communication - Speech, Language, Auditory, Visual Needs	Ed Aud	TODHH	SLP	Other

Educational Audiology Association   www.edaud.org   1-800-460-7EAA (7322)

Fig. 22.8 Suggested Roles of Educational Audiologists, Teachers of the Deaf and Hard of Hearing, and Speech-Language Pathologists (2018).

Continued on page 313

Resources to aid parent coaching and creation of a language-rich environment: See Resource 5.1

Coaching parents to use cognitive questions: See Resource 5.2

Sample Speech-Language Evaluation/Functional Listening Assessment: Preschool Case: See Resource 6.3

Sample Speech-Language Evaluation/Functional Listening Assessment: School-Aged Case: See Resource 6.4

Assessments to identify possible gaps in language and cognitive skills for evaluating hearing impaired students (ages 6+): See Resource 6.5

Functional Listening Checklists and Assessments: See Resource 6.6

Auditory Learning Guide in English: See Resource 7.1

Auditory Learning Guide in Spanish: See Resource 7.2

Current Level of Functioning (CLF)—Pre-Verbal: See Resource 7.5

Current Level of Functioning (CLF)—Verbal: See Resource 7.6

Expectations of Skill Development for HA & CI Users by Jane Madell, Joan Hewitt, and Sylvia Rotfleisch (2018): See Resource 7.7

Resources for additional learning on LSL Strategies: See Resource 10.1

	Ed Aud	TODHH	SLP	Other
14. Implementation of an appropriate therapy plan to develop speech, language, pragmatics, speechreading and auditory skills including strategies for generalization in the general education classroom.				
15. Self-advocacy instruction and support to enable students to advocate for their needs with peers, school personnel and other communication partners including: • Evaluation and inclusion of communication goals targeting identity, self-advocacy and communication repair strategies • Inclusion of language and communication goals related to classroom accommodations and modifications • Orientation and /or instruction for peers, families, and school staff regarding communication development, the impact of hearing loss, and communication repair strategies.				
16. Services that ensure opportunities for students to develop peer-to-peer social communication skills including: • Facilitated support groups for children who are deaf or hard of hearing or who have other auditory disorders. • Goals for communication repair strategies that will facilitate communication with peers. • Orientation to hearing peers that encourages social interactions and communication.				
17. Other:				
Student Assurances: Academic Needs	**Ed Aud**	**TODHH**	**SLP**	**Other**
18. Evaluation of educational performance in accordance with the requirements of IDEA 330.304 (b) that includes: • Use of a variety (no single measure) of assessment tools and strategies to gather functional, developmental and academic information. • Use of reliable and valid tools administered in the child's preferred language or other mode of communication to yield accurate information. • Measures administered by trained and knowledgeable personnel, according to procedures by the producers of the assessment tools.				
19. Assessment that distinguishes learning issues related to hearing status from those related to other cognitive, sensory or physical challenges.				
20. Specialized academic instruction to include preview and review of academic material to help optimize learning.		✓		
21. Specialized instruction including expanded core curricular areas such as communication, career education, self-determination and advocacy, social-emotional skills, technology and family education.				
Student Assurances: Academic Needs	**Ed Aud**	**TODHH**	**SLP**	**Other**

Fig. 22.8 Suggested Roles of Educational Audiologists, Teachers of the Deaf and Hard of Hearing, and Speech-Language Pathologists (2018).

Video examples of LSL strategies: See Resource 10.2

Suggested Materials for Use in Integrated Executive Function, Speech-Language and Auditory-Verbal Intervention Activities: See Resources 12.1, 12.2, and 12.3

Recommended website for information on how children learn to read, why some struggle, and how adults can help: See Resource 13.2

Recommended sources for children's books: See Resource 13.3

Children Who Are Deaf or Hard of Hearing with Additional Learning Needs by Susan Wiley: See Resource 15.1

Suggested websites for children with hearing loss and additional needs: See Resource 15.2

Section 5: Completing the Structure

Chapter 19: Music, Listening, and All That Jazz

Resource 19.1: Resources for parents and clinicians to encourage integrating music in intervention

- **Drum up Support**
- **AudiTunes**: A Music-Supported Approach to Spoken Language Development in Children with Hearing Loss. (2018): This is designed to be a resource for parents and professionals caring for children with hearing loss currently engaged in a spoken language program. Each short video targets a specific aspect of music development and provides novel ways (and encouragement) for novices to include music in a home or therapy setting. Printed materials for each lesson are available for download. The Learning to Listen Musical Sounds chart is also able to be printed. A core feature of AudiTunes is its use of multi-sensory music experiences within a diverse population and in a variety of settings. The series was developed by board certified music therapist, Christine Barton and speech pathologist, LSLS Cert. AVT, Amy McConkey Robbins. It is grounded on current research and evidence-based practice. AudiTunes is available at no cost to parents and professionals and is made possible through St. Joseph Institute for the Deaf, Indianapolis, WFYI and a private family foundation. Available at: www.sjid.org.
- **TuneUps**: A Music Program Designed to Foster Communication. (2008): Winner of the Therapy Times 2009, Most Valuable Product Award. Developed by these authors, this music CD and habilitation program engages children in a listening, language, and learning experience. Available for free from Advanced Bionics at www.thelisteningroom.com.

Resource 19.2: Industry Resources for encouraging music integration into intervention

- Advanced Bionics (AB), www.thelisteningroom.com Sponsored by AB and Phonak. Registration is free, but required. Here you will find "TuneUps," "BabyBeats," and "A Journey through a Rainforest," all musical programs for children.
- Cochlear, www.cochlear.com. The Communication Corner site has rehab activities from birth through adult, plus a music program for Teens and Tweens. Cochlear App: "Bring Back the Beat"
- MED-EL, www.med-el.com. Hosts a Blog called The Importance of Music in CI Rehabilitation for Adults.

Resource 19.3: Music Resources

- www.angelsound.emilyfufoundation.org/angelsound_music. html
- www.musictogether.com
- www.themusicplayhouse.com
- www.kindermusic.com
- www.little-folks-music.com
- www.westmusic.com. Quality instruments and musical games like Classroom Instrument Bingo by Harper and Instrument Lotto by Lavender

Chapter 20: Telepractice for Children with Hearing Loss

Resource 20.1: Suggested websites and readings

- Learning LSL through Telepractice (including several downloadable resources), retrievable from Hearing First at https://learn.hearingfirst.org/telepractice
- *Using Telepractice to Improve Outcomes for Children who are Deaf or Hard of Hearing & Their Families* (2018) by K. Todd Houston, Diane Behl, & Sabrina Mottershead, Chapter 17 in A Resource Guide for Early Hearing Detection & Intervention, retrievable from https://www.infanthearing.org/ehdi-ebook/2018_ebook/17%20Chapter17UsingTelepractice2018.pdf

Chapter 21: Working with Adults

Resource 21.1: Resources and websites to assist with listening practice

- Advanced Bionics / Sonova: The Listening Room: https://the-listeningroom.com/
- American English Pronunciation Practice: http://www.many-things.org/
- Angel Sounds: http://angelsound.tigerspeech.com/
- Cochlear Corporation: The Communication Corner: https://www.cochlear.com/us/communication-corner
- The English Listening Lounge: www.englishlistening.com/
- ESL Gold: http://eslgold.com/listening/
- MED-EL: Rehabilitation: https://www.medel.com/en-us/support/rehab/rehabilitation
- Randall's ESL Cyber Listening Lab: http://www.esl-lab.com/
- Spotify MED-EL Music Playlist for CI users: https://play.spotify.com/user/medelcochlearimplants/playlist/2USG4LCeBOZixFjRRtrIuB
- TED Talks: http://www.ted.com/

Index